Medical-Surgical Nursing Certification

Self-Assessment and Exam Review

Donna Martin, DNP, RN, CMSRN, CDE, CNE
Associate Professor
Faculty, College of Nursing and Health Professions
Lewis University
Romeoville, Illinois

Patricia Braida MSN, RN, AGPCNP-BC
Assistant Professor
Faculty, College of Nursing and Health Professions
Lewis University
Romeoville, Illinois

New York   Chicago   San Francisco   Athens   London   Madrid
Mexico City   Milan   New Delhi   Singapore   Sydney   Toronto

Medical-Surgical Nursing Certification

Copyright © 2019 by McGraw-Hill Education. All rights reserved. Printed in the United States of America. Except as permitted under the United States Copyright Act of 1976, no part of this publication may be reproduced or distributed in any form or by any means, or stored in a data base or retrieval system, without the prior written permission of the publisher.

1 2 3 4 5 6 7 8 9   LOV   23 22 21 20 19 18

ISBN 978-1-260-03137-9

MHID 1-260-03137-3

This book was set in Minion pro by MPS Limited.
The editors were Susan Barnes and Regina Y. Brown.
The production supervisor was Rick Ruzycka.
Project management was provided by Ruma Khurana, MPS Limited.
The illustrator was Kaitlyn Kruk.

This book is printed on acid-free paper.

Library of Congress Cataloging-in-Publication Data
Names: Martin, Donna Lynn, 1963- editor.
Title: Medical-surgical nursing certification / edited by Donna Martin, DNP,
    RN, CMSRN, CDE, CNE, Associate Professor, College of Nursing and Health
    Professions, Lewis University, Romeoville, IL, Patricia Braida, RN, MSN,
    AGPCNP-BC, Assistant Professor, Faculty, College of Nursing and Health
    Professions, Lewis University, Romeoville, IL.
Description: New York : McGraw-Hill Education, [2019] | Includes
    bibliographical references and index.
Identifiers: LCCN 2018032135 | ISBN 9781260031379 (paperback)
Subjects: LCSH: Nursing–Certification–Examinations, questions, etc. |
    Surgical nursing–Certification–Examinations, questions, etc.
Classification: LCC RT55 .M427 2019 | DDC 617/.0231076—dc23
    LC record available at https://lccn.loc.gov/2018032135

McGraw-Hill Education books are available at special quantity discounts to use as premiums and sales promotions or for use in corporate training programs. To contact a representative, please visit the Contact Us pages at www.mhprofessional.com.

Dedication

I would like to dedicate this book to all the nurses who have played a role in my 30+ years of nursing, with special thanks to the most influential nurse, my mom, Nancy J. Heerdt, RN.
Thank you for being an incredible role model and a source of support and endless encouragement.

This book would not be possible without the time, dedication, and expertise of all those that participated in the creation of this book; contributing authors and our illustrator Katie Kruk.

Donna (Heerdt) Martin

I am dedicating this book to my extraordinary colleagues, excellent students, inspiring patients—current and past—who have helped to shape me into the nurse that I am today. Special thanks go to my parents, husband, friends, and beautiful daughters Rebecca, Maggie, and Ellie for their encouragement, love, and support.

Patricia Braida

Contents

About the Editors

Donna L. Martin has been a registered nurse for over 30 years. She earned her Associate Degree in Nursing from Truman Junior College in Chicago, her BSN from Loyola University, a Master's Degree in Health Services Administration from St. Francis University, her MSN in Nursing Education from Lewis University, and her DNP in Nursing Leadership. Her specialties include medical-surgical nursing and diabetes. She has been a certified medical-surgical nurse and certified diabetes educator for more than 20 years. She currently teaches clinical and theory for medical-surgical nursing in a BSN program, and works as a Joint Commission Disease Specific Care reviewer for Advanced Inpatient Diabetes management, wound, sepsis, and orthopedic certification programs.

Patricia (Pat) Braida is an Assistant Professor of Nursing at Lewis University College of Nursing and Health Professions in Romeoville, Illinois. She is Lead Faculty for two Medical-Surgical courses and has taught clinical and didactic nursing courses to undergraduate nurses for over twenty years at Lewis. She received her Bachelor of Science in Nursing from Marycrest College in Davenport, Iowa, her Master of Science in Nursing as a Clinical Nurse Specialist in Critical Care from Loyola University of Chicago, and her Post Master's Certification as an Adult Geriatric Primary Care Nurse Practitioner from Lewis University. In over 30 years of practice in critical care and medical-surgical nursing, Pat has enjoyed various practice roles as a provider, educator, Clinical Nurse Specialist, and Nurse-Manager.

Contributors

Ida Anderson MSN, RN, ONC
Executive Director of Nursing Surgical Services
WellStar Kennestone Regional Medical Center
Marietta, Georgia

Barbara Bostelmann MS, RN
Assistant Professor
Elmhurst College Department of Nursing and Health Sciences
Elmhurst, Illinois

Patricia Braida MSN, RN, AGPCNP-BC
Assistant Professor
Lewis University College of Nursing & Health Professions
Romeoville, Illinois

Laura Brennan MS, RN
Assistant Professor/Director of Undergraduate Pre Licensure Program
Elmhurst College Department of Nursing and Health Sciences
Elmhurst Illinois

Stacie Elder PhD, RN, CNE
Professor
Lewis University College of Nursing & Health Professions
Romeoville, Illinois

Aliesha Emerson, MSN, RN-C
Nursing Professional Development Specialist
Wilmington, Delaware

Stephanie Gedzyk-Nieman, DNP, MSN, RNC-MNN
Assistant Professor
Lewis University College of Nursing & Health Professions
Romeoville, Illinois

Elizabeth Pepe Greenlee, DHA, MSN, BSN, RN
Associate Administrator of Quality Programs
Harris Health System
Houston, Texas

Amy Hagen, BSN, RN, CWS
Regional Director of Clinical Operations
Healogics, Inc.
Naperville, Illinois

Meritta Harris, BSN, RN, CWS, CHRN
Senior Director of Clinical Operations
Healogics, Inc.
Middletown, Ohio

Kaitlyn Kruk, Illustrator
Major: Illustration: Minor: Digital Media
Milwaukee Institute of Art and Design
Milwaukee, Wisconsin

M. Caitlin Kusnetzow, MSN, RN, CMSRN
Instructor
Lewis University College of Nursing & Health Professions
Romeoville, Illinois

Donna L. Martin DNP, RN, CMSRN, CDE, CNE
Associate Professor
Lewis University College of Nursing & Health Professions
Romeoville, Illinois

Katelyn S. Myroniak DNP(c), RN, CMSRN
Assistant Professor
Lewis University College of Nursing & Health Professions
Romeoville, Illinois

Nancy Paez, BSN, RN, CWCN, CHRN, LNC, CWS, DAPWCA
Chief Compliance and Training Officer
Shared Health Services
Johnson City, Tennessee

Nanci Reiland DNP, RN, PHNA-BC
Assistant Professor of Nursing/Coordinator of Continuing Education
Lewis University College of Nursing & Health Professions
Romeoville, Illinois

Jane Trainor MS, RN
Assistant Professor
Lewis University College of Nursing and Health Professions
Romeoville, Illinois

Foreword

Medical-Surgical Nursing is a specialty area in the field of nursing. Certification in this field demonstrates the critical importance and value of this area of nursing practice. This Medical-Surgical Nursing Certification review book was created to assist nurses seeking to be recognized in their area of specialty through the following certification exams:

The American Nurses Credentialing Center (ANCC) Medical-Surgical Nursing Board Certification Exam

The Academy of Medical-Surgical Nurses (AMSN) Medical-Surgical Nursing Certification Board (MSNCB) Exam

This book was developed using the test blueprints from both of these exams, providing content and domains of practice necessary for the medical-surgical nurse. Each chapter provides an overview, content, practice questions, case studies, and clinical considerations. Content experts were involved in the creation of this book, as contributing authors and as content reviewers. We hope that you find this to be an excellent resource as you prepare for the Medical-Surgical certification exam.

Preparing for the Exam

Donna Martin, DNP, RN, CMSRN, CDE, CNE
Patricia Braida MSN, RN, AGPCNP-BC

OVERVIEW

Congratulations for taking this important step to join your nursing colleagues who have also sought certification in a nursing specialty. Becoming certified demonstrates your professionalism and dedication to lifelong learning and to providing safe, high-quality care to your patients. Making the commitment to take any nursing certification exam can be intimidating, whether you are taking it for personal growth or because you are being asked/required to take it by an employer. This book was designed to be a self-assessment tool and study guide for medical-surgical nurses planning to take one of the medical-surgical nursing certification exams. The format of each chapter of this book was developed using the nursing process as the foundation. Assessment, diagnosis, planning, implementation, evaluation, and patient education are included for the various disorders that are presented in each chapter. In addition, practice questions and clinical considerations are interspersed throughout each chapter and a case study is located at the end of each chapter. Finally, a 150-question practice test is located in the last chapter.

Please do not take the certification exam lightly. Even though you may be a registered nurse (RN) who has been practicing in medical-surgical settings for many years, you should set aside ample time to review medical-surgical nursing content. Although this book provides information to help you prepare for the medical-surgical nursing certification exams, it is critical that you also be aware of the requirements and test blueprint for the specific medical-surgical certification exam that you are going to take.

Medical-surgical nursing was once thought of as the area in which new graduate nurses would work to develop their skills so they could be prepared to move to "specialty areas of nursing." Now, medical-surgical nursing is regarded as an increasingly complex specialty within the practice of nursing. Specific knowledge and skills are needed to provide care for patients and their families during all phases of their lives.

In 1972, the American Nurses Association (ANA) recognized medical-surgical nursing as a specialty and began to offer a certification exam. In addition, in 1990, the American Academy of Medical-Surgical Nurses (AMSN) was founded, and they also developed a certification exam.

CMSRN CERTIFICATION EXAM

▶ The following information was retrieved from the AMSN and the Medical-Surgical Nursing Certification Board (MSNCB; 2017) and was current as of March 2018. (amsn.org/certification/med-surg-certification and msncb.org)

▶ "The Certified Medical-Surgical Registered Nurse (CMSRN) incorporates current nursing science and evidence-based practices that the medical-surgical nurse consistently applies in practice to achieve desired patient outcomes across the continuum of care. This CMSRN exam validates the expertise and knowledge of the medical surgical nurse and promotes medical-surgical nursing as a unique specialty." (https://www.amsn.org/certification/med-surg-certification)

- Upon completion of eligibility requirements and successfully passing the exam, you are awarded the credential: Certified Medical-Surgical Registered Nurse (CMSRN).
- This credential is valid for 5 years.
- Maintaining your license to practice and meeting the renewal requirements are required at the time of your certification renewal.
- The CMSRN exam was granted accreditation by the Accreditation Board for Specialty Nursing Certification (ABSNC).

▶ Eligibility:
- RN with a current U.S. license
- Practiced a minimum of 2 years as a registered nurse in a medical-surgical setting
- Accrued a minimum of 2000 hours of practice (clinical, management, or education) within the past 3 years

▶ Certification application/testing process:
- Applications accepted year-round
- Choice of computer-based or paper-and-pencil testing format
- Computer-based testing format:
  - You will receive exam permit within 3 to 5 weeks after application
  - Permit contains:
    - 90-day testing window
    - Information on how to schedule exam
- Paper-and-pencil testing format:
  - You will receive permit approximately 2 weeks prior to exam date
  - Scheduling information is selected when you apply
- 150 multiple-choice questions
- Time allotted: 3 hours
- *Note:* Paper-and-pencil exam format also has 25 experimental questions (not scored) and one additional hour to test.

▶ Test blueprint:
- Content outline:
  - Based on 7 Domains of Practice (Table 1.1)

TABLE 1.1	MSNCB CERTIFICATION BLUEPRINT BY DOMAINS OF PRACTICE	
7 Domains of Practice	**Percent of Exam**
Therapeutic Intervention	23–25%
Assessing/Monitoring	23–25%
Helping Role	16–18%
Teaching/Coaching	16–18%
Managing Emergency	11–13%
Organizational/Work Role Competency	3–5%
Ensuring Quality	1–3%
(Retrieved from msncb.org)	

TABLE 1.2	MSNCB CERTIFICATION BLUEPRINT BY PATIENT PROBLEMS
Patient Problems	Percent of Exam
Gastrointestinal	16–18%
Pulmonary	15–17%
Cardiovascular	15–17%
Diabetes/Endocrine	14–16%
GU/Renal/Reproductive	14–16%
Musculoskeletal/Neuro	12–14%
Hematology/Immuno/Integumentary	7–9%

(Retrieved from msncb.org)

- Divided into Patient Problems (Table 1.2)
- Complete and detailed test blueprint can be located on the MSNBC and the AMSN websites
▶ Further information can be obtained at www.msncb.org.

ANCC CERTIFICATION EXAM

▶ The following information was retrieved from the American Nurses Credentialing Center (ANCC; nursingworld.org) and was current as of March 2018.

▶ "The ANCC Medical-Surgical Nursing board certification examination is a competency-based examination that provides a valid and reliable assessment of the entry-level clinical knowledge and skills of registered nurses in the medical-surgical specialty after initial RN licensure" (ANCC, 2018).

- Upon completion of eligibility requirements and successfully passing the exam, you are awarded the credential: Registered Nurse-Board Certified (RN-BC).
- This credential is valid for 5 years.
- Maintaining your license to practice and meeting the renewal requirements are required at the time of your certification renewal.
- The National Commission for Certifying Agencies and the Accreditation Board for Specialty Nursing Certification accredits this ANCC certification.

▶ Eligibility:

- Hold a current, active RN license within a state or territory of the United States or the professional, legally recognized equivalent in another country. *Note:* International applicants have additional requirements (refer to the ANCC website).
- Have practiced the equivalent of 2 years full-time as an RN.
- Have a minimum of 2000 hours of clinical practice in the specialty area of medical-surgical nursing within the past 3 years.
- Have completed 30 hours of continuing education in medical-surgical nursing within the past 3 years.

▶ Certification application/testing process:

- Applications accepted year-round
- Must test within 90 days of application approval
- Computer-based testing
- Time allotted: 3.5 hours
- 175 questions (150 scored plus 25 pretest questions that are not scored)

TABLE 1.3	ANCC CERTIFICATION BLUEPRINT
4 Domains of Practice	**Percent of Exam**
Assessment and Diagnosis	14.67%
Planning, Implementation & Outcomes Evaluation	33.33%
Professional Role	30%
Health Teaching and Health Promotion	22%
(Retrieved from nursecredentialing.org)	

▶ Test blueprint:

- Content outline (Table 1.3)

▶ Further information can be obtained at https://www.nursingworld.org/our-certifications/medical-surgical-nurse/.

STRATEGIES FOR SUCCESS

No matter which certification credential you choose to purse, there are some universal strategies that you will want to incorporate into your preparation for the exam.

▶ Carefully review the certification exam guideline, including the test blueprint.

▶ Complete a self-assessment of your current knowledge, application, and analysis of the information that could be covered on the exam.

- Practice exams are available for both certification exams
- Review content areas on the test blueprint

▶ Consider the following study strategies:

- Identify the way in which you learn best (reading, writing, or verbalizing) and use this technique as you study.
- Focus on content areas that you are not as familiar with, as well as patient problems that are not seen regularly in your nursing practice.
- Identify content areas that were challenging for you on the practice exams.
- Establish a routine to study. Do not wait until the week before to begin to review content for the exam.
- Prepare your "study" calendar to fit with other commitments in your life. Assign specific content to specific dates and times, and do not deviate from this schedule. Allow plenty of time to go back over content that is difficult or not as familiar.
- Consider studying with a colleague, if possible.
- Set short- and long-term study goals.
- Use effective time management. This can be done by using free time, such as waiting for an appointment or if you arrive early to work. Consider having study materials with you at all times (review book, index cards, notes, and so forth).
- Use all the materials that you have access to: certification website, content outlines, practice questions, and case studies.
- Look up content/terms/words you do not know or understand.

▶ Test-taking strategies:

- Ensure that you are well rested prior to the exam. Do not stay up late trying to cram for the test.
- Prepare the night before you take the exam by having all your clothes and supplies ready to go for the next day.
- Know which stress-management techniques work for you and practice them prior to the exam.

- Practice taking computer-based tests if you have not done so previously. They are different from paper-and-pencil tests!
- Arrive early for the exam; plan for the unexpected.
- Understand/read all directions prior to starting the exam.
- Manage allotted time effectively.
- Avoid reading into the question. Read the question carefully. Be sure to read the entire question and all answers prior to selecting a response. You may want to read the question again and think about what the question is asking. Then, re-read the answers briefly to search for clues. Select the best answer based only on the information that is provided.
- Trust your intuition; often the first answer you select is correct. Try not to change your answer unless you are certain the other answer is correct. The practice of changing answers often changes the answer from right to wrong.
- It is important to remain calm and positive as you are taking the exam. There may be answers that you don't know. Remember and try to visualize the material you studied. Some people can "see" tables in their mind or remember how they had their study notes arranged as they are taking an exam. Think of your many experiences and apply your background as a professional nurse. Logic, common sense, clinical judgment, and critical thinking are skills you apply in your daily practice. You must evaluate your answer according to established facts, guidelines, and criteria that you studied or that are reviewed in this book. Allow the knowledge, skills, and abilities to guide you as you take this next important step to validate your professionalism and commitment to excellent patient care.
- Key words may be underlined, *italicized*, or **bold**, but often they are not highlighted.
- Identify key words in the question or answer that:
  - Set a priority. Multiple answers may be correct, but you must use critical thinking to determine which answer is **most important** or is the priority. Examples of these terms include:
    - Best
    - First
    - Initial
    - Safest
    - Most important

Question	Discussion
The nurse would perform which of the following assessments initially for an elderly patient admitted with suspected hyperthyroidism? A. Assess for tremors B. Assess the heart rate and rhythm C. Weigh the patient D. Determine the body temperature	Answer: B The nurse must first assess for tachycardia and/or dysrhythmias. Tremors, weight loss and hyperthermia may also occur in patients experiencing hyperthyroidism. This style of question requires knowledge and critical thinking. The use of the word *initially* indicates that all of the interventions would need to be completed, but is asking that the interventions be prioritized and the intervention that should be performed first is chosen.

- **Negative polarity** requires that you detect exceptions, errors, or identify unacceptable interventions. Examples of these terms include:
  - Except
  - Not
  - Avoid
  - Contraindicated
  - Further
  - Violates

Question	Rationale
A patient with a diagnosis of right-sided stroke has been admitted from the emergency department to the medical-surgical floor. Which of the following interventions would be contraindicated for this patient? A. Keeping the head of the bed elevated B. Getting the blood pressure within the desired range quickly C. Administering 0.9% normal saline to ensure cerebral perfusion, if needed D. Placing sequential compression devices on both legs	Answer: B Carefully maintaining blood pressure according to guidelines is recommended for a patient experiencing a stroke. Hypertension may be common immediately after a stroke as the body tries to maintain cerebral perfusion. In the acute post-stroke setting, the brain is very sensitive to changes in blood pressure, and perfusion pressure. If it is necessary to lower the blood pressure, it must be done very carefully according to the guidelines. Adequate hydration must also be controlled carefully. This promotes cerebral perfusion and prevents further brain injury. Sequential compression devices are important for venous thromboembolism (VTE) prophylaxis. This style of questioning requires an understanding of the disease process and expected interventions. Using the word *contraindicated* indicates that there is an option listed that should not be considered for this medical problem. Not all answers may be correct but the intervention that could cause harm and should not be used would be the correct answer.

- Identify **all-inclusive terms,** as these words place limits or impose broad generalizations, which *often* make the statement/answer false. Examples of these terms include:
  - Always
  - Only
  - All
  - Never
  - Every
  - None

- It is important to remember that an all-inclusive term may also be used to stress an absolute, such as "Hand hygiene should always be done before and after patient contact."

Question	Rationale
The student nurse is asking his preceptor about confusion in the elderly. Which of the following statements will the preceptor share with the student? A. All elderly people become confused in the hospital. B. Older adults will always develop dementia. C. An older adult may present with cognitive impairment in the presence of infection. D. Opioids must never be withheld from elderly adults in acute care settings.	Answer: C Infection may cause some older adults to become cognitively impaired. The use of the words *all, always,* and *never* does not leave any room for a variation in practice. It is highly unusual that an answer using one of these words would be correct.

As you thoughtfully develop your study strategies and test-taking plan, we would like to commend you for demonstrating your commitment to this process. Your thirst for knowledge and willingness to seek certification prove that you are dedicated to providing excellent care to your patients and their families. By achieving certification as a medical-surgical nurse, you are demonstrating competency in the skills and knowledge needed to practice in this increasingly complex specialty area of nursing.

Bibliography

American Nurses Credentialing Center. (2018). *Medical-Surgical Nursing Certification.* Accessed January 25, 2018, from https://www.nursingworld.org/ancc/

Medical-Surgical Nursing Certification Board. (2017). *Medical-Surgical Nursing Certification.* Accessed January 25, 2018, from https://www.msncb.org/medical-surgical

2

Professional Role of the Nurse

Donna Martin, DNP, RN, CMSRN, CDE, CNE
Patricia Braida MSN, RN, AGPCNP-BC

OVERVIEW

Being a registered nurse (RN) is much more than just a job, it is a professional career. The professional role of the nurse involves more than just providing patient care; it also includes following legal, ethical, and regulatory expectations, as well as working collaboratively with others. In addition, nurses must participate in quality-improvement activities and use evidence-based practices to enhance patient care.

For the 16th consecutive year, America's ratings of the honesty and ethical standards of 22 occupations find nurses at the top of the list. More than 8 in 10 (82%) Americans describe nurses' ethics as "very high" or "high." Nurses have surpassed all other professions every year but one since Gallup first started this survey in 1999 (Brenan, 2017).

KEY ASPECTS OF PROFESSIONALISM

According to Yoder (2017), there are six key aspects of nursing professionalism:

▶ Acting in the best interest of the patient and family
▶ Maintaining high standards with regard to competence and knowledge
▶ Demonstrating high ethical standards
▶ Displaying caring empathy, humility, and compassion
▶ Being socially responsible
▶ Being sensitive to the cultures and beliefs of others

These key aspects of nursing professionalism mirror the expectations that are found in the American Nurses Association *Code of Ethics for Nurses* (2015).

AMERICAN NURSES ASSOCIATION (ANA) CODE OF ETHICS

"The Code of Ethics for Nurses with Interpretive Statements (The Code) was developed as a guide for carrying out nursing responsibilities in a manner consistent with quality in nursing care and the ethical obligations of the profession" (ANA, 2015). It consists of nine provisions.

<u>Provision 1</u>—"The nurse practices with compassion and respect for the inherent dignity, worth, and unique attributes of every person."

▶ For the professional nurse this means:

- It is expected that all patients are treated with respect and dignity, without bias or prejudice, regardless of lifestyle choices and/or behaviors.
- Nurses are expected to establish a trusting relationship with patients.
- An individualized plan of care is developed for each patient.
- The patient's right to make choices is respected, even if those choices are not consistent with those of the health care system or providers.
- The nurse develops a professional, respectful and collegial relationship with others. Bullying, harassment, intimidation, threats, and violence are always unacceptable behaviors.

<u>Provision 2</u>—"The nurse's primary commitment is to the patient, whether an individual, family, group, community, or population."

▶ For the professional nurse this means:

- The nurse needs to provide individualized care to the patient, which may include a family, group, community, and population.
- Nurses need to foster collaborative care based on trust, shared decision making, and open communication.
- Professional boundaries must be upheld within the nurse–patient relationship, to avoid the risk of boundary violations.

<u>Provision 3</u>—"The nurse promotes, advocates for, and protects the rights, health, and safety of the patient."

▶ For the professional nurse this means:

- Patient privacy and confidentiality must be maintained.
  - The Health Insurance Portability and Accountability Act (HIPAA) mandates standards for the protection of individually identifiable health information, as well as guidelines for the protection of electronic protected health information.
  - There must be appropriate utilization of informatics and the electronic health record.
- Protecting the rights of patients who are participating in research is ensured by:
  - Allowing individuals the ability to choose whether or not they wish to participate in research as a subject.
  - Protecting vulnerable populations and reporting to appropriate bodies if this right is violated.
- Nurses have a responsibility to promote a culture of safety.
  - ALWAYS use at least two patient identifiers to confirm that it is the correct patient.
  - Follow the 6 Rights of Medication Administration to prevent errors.
  - Be aware of The Joint Commission National Patient Safety Goals.
  - Report patient safety concerns. Serious reportable event (SREs), are called "never events."
  - Report errors and near misses to evaluate for system problems.
  - Report questionable or impaired practice of other nurses to appropriate leadership.
  - Promote and support a "Just Culture."

<u>Provision 4</u>—"The nurse has the authority, accountability, and responsibility for nursing practice; makes decisions; and takes action consistent with the obligation to promote health and provide optimal care."

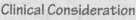

Clinical Consideration

6 Rights of Medication Administration
- Right patient
- Right medication
- Right dose
- Right time
- Right route
- Right documentation

Clinical Consideration

"Just Culture" involves frontline staff openly reporting errors, without fear of repercussions, for the goal of identifying system issues and preventing future errors.

Question	Rationale
After a very long, emotional day at work, which of the following would be acceptable for a nurse to post on social media? A. Do not post anything on social media about work or patients. B. "What a sad day at work, 25 years old is just too young to die from cancer." C. Posting a picture of her favorite patient that she took with her cell phone. D. "One of my favorite patients at Lewis Hospital passed away today. He was such a nice person."	Answer: A Sharing any information that could potentially identify a patient is prohibited and would be considered a HIPAA violation. Answers B, C, and D would be unacceptable. Sharing any information about the location, age, or diagnosis could lead to identification of the individual and is prohibited by HIPAA.

TABLE 2.1	ETHICAL/LEGAL PRINCIPLES
Term	**Definition**
Autonomy	Freedom to make one's own decisions.
Beneficence	Promote good; do what is best for the patient.
Justice	Give fair treatment.
Veracity	Provide truthful information so the person can make an informed decision.
Nonmaleficence	Avoid harm.
Fidelity	Be honest; do not deceive.
Loyalty	Be reliable; stay firm in a commitment.
Respect	Hold others in high regard and value their perspectives.
Informed consent	Full disclosure of risks, benefits, and alternatives; patient permission granted without coercion.
Living will	Statement of wishes regarding withholding and withdrawing life-sustaining treatments if the person is no longer able to make those decisions.
Durable power of attorney for health care	Names someone to make health care decisions, including termination of life support, in the event the person is no longer able to make those decisions. Wishes should be discussed with the designee so they are aware of the person's wishes.

▮ For the professional nurse this means:

- Nurses are accountable for their decisions and actions.
- Nurses must follow the moral principles of fidelity, loyalty, veracity, beneficence, and respect for patients (Table 2.1).
- Accurate and complete documentation of assessments and care is provided.
- Nurses need to seek the assistance of others when the needs of a patient exceeds their competencies.

- Nurses appropriately delegate tasks to unlicensed assistive personnel (UAP).
  - 5 Rights of Delegation:
    - Right task:
      - Is it an appropriate task to delegate?
      - Has the person been trained in performing this task?
    - Right circumstances:
      - Does the situation support delegation of the task?
    - Right person:
      - Is the person willing and able to do what is being delegated?
      - Is this task within the person's scope/job description and competency?
    - Right directions and communication:
      - Have directions for the task been clearly communicated?
      - Does the UAP understand what needs to be done?
    - Right supervision and evaluation:
      - Does the UAP require direct supervision for the task?

Provision 5—"The nurse owes the same duties to self as to others, including the responsibly to promote health and safety, preserve wholeness of character and integrity, maintain competence, and continue personal and professional growth."

▌ For the professional nurse this means:
- Nurses should be a role model for the health behaviors that they teach to others, in both their professional and personal identities.
- Nurses should be lifelong learners by:
  - participating in continuing education, not only for licensure requirements but for professional growth and to remain current in practice.
  - continuing their professional education through advanced nursing degrees.
- Obtaining certification in the area of specialty to demonstrate expertise and commitment.
- Maintaining professional nursing organization membership and involvement.
- Being politically aware and active with regard to nursing and health care issues.

Provision 6—"The nurse, through individual and collective effort, establishes, maintains, and improves the ethical environment of the work setting and conditions of employment that are conducive to safe, quality health care."

▌ For the professional nurse this means:
- Following institution policies and procedures.
- Using effective communication during transitions of care to provide safe, high-quality care:
  - SBAR format communication:
    - Situation—Describe the situation you want to discuss, with enough detail.
    - Background—Provide the background or circumstances leading up to the situation and any pertinent information.
    - Assessment—Include your assessment of the situation and what you think the problem is.
    - Recommendation/Request—Clearly state your recommendation to correct the problem or request.

Provision 7—"The nurse, in all roles and settings, advances the profession through research and scholarly inquiry, professional standards and development, and the generation of both nursing and health policy."

▶ For the professional nurse this means:

- Nurses participate in nursing research and scholarly activities.
- Evidence-based practice (EBP) is used whenever possible.
- Nurses research and share EBP with colleagues and their organizations.
- Nurses participate in shared governance whenever possible.
- Nurses assume an active role in patient outcomes by being aware of their role with regard to quality improvement through:
  - awareness of nursing-sensitive quality indicators.
  - dashboard data.
  - participating in root-cause analysis (RCA).
- Nurses must participate in local, regional, national, or global health care initiatives.

Provision 8—"The nurse collaborates with other health professionals and the public to protect human rights, promote health diplomacy, and reduce health disparities."

▶ For the professional nurse this means:

- Nursing care needs to be available for all, as health care is a universal right.
- Nurses are obligated to help advance the health and rights of all and reduce disparities that exist.

Provision 9—"The profession of nursing, collectively through its professional organizations, must articulate nursing values, maintain the integrity of the profession, and integrate principles of social justice into nursing and health policy."

▶ For the professional nurse this means:

- Being aware of professional nursing issues.
- Adhering to the code of ethics for nurses.
- Following your state Nurse Practice Act.
- Supporting professional nursing organizations to advocate for shaping health care and integrating social justice.

Question	Rationale
The nurse is caring for a patient who has just returned from surgery. Which task would be appropriate for the nurse to delegate to the UAP? A. Monitor the patient's pain level. B. Check the patients vital signs. C. Assess the patient's pedal pulses. D. Evaluate the dressing for drainage.	Answer: B Delegation of tasks must take into consideration the scope of practice and training of the UAP. The nurse is responsible for the assessment of the patient's pain level, pulses, and the incision site. The vital signs can be obtained by the UAP once competency has been established.

PRACTICE ROLES

There are several different roles that the medical-surgical nurse may assume: advocate, caregiver, change agent, coordinator, discharge planner, educator, and researcher (Figure 2.1). The medical-surgical nurses must also be knowledgeable about the stages of adult development (Table 2.2).

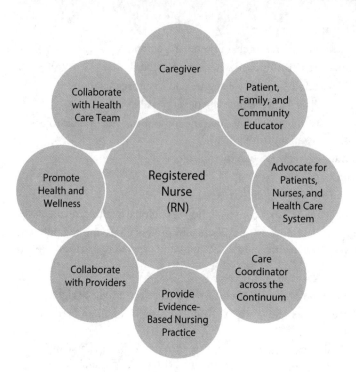

Figure 2.1 Practice Roles

TABLE 2.2	STAGES OF ADULT DEVELOPMENT	
Stage	Psychosocial Conflict	Physical and Cognitive Development
Young adulthood (ages 18–35)	**"Intimacy vs. Isolation"** *Intimacy*—develops satisfying intimate relationships *Isolation*—self-absorbed, unable to develop satisfying relationships	*Development*: peak of physical strength, physical growth completed, reproductive years, intellectual growth continues *Challenges:* assuming adult responsibilities (become financially independent, marriage, starting a family, prone to accidents and injuries, may suffer unemployment)
Middle adulthood (ages 36–65)	**"Generativity vs. Stagnation"** *Generativity*—productive and satisfied with family, work, and community *Stagnation*—dissatisfied with life roles, feeling stuck and stagnant	*Development*: slow decline in body functions with physical changes, intellectual abilities generally are not impacted *Challenges:* adjusting to physical decline and chronic diseases, preparing for retirement, helping children become independent, and helping aging parents
Older adulthood (ages 66 and above)	**"Integrity vs. Despair"** *Integrity*—feelings of accomplishment and fulfillment *Despair*—feelings of regret and hopelessness when reflecting on life	*Development*: increasing decline in body functions, decreasing mobility and strength *Challenges:* continued and increasing physical decline, development of additional chronic diseases, cognitive decline (memory loss, dementia, Alzheimer's disease)

Adapted from Erikson's Stages of Development (1963)

QUALITY AND PATIENT SAFETY

It is critical that the nurse take an active role in ensuring high-quality, safe patient care.

▶ Quality

- Quality assurance involves actions taken to ensure an expected standard of quality.
- Evidence-based practice (EBP) is defined as the integration of current research, clinical expertise, and the patient's values and preferences.

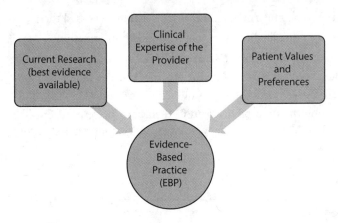

Figure 2.2 Evidence-Based Practice

- Performance improvement (PI) is the process of continually seeking out opportunities to improve the quality of care, clinical outcomes, and patient satisfaction.
- Some of the National Database of Nursing Quality Indicators (NDNQI) nurse-sensitive indicators reflect patient outcomes. These include:
  - Health-care–acquired infections
  - Patient falls
  - Patient falls with injury
  - Pressure ulcer rate (community-, hospital-, and unit-acquired)
  - Restraints
▶ Patient safety:
- Safety/Occurrence/Accident incidents need to be reported in an objective and timely manner.
- Ensure that all equipment is properly working and inspected (if required) to prevent patient harm.
- Suicide screening needs to be done for all patients; patients who are identified as being at risk need to have a comprehensive suicide risk assessment completed.
- Screening for abusive situations needs to be completed for all patients; a positive screen needs to be documented and reported to the appropriate authorities.

PATIENT'S BILL OF RIGHTS

The Patient's Bill of Rights (AHA, 2006) was developed to ensure that certain rights were afforded each person who receives medical care. Nurses need to be aware of, and respect, the patient's rights.

▶ Patients have the right to know their treatment options and to participate in decisions about treatment options.
- Informed consent—individuals have the right to be fully informed of illness, treatment options, and then be able to decide on treatment. It is important that diagnosis, prognosis, and treatment be explained in terms that the individual can understand. Translation services must be provided, if needed.
- Right to refuse treatment—individuals have the right to refuse treatment and to be informed of the consequences of their decision to refuse care.
- If patients are no longer able to make decisions, a living will and/or a durable power of attorney for health care can provide for their wishes to be known.
▶ Patients have the right to access to emergency care, whenever needed, regardless of the ability to pay for these services.
▶ Patients have the right to know who is interviewing, assessing, and caring for them.
▶ Patients have the right to choose and change their providers, for any reason.

❿ Patients have the right to respectful care that does not discriminate against them.

❿ Patients have the right to confidentiality/privacy of their health information:

- Requests to speak to their provider in private must be honored.
- Requests to view their medical records with the provider must be honored.
- Make a request to correct errors or omissions in the medical record.

❿ Patients also have a responsibility to be involved in their care, be respectful to the health care providers, and inform the provider of their current symptoms and history of illnesses, hospitalizations, and medications.

Question	Rationale
One of the roles of the registered nurse in terms of informed consent is to: A. Serve as the witness to the client's signature on an informed consent document. B. Get and witness the *Durable Power of Attorney for Health Care* signature before getting the informed consent. C. Explain the procedure and witness the client's signature on an informed consent document. D. None of the above.	Answer: A It is the responsibility of the provider doing the procedure to explain the procedure, risks, benefits, and alternatives to the patient. One of the roles of the nurse is to serve as a witness to the client's signature on an informed consent. A *Durable Power of Attorney for Health Care* is not required to be completed prior to getting informed consent.

Bibliography

American Nurses Association. (2015). *Code of ethics for nurses with interpretive statements.* Silver Spring, MD: American Nurses Association. Accessed February 5, 2018 from www.nursingworld.org

American Hospital Association (2006). Accessed June 15, 2017 from http://www.aha.org/advocacy-issues/communicatingpts/pt-car-partnership.shtml

Brenan, M. (2017). Nurses keep healthy lead as most honest, ethical profession. *Gallup News.* Accessed May 18, 2018, from http://news.gallup.com/poll/224639/nurses-keep-healthy-lead-honest-ethical-profession.aspx

Dean, E. (2017). Enabling professionalism in practice. *Nursing Management (2014+)* 24(4), 15. http://dx.doi.org/10.7748/nm.24.4.15.s18

Grove, S.K., Gray, J.R., and Burns, N. (2015). Understanding Nursing Research: Building an Evidence-Based Practice, 6th ed. (St. Louis: Elsevier).

Hutchinson, D. (2017). Professionalism and trust in general practice nursing. *Practice Nurse* 47(8), 12–16.

McLeod, S. (2017). Eric Erikson. *Simply Psychology.* Retrieved March 14, 2018 from https://www.simply psychology.org/Erik-Erikson.html

Promoting professionalism. (2017). *Community Practitioner, 90*(6), 15. Accessed February 5, 2018 from http://ezproxy.lewisu.edu/login?url=https://search.proquest.com/docview/1919074026?accountid=12073

Shepard, L.H. (2014). It takes a village to assure nurse professionalism. *I-Manager's Journal on Nursing* 3(4), 1-5.

Yoder, L. (2017). Professionalism in nursing. *MEDSURG Nursing, 26*(5), 293-294. Accessed February 5, 2018, from http http://www.medsurgnursing.net

3

Health Promotion, Disease Prevention, and Health Education

Nanci Reiland, DNP, RN, PHNA-BC

HEALTH PROMOTION AND DISEASE PREVENTION

In the areas of health and health care in the United States, the past century heralded many changes and new trends. As modern medicine has evolved, along with changes in society such as in technology, globalization, and economics, the United States has seen a swing from an emphasis on curative care to identifying that preventive care is more cost-effective and that it enhances the quality of life. In the past several decades, research has shown that prevention of chronic conditions, infectious diseases, and injuries is vital to managing the skyrocketing costs and availability of health care resources.

Emphasis on prevention should be part of the entire nursing process, not only in primary or community care but also in acute medical-surgical interventions. Enhancing individuals' ability to have control and impact over their own health is an important health promotion activity. The World Health Organization (WHO, 2017a) further explains that health promotion "covers a wide range of social and environmental interventions that are designed to benefit and protect individual people's health and quality of life by addressing and preventing the root causes of ill health, not just focusing on treatment and cure." Key areas for which all health care providers should have a basic understanding include behaviors that have the most impact on preventable conditions. Health care providers and their patients must focus on critical areas such as disorders associated with smoking and failure to follow appropriate dietary and exercise guidelines if lifelong changes are to be made.

LEVELS OF PREVENTION

Disease prevention measures related to specific interventions directed at individuals or populations can be implemented at various stages of the pathogenesis, or natural history, of a disease.

▶ Primary prevention: Strategies designed to prevent a disease or condition from occurring, such as seat belt use, immunizations, hand washing, and water fluoridation.

▶ Secondary prevention: Strategies meant to identify a disease or condition early to optimize treatment and positive outcomes. This includes screening for various conditions (i.e., depression, blood pressure, scoliosis) and treatment plans that may limit or reverse the course of the disease (i.e., diet education for a prediabetic patient).

▶ Tertiary prevention: Strategies focused on maximizing functionality and quality of life after an event has already occurred (e.g., cardiac rehabilitation after a myocardial infarction or the fitting of a prosthesis after amputation).

Question	Rationale
Teaching a group of adolescent girls about the importance of weight-bearing exercises to increase bone health is an example of: A. Primary prevention B. Secondary prevention C. Tertiary prevention	Answer: A The intervention occurs before an adverse outcome (osteopenia or osteoporosis) and is meant to prevent it from occurring.

HEALTHY PEOPLE

In 1976, to support and advise the nation regarding health promotion and disease prevention efforts, the U.S. Congress developed the Office of Disease Prevention and Health Promotion (ODPHP) as part of the Department of Health and Human Services. The ODPHP quickly became the coordinator of the important assessment, benchmarking, strategizing, and evaluation provided by the Healthy People initiative. Originating from the 1979 Surgeon General's *Healthy People: The Surgeon General's Report on Health Promotion and Disease Prevention* (ODPHP, 2017) and coupled with the vision for a society in which all people live long, healthy lives, this 10-year directive encompasses four overarching goals (Figure 3.1). The ODPHP website, www.heathlypeople.gov, is a valuable resource for information on the latest Healthy People–identified health indicators, the interagency collaborations working toward adressing these, and the progress being made to meet benchmarks during the 10-year cycle.

HEALTH, WELLNESS, DISEASE, ILLNESS AND THE ROLE OF THE NURSE

Similar to the WHO definition, O'Donnell (2009) defines health promotion as "the science and art of helping people change their lifestyle to move toward a state of optimal health." Important terms needed to ascertain how a person moves toward this optimal state and how nurses are involved in this dynamic process are provided below.

▶ **Health:** A state of complete physical, mental, and social well-being, and not merely the absence of disease or infirmity (WHO, 2017b).

▶ **Wellness:** The integration of many different components (mental, social, emotional, spiritual, and physical) that expands one's potential to live (quality of life) and work effectively and to make a significant contribution to society. Wellness reflects how one

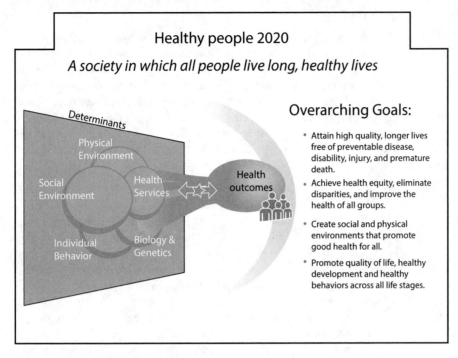

Figure 3.1 www.healthypeople.gov

feels (a sense of well-being) about life as well as one's ability to function effectively (Corbin, Welk, and Corbin, 2010).

▶ *Disease:* "The failure of a person's adaptive mechanisms to counteract stimuli and stresses adequately, resulting in functional or structural disturbances" (Edelman, Kudzma, and Mandle, 2014, 5–6).

▶ *Illness:* The sick feeling and/or symptoms associated with a disease or circumstances that upset homeostasis (Corbin, Welk, and Corbin, 2010).

▶ *Nursing:* The protection, promotion, and optimization of health and abilities, prevention of illness and injury, facilitation of healing, alleviation of suffering through the diagnosis and treatment of human response, and advocacy in the care of individuals, families, groups, communities, and populations (ANA, 2017).

HOLISTIC DIMENSIONS OF HEALTH

Even in its 1940s definition, the WHO (2017a) recognized that health was not just a physical state. The multiple dimensions that make up an individual were identified along with the need to address all of these in a holistic assessment. The holistic approach also emphasizes that individuals are greater than the sum of their parts. In general, the following are considered to be holistic dimensions:

▶ physical

▶ social

▶ psychological

▶ spiritual

HEALTH PROMOTION THEORY MODELS

Numerous theoretical models, within and complementary to nursing, provide a foundation to help understand basic health promotion and health behavior concepts. Several that are pertinent to health promotion are discussed here.

Health Belief Model

The Health Belief Model, used extensively to help understand behavior decisions related to unhealthy practices such as smoking or poor diet, looks at attitudes toward risk and benefit. If an individual feels that the risk for an event (e.g., lung cancer) is high, they are more likely to take action to avoid risks (e.g., quit smoking). Additionally, the perceived severity of a condition (e.g., amputation) impacts the individual's choice (e.g., diabetes control) along with the perceived benefits (e.g., I can play with my grandchildren) and perceived barriers (e.g., I can't give up sweets). This balance between the barriers to implementation and the benefits of change is a common base for many behavioral theories.

Social Cognitive Theory

An important variable that is also used within other models is one that was well developed in the earlier Social Cognitive Theory (SCT). Based on Bandura's social learning (Edelman, Kudzma, and Mandle, 2014) theory, when interpreted in health promotion situations, the concepts of observation and modeling of behaviors are key constructs. This psychologic model defines and points out the impact of self-efficacy, or one's confidence in being able to achieve an outcome. Self-efficacy is part of many health promotion and health behavior theories and identifies the need for support persons, such as nurses, to assess a patient's motivators and confidence level in making a change and increasing the chance of success. By encouraging realistic, short-term goals that a patient can successfully meet, a nurse can assist the patient in increasing self-efficacy with regard to a longer-term change. Recommending that an overweight patient cut out one high-calorie item, such as sugary drinks, may increase the success of losing a small amount of weight in a shorter period and enhance the feasibility of making more diet-change goals in the future.

Health Promotion Model

In the 1980s, nurse researcher Nola Pender did extensive work with adolescent girls and their physical activity behaviors. The resulting Health Promotion Model (HPM) highlights an individual's unique characteristics, life experiences, and motivators, including self-efficacy. The HPM stresses the impact nurses can have on the individual's action by identifying and helping modulate these variables. By developing a relationship and exploring the patient's history and stories, the nurse can assist with identifying positive behavior changes, barriers (perceived or real), and personal characteristics to help achieve the change. An example would be assisting a patient with chronic obstructive pulmonary disease (COPD) who continues to smoke in part because of a long family history of smoking to identify methods of overcoming this barrier. Encouraging self-reflection regarding values, beliefs, and goals will facilitate a plan to quit smoking.

CHANGE THEORIES

Lewin's Stages of Change

Lewin's 3–Stage Model of Change offers a simple framework of:

- Unfreezing: Developing motivators and removing obstacles to change
- Changing: Promoting communication, support, attitude, and environment to foster and sustain change
- Refreezing: Allow the change to become part of the new norm

Prochaska's Transtheoretical Change Theory

- Expands on the SCT, with an emphasis on identifying in which stage of change individuals are and on how to help them move forward to productive, long-term behavior change (Figure 3.2).
- Self-efficacy, or one's confidence that a task can be completed, plays a vital role in moving through the stages, and the possibility of relapse is addressed.

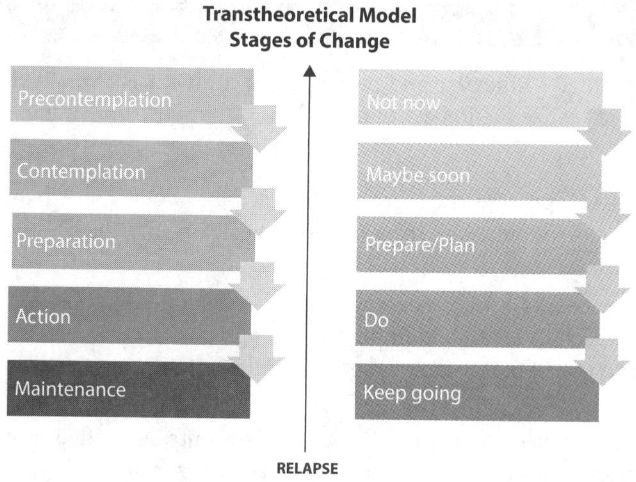

**Transtheoretical Model
Stages of Change**

RELAPSE

Figure 3.2 Prochaska's Change Model

Question	Rationale
Your patient has chosen a date at the end of the month when he will quit smoking. According to the Transtheorectical Change Model, what stage is he in? A. Precontemplation B. Contemplation C. Preparation D. Action	Answer: C The patient is in the preparation stage, as he has chosen a nearby date to begin his change.

DETERMINANTS OF HEALTH

Holistic health not only has multiple dimensions, but it is also impacted by numerous factors or determinants. Both Healthy People 2020 and the World Health Organization list many categories that can be assessed in relation to their impact on the health of individuals, groups, and society. Some of these areas include:

▶ *Social:* Social and cultural norms, economics, education, media, public safety, infrastructure and accessibility of needed resources

▶ *Physical*: Natural environment, environmental exposures, geography, climate, living and working conditions

▶ *Genetics*: Sex, inheritance

For many of these factors, individuals have little or no control over making a change. Society may have more of a collective impact on changing certain determinants (e.g., the environment). Public health initiatives are most effective when addressing these upstream determinants, or those that may be outside the control of individuals but have a great effect on the individual's outcomes (referred to as "downstream"). Pollution upstream that affects all those downstream of the pollutant is an example of this upstream–downstream theory. If the issue is addressed upstream, there will be a widespread and long-lasting impact for all those downstream. By addressing determinants that are beyond the control of single individuals, such as quality and accessible education, the impact will be beneficial to many and add to positive health outcomes into the future.

Clinical Consideration

The ANA *Code of Ethics* reminds nurses of the responsibility and commitment to the needs of society, including advocacy for those downstream of issues such as environmental impact, socioeconomic disparities, and violence.

EQUITY, DISPARITY, AND VULNERABLE POPULATIONS

As professional nurses committed to the care and protection of individuals and larger populations, it is important to realize the impact of inequities, disparities, and circumstances that increase vulnerability.

▶ *Equity*: The ability of all to optimize their health. An inequity would be a barrier that keeps individuals or populations from reaching health equity, such as in discrimination.

▶ *Health disparity*: A difference in a health outcome or status related to a population characteristic such as socioeconomic status, ethnicity, or geographic area. An example would be the increased risk of breast cancer mortality in black women over other races.

▶ *Vulnerable populations*: Those at increased risk of poor health outcomes often face inequities and disparities. Numerous factors can increase vulnerability including where one is born, what diseases they acquire, and what environmental factors they are exposed to. Examples of vulnerable populations may include:

- the very young and very old
- immigrants
- those with a diagnosis of human immunodeficiency virus infection
- the homeless
- pregnant teens

Nursing assessments that are comprehensive and holistic allow nurses to better identify needs of patients, especially the most vulnerable.

▶ A plan of care may need to include increased emphasis on interdisciplinary collaboration to connect patients and families with resources and services.

▶ Being aware of the environment that a patient came from and will likely return to better enables the nurse to investigate risks and foresee issues that require action. A child with recurrent asthma attacks may be living in a home with mold or other triggers that, if managed, may greatly improve the child's health status.

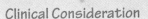

Clinical Consideration

The nursing role of advocate is especially important when working with vulnerable populations.

Question	Rationale
As a community health researcher, you have gathered data from a rural town where there is a larger-than-average number of cases of children with leukemia. This is an example of: A. Health equity B. Health disparity C. Vulnerable populations D. Genetics	Answer: B A difference in health outcomes in a population related to a geographic location refers to a health disparity in that population.

Culturally Sensitive Care

In meeting the holistic needs of patients, an important dimension is culture. In providing patient-centered culturally sensitive care, a nurse must be open to learning about and responding to the needs of culturally diverse patients.

Culture is the beliefs, customs, and traditions within a group. It may represent not only a person's ethnicity or race but also other subgroups based on similarities in lifestyle, hobbies, or place of residence.

With the increasing diversity of the global and U.S. population, health care providers will likely encounter a wide range of nationalities, languages, customs, and health care practices. Becoming proficient in all cultural aspects is unrealistic; however, a culturally competent organization strives to address the needs of varying cultures, whether ethnicities or minority populations, by being aware of policies, behaviors, and attitudes that impact care. The goal of such systems is to be aware of and sensitive to variations in needs in order to provide more patient-centered care with improved outcomes.

A nurse can be culturally sensitive and increase cultural competence by:

- being aware of his/her own customs, beliefs, and practices
- acknowledging past experiences, stereotypes, and biases
- being open to learning about the wide variety of cultural characteristics that patients bring

Communication and forming a trusting relationship is key to patients and families expressing their cultural needs. An open and welcoming nurse will assist and support in the accommodations that may be needed such as diet, time/space for prayer, birth/death rituals, and language interpretation. It is important for a nurse to be aware of cultural variations that are often met during a hospital stay. Care must also be taken to not assume a specific belief or custom based on a patient characteristics or a statement regarding ethnicity, culture, or religion. Being sensitive and anticipating the types of accommodations that *may* be needed includes knowledge about the following. (*Note:* This is a very brief description of only some of the subgroups and related traditions that may be encountered; not all members of the identified religions may follow the noted traditions.)

- *End-of-life practices* (see Chapter 20)
- *Religious dietary restrictions*
  - Catholic: No meat on Fridays and days of fasting during Lent (pre-Easter season); some may refrain from meat on all Fridays
  - Hindu: Most are vegetarian
  - Muslim: Prohibit non-halal meats (not slaughtered according to Islamic tradition), meat from pigs (e.g., pork, bacon); prohibit alcohol
  - Jewish: Prohibit non-kosher meats (not slaughtered according to Jewish tradition), meat from pigs
  - Mormon (Church of Jesus Christ of the Later-Day Saints): Prohibit alcohol, coffee, tea, tobacco; fasting once a month unless ill
  - Seventh Day Adventist: Restrict alcohol and caffeine
- *Prayer/worship rituals* (Healthcare Chaplaincy, 2014)
  - Baha'i Faith: Daily prayer and meditation
  - Buddhist: May include meditation and chanting
  - Catholic: Verbal and silent prayer, mass on Sundays, reception of Communion by priest or lay minister; rosary beads may be used in prayer
  - Christian: Prayer and scripture reading
  - Jewish: Strict adherence in Orthodox Jews, lesser with Reform Jews. Prayers three times a day, often in community; numerous holy days, including weekly Sabbath starting Friday evening and extending until Saturday evening
  - Hindu: Prayer, meditation and reading sacred scripture; must wash hands and feet and be barefoot during rituals
  - Muslim: Islamic prayers in Arabic are performed five times each day while facing Mecca; unless an emergency, do not interrupt or walk in front of those praying
- *Other cultural considerations*
  - Those of Asian background may, as a sign of respect, avoid eye contact with those considered to be in authority, such as a health care provider.

- Nodding of the head should not always be considered an affirmation of understanding or intent. The individual may not understand the conversation and nod as a sign of respect or to avoid conflict or embarrassment.
- Some cultures in which modesty is emphasized, such as Middle Eastern, may refuse a male caregiver for a female patient, or require a female family member to be present during exams.
- Some cultures follow a patriarchal view and require that a male family member, especially the eldest, be given instructions for a female patient and be a key figure in decision making. It is important for the nurse to clarify the wishes of the patient and to obtain appropriate release of information in order to respect the cultural traditions while ensuring the rights of the patient.

The Office of Minority Health offers a multitude of resources on cultural care along with implementation strategies for CLAS, the National Standards for Culturally and Linguistically Appropriate Services in Health and Health Care. The standards require that health care organizations offer quality assistance with communications needs, whether due to language differences or communication challenges, at no cost to patients. Nurses should be aware of the services and resources within their organization to assist patients and ensure that these measures meet the CLAS standards.

Question	Rationale
Your patient states that he is originally from Iran. Your first step in planning care includes: A. Arranging treatments around prayer time B. Ensuring that he has a male personal care giver C. Asking him about any religious practices D. Contacting dietary services to arrange a vegetarian diet	Answer: C The nurse should be careful not to assume any designation of religion or religious practices based on ethnicity or country of birth. Even if a particular religion is stated by a patient, the specifics as to how they practice and what should be considered when planning care may vary.

NURSES' ROLES IN HEALTH PROMOTION AND DISEASE PREVENTION AND HEALTH EDUCATION AND PATIENT TEACHING

As a vital role of a nurse, health education and patient teaching take place in all specialties, across the entire lifespan, and throughout the continuum of care. The primary purpose of health education (often used when referring to larger populations and in health promotion activities) and patient teaching (referring to more defined, direct interventions) is to empower others in their self-care and disease-management skills. Teaching patients and communities about health care needs has always been a hallmark of nursing, but with the trends toward decreased inpatient stays and increased responsibilities directed toward individuals and families, the need for effective, appropriate and timely education is all the more imperative.

Guided by the nursing process, the important stages of assessment, planning, implementation, and evaluation need to be followed to effectively engage in health education and patient education.

▶ *Assessment:* A thorough identification of learning needs includes evaluating:

- prior knowledge and past experiences
- level of motivation

- developmental stage
- physical state (e.g., fatigue, pain, sensory limitations)
- psychologic state (e.g., anxiety, fear)
- cognitive abilities (e.g., literacy level, preferred learning style)

▶ *Planning:*

- Identify goals of the education and learner-centered behavioral objectives that would indicate adequate meeting of goals.
- Be aware of the environment (e.g., timing, privacy, lack of distractions, proper lighting, collection of materials, etc.).

▶ *Implementation:*

- A comprehensive assessment will assist in being prepared to meet the individual learning needs of the patient(s) or other learners.
- In developing and delivering material, the learner's literacy level should be assessed. When these are unknown or when presenting to a larger group of people, the recommendation is to not use language beyond a sixth-grade reading level.
- Using a learner's preferred learning style is important but when it is unknown or when working with a group, a variety of styles should be addressed. These include visual (printed words, pictures, models, videos), oral (spoken word, repeating information), and kinesthetic, or physical (demonstration, role-play, simulation).
- Information should be delivered in manageable segments and prioritized to deliver the essentials. Especially while in a stressed situation, such as hospitalization, the learner may be able to retain only one or two new pieces of information at a time.
- Providing instruction to the patient, family, and other caregivers allows for support and reinforcement of the information.
- Offering visual or written take-aways gives learners something to refer back to for clarification.

▶ *Evaluation:*

- Assessing whether the learner has met the objectives may take a formal route or be evaluated more informally, depending on the type of teaching, setting, and time restraints.
- Attainment of objectives may be evaluated with a pre/post test, with a return demonstration, or using the teach-back method.

> **Clinical Consideration**
> Teach-back is a recommended patient-centered care strategy that provides evaluation of learning and skills while allowing the facilitator to offer correction of misinterpreted information.

OTHER CONSIDERATIONS IN HEALTH EDUCATION AND PATIENT TEACHING

Part of the assessment and development phase of the teaching/learning process is being aware of the developmental stage and needs of the learner.

▶ Attention span, although not always linked to age, generally is much shorter in children than in adults.

▶ Children are also more visual and physical learners, so demonstrations and learning through play is more effective.

▶ Depending on the age, technology may play a large role in gaining and practicing new knowledge and may be helpful in keeping the child's attention while introducing new information.

▶ Feedback and evaluation of learning is often built in to computer-based learning.

▶ Technology can also be used with those beyond childhood. Care must be given to the use of technology in a population that may be uncomfortable or unfamiliar with its use. This may include older adults or those with decreased exposure due to lack of education or lower socioeconomic status.

▶ With all ages, but especially prevalent in older ages, sensory challenges must be considered. The loss of vision and hearing can greatly impact an individual's ability to acquire or comprehend information.

▶ Cognitive changes may alter the ability to retain and retrieve details and confusion may cause frustration and fear.

▶ Multimodal instruction is key, with frequent reinforcement and reminders as well as identification of support people to assist with the long-term plan of care.

▶ The term *health literacy* refers not only to reading and writing abilities of individuals but also to the comprehension and application of health information. Having inadequate math skills that impair computation of medication doses is an example of decreased health literacy. Not being able to analyze the validity of health resource information can also be indicative of lower health literacy. According to the National Assessment of Adult Literacy, only 12% of U.S. adults are categorized as having proficient health literacy (OHPDP, n.d.). This data highlights that up to 9 out of 10 adults lack one or more of the skills needed to adequately manage and optimize their health.

The process of learning requires change, and often with patient teaching, a change in behavior. Being aware of the theories of change, some of which were described earlier, will assist the nurse in identifying the patient's attitudes, motivators, and barriers to change. This allows for a more individualized, patient-centered approach to the teaching–learning plan and process. Patients retain a choice as to whether they accept and commit to a change, and a well-developed, trusting nurse–patient relationship will improve the likelihood of success.

Other considerations when delivering new information, especially that related to consent, is the patient's ability to understand based on factors such as anxiety, fear, and pain.

▶ Being hospitalized or dealing with a new diagnosis escalates vulnerability and stressors and decreases the chance that new information might be correctly understood.

▶ Dealing with pain draws energy away from the task of information retention.

▶ Additionally, some analgesics, and other medications, may increase fatigue or decrease clarity and impair a patient's ability to learn.

Moving patients and consumers toward maximizing their ability for self-care is not only a goal of health education but also of the profession of nursing itself. Effective educational interventions enhance health outcomes, both of individual patients and communities, and also improve the trust relationship between nurse, patient, and caregivers. Other outcomes include:

▶ higher patient satisfaction

▶ improved continuum of care

▶ decreased readmissions

▶ more engaged health care consumers who are ready to advocate for their own and society's right to health

PATIENT EDUCATION AS A NURSING RESPONSIBILITY

Educating patients about their health care needs is not only a professional role of a nurse, but is also an ethical, moral, and legal requirement.

▶ The American Hospital Association's *Patient's Bill of Rights* of 1992, now updated in the Patient Care Partnership document (AHA, 2006) details the expectations that patients are involved in and adequately informed about their care, including diagnosis, treatments, possible complications, alternatives, and expected outcomes.

▶ Accreditors, such as The Joint Commission, also specify criteria related to meeting patient education needs, thereby also affecting possible third-party reimbursement related to accreditation status.

▶ Payer requirements, such as the Centers for Medicare and Medicaid Services (CMS) Meaningful Use, specify the type of entries expected in the electronic health record (EHR) to reflect provision of patient education, especially for patients with certain chronic conditions such as diabetes and hypertension.

▶ The use of patient self-management goals, especially for chronic disease, is expected for facilities engaging in a patient-centered continuum of care and emphasizes the intent that patients have the right and responsibilities to be active agents in their care decisions and behavior choices to meet outcomes.

> **Clinical Consideration**
> It is not only a nursing responsibility to meet all aspects of the teaching–learning process but also to clearly document the assessment, plan, implementation, and evaluation that takes place.

Question	Rationale
You are preparing a 90-year-old, low-income patient with COPD for discharge. Which patient education intervention would be least appropriate? A. Provide the patient with website information on breathing techniques. B. Allow for return demonstration of oxygen use by the patient and family. C. Prepare a simple written step-by-step list for how to use oxygen. D. Have the family bring their home scale in to show how to weigh the patient daily.	Answer: A Due to the economics and age of the patient, the use of and access to a computer is unlikely. The other interventions address the need for support systems and various types of learning styles and needs.

EPIDEMIOLOGY AND INFECTION CONTROL

Epidemiology is concerned with:

▶ what diseases or conditions impact individuals and society

▶ how do these occur and/or spread

▶ how can they be controlled or eradicated

Often this investigation relates to infectious diseases, like the spread of measles, but other conditions can also be studied, such as the factors related to developing diabetes. The common model of studying infectious diseases is the epidemiologic triangle that recognizes the interplay between host (patient), agent (pathogen), and environment.

Nurses should have a basic understanding of epidemiologic principles in order to identify risks and suspected cases, take measures to decrease transmission and institute measures that decrease the chance of recurrence. Infection control and bloodborne pathogen measures are a first line of defense, but nurses need to be aware of early signs and symptoms of infections that warrant prompt attention. With increased global travel and movement of vectors (organism that can transmit disease, such as a mosquito or tick), the ability to assess risk and identify infectious diseases is heightened. The Centers for Disease Control and Prevention (CDC), the World Health Organization (WHO), and local health departments offer a wealth of information on existing and emerging threats such as Zika, Ebola, and multidrug-resistant tuberculosis (MDR TB).

The most impactful primary prevention measure to control many infectious and communicable diseases is immunization. Since widespread vaccination programs began in the mid-1900s, the number of deaths from once-common diseases has greatly decreased, with some diseases, such as smallpox, having been eradicated. In the United States, children receive the vast majority of their recommended immunizations before starting school. Although the vaccination rate in the United States remains high, recent drops in coverage have been reported, and outbreaks of diseases such as measles and pertussis (whooping cough) have occurred in localized areas. Some parents resist vaccinating their children based on concerns about side effects or on religious or other beliefs that dissuade them. Most states allow for school immunization exemptions based on religious or personal belief objections (see your local state guidelines at http://www.ncsl. org/research/health/school-immunization-exemption-state-laws.aspx), although recent legislation has been moving toward more restrictions. Medical contraindications, such as for children with allergies or immunocompromised conditions, are supported in all states.

Nurses play an influential role in providing credible information, dispelling myths, and promoting evidence-based research on vaccination safety and efficacy. Herd immunity, or the theory that the more individuals who are immune to a disease (e.g., as through vaccination), the less likely the attributing pathogen is able to spread from person to person. Some pathogens, like measles, have high infectivity or easily spread from an infected individual to others. In these cases, high herd immunity is needed to protect the population. Not everyone can be made immune to a disease. Those who are too young or are outside the age for specific vaccinations are unprotected as well as those unable to receive the vaccine because of medical circumstances. Even among those properly vaccinated, some do not develop full immunity. Encouraging all those who can be vaccinated to do so will decrease the likelihood of disease spread or reemergence and is imperative to public and global health.

IMMUNIZATIONS

Outside of the childhood years, there are still opportunities to provide increased protection against infectious diseases. Current recommendations for adults include:

- Tdap (tetanus–diphtheria–acellular pertussis) or tetanus booster that also contains protection against pertussis for all adults. This is especially important for parents and caregivers of young infants who are not yet fully immunized against this highly contagious infection. After one Tdap dose, adults can return to the every 10-year Td (tetanus–diphtheria) vaccine.

- Influenza protection has been a key public health initiative over the past several decades. The WHO and CDC recommend annual vaccination for nearly all people 6 months of age or older, with special emphasis on the high-risk populations such as those who are pregnant and those who have chronic conditions. Health care professionals and those who live and work with vulnerable individuals are key to providing increased protection by receiving a yearly influenza vaccination.

- Other adult vaccinations that may be recommended are pneumococcal, human papillomavirus (HPV), meningitis, and shingles.

- Vaccines that were not received in childhood, like measles–mumps–rubella (MMR) or polio may be indicated for those with no evidence of immunity by titer. Those at higher risk for bloodborne disease exposure, such as health care providers, may also need the hepatitis B series vaccine.

- For those 65 years or older and those 19 years or older with high-risk conditions, two separate pneumococcal vaccines are recommended—PCV13 pneumococcal conjugate and PPSV23 pneumococcal polysaccharide vaccine, respectively.

The CDC website offers up-to-date recommendations for both pediatric and adult schedules along with special circumstances and contraindications for the various vaccines.

Question	Rationale
You are admitting a 40–year-old man with a puncture wound. You are asking about his immunization history. What immunization is of the most concern? A. Shingles B. Dtap C. Td D. Meningitis	Answer: C Because of an increased risk of infection of a wound with the bacterium *Clostridium tetani,* which is found in soil, the year of the last tetanus shot must be determined. Depending on the wound risks (e.g., type of injury and cleanliness), a tetanus shot may be given if it has been longer than 5 to 10 years since the previous immunization. Maintaining boosters every 10 years is recommended. Diphtheria and tetanus toxoids and acellular pertussis vaccine (Dtap) is a childhood immunization, while Tdap can be given to an adult to replace a Td if they have not had an adult immunization containing pertussis.

SCREENINGS

An important strategy for secondary prevention is screening. As technology advances, the possibility of discovering more conditions in the early, often asymptomatic, stages increases. The U.S. Preventive Services Task Force (USPSTF) is charged with collecting data and evidence on available screenings and prevention medications. The screening's benefit is weighed against any identified harm to make a recommendation, signified by a letter grade A (high evidence for benefit) to D (high evidence of no benefit or harm outweighs benefit) or I for inconclusive evidence. Nurses should be aware of the screening recommendations, especially related to the population for which they provide care, and assist patients with obtaining evidence-based recommendations such as the USPSTF website (www.uspreventivetaskforce.org). Differences in recommendations may be noted between certain specialty groups and the USPSTF, such as frequency of mammograms and prostate-specific antigen (PSA) testing, and providers should feel confident in explaining the various pros and cons of such screenings. An example of the USPSTF recommendation for hepatitis C screening is shown in Figure 3-3.

Population	Recommendation	Grade
Adults at High Risk	The USPSTF recommends screening for hepatitis C virus (HCV) infection in persons at high risk for infection. The USPSTF also recommends offering 1-time screening for HCV infection to adults born between 1945 and 1965.	B

Figure 3.3 USPSTF

Question	Rationale
You are assessing a 50-year-old woman for recommended screenings. The following screenings would be anticipated except: A. Mammogram B. Pap/HPV C. DXA scan D. Colonoscopy	Answer: C The dual-energy x-ray absorptiometry (DXA) scan is recommended for osteoporosis screening in men and women over 65 years of age; mammography is biennial for woman 50 to 74 years of age (under 50 screening is based on individual factors); cervical cancer screening for women ages 30 to 65 years is every 5 years with Pap/HPV or for ages 21 to 65 years, every 3 years with Pap alone; for those over 45 to 75 years old, a colonoscopy every 10 years is recommended.

Complementary and Alternative Medicine

Complementary and alternative medicine (CAM) approaches to many health conditions are becoming increasingly popular. Although many of these interventions have been used for centuries, mostly in Eastern medicine, more Western medicine patients and providers are becoming involved in their use.

- Complementary methods are those that are used in conjunction with traditional care.
- Alternative therapies replace mainstream care.
- Integrative medical systems are those that coordinate CAM methods with traditional approaches throughout the care process.

Common complementary care techniques include acupressure and use of natural products such as Echinacea. Evidence varies on the benefits of many CAM methods although most show only possible small benefits. Reviews of findings and recommendations can be found on the National Center for Complementary and Integrative Health website (https://nccih.nih.gov/health/atoz.htm). It is important for nurses to include assessment questions related to a patient's use of CAM and ask specific questions about any herbal or other supplements. Many common supplements are known to have interactions with prescription medications, such as interference with anticoagulants and antiplatelet medications from supplements like garlic, ginseng, feverfew, ginger, and others.

EMERGENCY AND DISASTER PREPAREDNESS

In addition to being prepared for the unexpected that may happen to an individual patient, the nurse must also be prepared for the unexpected that may happen in the workplace or the community. Workplace emergency plans should be available and practiced within the institution. Disaster drills should be held to mimic a variety of situations that the staff may need to respond to, ranging from natural disasters to bioterrorism to workplace violence. The key to emergency planning is identification of resources, including outside agencies and communication of roles and responsibilities. The first step a nurse should take in emergency preparedness is personal preparation. The Department of Homeland Security's Ready.gov provides extensive guides for individuals, families, and communities to assess their own preparedness. Knowing that one's family is prepared decreases stressors and anxiety for hospital staff that may be called away or asked to stay during a disaster situation.

Clinical Consideration

The ANA supports and encourages nurses in their personal preparedness and efforts to become involved in community and global emergency relief (http://www.nursingworld.org/disasterpreparedness).

CASE STUDY

As a medical-surgical staff nurse in a busy, urban hospital, you have been assigned to an interdisciplinary team to begin discharge plans for a patient with multiple recent hospitalizations. Mrs. C is a 60-year-old, Japanese, married woman whose most recent hospitalization is for exacerbation of heart failure (HF). She also has a history of arthritis and is hard of hearing. Your assessment of Mrs. C shows that she is a very quiet woman who relies heavily on her family for most of her needs. She ambulates slowly but steadily with a cane, but becomes short of breath after a few minutes. Her edema and weight have been stable for the past 2 days. When asked about any symptoms, Mrs. C usually smiles and nods and does not voice any concerns or questions. Her daughter, who lives with her parents, is in the hospital room most of the day and evening. She confides in you that she is afraid of losing her job because of the time she has taken off to care for her mother and that she is the primary breadwinner in the family. Mr. C, the patient's husband, is also quiet and asks little of the staff. He sits quietly in the room when he visits for a few hours each day. The health care team is working to identify barriers and challenges in Mrs. C's self-management at home to decrease instances of rehospitalizations and increase her quality of life.

1. **Related to her Asian culture, describe characteristics or traditions that might influence Mrs. C and her family's actions and interactions?**

   ▶ *Those of Asian culture may demonstrate a more reserved or quiet demeanor, especially when interacting with those considered to be in authority or when in unfamiliar situations.*

   ▶ *Family is often a central part of Asian culture, and care of one's elders may be highlighted.*

   ▶ *Family, especially male members, often are integral in decision making.*

2. **What might be factors related to Mrs. C's quiet and agreeable nature? Should Mr. C's decreased involvement be perceived as lack of interest in being involved?**

   ▶ *Along with possible cultural respect for authority and avoidance of disagreement or confrontations, Mrs. C's quiet nature and lack of questioning might be due to other factors. Her language abilities, literacy level, and diminished hearing capability may also be influencing her perceived lack of involvement.*

   ▶ *Mr. C's reserved nature may be culturally influenced and increased because of his lack of familiarity with the situation. Although not asking questions, he likely would be expected to be involved in decision making.*

   ▶ *The nurse should be open to involving the family and reflect with Mrs. C on her family's participation in care. In addition, the nurse should invite Mrs. C to offer guidance as to her family's involvement.*

3. **Should the nurse assume that Mrs. C. and her family are comprehending health education information because they are not asking questions? Why or why not?**

   ▶ *Multiple factors may impact Mrs. C's and her family's responses to information or interactions with health care providers; careful evaluation of learning is needed.*

   ▶ *The cultural tendency toward respect, along with not wanting to appear unknowledgeable, may prevent the patient or family from asking for further clarification or admitting to not understanding.*

   ▶ *Planning opportunities for Mrs. C and her husband and daughter to be part of the education is important. This must be offered in appropriate and multimodal formats (e.g., verbal, visual, written, and possibly in the native language).*

   ▶ *Allowing for teach-back of priority concepts and instructions will assist in evaluating effectiveness.*

4. **What considerations would be taken into account when planning and evaluating your education and discharge plan? How would you involve other disciplines?**

▶ *Along with assessing and addressing areas such as language, health literacy, and sensory challenges, the patient's and family's social situation need to be reviewed. Areas such as finances, the cost of medications, family stressors, and coping mechanisms can be addressed by the nurse and social services.*

▶ *Additionally, home health service referral would be indicated and can better assess the situation and family needs once at home.*

▶ *Nutritional needs and usual food practices, including shopping and preparation, should be part of a dietitian's assessment.*

▶ *Rehabilitation services, such as physical and respiratory therapies, can assess the patient's needs and home situation to offer suggestions for safety and comfort. The entire family must be included in medication teaching, focusing on the importance of adherence.*

▶ *Perhaps the patient would be evaluated for telehealth services to follow the response to treatment and progress at home. The use, availability, and comfort level with technology would need to be ascertained.*

Bibliography

American Hospital Association (2006). Accessed July 15, 2017 from http://www.aha.org/advocacy-issues/communicatingpts/pt-care-partnership.shtml

American Nurses Association (ANA). (2017). Accessed July 15, 2017 from http://www.nursingworld.org/EspeciallyForYou/What-is-Nursing

Corbin, C., Welk, R. L., and Corbin, W. (2010). *Concepts of Fitness and Wellness: A Comprehensive Lifestyle Approach*, 4th ed. (New York: McGraw–Hill).

Department of Homeland Security (2017). Accessed July 15, 2017 from https://www.ready.gov/

Edelman, C., Kudzma, E., and Mandle, C. (2014). *Health Promotion Throughout the Life Span*, 8th ed. (St. Louis: Elsevier).

Healthcare Chaplaincy (2013). Handbook of Patients' Spiritual and Cultural Values for Health Care Professionals. Accessed July 15, 2017 from http://www.healthcarechaplaincy.org/userimages/Cultural%20Sensitivity%20handbook%20from%20HealthCare%20Chaplaincy%20%20(3-12%202013).pdf

Healthy People 2020 (2017). Healthy People 2020 framework. Accessed July 15, 2017 from https://www.healthypeople.gov/sites/default/files/HP2020Framework.pdf

Hollingsworth, L., and Didelot, M. (2005). Illness: the redefinition of self and relationships. Paper presented at the 4th Global Conference—Making Sense of: Health, Illness and Disease, Mansfield College, Oxford: Great Britain.

O'Donnell, M. (2009) Definition of health promotion 2.0: embracing passion, enhancing motivation, recognizing dynamic balance, and creating opportunities. *American Journal of Health Promotion* 24(1), iv-vi

Office of Health Promotion and Disease Prevention (OHPDP). (2017). About OHPDP. Accessed July 15, 2017 from https://health.gov/about-us/

Office of Health Promotion and Disease Prevention (OHPDP). (n.d.). Quick Guide to Health Literacy. Accessed July 15, 2017 from https://health.gov/communication/literacy/quickguide/factsbasic.htm

World Health Organization (2017a). Accessed July 15, 2017 from http://www.who.int/topics/health_promotion/en/

World Health Organization (2017b). About WHO. Accessed July 15, 2017 from http://www.who.int/about/mission/en/

4

Adult Aging Process

Katelyn S. Myroniak DNP(c), RN, CMSRN

OVERVIEW

As the population begins to live longer and grow older at unprecedented rates, understanding the needs of the aging adult is more important than ever. The medical-surgical nurse should be aware of many considerations when taking care of the older adult. Understanding the normal aging process, health concerns of the older population, and the needs for health promotion and prevention are key to providing care for this population.

AGING STATISTICS

- The young old adult is 65 to 74 years of age, while the old old adult is 85 years or older.
- In 2014, 14.5% (46.3 million) of the U.S. population was aged 65 or older.
- It is projected that by 2060, those over 65 and older will reach 23.5% of the U.S. population (98 million).
- In 2012, 60% of older adults needed to manage two or more chronic conditions.
- The U.S. Census Bureau predicts life expectancy to continue to increase. It is estimated that those who reach 65 years of age will average an additional 19.2 years of life.
- About 6% of young old and 25% of old old adults live in nursing homes.
- The frail older adult is generally over the age of 75 years and has physical and cognitive conditions that interfere with performing activities of daily living (ADLs) independently.

(Lewis et al., 2017; Potter et al., 2016)

NORMAL AGING PROCESS AND PHYSIOLOGIC CHANGES

- Erikson's Developmental Stage: Integrity vs. Despair:
  - Older adults often engage in retrospective reflection on their lives.
  - They interpret lives as meaningful or experience regret for not achieving goals.
- Expected developmental tasks for older adults:
  - Adjusting to decreasing health and physical strength
  - Adjusting to reduced and fixed incomes and retirement
  - Coping with the death of loved ones

- Accepting self as an aging individual
- Maintaining satisfactory living arrangements
- Maintaining relationships with adult children
- Finding ways to maintain quality of life

▶ Functional changes:

- The functional status of an older adult refers to the capacity and safe performance of ADLs.
- It is a sensitive indicator of health or illness in the older adult.
- ADLs include bathing, dressing, toileting, grooming, and transfers.
- Instrumental activities of daily living (IADLs) include writing a check, making phone calls, preparing meals, shopping, and driving.
- When a decline in function is identified, focus nursing interventions on maintaining, restoring, and maximizing functional status to maintain independence and dignity (Table 4.1).

TABLE 4.1	COMMON PHYSIOLOGIC CHANGES WITH AGING
System	Common Changes
Integumentary	Loss of skin elasticity; pigmentation changes; glandular atrophy (less oil and sweat production); thinning and graying hair; slower nail growth
Respiratory	Decreased cough reflex and cilia; increased anterior–posterior chest diameter; chest wall rigidity is increased; fewer alveoli; increased airway resistance; increased risk of respiratory infections
Cardiovascular	Lower cardiac output; decreased number of heart muscle fibers; calcification of heart valves; thickening of blood vessels, loss of elasticity and narrowing of lumens; decreased baroreceptor sensitivity; less-efficient venous valves; increased pulmonary vascular tension; increased systolic blood pressure; decreased peripheral circulation/perfusion
Gastrointestinal	Decreased saliva and gastric secretions; decreased pancreatic enzymes; decreased peristalsis and intestinal mobility; gastric atrophy; increased stomach pH; hemorrhoids; periodontal disease; impaired rectal sensation
Musculoskeletal	Decreased muscle mass and strength; weakening and decalcification of bones; degenerative joint changes; increased fat tissue
Neurologic	Decreased rate of nerve impulses; decreased neurotransmitters; nerve-cell degeneration
Sensory	Eyes: vision changes and decreased accommodation to near/ vision (presbyopia); difficulty adjusting from light to dark; yellowing of lens; altered perception of color; smaller pupils Ears: Loss of hearing for high-pitched tones; build-up of earwax; thickening of tympanic membrane Taste: Fewer taste buds; taste often diminished Smell: Often diminished Touch: Fewer skin receptors
Genitourinary	50% decrease in renal blood flow by age 80; decreased bladder capacity; enlarged prostate for males; reduced sphincter tone for females
Reproductive	Male: decreased sperm count; smaller testes; erections less firm and slow to develop Female: decreased estrogen production; smaller ovaries; atrophy of vagina, uterus, and breasts
Endocrine	Various alterations in hormone production; decreased ability to respond to stress; diminished thyroid secretion; increased antiinflammatory hormones; decreased sensitivity to insulin; decreased secretion of pancreatic enzymes and hormones
Immune	Decreased core temperature; decreased T-cell function; decreased thymus size

Question	Rationale
In performing a physical assessment for an older adult, the nurse anticipates finding which of the following normal physiologic changes of aging? A. Increased perspiration B. Increased airway resistance C. Increased salivary secretions D. Increased pitch discrimination	Answer: B Rationale: Normal physiologic changes of aging include increased airway resistance in the older adult. Older adults would be expected to have decreased perspiration and drier skin as they experience glandular atrophy (oil, moisture, sweat glands) in the integumentary system. The older adult would be expected to have a decrease in saliva. A normal physiologic change of the older adult related to hearing is a loss of acuity for high-frequency tones (presbycusis).

HEALTH PROMOTION AND PREVENTION

▶ Preventive measures to recommend to the older adult:
- Participate in screening activities:
  - Blood pressure
  - Mammography:
    - Women ages 50 to 74 years old should have a screening mammogram every 12 to 24 months
  - Papanicolaou (Pap) smears:
    - Women every 5 years with human papillomavirus (HPV) co-test (Pap + HPV test) or every 3 years with cytology until age 65
    - No screening needed past age 65 if adequate prior screening results can be accessed and not otherwise at high risk for cervical cancer
  - Depression screening
  - Vision and hearing
  - Colonoscopy screening every 10 years between the ages of 45 and 75
- Regular exercise
- Weight reduction if overweight
- Eating a low-fat and well-balanced diet
- Moderate alcohol use
- Regular dental visits
- Smoking cessation
- Stress management
- Socialization
- Good handwashing
- Regular checkups with primary care providers

▶ Immunization recommendations:
- Yearly seasonal flu vaccine is recommended.
- Tetanus–diphtheria–acellular pertussis (Tdap) vaccination is recommended once if not received as an adolescent.
- Tetanus–diphtheria (Td) booster shot every 10 years is recommended.
- Shingles vaccine is recommended for adults 50 years of age or older.

Clinical Consideration
Women over 75 years old can continue mammogram screening every 2 years if in good health with a life expectancy of 5 to 10 more years.

Clinical Consideration
Screening (Pap) after the age of 75 should be made on an individual basis.

Clinical Consideration
Those who die from influenza each year are mostly older adults.

- Pneumococcal vaccine is recommend for all adults over the age of 65 (and for those who have certain chronic health conditions):
  - PCV13 (pneumococcal conjugate vaccine)
  - PPSV23 (pneumococcal polysaccharide vaccine)

HEALTH CONCERNS FOR THE AGING ADULT

▶ Falls (see section on "Geriatric Syndromes")

▶ Cognitive changes (see section on "Geriatric Syndromes"):
- Delirium
- Dementia
- Depression

▶ Sleep:
- Older age is associated with shorter sleep time, decreased adequate sleep, and more awakenings.
- Insomnia symptoms often appear with depression, cardiovascular disease, pain, and cognitive problems.
- Medications (pseudoephedrine, caffeine-containing drugs, nicotine) can contribute to poor sleep.
- Awakening in the middle of the night to use the bathroom increases the risk of falls.
- Use a sleep assessment to detect sleep disturbances in older adults.
- Sleep medications should be used with caution.

▶ Safe medication use and polypharmacy:
- Safe medication use in the older adult can be a great challenge.
- Causes of medication errors by older adults:
  - Decreased vision
  - Use of various nonprescription and over-the-counter medications
  - Forgetting to take medications
  - Use of medications prescribed for someone else
  - Lack of financial resources to obtain needed medications
  - Failure to understand directions and instructions for drug treatments
  - Refusal to take medication because of undesirable side effects
- Polypharmacy is the use of multiple medications by a person who has more than one health problem.
- Evaluate medications using the Beers criteria for potentially inappropriate medication use in older adults.
  - The Beers criteria are guidelines that emphasize deprescribing medications that are unnecessary to reduce the use of polypharmacy and to reduce drug interactions.
- The effects of aging on drug metabolism:
  - Brain receptors become sensitive.
  - Hepatic blood flow declines and liver mass shrinks.
  - Metabolism drops to half to two-thirds the rate in young adults.
  - Gastric emptying slows and absorption rate declines.
  - Vascular nerve control is less stable.
  - Renal blood flow decreases and number of functional nephrons decreases.
  - Half-life of many medications is increased.
  - Lean mass decreases while adipose tissues increases.
  - Total body water declines, raising concentrations of water-soluble drugs.
  - Plasma protein levels decrease, reducing number of available sites for protein-bound drugs and raising blood levels of free drug.

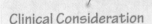

Clinical Consideration

Metabolism of hypnotic drugs decreases, and sensitively increases, with age.

Clinical Consideration

Because of decreased liver and kidney function, the most dramatic change related to aging and medication is decreased drug metabolism.

- Measures to prevent medication errors in older adults:
    - Assess closely for cognitive or motor changes.
    - Encourage the use of one pharmacy.
    - Collaborate with primary care providers (PCPs) and pharmacy to establish medication profiles for all older adults.
    - Reduce number of nonessential medications by contacting the PCP or pharmacist.
    - Assess patient's ability to self-administer medications.
    - Encourage the use of pill organizers and reminder systems.
    - Assess alcohol and illicit drug use.
- Atypical presentations in the older adult:
    - Illness in the older adult is complicated by physical aging, multiple comorbidities, and multiple health problems. Because of this, there are some commonly seen atypical presentations of illness that the nurse must recognize to prevent further complications (Table 4.2).
    - Risk factors for atypical presentations:
        - Over the age of 85
        - Multiple comorbidities
        - Multiple medications
        - Cognitive or functional impairments
    - Common nonspecific signs and symptoms that represent specific illness:
        - Confusion
        - Self-neglect
        - Falling
        - Incontinence
        - Apathy
        - Anorexia
        - Dyspnea
        - Fatigue

TABLE 4.2   ALTERED PRESENTATION OF ILLNESS IN ELDERLY PERSONS

Illness	Atypical Presentation
Infectious disease	Absence of fever; sepsis without leukocytosis and fever; change in functional status; confusion; increase in falls; decreased appetite and fluid intake; incontinence
Acute abdomen	General absence of symptoms; mild constipation or abdominal discomfort; some vague respiratory symptoms or tachypnea
Malignancy	Back pain secondary to slow-growing metastases
Myocardial infarction	Absence of chest pain; vague symptoms including fatigue, decrease in functional status, and nausea; shortness of breath is more common than chest pain
Pulmonary edema	Usually does not present with typical nocturnal dyspnea or coughing; changes in function, confusion, changes in food or fluid intake
Thyroid disease	Hyperthyroidism can present as fatigue and slowing down; hypothyroidism can present with confusion and agitation
Depression	Somatic symptoms such as appetite changes, gastrointestinal (GI) symptoms, and sleep disturbance; lack of sadness; hyperactivity; sadness is often interpreted as a normal sign of aging; medical problems may mask depression.
Illness that presents as depression	Hypothyroid and hyperthyroid disease can present as diminished energy or apathy, which is mistaken for depression.

Question	Rationale
The nurse is admitting a patient for the first time. While assessing the medication history, it is noted that the patient has been taking 19 prescription and several over-the-counter medications. Which intervention should the nurse undertake first? A. Check for medication interactions. B. Determine whether there are medication duplications. C. Call the prescribing health care provider (HCP) and report polypharmacy. D. Determine whether a family member supervises medication administration.	Answer: B Polypharmacy is a concern in the older client. Duplication of medications needs to be identified before medication interactions can be determined because the nurse needs to know what the client is taking. Asking about medication administration supervision may be part of the assessment, but it is not a first action. The phone call to the HCP is the intervention after all other information has been collected.

ELDER MISTREATMENT

Elder mistreatment is an intentional action that can cause harm to a vulnerable elder by a caregiver. Types of elder mistreatment include (Table 4.3):

- Physical: slapping, striking, hitting, restraining
- Neglect: refusing to provide basic life needs (food, water, medications, hygiene)
- Psychologic: verbally harassing, intimidating threatening punishment, treating like a child
- Sexual: nonconsensual sexual contact, touching inappropriately
- Financial: denying access to personal resources, coercing to sign contracts or durable power of attorney, making changes to a will or trust without consent
- Violation of personal rights: denying right to privacy or making decisions
- Abandonment: desertion by someone who had assumed responsibility

Clinical Consideration

Although underreported, about 10% of older adults in the United States experience elder mistreatment.

TABLE 4.3	TYPES OF ELDER MISTREATMENT
Type	**Manifestations**
Physical	Bruises, upper arm injuries, bruises and injuries in various stages of healing, oversedation, use of multiple emergency departments
Neglect	Patient's report of feeling neglected, untreated pressure injuries, malnutrition, poor hygiene, lab values compatible with dehydration
Psychologic	Depression, withdrawn, agitated, flat affect toward caregiver or family
Sexual	Patient's report of sexual abuse, vaginal or anal bleeding, bruised breasts, unexplained sexually transmitted infections (STIs)
Financial	Sudden change in finances, living situation below level of personal resources
Violation of personal rights	Sudden change in living situation, confusion
Abandonment	Patient's report of being abandoned; desertion of older adult at hospital, nursing facility, or public place

◗ Interventions:
- Follow organizational protocols for screening and interventions.
- Registered nurses are mandated reporters to Adult Protective Services.
- Perform a thorough history and physical, and interview the patient alone.
- Be attentive to explanations about injuries that are not consistent with what is observed.
- After obtaining consent, collect physical evidence and photographs per protocol.
- Know the legal responsibilities and resources in your state.

NURSING DIAGNOSIS

Various nursing diagnosis are appropriate for the older adult. Some examples include:

◗ Frail elderly syndrome related to altered cognitive function, chronic illness, history of falls, living alone, prolonged hospitalization, and malnutrition

◗ Self-care deficit related to memory deficit, cognitive impairment, neuromuscular impairment, sensory deficits, deconditioning

◗ Risk for injury related to alteration in cognitive or psychomotor function, alteration in orientation, alteration in sensation

◗ Impaired skin/tissue integrity related to mechanical factors, immobilization, impaired circulation, imbalanced nutritional intake

◗ Impaired memory or confusion related to effects of delirium or dementia

◗ Incontinence related to alteration in cognitive function, immobility, generalized decline in muscle and sphincter tone, neuromuscular impairment, weakened pelvic structure

◗ Impaired physical mobility related to alteration in bone structure, altered cognitive function, decrease in endurance, decrease in muscle mass and strength, disuse, joint stiffness, deconditioning, sensory-perceptual impairment

◗ Activity intolerance related to bed rest, generalized weakness, immobility

◗ Social isolation related to alterations in mental status, altered state of wellness, insufficient personal resources, pain, illness, disabling condition

GERIATRIC SYNDROMES

◗ *Falls and Gait Impairment*
- Approximately 23% of those over the age of 65 fall.
- In 2013, there were 2.5 million emergency department visits for nonfatal falls and approximately 734,000 of these patients were hospitalized (Potter, 2016).
- *Assessment/Intervention/Education*
  - Medical history and risk factors (Table 4.4)
  - Clinical manifestations:
    - The most common injuries from falls are fractures of the spine, hip, forearm, leg, ankle, pelvis, upper arm, and hand.
    - Bruises, hematomas, contusions.
    - Those who have fallen often develop a fear of falling again, which can often cause them to walk less naturally. This will limit their activities and lead to reduced mobility and loss of fitness.
  - Treatment:
    - Treat fractures and other injuries as ordered.
    - Monitor and assess for signs of agitation, delirium, incontinence, and postural hypotension.
    - Follow fall prevention protocols: bed alarms, nonskid socks, frequent rounding, etc.

TABLE 4.4	RISK FACTORS FOR FALLS IN OLDER ADULTS

Intrinsic Factors
- History of previous fall
- Impaired vision
- Syncope and postural hypotension
- Any condition affecting mobility (arthritis, neuropathies, foot problems, weakness)
- Conditions affecting balance and gait
- Frequency and urge incontinence
- Cognitive impairment
- Medication side effects, especially when taking antihypertensives/vasodilators, sedatives, hypnotics, anticonvulsants, and opioids
- Slower reaction times
- Deconditioning

Extrinsic Factors
- Environmental hazards: poor lighting, slippery surfaces, trip hazards, clutter, furniture placement, stairs
- Inappropriate footwear
- Unfamiliar environments
- Improper use of assistive devices

- Encourage physical therapy and exercise as ordered.
- Orient the patient to the environment and make sure the room is free from clutter.
- Patient teaching:
  - Stress the importance of wearing shoes that have stable soles and heels.
  - Safety precautions at home:
    - Make sure stairwells are well lit.
    - Have patient grasp handrails on stairs, and install handrails in the bath and by the commode.
    - Remove throw rugs.
    - Use nonskid mats in showers and tubs.
    - Use glasses and hearing aids as ordered.
    - Use mobility/assistive devices as ordered/recommended.

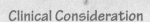

Clinical Consideration

In older adults, delirium is precipitated by systemic infections, environmental factors, sleep deprivation, or emotional distress.

▶ **Delirium**

- Delirium is the state of acute mental confusion.
- As many as 50% of people older than 65 who are hospitalized experience delirium (Lewis, 2017).
- In most cases, delirium is preventable and/or reversible. It is a medical emergency that requires prompt intervention.
- The pathophysiology of delirium is poorly understood. It is believed that the brain gets less oxygen and has problems using it; it is possible that other neurotransmitter abnormalities may also be involved.
- *Assessment/Intervention/Education*
  - Medical history and risk factors
  - Clinical manifestations:
    - There can be a variety of signs and symptoms of delirium.
    - Early manifestations include:
      - Inability to concentrate
      - Loss of appetite
      - Insomnia
      - Irritability

- Disorganized thoughts
- Restlessness
- Confusion
- Later manifestations include:
  - Agitation
  - Misperceptions and interpretations
  - Hallucinations
- Diagnosis involves:
  - A detailed medical and psychologic history and physical examination
  - Careful examination of all medications, including over-the-counter medications.
  - The Confusion Assessment Method tool has been found to be a reliable tool in assessing for delirium (Inouye et al., 1990).
  - Once delirium is diagnosed, potential causes must be explored.
  - Delirium is correlated with increased mortality rates (Kiely et al., 2009).
  - Various laboratory and diagnostic tests can be used to determine underlying causes:
    - Electrolyte, kidney, liver function, thiamine, B_{12}, folate
    - Blood counts
    - Blood glucose
    - Urinalysis
    - Cerebrospinal fluid (CSF) fluid analysis
    - Electroencephalography (EEG)
    - Electrocardiography (ECG)
    - Thyroid levels
    - Arterial blood gas (ABG) and oxygen levels
    - Drug and alcohol levels
    - Head and brain x-rays, computed tomographic (CT) and magnetic resonance imaging (MRI) scans
- Treatment:
  - The nurse's role includes prevention, early recognition, and treatment of delirium.
  - Monitor high-risk groups and eliminate precipitating factors.
  - Treat the underlying cause of the delirium.
  - Protect the patient from harm:
    - Create a calm and safe environment.
    - Encourage family to stay at the bedside.
    - Provide the patient with familiar photos and objects.
    - Consistently reorient the patient.
    - Provide reassurance.
    - Reduce environmental stimuli.
    - Avoid the use of restraints.
    - Address issues related to polypharmacy.
- Patient teaching:
  - Educate the family and caregivers about the factors that precipitated the delirium (Table 4.5).
  - How family/friends can help patients:
    - Speak softly and use simple words or phrases.
    - Remind the patient of the day and date.

Clinical Consideration

A key distinction of delirium is the sudden and acute onset of confusion; this differentiates it from dementia.

TABLE 4.5	FACTORS THAT CAN TRIGGER DELIRIUM

Demographics
- Older than 65, male sex

Cognitive Status
- Dementia, depression, other cognitive impairment, history of delirium

Environmental
- Emotional stress, pain, sleep deprivation, use of physical restraints

Functional and Nutritional Status
- Functional dependence, history of falls, immobility
- Dehydration and malnutrition

Sensory
- Visual or hearing impairment, sensory deprivation or overload

Drugs
- Alcohol or drug abuse, aminoglycosides, anticholinergics, opioids, sedatives, hypnotics, use of multiple drugs

Medical Conditions
- Acute infection, kidney or liver disease, electrolyte imbalance, fracture/trauma, history of stroke, neurological disease, terminal illness

Surgery
- Previous surgical procedure, prolonged cardiopulmonary bypass

- Talk about family and friends.
- Bring glasses, hearing aids, or other assistive devices.
- Bring familiar items that might be reminders of home.
- Provide the patient with favorite music or TV shows.
- Family/friends might be asked to sit and help calm them.

Question	Rationale
In reviewing changes in the older adult, the nurse recognizes that which of the following statements related to cognitive functioning in the older patient is true? A. Delirium is usually easily distinguished from irreversible dementia. B. Therapeutic drug intoxication is a common cause of senile dementia. C. Reversible systemic disorders are often implicated as a cause of delirium. D. Cognitive deterioration is an inevitable outcome of the human aging process.	Answer: C Rationale: Delirium is a potentially reversible cognitive impairment that is often due to a physiologic cause such as an electrolyte imbalance, cerebral anoxia, hypoglycemia, medications, tumors, cerebrovascular infection, or hemorrhage.

▶ *Functional Decline*

- Functional status includes activities of daily living (ADLs) and instrumental activities of daily living (IADLs) that are involved in activities of the physical, psychologic, cognitive, and social domains.
- A decline of function in the older adult is usually due to illness or disease and the degree of its chronicity.
- *Functional status* refers to the capacity to safely perform ADLs and IADLs.
- Deconditioning occurs because of unstable medical conditions, lack of assistive devices, and a lack of motivation to stay active.
- *Assessment/Intervention/Education*
  - Assessment:
    - Any medical history of mobility, sensory, or cognitive impairments may lead to a decrease in functional ability.
    - Chronic inactivity and immobility lead to decreases in functional ability.
    - Assess the patient's ability to perform ADLs (bathing, dressing, toileting, eating, grooming).
    - Assess the patients' ability to perform IADLs (ability to write a check, make phone calls, or prepare a meal).
    - A sudden change in function could be the sign of an acute illness.
    - Use functional assessment tools.
  - Interventions/treatment:
    - Focus interventions on maintaining, restoring, and maximizing functional status.
    - Consult with physical, occupational, and speech/language therapists.
    - Rehabilitation:
      - This treatment may occur in acute inpatient, subacute, or long-term care settings.
      - Preexisting conditions that affect reaction time, visual acuity, fine motor skill, physical strength, and cognitive function affect the length of rehabilitation for an older adult.
      - Older adults can improve strength, flexibility, and aerobic capacity even into very old age.
      - Active rehabilitation can prevent deconditioning and functional decline.
      - The goal of rehabilitation is to achieve maximal functioning and physical capabilities of an individual.
    - Assistive devices:
      - Dentures
      - Glasses
      - Hearing aids
      - Walkers
      - Wheelchairs
      - Adaptive utensils
      - Elevated toilet seats
      - Skin protective devices
      - Handrails
      - Electronic monitoring equipment
      - GPS and medical alert devices

- Patient teaching:
  - Promote understanding of age-related changes.
  - Teach appropriate lifestyle adjustments.
  - Encourage healthy diets, appropriate activity, regular visits with health care providers, participation in meaningful activities, stress management, and avoidance of drugs and alcohol.

Question	Rationale
When developing the plan of care for an older adult who is hospitalized for an acute illness, the nurse should: A. use a standardized geriatric nursing care plan. B. plan for likely long-term–care transfer to allow additional time for recovery. C. consider the preadmission functional abilities when setting patient goals. D. minimize activity level during hospitalization	Answer: C The plan of care for older adults should be individualized and based on the patient's current functional abilities. A standardized geriatric nursing care plan is unlikely to address individual patient needs and strengths. A patient's need for discharge to a long-term–care facility is variable. The activity level should be designed to allow the patient to retain functional abilities while hospitalized and also to allow any additional rest needed for recovery from the acute process.

▶ *Pressure Injuries*

- A pressure injury is a localized skin injury resulting from pressure in combination with shear forces.
- The most common site for pressure injuries is the sacrum, followed by the heels.
- Factors that influence the development of a pressure injury are amount of pressure, length of time the pressure is exerted, and the ability of tissue to tolerate the applied pressure.
- *Assessment/Intervention/Education*
  - Medical history and risk factors:
    - Advanced age
    - Anemia
    - Contractures and immobility
    - Diabetes mellitus
    - Obesity
    - Vascular disease and diseases affecting circulation
    - Incontinence
    - Low blood pressure
    - Cognitive impairment and neurologic disorders
    - Prolonged surgery
    - Poor nutrition
    - Presence of infection
  - Clinical manifestations:
    - The manifestations are dependent on the extent of the tissue involved based on the National Pressure Ulcer Advisory Panel guidelines (see Chapter 18).
    - Infected pressure injuries may lead to leukocytosis and fever.

- Untreated pressure injuries can lead to increases in size, odor, and drainage, necrotic tissue, excessive warmth, and pain.
  - Chronic infections can lead to sepsis and death.
- Treatment:
  - Relieve pressure and keep patient off of the wound.
  - Reposition patient frequently and use lift sheets/life devices to prevent shear.
  - Carefully measure and document the wound.
  - Clean wound and apply dressings per orders.
  - Clean wounds with noncytotoxic solutions.
  - Surgical, mechanical, enzymatic, or autolytic debridement may be ordered.
  - Surgical reconstruction may be done using skin grafts and flaps.
  - Continually monitor for signs and symptoms of infection.
  - Provide adequate nutrition with plenty of protein.
- Patient teaching:
  - Explain etiology and risk factors.
  - Teach the caregiver how to care for incontinence.
  - Demonstrate correct positioning.
  - Assess resources of patient and caregiver if wound care will occur at home.
  - When choosing dressings, consider cost and caregiver time required.
  - Teach how to change dressings using sterile or clean technique as ordered.
  - Teach how to inspect skin daily and to report significant changes to the provider.
  - Teach about the importance of good nutrition.

Question	Rationale
Which one of the orders should a nurse question in the plan of care for an elderly immobile patient with a stage III pressure injury? A. Pack the wound with foam dressing. B. Turn and position the patient every hour. C. Clean the wound with Dakin's solution. D. Assess for pain and medicate before the dressing change.	Answer: C Rationale: Dakin's solution is cytotoxic and should not be used to clean pressure injuries because it will destroy and damage cells.

▶ *Incontinence*
- Urinary incontinence (UI) is the involuntary leakage of urine.
- When bladder pressure exceeds urethral closure pressure, incontinence occurs.
- Anything that interferes with the bladder or urethral sphincter can result in UI.
- Fecal incontinence is the involuntary passage of stool.
- Problems with motor or sensory function can result in fecal incontinence.
- Types of urinary incontinence include:
  - Stress
  - Urge
  - Overflow
  - Reflex

Clinical Consideration

Incontinence is not a natural consequence of the process of aging.

- Posttrauma or postsurgery
- Functional
- *Assessment/Intervention/Education*
  - Medical history and risk factors:
    - Use the acronym DRIP to identify causes of UI:
      - D: delirium, dehydration, depression
      - R: restricted mobility, rectal impaction
      - I: infection, inflammation, impaction
      - P: polyuria, polypharmacy
    - Causes of fecal incontinence include:
      - Trauma to the perineal and rectal area
      - Infection, inflammatory bowel disease
      - Radiation
      - Pelvic floor dysfunction due to medications or prolapse
      - Functional impairment affecting toileting ability
      - Neurologic impairments
      - Chronic constipation, fecal impaction
      - Loss of rectal or pelvic muscle elasticity
      - Rapid transit of large diarrheal stools
  - Clinical manifestations:
    - Involuntary leakage of urine or stool.
    - Continual leakage can lead to skin breakdown, wounds, and infection.
    - If pressure injuries are already present, incontinence may continue to exacerbate the wound and lead to wound growth and infection.
  - Diagnosis:
    - A focused history, physical, bladder log or voiding record, or fecal log
    - A pelvic examination, urinalysis, or urinary ultrasound
    - A rectal examination, stool samples, x-ray or CT scan, colonoscopy, or other imaging
  - Treatment:
    - Treatment for UI is individualized, based on patient preference, the type of severity of UI, and any anatomic defects:
      - Pelvic floor training (Kegel exercises) and biofeedback.
      - Alpha-adrenergic agonists increase bladder sphincter tone (e.g., doxazosin [Cardura], tamsulosin [Flomax]).
      - Muscarinic receptor blockers relax bladder muscle and inhibit detrusor muscle contractions (e.g., oxybutynin [Ditropan], tolterodine [Detrol]).
      - Surgical techniques vary depending on type of UI.
    - Treatment of fecal incontinence depends on the underlying cause:
      - Removal of fecal impaction
      - High-fiber diet and bulk-forming laxatives
      - Antidiarrheal agents
      - Kegel exercises
      - Surgery can be used for prolapse and repair of anal sphincter
  - Patient teaching:
    - Lifestyle modifications:
      - Smoking cessation
      - Weight reduction
      - Good bowel regimen

- Reduction of bladder irritants (caffeine, citrus juice, artificial sweeteners, alcohol)
- Fluid modification
- Schedule voiding regimens; bladder and bowel training.
- Pelvic floor muscle rehabilitation.
- Avoid foods that may trigger fecal incontinence episodes.
- Demonstrate proper perineal and perianal care and hygiene practices.
- Educate patient about the use of incontinence and absorbent products.
- Teach strategies to use when incontinence episodes do occur.

CASE STUDY

Mrs. H. is a 75-year-old female brought to her family doctor's office by her son. They had been to the emergency department (ED) 2 nights ago when Mrs. H. sustained a mechanical fall from standing while going to the washroom at night and fractured her shoulder. She was able to call her son, who took her to the ED for x-rays. After a bit of a wait, she was given a sling for her arm, a prescription for analgesics, and a follow-up appointment with orthopedics. The ED doctor suggested that she go see her family doctor "in a few days." When Mrs. H.'s son John visits her at home to take her to her family doctor, she doesn't seem to be managing well at home. She is not eating right, her house is unkempt, and John isn't sure that she's changed her clothes since that night in the ED. John can't take care of her, as he works two jobs and is a single dad.

Current medications include calcium carbonate 500 mg daily; vitamin D 2000 IU daily; furosemide (Lasix) 40 mg daily, docusate (Colace)100-mg capsule daily; and acetaminophen/hydrocodone (Norco) 325/5 mg, 1 to 2 tabs, every 4 hours as needed for pain.

At the office, the nurse calls back the patient and notices that she looks a little disheveled. The nurse asks a few questions about her fall and the ED visit. Mrs. H. seems vague, distracted, and confused. She is able to tell the nurse that she lives alone. The nurse decides to call John into the room for more information about the situation. John has had no concerns about his mom up until she fell and broke her shoulder. He says that she was managing just fine, and was "sharper than I am."

1. **Based on assessment findings what diagnosis might you expect?**
   - *The patient is demonstrating symptoms of delirium. It is apparent that the confusion is acute and was precipitated by trauma, which resulted in a fracture. A new medication for pain was also prescribed.*
   - *The patient is not eating well, her house is cluttered and messy, and she seems vague, distracted, and confused.*

2. **What other information would be important to know?**
   - *How long has the patient been confused like this?*
   - *Has the patient been taking all of her medications as ordered?*
   - *Has the shoulder pain been managed and controlled?*
   - *How has the patient been sleeping?*
   - *Any other signs/symptoms of infection?*
   - *Possibly a more thorough neurologic/musculoskeletal assessment needs to be performed?*
   - *Has she fallen again?*

▶ *In relation to the fall: Did she hit her head with her original fall? Did she lose consciousness before or after the fall? Was she dizzy before she fell? Did she require a CT of the head with the original fall?*

3. **What diagnostic tests would you anticipate the provider to order?**

▶ *Comprehensive metabolic panel (CMP) to check electrolyte balance, kidney, and liver function since she has not been eating well*

▶ *White-cell count with differential to rule out infection*

  · *If elevated or febrile, blood cultures and urine culture may be ordered*

▶ *Thyrotropin (TSH), vitamin B_{12}, syphilis/rapid plasma reagin (RPR), folate levels*

▶ *CT scan of the head if she reports dizziness, loss of consciousness, syncope/near-syncope signs and symptoms*

▶ *A reliable tool for assessing delirium*

4. **What education would you want to provide to this patient?**

▶ *Treatment of delirium:*

  · *Take a close look at all medications, and perform a physical exam looking for possible causes for her acute confusion.*

  · *Eliminate precipitating factors and treat the underlying cause.*

  · *Explore her pain medication regimen. Recommend a nonopioid medication and a decrease in the opioid dosage.*

▶ *Prevention:*

  · *Educate the patient and family about what can precipitate delirium*

  · *When the patient is experiencing delirium:*

    · *Speak softly and use simple words or phrases.*

    · *Remind the patient of the day and date.*

    · *Talk about family and friends.*

    · *Bring familiar items that might be reminders of home.*

    · *Provide the patient with favorite music or TV shows.*

  · *Use glasses, hearing aids, and other assistive devices.*

  · *Provide a safe environment, bed alarm, and/or home companion.*

5. **What considerations would you make based on this patient's age?**

▶ *Metabolism of drugs in the older adult decreases and sensitivity increases. Because of decreased liver and kidney function, the most dramatic change related to aging and medication is decreased drug metabolism. The patient's pain medication may have been a precipitating factor of her delirium.*

▶ *In the older adult, infectious diseases can present as a change in functional status, confusion, and a decrease in appetite and fluid intake.*

▶ *A social worker may need to be consulted, since the patient lives alone and the son is unable to care for her. A home health care aid may be needed in order for the patient to safely return home.*

Discussion

Risk factors for delirium include age 65 years or older, as well as various other factors. In the older adult, complete a thorough assessment when cognitive changes occur. This is usually a sensitive indicator that some other illness is occurring. An older adult in an acute care setting is at higher risk of delirium because of predisposing factors mixed with multiple underlying conditions. An abrupt change in medications can also lead to delirium because of the metabolic changes in the older adult. Rule out all possible causes of delirium before assuming that the cognitive change is reflective of dementia. The older adult exhibits atypical presentations for many underlying conditions, and delirium is one of these presentations.

Bibliography

Centers for Disease Control and Prevention. (2018). *Breast cancer screening guidelines for women.* Accessed February 6, 2018 from https://www.cdc.gov/cancer/breast/pdf/breastcancerscreeningguidelines.pdf

Centers for Disease Control and Prevention. (2015, September 16). *Cervical cancer: Screening recommendations and consideration.* Accessed February 6, 2018 from https://www.cdc.gov/cancer/knowledge/provider-education/cervical/recommendations.htm

Centers for Disease Control and Prevention. (2017, March 24). *Colorectal cancer screening tests.* Accessed February 6, 2018 from https://www.cdc.gov/cancer/colorectal/basic_info/screening/tests.htm

Centers for Disease Control and Prevention. (2018, January 25). *What vaccines are recommended for you.* Accessed February 6, 2018 from https://www.cdc.gov/vaccines/adults/rec-vac/index.html

Flaherty, E., & Zwicker, D. (2005). *Nursing standard of practice protocol: Atypical presentation.* Accessed March 7, 2018 from https://consultgeri.org/geriatric-topics/atypical-presentation

ICU Delerium.org. (2013). *For patients and families.* Accessed March 7, 2018 from http://icudelirium.org/patients.html

Inouye S.K., van Dyck, C.H., Alessi, C.A., Balkin, S., Siegal, A.P., and Horwitz, R.I. (1990). Clarifying confusion: the confusion assessment method. *Annals of Internal Medicine* 113(12), 941–948.

Kiely, D.K. et al. (2009). Persistent delirium predicts increased mortality. *Journal of the American Geriatric Society* 57(1), 55–61.

Lewis, S.L., Bucher, L., Heitkemper, M., and Harding, M.M. (2017). *Medical-Surgical Nursing: Assessment and Management of Clinical Problems,* 10th ed. (St. Louis: Elsevier).

Office of Disease Prevention and Health Promotion. (2018). *Older adult.* Accessed February 6, 2018 from https://www.healthypeople.gov/2020/topics-objectives/topic/older-adults#1

Potter, P.A., Perry, A.G., Stockert, P.A., and Hall, A.M. (2016). *Fundamentals of Nursing,* 9th ed. (St. Louis: Elsevier).

5

Perioperative Nursing

Patricia Braida MSN, RN, AGPCNP-BC

OVERVIEW

Perioperative nurses have the responsibility and privilege of guiding the patient and family through the surgical experience. Perioperative nurses care for patients during the preoperative, intraoperative, and postoperative phases. This may be the patient and family's first experience with the surgical process, anesthesia, and a health care setting. The surgical or invasive procedure may be performed in the traditional operating room (OR), an ambulatory care surgical center, the provider's office, the radiology department, or in other areas where invasive or operative procedures are performed. Surgery is considered an uncomfortable and stressful situation for most people. Monitoring the patient's response to the stress of surgery is critical. Perioperative nurses play a crucial role in caring for patients as part of the interdisciplinary team, guiding them through the surgical journey.

PREOPERATIVE PHASE

▶ Begins when the decision for surgery is made and ends when the patient is transferred to the surgical suite.

- Assessment and preoperative interview may occur prior to, and/or on the day of surgery.
  - Psychosocial—Identify patient name, birthday, readiness for surgery, expectations about surgical outcomes, understanding of what the plan is, and sources of anxiety or fear.
    - Culture—Identify religious beliefs, language spoken, traditions or other specific needs.
  - History of present problem:
    - Why is the patient here? What is the patient's understanding of the procedure to be performed and the rationale for performing it?
  - Health history—The Joint Commission requires that all patients admitted to the OR have a documented history and physical (H&P) in their medical record (The Joint Commission, n.d.b), including the following information:
    - Allergies to surgical preparation solutions, soaps, adhesive tape, latex, drugs, and foods

> **Clinical Consideration**
> Patients allergic to bananas, avocado, and kiwi may also be allergic to latex because the food proteins are similar to the proteins in latex.

- Medical and surgical history:
  - Any complications during or after previous surgeries: infections; reaction to drugs or anesthesia; venous thromboembolism; postoperative nausea and vomiting
  - Obstructive sleep apnea (OSA)
  - Cardiac, pulmonary, liver, renal, gastrointestinal, endocrine, vascular, or hematologic diseases
- Smoking, alcohol, opioids, use of recreational drugs:
  - Chronic alcoholism and substance abuse can affect liver function and nutritional status. If liver function is decreased, metabolism of anesthesia agents can be prolonged. Helpful to know the last time patient used alcohol or drugs, as they may experience withdrawal symptoms, which can be life-threatening during or after surgery.
- Implanted devices, pumps, pacemakers, any metal, prosthetics, body jewelry
- Medications: prescription and over the counter; herbals and dietary supplements; and last time taken:
  - Specific instructions need to be given about certain medications, such as when to stop taking the medication, whether the patient should decrease the dosage, and whether any medications should be taken the morning of surgery with sips of water:
    - Antiplatelet medications, anticoagulants
    - Insulin and antidiabetes medications
    - Steroids
    - Antihypertensives
- Diet and time last food eaten
- Family history of cardiac, pulmonary, endocrine disease; adverse reaction to anesthesia, such as malignant hyperthermia (MH)
- Review of systems:
  - Ask specific questions about current health problems to identify systems that should be more thoroughly assessed during the physical exam.
- Physical exam:
  - Baseline: height, weight, vital signs, pain, and assessment of cognition.
  - Complete baseline exam.
  - Identify any cognitive or sensory impairments that require special planning or interventions (hearing, vision, paralysis, etc.).
  - Identify loose teeth, caps, or dentures.
  - Identify any skin lesions, breakdown, or rashes.
  - Findings from H&P will be used by the anesthesia care provider (ACP) to assign a physical status rating for anesthesia administration. This is an indicator of the patient's perioperative risk and can guide treatment decisions (Table 5.1).
- Diagnostic studies—obtain and assess results:
  - If patient is taking antiplatelet medication or anticoagulant, a coagulation profile is ordered.
  - If patient is on diuretic therapy, measurement of blood urea nitrogen (BUN), creatinine, and electrolytes will be ordered.

Clinical Consideration

Administration of opioids and sedatives can worsen OSA by depressing respiration. Patients may be asked to bring in their home OSA devices.

Clinical Consideration

Recreational drug use and regular use of prescribed opioids may affect the type and amount of anesthesia required.

Clinical Consideration

MH is a rare but potentially life-threatening disorder with a genetic predisposition.

Clinical Consideration

Dentures will be removed, but loose teeth and caps/crowns may be an aspiration risk during intubation and during general anesthesia.

TABLE 5.1   AMERICAN SOCIETY OF ANESTHESIOLOGISTS (ASA) PHYSICAL CLASSIFICATION SYSTEM

ASA PS Classification	Definition	Examples
ASA I	A normal, healthy patient	Healthy, nonsmoking, no or minimal alcohol use
ASA II	A patient with mild systemic disease	Mild diseases only, without substantive functional limitations. Examples include (but are not limited to) current smoker, social alcohol drinker, pregnancy, obesity (>30 and <40 BMI), well-controlled DM/HTN, mild lung disease.
ASA III	A patient with severe systemic disease	Substantive functional limitations; One or more moderate to severe diseases. Examples include (but are not limited to) poorly controlled DM or HTN, COPD, morbid obesity (BMI ≥40), active hepatitis, alcohol dependence or abuse, implanted pacemaker, moderate reduction of ejection fraction, ESRD with regularly scheduled dialysis, premature infant PCA <60 weeks, history (>3 months) of MI, CVA, TIA, or CAD/stents.
ASA IV	A patient with severe systemic disease that is a constant threat to life	Examples include (but not limited to): recent (<3 months) MI, CVA, TIA, or CAD/stents, ongoing cardiac ischemia or severe valve dysfunction, severe reduction of ejection fraction, sepsis, DIC, ARD, or ESRD with no regularly scheduled dialysis.
ASA V	A moribund patient who is not expected to survive without the operation	Examples include (but are not limited to) ruptured abdominal/thoracic aneurysm, massive trauma, intracranial bleed with mass effect, ischemic bowel in the face of significant cardiac pathology or multiple organ/system dysfunction.
ASA VI	A patient declared brain-dead whose organs are being removed for purposes of donation	

(American Society of Anesthesiologists; https://www.asahq.org/resources/clinical-information/asa-physical-status-classification-system)

Question	Rationale
The nurse is admitting the patient for surgery who will receive general anesthesia. Which of the following statements would generate alarm and warrant immediate notification of the surgical team? A. "I am very nervous about this surgery because I think it is cancer." B. "I smoke a pack of cigarettes a day and I wasn't able to stop before surgery as they suggested." C. "I have had several family members who have had complications from surgery and anesthesia, so I am nervous about this." D. "I forgot to do my shower this morning with the Chlorhexadine Gluconate (CHG) wipes."	Answer: C The surgical team should be notified immediately about this statement. A history of complications associated with surgery that occurs in families can represent malignant hyperthermia (MH). This is a potentially life-threatening disorder characterized by a hypermetabolic state with hyperthermia and rigidity of skeletal muscles that can result in death. It occurs in susceptible people when they are exposed to anesthetic agents, such as succinylcholine and some inhaled agents. The other statements are important also and should be noted by the team. Someone should talk to the patient a bit more so he can express feelings about the surgery and ask more questions of the provider if necessary. If all members of the team are aware of the patient's smoking history, appropriate intraoperative/postoperative measures must be incorporated (choice of anesthesia, early ambulation, use of incentive spirometer, coughing, deep breathing, etc.). The skin preparation is important, but the family history of surgical complications is the most alarming of these statements.

- If a female patient is of childbearing age, a pregnancy test may be ordered.
- Chest x-ray may be ordered for a patient with a cardiopulmonary disorder.
- Liver-function tests may be ordered for patients with liver disease.
- 12-Lead electrocardiogram (ECG) may be ordered for a patient over age 40 or for those with cardiac disease or dysrhythmias.
- Complete blood count (CBC) may be ordered for those with anemia or infection.
- Blood glucose test will be ordered before, during, after surgery for diabetic patients.
- Arterial blood gas (ABG) measurement and pulmonary-function tests (PFTs) may be ordered for patients with pulmonary disorders.
- Disease-specific diagnostic procedures/tests/imaging may be ordered.
- Type and screen/cross-match may be ordered for a patient undergoing major surgery with anticipated blood loss.
- Baseline CBC, electrolytes, BUN, and creatinine measurements may be ordered for any patient undergoing major surgery.
- Methicillin-resistant *Staphylococcus aureus* (MRSA) screening may be performed.
- Preoperative teaching (Table 5.2)
- Informed consent—surgical procedure and blood transfusion (Table 5.3)

TABLE 5.2	PREOPERATIVE TEACHING FOR THE PATIENT AND FAMILY
Preparation	• Testing, procedures before surgery such as enemas, cleaning/shower with antimicrobial soap/wipes • Diet; when to start nothing by mouth • Stop smoking and consuming alcohol for 48 hours before surgery • Which medications to take; which to hold • Special instructions for antidiabetes medication, insulin, antihypertensive agents for day of surgery • If on long-term steroids, may be given "stress dose" IV the day of surgery • Consult with specialists about anticoagulation, antiplatelet medications, or use of antibiotics for some patients who have prosthetic valve? • Cardiology clearance needed before surgery? • What to wear or bring day of surgery • Driver must be present if being discharged same day • Will sign informed consent before day of surgery or day of surgery before receiving sedatives
Procedure	• Time/place to check in • Admission area, holding area, OR, PACU, transfer to clinical unit, or home • Approximate procedure length • Family will be in waiting room and will be notified when you are finished; surgeon usually talks to family after procedure • Will have to take off own clothes and put on a surgical gown • IV, warming blanket, monitors, other special equipment • Noisy, busy, lots of equipment, monitors that make noise • Surgical site will be marked and explain that "time outs" will occur • OR will be cold, bright; odorous skin prep solutions • Anesthesia administration (specifics from ACP) • Monitors, compression devices, IVs etc. that will be in place upon waking, and recovery process
General Preoperative Teaching Points	• Frequent vital signs • Presence of pain, pain management • Coughing and deep breathing, splinting • Probable post op course • Progression of activity and diet • Incision care • Presence of drains, specialized equipment
ACP = anesthesia care-provider; IV = intravenous; OR = operating room; PACU = post anesthesia care unit	

TABLE 5.3 ELEMENTS OF INFORMED CONSENT

Condition	Description
1. Disclosure of the following must be included/discussed:	• Diagnosis being addressed with this proposed treatment • Description and purpose of proposed treatment • Risks and consequences of proposed treatment • Probability of a successful outcome • Availability of alternative treatments? Risks? Benefits? • Prognosis if this treatment is not initiated
2. Must demonstrate understanding of the information being provided	• Must occur before receiving preoperative drugs or sedatives, opioids, etc.
3. Voluntary	• Must give consent freely without being coerced by anyone
Other considerations	• The surgeon or person doing the procedure is responsible for obtaining informed consent from the patient. • The nurse may be asked to witness the patient signing the consent. • Nurse may need to act as advocate to notify surgeon if patient does not understand anything related to the surgery or needs further explanation. • The consent is dynamic—it can be withdrawn at any time. • If the surgery is considered lifesaving and is an emergency, consent is not required. • If the patient is a minor, incompetent, or unconscious, a family member or legally appointed person may sign the consent. • The patient may be an emancipated minor and may be legally able to sign the consent. Nurses must be aware of the state's Nurse Practice Act and state law surrounding informed consent.

Question	Rationale
Which of the following is included in the preoperative teaching plan for a patient who will undergo a total hip arthroplasty? A. Postoperative nursing interventions B. Risk for postoperative complications C. Risks and benefits of the arthroplasty D. Rationale for why the patient should have spinal anesthesia	Answer: B The preoperative teaching must include what a patient may experience in the surgical journey: feelings, interventions, expected course of recovery, etc. The risks and benefits of the surgery and anesthesia techniques are discussed by the anesthesia and surgical teams.

- Upon admission to the preoperative area, the patient is given an identification wrist band; the time-out procedure includes the patient and the nurse:
  - Two patient identifiers, correct procedure, and correct surgical site are verified (The Joint Commission, 2018)
- Preoperative checklist ensures patient safety (Table 5.4)
- Preoperative and intraoperative medications that may be given (Table 5.5)
- Nursing diagnosis:
  - Knowledge deficit related to preoperative procedures
  - Anxiety related to change in health status
  - Readiness for enhanced knowledge: shows understanding of perioperative and postoperative expectation for self-care

TABLE 5. 4	COMPONENTS OF THE PREOPERATIVE/PREPROCEDURE CHECKLIST

✓ Patient demographics
✓ ID and allergy band: two identifiers verified
✓ Time out
  • Planned procedure
  • Operative site
  • Is the site marked?
✓ Home meds
✓ BMI
✓ Vital signs
✓ Isolation status
✓ Difficult airway?
✓ Preprocedure preparation ordered/completed (e.g., bowel preparation, wash with wipes, shower with specific soap)
✓ Last food and drink
✓ IV access
✓ Gown on
✓ Warming blanket
✓ Cardiac monitor, SCD
✓ Presence of any pumps, retained metal, internal devices, pacemakers, tubes, catheters, artificial airway
✓ Jewelry, dentures, partials, contact lenses, glasses, hearing aids, artificial nails, wigs, nail polish removed and given to family
✓ Location/contact information for family
✓ Consent for procedure and for blood transfusion
✓ History and physical
✓ Lab results, diagnostic procedures (patient name on any x-rays, brought to OR)
✓ HCG if applicable
✓ Type and cross match if applicable
✓ Preoperative medications given
✓ Preoperative skin preparation
✓ Patient is asked to void

BMI = body-mass index; HCG = human chorionic gonadotropin; IV = intravenous; SCD = sequential compression device.

TABLE 5. 5	PERIOPERATIVE MEDICATIONS AND ADJUNCTS TO GENERAL ANESTHESIA

Drug	Type and Use	How It Works	Side Effects
Antibiotic • **Cefazolin (Ancef)**	Antiinfective–bactericidal; given 30-60 minutes before incision is made	Prevent SSI	• Rash • Diarrhea • Urticaria • Nausea/vomiting
Anticholinergic • **Atropine** • **Glycopyrrolate (Robinul)** • **Scopolamine**	Anticholinergic to dry oral and respiratory secretions; prevents nausea and vomiting	Antagonizes acetylcholine receptors	• Xerostomia • Constipation • Flushing • Urinary retention • Blurred vision • Tachycardia
Metoclopramide (Reglan)	Prokinetic agent to prevent postoperative nausea and vomiting by increasing peristalsis and gastric emptying	Increases the effect of acetylcholine on the GI system by stimulating motility; acetylcholine is responsible for normal GI function	• Drowsy • Restless • Fatigue • Anxiety • Insomnia • Headache • Dizziness • Extrapyramidal symptoms • Tardive dyskinesia

(continued)

TABLE 5.5 (*Continued*)

Drug	Type and Use	How It Works	Side Effects
Ondansetron (Zofran)	Antiemetic; used to treat and prevent post op nausea and vomiting	Selectively antagonizes serotonin 5-HT3 receptors in the CTZ zone	• Headache • Constipation • Fatigue • Diarrhea • Urinary retention • Dizziness
Famotidine (Pepcid) or ranitidine (Zantac)	H_2 receptor antagonist used to prevent heartburn, indigestion, GERD	Blocks H_2 receptors and decreases gastric acid production	• Dizziness • Headache • Constipation • Diarrhea • Vitamin B_{12} deficiency with long-term use
Midazolam (Versed)	Benzodiazepine used for antianxiety, sleep, and anesthesia induction and maintenance; used as sedation in local, regional anesthesia and MAC	Binds to benzodiazepine receptors and enhances GABA effects	• Sedation • Respiratory depression • Hypotension • Dystonia • Amnesia • Diplopia
Beta-blockers	Beta-adrenergic antagonist may be used to block SNS response to stress of surgery, or to treat hypertension before or during surgery	Antagonizes beta receptors	• Hypotension • Bradycardia • Dizziness • Fatigue
Opioids (morphine; fentanyl (Sublimaze)	Opioids to relieve pain and anxiety during preoperative procedures and after surgery; anesthesia adjunct to help induce and maintain anesthesia	Binds to various opioid receptors, producing analgesia and sedation	• Respiratory depression • Somnolence • Nausea/vomiting • Confusion • Constipation • Asthenia • Xerostomia • Diaphoresis • Dizziness • Urinary retention • Pruritus • Hypotension
Succinylcholine (Anectine)	Depolarizing neuromuscular blocking agent used to facilitate endotracheal intubation, skeletal muscle relaxation and paralysis	Stimulates motor end plate acetylcholine receptors	• Hypotension • Hypersensitivity reaction • Dysrhythmias • Myalgia • Jaw rigidity • Bradycardia • Tachycardia • Muscle fasciculation • MH (rare)
Rocuronium (Zemuron)	Nondepolarizing neuromuscular blocking agent that induces paralysis and skeletal muscle relaxation	Antagonizes motor end plate acetylcholine receptors	• Transient hypotension • Hypertension • Tachycardia • Effects usually reversed toward end of surgery with anticholinesterase agents such as neostigmine (Bloxiverz), pyridostigmine • Must monitor respirations, muscle strength, and ability to protect airway

CTZ = chemoreceptor trigger zone; H_2 = histamine H_2; GABA = gamma-aminobutyric acid; GERD = gastroesophageal reflux disease; GI = gastrointestinal; 5-HTD = 5-hydroxytryptamine; MAC = monitored anesthesia care; MH = malignant hyperthermia; SNS = sympathetic nervous system; SSI = surgical site infection. (Burcham & Rosenthal, 2016; Epocrates, 2018)

INTRAOPERATIVE PHASE

▶ Begins when the patient is transferred to the operating table and ends when the patient is transferred to the postanesthesia care unit (PACU).

▶ Another time-out occurs with surgical team: confirming correct patient, correct procedure, correct site; surgeon marks correct site

▶ Anesthesia techniques (Table 5.6 and Table 5.7)

▶ Catastrophic events in the operating room
- Anaphylactic reactions:
  - Latex, antibiotics, anesthesia agents, blood products
  - Hypotension, tachycardia, bronchospasm, possible pulmonary edema
- Malignant hyperthermia (MH)—inherited, rare disorder
  - Occurs in susceptible people when they are exposed to anesthetic agents—succinylcholine (Anectine) given with inhalation agents

TABLE 5.6	ANESTHESIA TECHNIQUES
Technique	Description
Moderate sedation	• Sedatives, analgesics, anxiolytics used to control pain and anxiety during minor diagnostic or therapeutic procedure; no inhalation agents used • Not expected to induce deep sedation that would impair ability to maintain own airway • Continuous monitoring of effects on LOC, cardiac, and respiratory function
MAC	• Administration of sedatives, analgesics and anxiolytics used in moderate sedation (above); usually no inhalation agents used • Decreased level of consciousness, maintains own airway, responds appropriately to verbal commands and physical stimulation; may have some amnesia; quick, safe return to baseline functioning • If sedation to a deeper level or transition to general anesthesia is required, the ACP must be able to provide this and airway support as needed • ACP must assure full return to consciousness, relief of pain, and management of any side effects • May be used in conjunction with local anesthesia or regional anesthesia
General anesthesia	• Administration of inhalation gases, IV agents, hypnotics, anxiolytics, and adjuncts (neuromuscular blocking agents, opioids, benzodiazepines, antiemetics) to induce a reversible unconscious state, neuromuscular relaxation, and loss of sensation and awareness • Patient unable to maintain or protect airway, must have advanced airway management and continuous monitoring
Regional anesthesia	• Administration of a local anesthetic to provide loss of sensation over a specific body area • No loss of consciousness, but may be used in conjunction with MAC or moderate sedation • Used safely in patients with multiple comorbidities (perhaps instead of general anesthesia) • Includes spinal, epidural, caudal anesthesia and nerve blocks • Spinal anesthesia for surgeries/procedures involving lower extremities in combination with MAC • Epidural anesthesia by itself for surgeries/procedures, or in combination with MAC or general anesthesia, and/or as postoperative analgesia (in lower doses) • Peripheral-nerve blocks (axillary, infraclavicular, interscalene, popliteal, etc.) obstruct a specific nerve or nerve plexus; used in surgery and can provide continued pain relief after surgery if indwelling catheter is left in for up to 72 hours postoperatively
Local anesthesia	• Administered topically, nebulized, or infiltrated intracutaneously or subcutaneously • Nerve impulses blocked and analgesia produced over a limited area • No sedation or loss of consciousness

ACP = anesthesia care provider; IV = intravenous; LOC = level of consciousness; MAC = monitored anesthesia care. (http://asahq.org/quality-and-practice-management/standards-guidelines-and-related-resources/distinguishing-monitored-anesthesia-care-from-moderate-sedation-analgesia; http://anesthesiology.pubs.asahq.org/article.aspx?articleid=2670190)

- Hyperthermia to core temperature of 105°F with rigidity of skeletal muscle
- Hypoxemia
- Increased creatine kinase levels, myoglobinuria
- Lactic acidosis
- Hypermetabolic state
- Cardiac arrest:
  - Treatment for MH is dantrolene (Dantrium)
  - Cool the patient
  - Protect patient from injury; treat acid–base imbalances

Clinical Consideration
Although rare, MH occurs usually during general anesthesia, but can also occur during recovery period.

TABLE 5.7 GENERAL ANESTHESIA

Drug	Type and Use	How It Works	Side Effects
Methohexital (Brevital)	Barbiturate for rapid induction of general anesthesia and maintenance of general anesthesia	Alters sensory cortex, cerebellar and motor activities; produces sedation, hypnosis, and anesthesia	• Hypotension • Excitatory phenomena • Thrombophlebitis • Tachycardia • Bradycardia • Dyspnea • Respiratory depression
Etomidate (Amidate)	Nonbarbiturate hypnotic used for general anesthesia induction and maintenance	May have GABA-like effects, depresses brain stem, reticular formation activity, and produces hypnosis	• Myoclonic movements • Injection-site pain • Tonic movements • Nausea • Vomiting • Apnea
Propofol (Diprivan)	Nonbarbiturate hypnotic for general anesthesia induction and maintenance; also for sedation for short procedures	Promotes release of GABA causing CNS depression	• Injection-site reaction • Hypotension • Involuntary muscle movements • Rash • Pruritus • Bradycardia • Nausea • Vomiting
Isoflurane (Forane); desflurane (Suprane); sevoflurane (Ultane)	Inhalation agents, volatile liquids used for skeletal relaxation and general anesthesia induction and maintenance	Alters neuronal ion channels such as GABA, glutamate, and glycine receptors, resulting in decreased tissue excitability	• Respiratory depression • Hypotension • Myocardial depression • Nausea • Vomiting • Increased cough
Nitrous oxide	Gaseous agent potentiates volatile agents and reduces amount needed; reduces side effects from volatile agents	Weak anesthetic; usually used with other agents; given with oxygen	• Nausea • Vomiting
Ketamine (Ketalar)	Dissociative agent that causes sedation, immobility, analgesia, amnesia	Acts on cortex and limbic receptors, producing dissociative analgesia and sedation	• Nausea • Vomiting • Hypertension • Tachycardia • Nystagmus • Hallucination • Diplopia • Respiratory depression

(Burcham & Rosenthal, 2016; Epocrates, 2018)

CNS = central nervous system; GABA = gamma-aminobutyric acid.

- Wrong-site surgery
- Fire (rare):
  - Can occur secondary to the use of electrocautery, lasers, and surgical probes in an oxygen-enriched environment.
  - Skin, tissues, hair, drapes, tubes, skin preparation solutions can serve as fuel for a surgical fire.
▶ Nursing diagnosis:
  - Risk for imbalanced fluid volume related to surgery
  - Risk for perioperative hypothermia related to cold surgical room
  - Risk for perioperative positioning injury related to prolonged surgery, immobility

POSTOPERATIVE PHASE

▶ Begins when the surgery is completed and ends when the patient is discharged from medical care:
  - PACU nurse receives situation, background, assessment, recommendation (SBAR) report from the ACP and the OR nurse(s)
  - PACU nurse frequently assesses and monitors recovery from sedation and anesthesia
  - Frequent monitoring of vital signs, airway, pain management, neurologic function, surgical drains, and surgical site(s)
  - PACU nurse may discharge patient home with family or may give SBAR hand-off report to another clinical unit
▶ Potential postoperative complications:
  - Respiratory problems—airway obstruction, hypoxemia, hypoventilation
    - Nursing diagnosis:
      - Ineffective airway clearance related to ineffective cough, pain, use of opioids
      - Ineffective breathing pattern related to use of opioids, anesthesia agents
      - Impaired gas exchange related to hypoventilation:
        - Interventions:
          - Assess airway; oxygen therapy; patient positioning; evaluate use of opioids and response; incentive spirometry; increased activity, cough, deep breathe; venous thromboembolism (VTE) prophylaxis
  - Cardiovascular problems—most common are hypotension, hypertension, dysrhythmias, fluid overload (especially days 1 to 3) due to intraoperative and postoperative fluids and activation of stress response; VTE.
    - Nursing diagnosis:
      - Decreased cardiac output related to hypervolemia
      - Ineffective peripheral perfusion related to prolonged immobility, venous stasis
      - Risk for impaired cardiovascular status
        - Interventions:
          - Intake and output (I & O), daily weights; lung, heart sounds/cardiac, peripheral vascular assessment; blood urea nitrogen (BUN), creatinine, electrolytes; VTE prophylaxis—possible anticoagulant, antiplatelet, sequential compression devices, early ambulation
  - Neurologic and psychologic problems—emergence delirium in PACU (thrashing about, agitation, disorientation); postoperative delirium:
    - Must rule out hypoxia, hypoperfusion, hypo/hyperglycemia, pain, and other emergent problems first
    - Associated with infections, duration of anesthesia, intraoperative complications, and postoperative complications

Clinical Consideration
At high risk for VTE are those with a history of previous thrombosis, blood clotting disorders, cancer, obesity, heart failure, and chronic obstructive pulmonary disease (COPD).

Clinical Consideration
When emergence delirium occurs, assess for hypoxia first. Other causes are pain, prolonged surgery, non per os (NPO; nothing by mouth) status, presence of tubes, devices, and fluid and electrolyte imbalances.

Clinical Consideration
Postoperative delirium is more common in older adults and in patients with existing cognitive impairments.

- Nursing diagnosis:
  - Acute confusion related to hypoxia, anesthesia agents, delirium, age, and/or sensory impairment
  - Anxiety related to change in health, new environment, pain
    - Interventions:
    - Always assess for hypoxemia first; treat pain; frequent assessment/reassessment; provide safe, reassuring, calm environment

Question	Rationale
An elderly patient has just arrived in the PACU after undergoing open reduction internal fixation (ORIF) of her left hip with spinal anesthesia and MAC. She has a history of mild cognitive impairment and lives with her son. The patient's vital signs are: temperature 98.7°F, pulse 110 beats/min and regular, respirations 24 breaths/min and blood pressure 150/80 mm Hg. The patient becomes agitated, anxious, and is pulling at the covers. The nurse's priority intervention is to: A. Administer the ordered lorazepam (Ativan) for agitation B. Assume that this is an exaggeration of her baseline cognitive status C. Check the blood glucose D. Assess the oxygen saturation and perform a thorough airway and lung assessment	Answer: D When a patient is anxious or agitated after surgery, always assume it is due to hypoxia until proven otherwise. The nurse should assess the oxygen saturation and airway and perform a thorough lung assessment and bedside neurocognitive assessment. If the oxygen saturation was low, oxygen would be started. The patient can be repositioned for optimal lung excursion, and the nurse would assess for possible reasons for low oxygen saturation (airway, anesthesia, pain, etc.). The nurse would ask the patient to cough, deep breathe, and use the incentive spirometer. Staying with the patient, calmly reorienting her, keeping her warm, and allowing her son to be at the bedside will help also. There is no history of other diseases that would suggest performing a blood glucose test.

- Uncontrolled pain—incisional; nausea, vomiting, fear, and anxiety can make worse; does patient have chronic pain?
  - Nursing diagnosis:
    - Acute pain related to surgical incision
    - Chronic pain related to preexisting conditions
      - Interventions:
        - Everyone on the team should know pain management plan; use pain scale; and evaluate vital signs and LOC; use of two or more analgesics post operatively for some surgeries; possible use of patient-controlled analgesia (PCA) pump; epidural analgesia; local anesthesia—infiltration of nonopioid drug into surgical site with effects lasting several days; typical postoperative progression is to wean off parenteral drug(s) and convert to oral agent(s); use of nondrug approaches (positioning, alternative and complementary therapies) in conjunction with analgesia

Clinical Consideration

It is important to assess what type of pain and location. Many patients have chronic pain, for which special considerations and adjustments to the pain plan may need to be made.

Question	Rationale
The nurse is completing the assessment on a patient recovering from abdominal surgery who has a PCA pump. The patient has shallow respirations and refuses to breathe deeply. Which of the following should the nurse do first? A. Insist that the client take deep breaths B. Notify the surgeon to request a chest x-ray C. Determine the last time the patient used the PCA pump D. Administer oxygen 2 L/min via nasal cannula	Answer: C Assessing when the PCA pump was last used is very important. Perhaps the patient is not able to take deep breaths because they are in pain and have not used the PCA pump recently. There is no information presented in the question about breath sounds, temperature, signs and symptoms of infection, or oxygen saturation, so B and D would not be appropriate answers.

- Alterations in temperature (see section on MH)—perioperative hypothermia (core temperature less than 96.8°F) can be associated with surgical-site infections (SSIs), bleeding, hypertension, lactic acidosis, altered drug metabolism, shivering, and postoperative pain; shivering is uncomfortable, but can also lead to increased oxygen consumption, tachycardia, and cardiac events.
  - If the patient has a fever, the provider must rule out normal inflammatory response, SSI, respiratory infection, and catheter-associated urinary-tract infection (CAUTI).
  - Consider sepsis in the presence of high fever, shaking chills, hypotension, tachycardia, or increased respiratory rate.
- Nursing diagnosis:
  - Hypothermia related to long procedures, spinal and epidural anesthesia, and use of cold irrigants
  - Hyperthermia related to infection; hypermetabolic state (see section on MH):
    - Interventions:
      - Frequent monitoring; sepsis screening; possible infection workup; increase fluid intake; CAUTI prevention (see Chapter 17); use of pulmonary hygiene, incentive spirometer, early ambulation; aseptic technique; frequent oral care; warming devices; shivering treated with oxygen and opioids
- Gastrointestinal problems—postoperative nausea and vomiting (PONV) most common; postoperative ileus; constipation
- Nursing diagnosis:
  - Nausea related to anesthesia medications, opioids
  - Imbalanced nutrition: less than body requirements related to vomiting, decreased peristalsis

- Constipation related to anesthesia medications, opioids, decreased activity, and/or change in food and fluid intake
- Risk for imbalanced fluid volume:
  - Interventions:
    - Prevention of aspiration; antiemetics; prokinetic drugs (see Table 5.5); ambulation, repositioning; laxative/stool softener for constipation; if ileus, also may need NPO status, possible nasogastric tube with suction; progression to oral fluids, food as tolerated
- Urinary problem—low urine output related to stress response and NPO status; acute urinary retention; perhaps acute kidney injury; CAUTI
  - Nursing diagnosis:
    - Urinary retention related to anesthetic agents, anticholinergics, spinal anesthesia, low abdominal or pelvic surgery
    - Risk for infection
      - Interventions:
        - I&O; remove Foley catheter as soon as possible after surgery to avoid infection; sit on toilet or stand to void; ambulate; drink water; scan the bladder with portable ultrasound to assess for urinary retention; if no void after 6 to 8 hours and excessive urine in bladder, may have to perform straight catheterization
- Integumentary problems—SSI (the most common health-care–acquired infection) and associated with prolonged hospitalization, increased cost of care and poor outcomes (CDC, 2018); continuously assess for injuries to skin related to medical devices, surgical procedure, or prolonged immobilization; may notice surgical incision infection on day 3 to day 5 postoperatively
  - Nursing diagnosis:
    - Impaired skin integrity related to surgical incision, medical devices, and/or prolonged immobility
    - Risk for infection: SSI related to malnutrition, emergency surgical procedures, underlying medical problems, immunocompromised state, and/or age
      - Interventions:
        - Assess for signs/symptoms of any injury to skin from equipment or immobility; assess for signs/symptoms of drainage or infection on the skin and in the incision; assess the dressing covering surgical wound for drainage; judicious use of antibiotics (usually given 30 to 60 minutes before the surgical incision is made); aseptic technique when reinforcing dressings, emptying drains; enhance nutrition and ensure adequate fluid intake; assess electrolytes, BUN, creatinine, CBC, and blood glucose levels; assess for wound dehiscence (separation of primary incision and wound edges); Evisceration occurs if the wound edges open and underlying tissue protrudes through the incision (e.g., intestine, bone)—a surgical emergency; notify the surgeon (see Chapter 18).

▶ Discharge and follow-up care teaching:
- Assess patient and family readiness for self-care and discharge.
- Interdisciplinary team may be required to assist with complex discharge needs.
- Patient may not be going to own home.
- Need to ensure safe transition from hospital-based care to community-based care or to home care (Table 5.8).

Clinical Consideration

Evidence-based practice for prevention of SSI includes appropriate antibiotic selection, timing, and duration; skin preparation with antimicrobial agents; and perioperative blood glucose monitoring.

Clinical Consideration

Assess for injuries to skin from tape or medical devices used during/after surgery. Antiseptic agents used to prepare the skin can pool under or next to the patient and cause injury to the skin if not contained and allowed to dry.

Clinical Consideration

Wound infections can occur from contamination due to flora in the environment and on the skin, from oral flora, and from intestinal flora.

Clinical Consideration

If evisceration occurs, assess the patient, cover the exposed tissue with sterile saline gauzes, and notify the surgeon.

| TABLE 5.8 | POSTOPERATIVE DISCHARGE INSTRUCTIONS |

Meet with the patient and significant other(s) and give them written instructions about:

Signs and symptoms to report to provider
• Fever, increased unrelieved pain, incision looks red, has increasing drainage, or is pulling apart

Medication list reconciled
• Written instructions about when to take, what they are used for, and possible side effects

Diet
Activity
• What is permitted? What is to be avoided?
• Lifting restrictions?
• Physical therapy?
• Driving? Return to work? Return to school? Return to sports? Sexual activities?

Incisions/wounds/drains
• How to care for? Hygiene?
• Other procedures to perform at home or new equipment?

Follow-up appointment(s)
• Call for appointment. When and where will appointment be held?

Any in-home therapies?
• Physical, occupational, and intravenous therapies
• Home health

Who does the patient call if there are questions?

Provide written instructions
Document discharge instructions in the medical record and the patient response.

Question	Rationale
The nurse is caring for a patient who underwent a bowel resection 2 days ago. The patient is reporting pain. What is a priority in the plan of care for this patient? A. Suggest that the patient use the PCA pump for pain relief. B. Reposition the patient on her side. C. Encourage the patient to ambulate, as this will probably help. D. Perform a thorough assessment of the patient's pain.	Answer: D It is a priority to first assess the patient's pain by determining the following: P: provocation/palliation Q: quality/quantity R: region/radiation S: severity T: timing: when did it start? (Crozer Keystone Center for Nursing Excellence, n.d.). A thorough assessment of the patient's pain will guide the nurse's interventions. A patient who had a bowel resection may have postoperative incisional pain, but may also have pain due to gas. If the patient confirms gas pain, the nurse would perform a thorough physical assessment and perhaps recommend that the patient walk in the hallway to help mobilize the gas. If the patient is reporting pain in the right lower leg for example, the nurse would be guided to more thoroughly assess the patient's leg.

GERONTOLOGIC CONSIDERATIONS

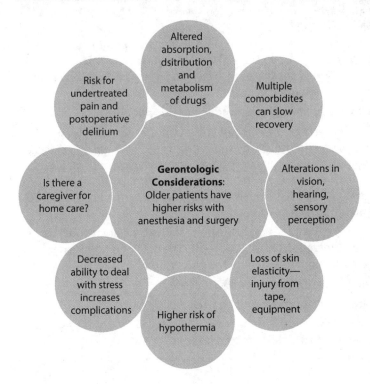

Figure 5.1 The Older Adult Undergoing Surgery

CASE STUDY

A 53-year-old female patient presents for an elective laparoscopic cholecystectomy. In the past 3 months she has had several bouts of right-upper-quadrant pain, feelings of fullness and bloating, and diarrhea after eating. She had an endoscopic retrograde cholangiopancreatography (ERCP) and it was determined that surgery was needed. She has a 5-year history of type 2 diabetes and a 3-year history of hyperlipidemia.

Home Medications:

Metformin (Glucophage) 1000 mg twice daily

Atorvastatin (Lipitor) 40 mg daily

The laparoscopic cholecystectomy goes as planned, and she is extubated and admitted to the recovery room. In the recovery room, she is sleepy, but oriented X 4 (person, place, time, and situation). She has three vomiting episodes and ondansetron (Zofran) provides some relief. Her vital signs are: temperature 98.9°F, pulse 101 beats/min, respirations 24 breaths/min, blood pressure 92/62 mm Hg, and SaO_2 94% on 2 L by nasal cannula. The pain level is 6 of 10 in her midabdominal area and in her back. Capillary blood glucose upon arrival in the PACU is 178 mg /dL. It is decided that she will be admitted to the hospital for overnight monitoring because of vomiting and hypotension.

1. **What are priority assessments for the nurse in the PACU?**

   Frequent assessment of vital signs, including pain assessment and oxygen saturation with careful attention to airway, breathing, circulation, and cognition would be critical. The nurse would assess the lung sounds, breathing pattern, heart rhythm/rate, and assess for chest pain. Skin color/temperature and peripheral pulses would be assessed. The nurse would assess for bowel sounds, distention, incisional drainage, drainage on dressings, any signs of bleeding, and color/amount of drainage in any wound evacuation devices, if applicable. It is important to ask if the patient is passing gas, feels nauseated, or if she has the hiccups. This patient does not have an indwelling Foley catheter, and she may or may not urinate while in the recovery room. The recovery room nurse would monitor the vital signs continuously and possibly need to give a fluid bolus of isotonic solution for the vomiting and hypotension.

2. **Would the nurse anticipate any other orders for this patient?**

   Blood glucose may be rechecked. Hemoglobin level may be ordered, since she did experience some hypotension and tachycardia. In addition, a 53-year-old diabetic woman with hyperlipidemia may possibly be displaying atypical signs of myocardial ischemia (nausea, hypotension, back pain, and epigastric pain). Surgery is a stressful event, and untoward cardiac events can occur. So, perhaps a 12-lead ECG and serial troponins will be checked.

The cardiac enzymes and the 12-lead ECG are normal. The capillary blood glucose on admission to the observation unit is 186 mg/dL. The patient is admitted to the observation unit for overnight monitoring. The orders are:

- Fluid bolus of 500 ml of 0.9% normal saline (0.9 NS)
- IV fluid of 0.9 NS at 100 ml/hr; discontinue when taking oral fluids
- Acetaminophen 325 mg/hydrocodone 5 mg—1 tablet every 4 hours as needed for pain that reaches 4 to 6 on a 10-point pain scale
- Morphine 2 mg IV push every 2 hours as needed for pain level that reaches 7 to 10 on the pain scale
- Ondansetron (Zofran) 4 mg IV push every 8 hours as needed for nausea
- Controlled carbohydrate diet
- Ambulate at least four times daily
- Blood glucose before meals and at bedtime

3. **Are there any other orders the nurse would discuss with the provider?**

   The nurse spoke to the surgeon, using the SBAR format, about other interventions for the patient. She obtained the orders for sequential compression devices and an incentive spirometer. The nurse asked the surgeon if she wanted to order insulin to control blood sugar. The nurse also noted that the surgeon did not order enoxaparin (Lovenox) for the patient. This was an oversight and the surgeon added it to the orders for VTE prophylaxis.

4. **What would be included in the postoperative teaching?**

   The nurse would include coughing/deep breathing/splinting; taking plenty of fluids; and the rationale for ambulation, SCDs (sequential compression device), and daily enoxaparin (Lovenox) in the postoperative teaching. The need for frequent assessment of vital signs, ensuring pain management/control, and assessing the incision/surgical wound for drainage or discoloration will be reviewed. Monitoring the I&O is also important because anesthesia, immobility, prolonged time without food/drink, and opioids can contribute to urinary retention and constipation. The patient would be encouraged to ambulate, as this is important to help clear any retained CO_2 gas from the laparoscopic surgery. Retained CO_2 can cause excruciating pain, and it can be mobilized when the patient walks. It can also cause nausea and back pain. With pain from the retained gas, it is much more beneficial to ambulate, rather than take opioids. The opioids can further decrease GI motility and worsen the gas pain.

   Hygiene and home care for the patient's surgical wounds from the laparoscopic procedure will be explained. Signs and symptoms of SSI will be reviewed with the patient. Because of her diabetes, she is at risk of impaired wound healing. Important signs and symptoms that the patient must report to the surgeon will be reviewed before discharge.

Bibliography

American Association of periOperative Registered Nurses. (2015). *2015 guidelines for perioperative practice.* Accessed January 19, 2018 from https://www.aorn.org/-/media/aorn/guidelines/...standards/ii-01_standards_2015

American Society of Anesthesiologists. (2012). Practice guidelines for acute pain management in the perioperative setting: An updated report by the American Society of Anesthesiologists task force on acute pain management. *Anesthesiology 116,* 248–273.

American Society of Anesthesiologists. (2013). Distinguishing monitored anesthesia care (MAC) from moderate sedation/analgesia (conscious sedation. Accessed January 19, 2018 from http://www.asahq.org/quality-and-practice-management/standards-guidelines-and-related-resources/distinguishing-monitored-anesthesia-care-from-moderate-sedation-analgesia

American Society of Anesthesiologists. (2014). ASA physical status classification system. Accessed January 19, 2018 from https://www.asahq.org/resources/clinical-information/asa-physical-status-classification-system

American Society of Anesthesiologists. (2018). Practice guidelines for moderate procedural sedation and analgesia 2018: A report by the American Society of Anesthesiologists task force on moderate procedural sedation and analgesia, the American Association of Oral and Maxillofacial Surgeons, American College of Radiology, American Dental Association, American Society of Dentist Anesthesiologists, and Society of Interventional Radiology. *Anesthesiology* 128 (3), 437–439. doi:10.1097/ALN.0000000000002043

Burchum, J.R., and Rosenthal, L.D. (2016). *Lehne's Pharmacology for Nursing Care.* 9th ed. (St. Louis: Elsevier).

Crozer Keystone Center for Nursing Excellence. (n.d.). Best practices: PQRST method facilitates accurate pain assessment. Accessed March 18, 2018, from http://www.crozerkeystone.org/healthcare-professionals/nursing/pqrst-pain-assessment-method/

Epocrates Plus for Apple iOS (Version 18.2.1). (2018). General anesthesia. [Mobile application software]. Accessed January 19, 2018 from http://www.epocrates.com/mobile/iphone/essentials

Hanning, C.D. (2005). Postoperative cognitive dysfunction. *British Journal of Anesthesia* 95, 82–87.

Hooper, V.D., Chard, R., Clifford, T., Fetzer, S., Fossum, S., Godden, B. ...Wilson, L. (2010). ASPAN's evidence-based clinical practice guideline for the promotion of perioperative normothermia: second edition. *Journal of PeriAnesthesia Nursing* 25, 346–365.

Lewis, S.L., Bucher, L., Heitkemper, M.M., Harding, M.M., Kwong, J., and Roberts, D. (2017). *Medical-Surgical Nursing: Assessment and Management of Clinical Problems,* 10th ed. (St. Louis: Elsevier).

Malignant Hyperthermia Association of the United States. (2018). Managing a crisis. Accessed January 19, 2018 from https://www.mhaus.org/healthcare-professionals/managing-a-crisis

Mohanty, S., Rosenthal, R.A., Russell, M.M., Neuman, M.D., Ko, C., and Esnaola, N.F. *Optimal Perioperative Management of the geriatric patient: best practices guideline from ACS NSQIP®/American Geriatrics Society.* Accessed January 19, 2018, from https://www.facs.org/.../geriatric/acs%20nsqip%20geriatric%202016%20guidelines.ashx

The Joint Commission. (2018). 2018 Hospital national patient safety goals. Accessed January 19, 2018 from https://www.jointcommission.org/hap_2017_npsgs/

The Joint Commission (n.d.a). History and physical update requirements. Accessed March 26, 2018, from https://www.jointcommission.org/standards_information/jcfaqdetails.aspx?StandardsFAQId=1422

The Joint Commission. (n.d.b). Surgical care improvement project. Accessed January 19, 2018, from https://www.jointcommission.org/assets/1/6/Surgical _Care_ Improvement_ Project.pdf

The Joint Commission. (n.d.c). The Universal Protocol for preventing wrong site, wrong procedure, and wrong person surgery: Guidance for health care professionals. Accessed January19, 2018, from https://www.jointcommission.org/assets/1/18/UP_Poster1.PDF

Xará, D., Silva, A., Mendonca, J., and Abelha, F. (2013). Inadequate emergence after anesthesia: emergence delirium and hypoactive emergence in the post anesthesia care unit. *Journal of Clinical Anesthesia* 25, 439–446.

6

Fluid, Electrolyte, and Acid–Base Imbalances

M. Caitlin Kusnetzow, MSN, RN, CMSRN

OVERVIEW

Homeostasis is the term used to describe the stable internal environment in the body. The body's ability to maintain the proper balance of fluid and electrolytes within specific parameters is essential to maintain homeostasis. This is achieved through many regulatory mechanisms and compensatory responses. Numerous factors can alter the fluid and electrolyte balance, including health conditions and treatments. Alterations in electrolytes can present as excesses or deficits and are described as hyper- (high) or hypo- (low). Fluid imbalances that occur in extracellular or intracellular spaces are described as excesses, deficits, or fluid shifts.

Homeostasis is also dependent on the body's ability to maintain the proper ratio between acids that result from processes of metabolism and the bases that neutralize those acids and aid in their elimination. Acid–base imbalances result from underlying health problems. Arterial blood gas (ABG) levels are interpreted to identify specific imbalances. Components used to interpret ABGs include pH, carbon dioxide ($PaCO_2$), bicarbonate (HCO_3^-), oxygen (PaO_2), and oxygen saturation (SaO_2). The categories of acid–base imbalances are respiratory acidosis, respiratory alkalosis, metabolic acidosis, and metabolic alkalosis. Imbalances can be acute or chronic, and it is possible to have mixed disorders.

The primary treatment for fluid, electrolyte, and acid–base imbalances is aimed at identifying and correcting the underlying cause.

ANATOMY AND PHYSIOLOGY: FLUIDS

The body has two main fluid compartments:

▶ Intracellular space contains intracellular fluid (ICF) that makes up approximately two thirds of the body's water .

▶ Extracellular space contains extracellular fluid (ECF) that makes up about one third of the body's water.

- Two primary extracellular compartments contain ECF:
  - Interstitial fluid—fluid contained in spaces between cells
  - Intravascular fluid—plasma
  - Other ECF:
    - Lymph fluid
    - Transcellular fluid: cerebrospinal fluid, gastrointestinal tract fluid, synovial fluid
    - Fluids in the pleural cavity, peritoneal cavity, pericardial cavity, and intraocular spaces

▌ The movement of fluids between the intracellular and extracellular spaces is controlled by osmosis, hydrostatic pressure, and oncotic pressure (Table 6.1).

▌ Mechanisms of intake and fluid loss maintain fluid balance:
- Water intake:
  - Oral fluid makes up the majority
- Water loss:
  - Urination
  - Insensible losses:
    - Vaporization from lungs
    - Vaporization from skin

TABLE 6.1	MECHANISMS OF FLUID AND ELECTROLYTE MOVEMENT
Mechanism	Action
Diffusion	Movement of molecules from an area of high concentration to an area of low concentration. *Example:* A lump of sugar dissolves in a glass of water.
Facilitated diffusion	Movement of molecules from an area of high concentration to an area of low concentration using a protein carrier in the cell membrane. *Example:* Protein carrier molecules facilitate the diffusion of large glucose molecules across the cell membrane to enter the cell.
Active transport	Movement of molecules against the concentration gradient with use of external energy. *Example:* The sodium–potassium pump uses energy in the form of adenosine triphosphate (ATP) for the movement of sodium out of and potassium into the cell.
Osmosis	Movement of water from an area of low solute concentration to an area of high solute concentration across a semipermeable membrane. *Example:* If a glass of water is separated into halves by a semipermeable membrane and solute is added to one side, water will move to the side with the solute to establish an equilibrium—the two halves have equal concentrations.
Hydrostatic pressure	Force of fluid pushing against a cell membrane or vessel wall. In the vascular system, at the level of the capillaries, forces water out of the vessel and into the interstitial space. *Example:* With a rise in venous hydrostatic pressure in a case such as heart failure, fluid movement back into the capillary will be inhibited, which results in edema.
Oncotic pressure (colloid osmotic pressure)	Osmotic pressure created by plasma colloids (proteins) in a solution. In plasma, those protein molecules attract water, pulling it into the vascular space from the interstitial space. *Example 1:* Increased interstitial oncotic pressure, such as in trauma, can damage capillaries so that plasma proteins are able to accumulate in interstitial space and attract fluid. *Example 2:* Decreases in plasma oncotic pressure, such as in protein malnutrition, result in the inability to pull fluid back into the capillary from the interstitial space.

▶ Body systems and hormonal regulation play a role in fluid balance:
- Hypothalamic–pituitary regulation:
  - Hypothalamus activated by fluid deficit or increased plasma osmolality:
    - Thirst mechanism stimulated
    - Pituitary gland stimulated to release antidiuretic hormone (ADH):
      - Kidneys become more permeable to water because of:
        - Increased water reabsorption
        - Decreased excretion of water in urine:
          - Increased free body water
          - Decreased plasma osmolality
          - Restoration of fluid volume
    - Other factors can stimulate ADH release:
      - Hypotension
      - Nausea
      - Pain
      - Hypoglycemia
      - Hypoxemia
      - Stress response
- Renal regulation:
  - The kidneys adjust the volume of urine and excretion of electrolytes to maintain fluid and electrolyte balance
  - ADH, aldosterone, and other hormones cause reabsorption and secretion of water and electrolytes
  - Impaired renal function can cause inability to maintain fluid and electrolyte imbalance
- Adrenocortical regulation:
  - The adrenal cortex releases glucocorticoids and mineralocorticoids to help maintain fluid and electrolyte balance:
    - Glucocorticoids (e.g., cortisol) have antiinflammatory effects and increase serum glucose.
    - Mineralocorticoids (e.g., aldosterone) increase sodium retention and potassium excretion:
      - Aldosterone increases sodium and water reabsorption in the renal tubules.
      - Many factors stimulate aldosterone release:
        - Decreased renal perfusion
        - Decreased sodium in the distal renal tubule
        - Activation of the renin-angiotensin-aldosterone system (RAAS)
        - Increased serum potassium
        - Decreased serum sodium
        - Adrenocorticotropic hormone (ACTH)
- Cardiac regulation:
  - Natriuretic peptides are hormones produced in reaction to increased atrial pressure from increased intravascular volume and elevated serum sodium levels.
  - Natriuretic peptides consist of atrial natriuretic peptide (ANP) and B-type natriuretic peptide (BNP):
    - Antagonize the RAAS
    - Suppress aldosterone, renin, ADH, and action of angiotensin II
    - Promote excretion of sodium and water in the renal tubules

Clinical Consideration
Patients without an intact thirst mechanism are at higher risk for dehydration.

Clinical Consideration
Decreased renal blood flow, glomerular filtration, and ability to conserve water increase the older adult's risk for fluid and electrolyte imbalances.

Osmolality is the preferred method to describe the concentration of body fluids and measure the amount of molecules per weight of water (mOsm/kg).

▶ Plasma osmolality typically measures between 280 and 295 mOsm/kg:

- High osmolality (>295 mOsm/kg) means high concentration of solute or low water content, also known as "water deficit."
- Low osmolality (<275 mOsm/kg) means high water content or low solute, also known as "water excess."

▶ Osmolality of the ECF can affect the cells that it surrounds (Table 6.2):

- Isotonic fluid has the same osmolality as the fluid in the cell:
  - Under normal conditions, ECF and ICF are isotonic.
  - No net movement of water will occur.
- Hypotonic fluid (hypoosmolar) has lower osmolality than the fluid in the cell:
  - Hypotonic fluid surrounding the cell results in water moving into the cell:
    - Cellular swelling progressing to the cell bursting can occur.
- Hypertonic fluid (hyperosmolar) has higher osmolality than the fluid in the cell:
  - Hypertonic fluid surrounding the cell results in water moving out of the cell, and cell shrinkage progressing to cell death can occur (Figure 6.1).

TABLE 6.2	INTRAVENOUS FLUIDS SUMMARY		
	Examples	Movement of Fluid	Uses
Isotonic	0.9% Normal saline (NS) Lactated Ringer's (LR)	No shifts will occur, as fluid will expand the intravascular compartment only.	Intraoperatively Trauma Dehydration Hypotension
Hypotonic	0.45% saline 0.33% saline 0.22% saline 5% dextrose in water (D5W) (once infused)	Fluid shifts out of intravascular space into intracellular and interstitial spaces (will hydrate cell and interstitial compartments).	Diabetic ketoacidosis (DKA) Depletion from diuretics Patients who need cellular hydration
Hypertonic	5% dextrose in 0.9% NS (D5.9) 5% dextrose in LR (D5LR) 5% dextrose in 0.45% saline (D5.45)	Fluid shifts out of intracellular and interstitial spaces into intravascular space (will dehydrate cell and interstitial compartments).	Postoperatively (reduces postoperative edema, stabilizes blood pressure, maintains urinary output) Third spacing.

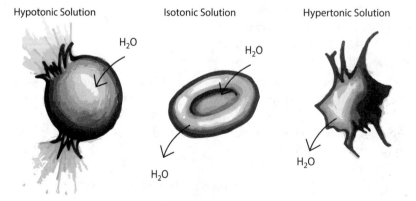

Hypotonic Solution   Isotonic Solution   Hypertonic Solution

H$_2$O   H$_2$O   H$_2$O

H$_2$O

Figure 6.1 Effects of Osmolality on the Cell

FLUID VOLUME IMBALANCES

Fluid imbalances can result from illness, injury, therapeutic measures, and surgical procedures, and they are classified as deficits and excesses that are intracellular, extracellular, or related to fluid shifts.

▶ **Extracellular fluid volume deficit (ECFVD)**

- Dehydration
- Causes:
  - Loss of body fluid:
    - Increased insensible water loss/perspiration from fever, heatstroke
    - Diabetes insipidus
    - Osmotic diuresis
    - Hemorrhage
    - Gastrointestinal (GI) losses through vomiting, nasogastric (NG) suction, diarrhea, fistula drainage
    - Overuse of diuretics
  - Inadequate fluid consumption
  - Fluid shift of plasma from the intravascular to interstitial space (third spacing) from conditions such as burns or pancreatitis
- Manifestations:
  - Neurologic:
    - Restlessness, drowsiness, lethargy, confusion, weakness, dizziness, seizures, coma
  - Skin and mucous membranes:
    - Thirst, dry mucous membranes, cold and clammy skin, decreased skin turgor
  - Cardiovascular:
    - Decreased capillary refill, postural hypotension, bradycardia, decreased central venous pressure (CVP)
  - Genitourinary:
    - Decreased urine output, concentrated urine
  - Respiratory:
    - Increased respiratory rate
  - General:
    - Weight loss
  - Lab values indicate hemoconcentration (elevated serum osmolality, sodium, blood urea nitrogen (BUN), creatinine, hematocrit, urine specific gravity)
- If ECFVD is allowed to progress, intracellular fluid volume deficit (ICFVD) can occur. This results in cellular shrinkage and dehydration.
  - Fluid moves out of the cells in response to the hyperosmolarity in the vascular space, and manifestations result from this attempt to restore equilibrium.
  - Central nervous system (CNS) symptoms arise from the effects of cellular shrinkage on the cerebral cells and can progress from confusion to coma. General symptoms like thirst and oliguria may also be noted.
  - Treatment of ICFVD is also focused on identifying and treating the underlying cause. Fluid replacement is necessary and hypotonic IV fluids such as 5% dextrose in water (D5W) or 0.45% normal saline (NS) may be administered in order to hydrate the cells.
- Treatment:
  - Identify and treat the underlying cause

> **Clinical Consideration**
> To maintain fluid balance, daily water intake for the average adult should be 2 to 3 L.

> **Clinical Consideration**
> Unconsciousness or cognitive impairment limits ability to express thirst or obtain water.

> **Clinical Consideration**
> Skin turgor may not be reliable in the older adult because of loss of tissue elasticity.

- Replace fluid and electrolytes as needed:
  - Depends on severity and type of volume loss
  - Mild losses can be treated with oral rehydration:
    - Assess patient's ability to obtain fluids, express thirst
    - Assess patient's ability to swallow
  - Severe losses or deficits require volume replacements:
    - Administer intravenous (IV) fluids as ordered
    - Choice of fluid depends on cause and electrolyte status:
      - 0.9% NS
      - Lactated Ringer's
      - Blood products if deficit is due to blood loss
- Monitoring:
  - Patient assessment to identify changes in condition and prevent overcorrecting
  - Vital signs
  - Daily weights
  - Intake and output
  - Laboratory results
  - Cardiovascular care:
    - Monitor the patient's cardiovascular status with a thorough assessment as needed.
    - Assess for orthostatic changes in vital signs.
  - Respiratory care:
    - Pulse oximetry
    - Administer oxygen as ordered
  - Skin care:
    - Assessment of skin turgor
    - Frequent skin care
    - Frequent changes in position to prevent skin breakdown
    - Application of moisturizing creams or oils unless contraindicated
    - Protect from trauma and extremes in temperature
  - Safety:
    - Assess level of consciousness, gait, and muscle strength.
    - Institute fall precautions if needed, including use of alarm monitors.
    - Educate patient regarding fall prevention.
  - Educate patient on plan of care.
- Nursing diagnosis:
  - Many nursing diagnoses are appropriate for the patient experiencing ECF volume deficit. Some diagnoses include:
    - Deficient fluid volume related to extracellular fluid loss or decreased fluid intake
    - Decreased cardiac output related to excess extracellular fluid losses or decreased fluid intake
    - Risk for impaired oral mucous membrane related to fluid volume deficit
    - Risk for injury related to decreased cardiac output, hypotension, weakness

▶ **Extracellular Fluid Volume Excess (ECFVE)**

- Causes:
  - Excess intake of fluid:
    - Excessive isotonic or hypotonic IV fluid
    - Primary polydipsia

- Abnormal retention of fluid:
  - Congestive heart failure (CHF)
  - Renal failure
  - Syndrome of inappropriate ADH (SIADH)
  - Cushing's syndrome
  - Long-term use of corticosteroids
- Fluid shift from interstitial space into intravascular space
- Manifestations:
  - Neurologic:
    - Headache, confusion, lethargy, seizures, coma
  - Cardiovascular:
    - Peripheral edema, jugular venous distention (JVD), S3 heart sound, bounding pulse, hypertension, increased CVP
  - Genitourinary:
    - Polyuria
  - Respiratory:
    - Dyspnea, crackles, pulmonary edema
  - Neuromuscular:
    - Muscle spasms
  - General:
    - Weight gain
  - Lab values indicate hemodilution (decreased serum osmolality, sodium, BUN, creatinine, hematocrit, urine specific gravity)
- Treatment:
  - Identification and treatment of underlying cause
  - Removal of fluid without altering electrolyte balance or ECF osmolality
  - Primary forms of therapy:
    - Diuretics
    - Fluid restriction
    - Sodium restriction
  - Alternative therapies may be necessary, depending on the patient situation
    - Paracentesis for ascites
    - Thoracentesis for pleural effusion
- Monitoring:
  - Patient assessment to identify changes in condition and prevent overcorrecting
  - Daily weights
  - Vital signs
  - Intake and output
  - Laboratory results
  - Cardiovascular care:
    - Monitor the patient's cardiovascular status with a thorough assessment as needed.
  - Respiratory care:
    - Assess for crackles and shortness of breath, which may indicate pulmonary congestion and edema.
    - Pulse oximetry
    - Administer oxygen as ordered

Clinical Consideration
Weight gain is the most consistent manifestation of fluid volume excess.

- Skin care:
  - Assess for edema
  - Frequent skin care
  - Frequent changes in position to prevent skin breakdown
  - Elevate edematous extremities
  - Ensure protection from trauma and extremes in temperature
- Safety:
  - Assess level of consciousness, gait, muscle strength.
  - Institute fall precautions if needed, including use of alarm monitors.
  - Educate patient regarding fall prevention.
- Ensure compliance with fluid and/or sodium restriction.
- Administer prescribed diuretics as ordered.
- Educate patient on the plan of care.
- Nursing diagnosis:
  - Many nursing diagnoses are appropriate for the patient experiencing ECFVE. Some diagnoses include:
    - Excess fluid volume related to increased water retention and/or sodium retention
    - Impaired gas exchange related to water retention presenting as pulmonary edema
    - Risk for impaired skin integrity related to edema

Question	Rationale
A patient receiving diuretic therapy has lost 4.4 lb over the course of 24 hours. The nurse is aware that this is equivalent to a loss of approximately how much fluid volume? A. 4 Liters B. 2.2 Liters C. 2 Liters D. 4.4 Liters	Answer: C A body weight loss of 1 kg, or 2.2 lb, is equivalent to a fluid volume loss of 1 liter. Therefore, this patient has lost approximately 2 liters of fluid.

▶ **Intracellular Fluid Volume Excess (ICFVE)**

- Water intoxication
- Causes:
  - Water excess:
    - Excessive water intake
    - Compulsive water drinking (psychogenic polydipsia):
      - Can be associated with mental illness
    - Increased secretion of ADH
  - Administration of excessive intravenous hypotonic solution
  - Renal dysfunction:
    - Inability to excrete excess water
  - Solute (sodium) deficit
- Manifestations:
  - Result from cellular swelling that occurs with fluid movement into the cell in response to hypoosmolarity in the vascular space as the body attempts to restore the equilibrium. Cerebral cells are generally the first to experience this fluid shift.

- Neurologic:
  - Headache (early), irritability, confusion, increased ICP, altered level of consciousness
- Gastrointestinal:
  - Nausea and vomiting (early)
- Cardiovascular and respiratory (symptoms of progressive ICFVE):
  - Increased blood pressure and pulse
  - Increased respirations
- Lab values indicate hemodilution (decreased hematocrit, serum sodium level less than 125 mEq/L)

- Treatment:
  - Identify and treat the underlying cause.
  - Ensure compliance with fluid restriction as ordered.
  - Administer medications and IV fluids as ordered.
    - Sodium administration
    - Hypertonic solution, 3% NaCl:
      - Hypertonic solutions must be administered slowly.
    - Osmotic diuretics (e.g., mannitol [Osmitrol])
  - Decrease intracranial pressure:
    - Elevate head of the bed.
    - Keep neck in neutral position.
    - Maintain normal body temperature.
    - Ensure proper oxygenation.
  - Safety:
    - Assess level of consciousness.
    - Institute fall precautions, if needed, including use of alarm monitors.
    - Educate patient regarding fall prevention.
  - Educate patient on the plan of care.
- Monitoring:
  - Patient assessment to identify changes in condition and prevent overcorrecting
  - Vital signs
  - Laboratory results
  - Daily weights
  - Intake and output

▶ Third Spacing

- Results from an extracellular fluid volume shift into the nonfunctional area between cells
- Causes:
  - Increased capillary permeability:
    - Tissue injury
    - Burns
    - Sepsis
  - Decreased serum protein/albumin levels:
    - Protein malnutrition
    - Liver disease
  - Obstructed lymphatic drainage
  - Increased capillary hydrostatic pressure
- Manifestations:
  - Reflect hypovolemia resulting from fluid shifting out of vascular space and into the interstitial space or tissues

- Cardiovascular:
  - Weak pulse, hypotension, tachycardia, low central venous pressure, pallor
- CNS:
  - Decreased level of consciousness
- Oliguria
- Increased body weight
- Labs indicate elevated BUN, hematocrit, urine specific gravity
- Treatment:
  - Identify and treat the underlying cause.
  - Promote vascular repletion:
    - Possible administration of hypertonic IV fluid
- Monitoring:
  - Patient assessment to identify changes in condition and prevent overcorrecting
  - Vital signs
  - Daily weights
  - Intake and output
  - Laboratory results
  - Skin care:
    - Assess for edema
    - Frequent skin care
    - Frequent changes in position to prevent skin breakdown
    - Elevate edematous extremities
    - Protect from trauma and extremes in temperature
  - Safety:
    - Assess level of consciousness.
    - Institute fall precautions, if needed, including use of alarm monitors.
    - Educate patient regarding fall prevention.
  - Educate patient on plan of care.
- Nursing diagnosis:
  - Many nursing diagnoses are appropriate for the patient experiencing third spacing. Some diagnoses include:
    - Decreased cardiac output related to extracellular fluid shift
    - Risk for impaired skin integrity related to edema
    - Risk for injury related to decreased cardiac output, decreased level of consciousness

> **Clinical Consideration**
> Do not administer hypotonic IV fluids to patients at risk for third spacing.

Question	Rationale
A patient who has an extracellular fluid volume deficit that results in hyperosmolality of the fluid in their vascular space will experience which of the following in terms of fluid movement? A. Movement of fluid from the intracellular space to the vascular space B. No fluid movement C. Movement of fluid from the vascular space to the intracellular space D. Third spacing	Answer: A Hyperosmolality of the intravascular fluid indicates that there is too much solute in comparison to fluid. This will cause a shift of fluid out of the intracellular space and into the vascular space in order to restore the equilibrium.

TABLE 6.3	NORMAL SERUM ELECTROLYTE VALUES
Electrolyte	Reference Range
Anions	
Bicarbonate (HCO_3^-)	22–26 mEq/L (22–26 mmol/L)
Chloride (Cl^-)	96–106 mEq/L (96–106 mmol/L)
Phosphate (PO_4^{3-})	2.4–4.4 mg/dL (0.78–1.42 mmol/L)
Cations	
Potassium (K^+)	3.5–5.0 mEq/L (3.5–5.0 mmol/L)
Magnesium (Mg^{2+})	1.5–2.5 mEq/L (0.75–1.25 mmol/L)
Sodium (Na^+)	135–145 mEq/L (135–145 mmol/L)
Calcium (Ca^{2+}) (total)	8.6–10.2 mg/dL (2.15–2.55 mmol/L)
Calcium (ionized)	4.6–5.3 mg/dL (1.16–1.32 mmol/L)

ANATOMY AND PHYSIOLOGY: ELECTROLYTES

▶ Electrolytes are substances that have molecules that separate into ions when placed in water:
  - Cations are positively charged ions and include sodium (Na^+), potassium (K^+), calcium (Ca^{2+}), and magnesium (Mg^{2+}).
  - Anions are negatively charged ions and include bicarbonate (HCO_3^-), chloride (Cl^-), and phosphate (PO_4^{3-}).
▶ Electrolyte levels are expressed in milliequivalents per liter (mEq) (Table 6.3).
  - In the ECF, the most abundant cation is sodium and the most abundant anion is chloride.
  - In the ICF, the most abundant cation is potassium and the most abundant anion is phosphate.
▶ The movement of electrolytes between the ICF and ECF is controlled by diffusion, facilitated diffusion, and active transport (Table 6.1).

ELECTROLYTE IMBALANCES: SODIUM

▶ Sodium (Na^+):
  - Has many roles:
    - Aids in regulating the concentration and volume of the ECF
    - Effects water distribution between ECF and ICF
    - Important for nerve and muscle function and regulation of acid–base balance
  - Changes in serum sodium level can result from multiple factors:
    - Primary water imbalance
    - Primary sodium imbalance
    - Both primary water and primary sodium imbalances
  - Absorbed from oral intake through the GI tract
  - Excreted from the body through urine, sweat, and feces
  - Balance is regulated by the kidneys:
    - ADH controls excretion or retention of water.
    - Aldosterone enhances sodium reabsorption from the renal tubules.

▶ **Hyponatremia**
- Sodium <135 mEq/L
- Causes a fluid shift out of the ECF and into the cells:
  - Leads to cellular edema, cells bursting
- Causes:
  - Excessive loss of sodium:
    - GI:
      - Diarrhea
      - Vomiting
      - Fistulas
      - NG suction
    - Renal:
      - Diuretics
      - Adrenal insufficiency
      - Sodium wasting renal disease
    - Skin:
      - Burns
      - Wound drainage
  - Inadequate sodium intake:
    - Fasting diets
  - Excessive water gain:
    - Excessive sodium-free or hypotonic IV fluids
    - Primary polydipsia
  - Disease processes:
    - SIADH
    - Heart failure
    - Primary hypoaldosteronism
    - Cirrhosis
- Manifestations:
  - Result from cellular swelling and depend on the severity of the hyponatremia from mild to severe
  - Hyponatremia with decreased ECF volume:
    - Neurologic:
      - Irritability, apprehension, difficulty concentrating, dizziness, confusion, personality changes, tremors, seizures, coma, brain herniation, which causes irreversible damage or death
    - Skin/mucous membranes:
      - Dry mucous membranes, cold and clammy skin
    - Cardiovascular:
      - Postural hypotension, decreased CVP, decreased jugular venous filling, tachycardia, thready pulse
  - Hyponatremia with normal or increased ECF volume:
    - Neurologic:
      - Headache, apathy, confusion, seizures, coma
    - Gastrointestinal:
      - Nausea, vomiting, diarrhea, abdominal cramps
    - Cardiovascular:
      - Hypertension, increased CVP
    - Neuromuscular:
      - Muscle spasms

- General:
  - Weight gain
- Treatment:
  - Identify and treat the underlying cause
  - Hyponatremia from fluid loss:
    - Fluid therapy:
      - Administer isotonic, sodium-containing solutions.
      - Encourage oral intake.
  - Hyponatremia from water excess:
    - Fluid restriction
  - Acute and/or severe hyponatremia:
    - Fluid therapy:
      - Administration of small amounts of hypertonic saline (3% sodium chloride) solution infused slowly
    - Medication:
      - Vasopressor receptor antagonists:
        - Block actions of ADH
        - Used for treatment of severe symptoms and when fluid restriction is not possible
        - Examples:
          - Conivaptan (Vaprisol) given IV
          - Tolvaptan (Samsca) given PO
    - Educate patient on plan of care.
  - Monitoring:
    - Patient assessment to avoid correcting too rapidly or overcorrecting
    - Serum sodium levels:
      - Rapid increases can cause osmotic demyelination syndrome, permanently damaging nerve cells in the brain.
    - Intake and output
    - Seizure precautions
- Nursing diagnosis:
  - Many nursing diagnoses are appropriate for the patient experiencing hyponatremia. Some diagnoses include:
    - Risk for electrolyte imbalance related to excess sodium loss and/or excess water intake/retention
    - Risk for injury related to decreased level of consciousness
    - Risk for acute confusion related to electrolyte imbalance

> **Clinical Consideration**
> Sodium level should not be increased by more than 8 to 12 mEq/L in 24 hours.

▌ **Hypernatremia**
- Sodium level >145 mEq/L
- Causes hyperosmolality, fluid shift out of the cells into the ECF, leading to cellular dehydration, cell death
- Prevented by thirst mechanism
- Causes:
  - Inadequate water intake:
    - Altered level of consciousness
    - Cognitive impairment
  - Excess water loss:
    - ADH deficiency
    - Decreased response of the kidneys to ADH
    - Diarrhea

> **Clinical Consideration**
> Inability to swallow, sense thirst, or obtain fluids increases the risk of hypernatremia.

- Osmotic diuretic therapy (e.g., mannitol [Osmitrol])
- Increased insensible losses:
  - High fever, heatstroke, excessive hyperventilation
- Sodium gain (rare):
  - Excess sodium intake without adequate water intake:
    - Hypertonic saline, sodium bicarbonate, or excessive normal saline per IV
    - Sodium-containing medications
    - Hypertonic enteral feedings without water supplements
    - Excessive oral intake of sodium:
      - Ingestion of saltwater in near-drowning incidents
    - Hypersecretion of aldosterone:
      - Primary aldosteronism caused by adrenal gland tumor.
- Disease processes:
  - Diabetes insipidus
  - Cushing syndrome
  - Uncontrolled diabetes mellitus
- Manifestations:
  - Result from cellular dehydration and shrinkage and depend on the severity of the hypernatremia from mild to severe
  - Hypernatremia with decreased ECF volume:
    - Neurologic:
      - Restlessness, agitation. lethargy, seizures, coma
    - Neuromuscular:
      - Weakness, muscle cramps
    - Skin/mucous membranes:
      - Dry and swollen tongue, sticky mucous membranes
    - Cardiovascular:
      - Postural hypotension, decreased CVP, tachycardia
    - General:
      - Intense thirst, weight loss
  - Hypernatremia with normal or increased ECF volume:
    - Neurologic:
      - Restlessness, agitation, twitching, seizures, coma
    - Skin/mucous membranes:
      - Flushed skin
    - Cardiovascular:
      - Peripheral edema, hypertension, increased CVP
    - Respiratory:
      - Pulmonary edema
    - General:
      - Intense thirst, weight gain
- Treatment:
  - Identify and treat the underlying cause.
  - Primary water deficit:
    - Provide fluid replacement as ordered:
      - Orally
      - Isotonic IV fluids
  - Sodium excess:
    - Administer sodium-free IV fluids as ordered.
    - Administer diuretics as ordered to promote sodium excretion.

- • Implement sodium restrictions as ordered.
      - • Initiate seizure precautions.
    - • Educate patient on plan of care.
  - • Monitoring:
    - - Patient assessment to avoid correcting too rapidly or overcorrecting
    - - Serum sodium levels:
      - • Rapid reduction can cause water to shift back into the cells too quickly, causing cerebral edema and adverse neurologic outcomes
    - - Intake and output
  - • Nursing diagnosis:
    - • Many nursing diagnoses are appropriate for the patient experiencing hypernatremia. Some diagnoses include:
      - - Risk for electrolyte imbalance related to inadequate water intake, excess sodium intake, and/or water loss
      - - Risk for fluid volume deficit related to inadequate water intake or water loss
      - - Risk for injury related to altered sensorium and seizures

> **Clinical Consideration**
> Sodium level should not be reduced by more than 8 to 15 mEq/L in 8 hours.

ELECTROLYTE IMBALANCES: POTASSIUM

- ▶ Potassium (K^+):
  - • Is obtained from the diet:
    - • Many salt substitutes contain potassium
  - • Most of the potassium in the body is intracellular.
  - • Concentration differences in the cells are maintained by the sodium–potassium pump:
    - • Insulin stimulates the sodium–potassium pump
  - • Has many roles:
    - • Important for nerve and muscle function:
      - - ECF-to-ICF ratio contributes to resting membrane potentials of nerve and muscle cells.
      - - Neuromuscular and cardiac function are affected by imbalances.
    - • Aids in regulation of acid–base balance
    - • Helps regulate intracellular osmolality
    - • Promotes cell growth
    - • Required for glycogen deposition in muscle and liver cells
  - • Is excreted by the kidneys:
    - • Approximately 90% of daily intake is eliminated.
    - • Excretion is dependent on several factors:
      - - Serum potassium level:
        - • When high (>5.0 mEq/L), excretion increases
        - • When low (<3.5 mEq/L), excretion decreases
      - - Urine output:
        - • Large amounts of output can cause excess losses.
      - - Renal function:
        - • Impaired renal function can cause retention.
- ▶ **Hypokalemia**
  - • Potassium level <3.5 mEq/L
  - • Causes
    - • Increased loss of potassium:
      - - Most common causes are abnormal kidney and GI tract losses

> **Clinical Consideration**
> Hypovolemia, hyponatremia, and aldosterone secretion cause Na^+ retention and K^+ excretion.

- Kidneys:
  - Diuretics
  - Hyperaldosteronism
  - Low magnesium levels:
    - Stimulate renin and aldosterone release
- GI tract:
  - Diarrhea
  - Laxative misuse
  - Vomiting
  - NG suction
  - Ileostomy drainage
  - Fistulas
- Other losses:
  - Diaphoresis
  - Dialysis
- Increased shift from ECF to ICF:
  - Alkalosis:
    - Potassium shifts into cells in exchange for hydrogen (H^+) ions
  - Insulin therapy
  - Increased insulin release:
    - IV dextrose loading
  - Beta-adrenergic stimulation:
    - Stress
    - Coronary ischemia
- Deficient intake (rare):
  - Starvation
  - Low-potassium diet
  - Lack of potassium in parenteral fluids for non per os (NPO; nothing by mouth) status
- Manifestations:
  - Depend on the severity of the hypokalemia and reflect the resulting hyperpolarization of the cells and impaired muscle contraction
  - The most serious problems that arise are cardiac changes (as listed in the following).
  - Neurologic:
    - Fatigue
  - Cardiovascular:
    - Weak, irregular pulse, lethal dysrhythmias, ECG changes (Table 6.4)
  - Respiratory:
    - Shallow respirations, respiratory arrest with severe hypokalemia due to paralysis

TABLE 6.4	ECG CHANGES WITH POTASSIUM IMBALANCES
Hypokalemia	Hyperkalemia
Flattened T wave	Tall, peaked T wave
Presence of U wave	Prolonged PR interval
ST-segment depression	ST-segment depression
Prolonged QRS	Widening QRS
Peaked P wave	Loss of P wave
Ventricular dysrhythmias	Ventricular fibrillation
First- and second-degree heart blocks	Ventricular standstill

- Gastrointestinal:
  - Constipation, nausea, paralytic ileus
- Neuromuscular:
  - Muscle weakness, leg cramps, soft, flabby muscles, paresthesias, decreased reflexes, paralysis with severe hypokalemia
- General:
  - Hyperglycemia, glucose intolerance
- Treatment:
  - Identify and treat the underlying cause
  - Replace potassium:
    - Dependent on severity:
      - Significant hypokalemia:
        - Oral potassium chloride supplements
        - IV potassium chloride
      - Mild hypokalemia:
        - Increase consumption of foods high in potassium
  - Educate patient about:
    - Plan of care
    - Signs and symptoms of hypokalemia, when to report
    - Importance of regularly having serum potassium levels checked
    - Potassium-rich foods to include in diet (e.g., many fruits and vegetables, nuts and seeds, bananas, milk)
    - Importance of moderating alcohol consumption
    - Avoiding consumption of licorice in large quantities
    - Importance of adhering to medication regimen as prescribed
    - Importance of taking oral potassium supplements whole with a full glass of water
- Monitoring:
  - Continuous electrocardiographic (ECG) monitoring to detect cardiac changes (Figure 6.2)
  - Patient assessment to avoid correcting too rapidly or overcorrecting
  - Serum potassium levels
  - Intake and output
  - Appropriate administration of potassium chloride:
    - IV potassium chloride (KCl):
      - Must be diluted
      - Should not be given as IV push or as a bolus
      - Bag of solution should be inverted multiple times to ensure even distribution
      - Must be infused on a pump

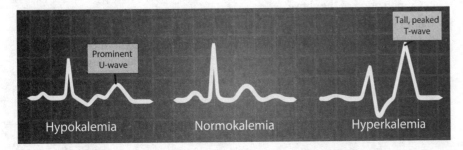

Figure 6.2 Electrocardiographic Changes with Potassium Imbalances

- Infuse at a rate no higher than 10mEq/hr (exceptions in critical care settings)
- IV site should be assessed at least once an hour during infusions because of irritating nature of KCl to the vein and potential effects of infiltration
  - Assess patients being treated with digitalis for digoxin toxicity.
- Nursing diagnosis:
  - Many nursing diagnoses are appropriate for the patient experiencing hypokalemia. Some diagnoses include:
    - Risk for electrolyte imbalance related to excess potassium loss
    - Imbalanced nutrition: less than body requirements related to insufficient intake of potassium-rich foods
    - Risk for activity intolerance related to muscle weakness
    - Risk for injury related to muscle weakness and hyporeflexia
    - Risk for decreased cardiac output related to ECG changes, dysrhythmias

▶ **Hyperkalemia**
- Potassium level >5.0 mEq/L
- Causes:
  - Most common is renal failure
  - Failure to eliminate potassium:
    - Impaired renal excretion
    - Adrenal insufficiency with resulting aldosterone deficiency
    - Medications:
      - Angiotensin II receptor blockers
      - Angiotensin-converting enzyme (ACE) inhibitors
      - Heparin
      - Potassium-sparing diuretics (e.g., spironolactone [Aldactone])
      - Nonsteroidal antiinflammatory drugs (NSAIDs)
  - Massive intake of potassium:
    - Excessive or rapid parenteral administration
    - Potassium-containing drugs (e.g., potassium penicillin [penicillin VK])
    - Potassium-containing salt substitutes
  - Potassium shifts from ICF to ECF:
    - Massive cell destruction:
      - Trauma, burn, crush injury
      - Tumor lysis
      - Severe infections, sepsis
    - Intense exercise
    - Acidosis:
      - Potassium will move from the ICF into the ECF in exchange for hydrogen ions.
  - Combination of the above
- Manifestations:
  - Depend on severity of hyperkalemia and reflect the increased cell excitability and resulting changes in impulse transmission to nerve and muscle cells
  - The most serious problems that arise are disturbances in cardiac conduction (as listed in the following)
  - Neurologic:
    - Fatigue, irritability, confusion

- Cardiovascular:
  - Irregular pulse, ECG changes (see Table 6.4), lethal dysrhythmias, cardiac standstill, failure to capture in individuals with a pacemaker
- Respiratory:
  - Weakness of respiratory muscles, respiratory arrest with severe hyperkalemia due to paralysis
- Neuromuscular:
  - Muscle weakness, cramps, loss of muscle tone, paresthesias, decreased reflexes, tetany
- Gastrointestinal:
  - Abdominal cramping, diarrhea, vomiting
- Treatment:
  - Identify and treat the underlying cause.
  - Mild hyperkalemia in the setting of normal kidney function:
    - Eliminate intake of oral and parenteral potassium.
    - Increase potassium elimination:
      - Diuretics:
        - Loop (e.g., furosemide [Lasix])
        - Thiazide (e.g., hydrochlorothiazide [Microzide])
      - Patiromer (Veltessa):
        - Binds potassium in the GI tract
        - Best for use in chronic hyperkalemia
        - Administration must occur apart from other oral drugs by 6 hours
      - Sodium polystyrene sulfonate (Kayexalate):
        - Oral or rectal
        - Binds potassium in the bowel
        - Used for acute hyperkalemia
      - Hemodialysis:
        - Treatment in cases of renal failure
  - Symptomatic or severe hyperkalemia:
    - Cause potassium to move from ECF to ICF:
      - Activate the sodium–potassium pump to shift potassium into cells:
        - Regular insulin:
          - Administered with dextrose 50% IV
        - Beta-adrenergic agonist (e.g., nebulized albuterol)
      - IV sodium bicarbonate:
        - Used in acidosis
    - Stabilize cardiac membranes and protect from dysrhythmias:
      - Reverse effects on the membrane potential and restore electrical gradient:
        - IV calcium chloride
        - IV calcium gluconate
  - Educate patient about:
    - Plan of care
    - Signs and symptoms of hyperkalemia, when to report
    - Importance of having serum potassium levels checked regularly
    - Diet:
      - Foods low in potassium to include in diet (e.g., apples, corn, lettuce, pasta, non–whole grain bread products)

- Foods high in potassium to avoid (e.g., many fruits and vegetables, nuts and seeds, bananas, milk)
    - Avoiding salt substitutes that contain potassium
    - Importance of adhering to medication regimen as prescribed
- Monitoring:
    - Patient assessment to avoid correcting too rapidly or overcorrecting
    - Continuous ECG monitoring to detect cardiac changes
    - Serum potassium levels
    - Blood pressure (BP) during administration of IV calcium:
      - May cause hypotension
    - Blood glucose during administration of insulin:
      - May cause hypoglycemia
    - Intake and output
- Nursing diagnosis:
    - Many nursing diagnoses are appropriate for the patient experiencing hyperkalemia. Some diagnoses include:
    - Risk for electrolyte imbalance related to excessive retention of potassium or cellular release of potassium
    - Risk for activity intolerance related to muscle weakness
    - Risk for injury related to muscle weakness, seizures
    - Risk for decreased cardiac output related to ECG changes, dysrhythmias

Question	Rationale
A patient is admitted with a potassium level of 6.0 mEq/L. Which of the following findings may be noted on ECG monitoring? A. Inverted P waves B. Large Q waves C. U waves D. Peaked T waves	Answer: D This patient is experiencing hyperkalemia. Symptoms of hyperkalemia include ECG changes such as the presence of tall, peaked T waves.

ELECTROLYTE IMBALANCES: CALCIUM

▸ Calcium (Ca^{2+})
- Necessary electrolyte for numerous metabolic processes:
    - Major component of bones and teeth
    - Contributes to blood clotting
    - Aids in transmission of nerve impulses
    - Plays a role in myocardial and muscle contractions
- Is obtained from the diet:
    - Requires vitamin D for absorption
- The majority of the calcium in the body is stored in the bones (99%) (Lewis et al., 2017); plasma and body cells contain remainder
- In the plasma, 40% of calcium is in an ionized (free) form and 50% binds with plasma proteins like albumin (Lewis et al., 2017)

- Low serum pH or acidosis increases ionized calcium, decreases binding to albumin.
- High serum pH or alkalosis decreases ionized calcium, increases binding to albumin.
- Serum calcium levels measure total of all forms of plasma calcium:
  - Serum albumin levels affect interpretation,
  - Total calcium levels are directly associated with increased or decreased albumin levels (e.g., serum calcium may be low because of low albumin level, in which case evaluation of the ionized (free) calcium may be helpful).
- Regulated by parathyroid hormone (PTH) and calcitonin:
  - Low serum calcium levels stimulate PTH release from the parathyroid glands:
    - Increases bone resorption and moves calcium out of bones
    - Increases GI absorption of calcium
    - Increases calcium reabsorption in renal tubules
  - High serum calcium levels trigger the thyroid gland to secrete calcitonin:
    - Opposite effect of PTH
    - Increases calcium deposition into bone
    - Increases renal excretion of calcium
    - Decreases GI absorption of calcium

▶ Hypocalcemia

- Serum calcium level <8.6 mg/dL
- Causes:
  - Decreased total calcium:
    - Any process that causes PTH deficiency:
      - Primary hypoparathyroidism
      - Removal of parathyroid glands during surgery
      - Injury to parathyroid glands:
        - May result from surgeries near the parathyroid glands
      - Neck radiation
    - Kidney disease
    - Acute pancreatitis
    - Elevated phosphorus
    - Vitamin D deficiency
    - Malnutrition
    - Magnesium deficiency
    - Medications:
      - Bisphosphonates (e.g., alendronate [Fosamax])
      - Loop diuretics (e.g., furosemide [Lasix])
    - Tumor lysis syndrome
    - Chronic alcoholism
    - Diarrhea
    - Decreased serum albumin
  - Decreased ionized calcium:
    - Alkalosis
      - High pH increases calcium-to-protein binding.
    - Excess administration of citrated blood:
      - Citrate in blood products binds with calcium.

> **Clinical Consideration**
> Assess for hypocalcemia symptoms in patients who have undergone neck surgery.

TABLE 6.5	ECG CHANGES WITH CALCIUM IMBALANCES
Hypocalcemia	Hypercalcemia
Elongated ST segment Prolonged QT interval Ventricular tachycardia	Shortened ST segment Shortened QT interval Ventricular dysrhythmias Heart block Increased digitalis effect

- Manifestations:
  - Result from decreased threshold for activating the sodium channels responsible for cell membrane depolarization and reflect increased nerve excitability and prolonged muscle contraction
  - Neurologic:
    - Weakness, fatigue, depression, irritability, confusion, seizures
  - Neuromuscular:
    - Hyperreflexia, muscle cramps, numbness and tingling in extremities and around mouth, tetany
    - Chvostek sign:
      - Tapping the facial nerve in front of ear causes contraction of facial muscles
    - Trousseau sign:
      - Inflating a blood pressure cuff above the systolic pressure causes carpal spasms within 3 minutes.
  - Cardiovascular:
    - Hypotension, ECG changes (Table 6.5)
  - Respiratory:
    - Laryngeal stridor and spasms, bronchial spasms
- Treatment:
  - Identify and treat the underlying cause.
  - Mild or asymptomatic hypocalcemia:
    - High-calcium diet
    - Calcium and vitamin D supplements
  - Symptomatic hypocalcemia:
    - IV calcium gluconate
    - Control muscle spasms and tetany:
      - Promote CO_2 retention:
        - Have patient breathe into a paper bag
        - Sedation
  - Decrease urinary calcium excretion:
    - Evaluate need to switch patient from loop diuretic to thiazide diuretic
  - Treat pain and anxiety:
    - Respiratory alkalosis from hyperventilation can cause hypocalcemic symptoms.
  - Educate patient about:
    - Plan of care
    - Signs and symptoms of hypocalcemia
    - High-calcium foods (e.g., dairy products, fortified foods, collard greens, kale, etc.)
    - Importance of taking medications and supplements as instructed

- Monitoring:
  - Patient assessment to identify changes in condition and avoid overcorrecting
  - Continuous ECG monitoring to detect cardiac changes
  - Serum calcium levels
  - Appropriate administration of calcium gluconate
- Nursing diagnosis:
  - Many nursing diagnoses are appropriate for the patient experiencing hypocalcemia. Some diagnoses include:
    - Risk for electrolyte imbalance related to decreased parathyroid hormone level
    - Ineffective breathing pattern related to laryngospasm
    - Acute pain related to sustained muscle contractions
    - Risk for injury related to tetany and seizures
    - Risk for decreased cardiac output related to ECG changes, hypotension

▷ **Hypercalcemia**
- Serum calcium level >10.2 mg/dL
- Causes:
  - Increased total calcium:
    - Hyperparathyroidism:
      - Accounts for around two thirds of cases (Lewis et al., 2017)
    - Malignancies:
      - Hematologic, breast, and lung
      - Malignancies with metastasis to the bones
    - Prolonged immobilization
    - Overdose:
      - Vitamin A
      - Vitamin D
    - Paget disease
    - Adrenal insufficiency
    - Thyrotoxicosis
    - Medications:
      - Thiazide diuretics
      - Calcium-containing antacids
    - Milk-alkali syndrome
    - Mycobacterium infection
  - Increased ionized calcium:
    - Acidosis
- Manifestations:
  - Related to the effects of excess calcium, which are similar to those of a sedative, and reflect the reduced excitability of muscles and nerves
  - Neurologic:
    - Lethargy, weakness, fatigue, decreased memory, confusion, psychosis, hallucinations, seizures, coma
  - Neuromuscular:
    - Depressed reflexes
  - Cardiovascular:
    - Hypertension, ECG changes (Table 6.5)
  - Gastrointestinal:
    - Anorexia, nausea, vomiting

- Genitourinary:
  - Polyuria, nephrolithiasis
- General:
  - Bone pain, fracture, dehydration
- Treatment:
  - Depends on severity of hypercalcemia and patient condition
  - Identify and treat underlying cause
  - Mild hypercalcemia:
    - Discontinue use of medications related to hypercalcemia.
    - Low-calcium diet
    - Increase weight-bearing activity.
    - Maintain adequate hydration and prevent kidney stone formation:
      - Increase fluid intake
      - Promote urine acidity:
        - Encourage consumption of cranberry and prune juices
  - Severe hypercalcemia:
    - Administer saline:
      - IV isotonic saline should be administered to maintain urine output of 100 to 150 mL/hr
    - Administer a bisphosphonate (e.g., pamidronate [Aredia], zoledronic acid [Reclast]):
      - Most effective agents to treat hypercalcemia:
        - Frequently used when cause related to malignancy
      - Interfere with osteoclasts, which break down bone
      - Will take several days to be therapeutic:
        - Administer calcitonin for immediate effect
          - Quickly increases renal calcium elimination
          - Effective for only a few days
          - Can cause tachycardia
  - Life-threatening situations:
    - Dialysis
  - Educate patient about:
    - Plan of care
    - Signs and symptoms of hypercalcemia
    - Low-calcium foods
    - Proper fluid intake
    - Importance of taking medications as instructed
- Monitoring:
  - Patient assessment to identify changes in condition and avoid overcorrecting
  - Continuous ECG monitoring to detect cardiac changes
  - Correct administration of ordered fluids and medications:
    - Monitor for fluid overload with administration of IV fluids
  - Serum calcium levels
- Nursing diagnosis:
  - Many nursing diagnoses are appropriate for the patient experiencing hypercalcemia. Some diagnoses include:
    - Risk for electrolyte imbalance related to increased parathyroid hormone, excessive bone destruction

---

Clinical Consideration

3 to 4 L of fluid daily promotes elimination of Ca+ and reduces the incidence of kidney stones.

- Risk for activity intolerance related to muscle weakness
- Risk for injury related to neuromuscular and sensorium changes
- Risk for decreased cardiac output related to ECG changes, dysrhythmias

Question	Rationale
Headache, confusion, muscle spasms, and weight gain are symptoms consistent with which electrolyte imbalance? A. Hypernatremia B. Hyponatremia C. Hypercalcemia D. Hypokalemia	Answer: B Headache, confusion, muscle spasms, and weight gain are all symptoms of hyponatremia, which occurs with normal or increased extracellular fluid volume.

ELECTROLYTE IMBALANCES: PHOSPHATE

- Phosphorus (PO_4^{3-})
  - Mostly found in bones and teeth as calcium phosphate
  - Remaining phosphorus is essential for various metabolic activities:
    - Muscle, red cell, and nervous system function
    - Acid–base buffering system functions
    - Mitochondrial formation of adenosine triphosphate (ATP)
    - Glucose uptake and use by cells
    - Metabolism of carbohydrates, protein, and fat
  - Serum levels are maintained by PTH:
    - Low serum calcium level stimulates PTH release, which decreases reabsorption of phosphorus to lower phosphorus level
  - Excretion occurs through the kidneys:
    - Proper renal function is essential to maintain phosphate balance.
    - Low phosphate level in glomerular filtrate or low PTH level causes kidneys to reabsorb phosphorus.
- **Hypophosphatemia**
  - Phosphate level <2.4 mg/dL
  - Causes:
    - Nutritional deficiencies:
      - Malabsorption syndromes
      - Decreased intestinal absorption:
        - Chronic diarrhea
      - Malnutrition
      - Vitamin D deficiency
      - Parenteral nutrition:
        - With inadequate phosphorus replacement
    - Increased urinary excretion
    - Chronic alcoholism
    - Phosphate-binding antacids (e.g., calcium carbonate [Tums])
    - Diabetic ketoacidosis
    - Hyperparathyroidism

- Refeeding syndrome
- Respiratory alkalosis
- Manifestations:
  - Result from low levels of cellular ATP and 2,3-diphosphoglycerate (2,3-DPG), which facilitates oxygen delivery to tissues, and reflect impaired oxygen delivery and impaired cellular energy
  - Acute manifestations:
    - Neurologic:
      - CNS depression, confusion, polyneuropathy, seizures, coma
    - Neuromuscular:
      - Muscle weakness, muscle pain, rhabdomyolysis
    - Respiratory:
      - Respiratory failure (from respiratory muscle weakness)
    - Cardiac:
      - Dysrhythmias, heart failure
  - Chronic hypophosphatemia:
    - Alters bone metabolism:
      - Rickets
      - Osteomalacia
  - Severe hypophosphatemia:
    - Can be fatal because of decreased cellular function
- Treatment:
  - Identify and treat the underlying cause.
  - Mild phosphorus deficiency:
    - Increase oral intake:
      - Dairy products:
        - May be preferred method of oral replacement, better tolerated
      - Phosphate supplements:
        - Can cause adverse GI effects
  - Symptomatic hypophosphatemia:
    - IV administration of sodium phosphate or potassium phosphate
  - Educate patient about:
    - Plan of care
    - Signs and symptoms of hypophosphatemia
    - Importance of taking medications as instructed
- Monitoring:
  - Frequent monitoring during IV therapy for complications:
    - Hypocalcemia, hyperkalemia, hypotension, and dysrhythmias can result
  - Patient assessment to identify changes in condition and avoid overcorrecting
  - Serum phosphate levels
- Nursing diagnosis:
  - Many nursing diagnoses are appropriate for the patient experiencing hypophosphatemia. Some diagnoses include:
    - Risk for electrolyte imbalance related to increased elimination or decreased absorption of phosphate, treatment of hypophosphatemia
    - Risk for activity intolerance related to muscle weakness
    - Risk for injury related to muscle weakness, altered mental status
    - Risk for decreased cardiac output related to dysrhythmias, heart failure

▶ **Hyperphosphatemia**
- Phosphate level >4.4 mg/dL
- Causes:
  - Altered excretion of phosphate by the kidneys
    - Acute kidney injury
    - Chronic kidney disease
  - Excess phosphate intake:
    - Phosphate-containing laxatives (e.g., sodium biphosphate and sodium phosphate [Osmoprep])
    - Phosphate-containing enemas (e.g., sodium phosphate enema [Fleet Enema])
  - Increased renal phosphate reabsorption:
    - Hypoparathyroidism
    - Vitamin D intoxication
  - Shifts of phosphate from ICF to ECF:
    - Tumor lysis syndrome
    - Rhabdomyolysis
  - Thyrotoxicosis
  - Hyperthermia
  - Sickle cell and hemolytic anemias
- Manifestations:
  - Generally asymptomatic unless calcium binds with phosphate, which causes symptoms of hypocalcemia:
    - Paresthesias, muscle cramps, tetany, seizures
  - Chronically elevated phosphate levels lead to calcified deposits outside of the bones in areas such as the joints, blood vessels, skin, corneas, kidneys, etc.
    - Organ dysfunction related to the deposits, such as renal failure
- Treatment:
  - Identify and treat the underlying cause.
  - Decrease intake of phosphate.
    - Limit foods and fluids high in phosphate (e.g., dairy).
  - Administer oral phosphate-binding agents (e.g., calcium carbonate [Tums], sevelamer [Renvela]):
    - Will limit phosphate absorbed through intestines and increase intestinal phosphate secretion
  - Severe hyperphosphatemia:
    - Hemodialysis
  - Increase phosphate excretion:
    - Volume expansion and forced diuresis using a loop diuretic (e.g., furosemide [Lasix])
  - Correct hypocalcemia if present.
  - Educate patient about:
    - Plan of care
    - Signs and symptoms of hyperphosphatemia
    - Limiting high-phosphorus foods
    - Importance of taking medications as instructed, usually with meals and snacks
- Monitoring:
  - Patient assessment to identify changes in condition and avoid overcorrecting
  - Correct administration of ordered fluids and medications

- Serum phosphate levels
- Serum calcium levels
- Nursing diagnosis:
  - Many nursing diagnoses are appropriate for the patient experiencing hyper-phosphatemia. Some diagnoses include:
    - Risk for electrolyte imbalance related to decreased excretion of phosphate, excessive phosphate intake
    - Risk for injury related to seizures

ELECTROLYTE IMBALANCES: MAGNESIUM

▶ Magnesium (Mg^{2+})

- Most (50 to 60%) stored in muscle and bone, with approximately 30% in the cells and very little (1%) in the ECF (Lewis et al., 2017)
- Cofactor in various enzyme systems and has a role in essential cellular processes:
  - Carbohydrate metabolism
  - DNA and protein synthesis
  - Blood glucose control
  - Blood-pressure regulation
- Required for synthesis and use of ATP
- Required for neuromuscular functions:
  - Muscle contraction and relaxation
  - Normal neurologic function
  - Neurotransmitter release
- Regulation occurs through the intestines and kidneys:
  - GI absorption increases with low magnesium levels
  - Renal regulation occurs as the kidneys control magnesium reabsorption

▶ **Hypomagnesemia**

- Serum magnesium level <1.5 mEq/L
- Causes:
  - Limited magnesium intake:
    - Prolonged fasting, malnutrition
    - Starvation
    - Chronic alcoholism
    - Extended parenteral nutrition without magnesium supplementation
  - Increased GI or renal losses/decreased magnesium absorption:
    - GI fluid loss:
      - Nasogastric suction
      - Diarrhea
      - Fistulas
    - Malabsorption syndromes
    - Inflammatory bowel disease
    - Proton-pump inhibitors (PPIs) (e.g., pantoprazole [Protonix])
    - Increased urine output:
      - Diuretics
      - Hyperglycemia:
        - Causes osmotic diuresis
- Manifestations:
  - Signs and symptoms resemble hypocalcemia

- Neuromuscular (common):
  - Muscle cramps, tremors, hyperactive deep tendon reflexes, Chvostek sign, Trousseau sign
- Neurologic:
  - Confusion, vertigo, seizures
- Cardiovascular:
  - Tachycardia, hypertension, digitalis toxicity, dysrhythmias including Torsades de pointes and ventricular fibrillation
- Treatment:
  - Dependent on patient symptoms
  - Identify and treat the underlying cause
  - Mild hypomagnesemia:
    - Increase magnesium intake:
      - Oral supplements
      - Increased intake of high-magnesium foods (e.g., dark chocolate)
  - Severe hypomagnesemia or hypomagnesemia with hypocalcemia:
    - IV administration of magnesium (e.g., magnesium sulfate):
      - Infused by pump
      - Rapid infusion can cause hypotension and cardiac or respiratory arrest.
  - Educate patient about:
    - Plan of care
    - Signs and symptoms of hypomagnesemia
    - Foods high in magnesium (e.g., dark chocolate, avocados, nuts, tofu, etc.)
    - Importance of taking medications as instructed
- Monitoring:
  - Patient assessment to identify changes in condition and avoid overcorrecting:
    - Vital signs and cardiac/respiratory status
  - Correct administration of ordered medications
  - Serum magnesium levels
  - Serum calcium levels
- Nursing diagnosis:
  - Many nursing diagnoses are appropriate for the patient experiencing hypomagnesemia. Some diagnoses include:
    - Risk for electrolyte imbalance related to deficient intake of magnesium or increased loss of magnesium
    - Risk for injury related to altered mental status, seizures
    - Risk for decreased cardiac output related to dysrhythmias

Hypermagnesemia
- Serum magnesium level >2.5 mEq/L
- Causes:
  - Increased magnesium intake:
    - Medications:
      - Laxatives containing magnesium:
        - Milk of magnesia
      - Antacids containing magnesium:
        - Maalox
      - IV magnesium:
        - Treatment for preeclampsia in pregnancy
  - Renal insufficiency/renal failure

- Tumor lysis syndrome
- Metastatic bone disease
- Adrenal insufficiency
- Hypothyroidism
- Manifestations:
  - Reflect impaired nerve and muscle function from inhibition of acetylcholine release at the myoneural junction and calcium movement into cells
  - Initial:
    - Cardiac:
      - Hypotension, bradycardia, facial flushing
    - Neurologic:
      - Lethargy, drowsiness
    - Neuromuscular:
      - Muscle weakness
    - Genitourinary:
      - Urinary retention
    - Gastrointestinal:
      - Nausea, vomiting
  - Moderate to severe:
    - Neuromuscular:
      - Loss of deep tendon reflexes
      - Muscle paralysis
    - Neurologic:
      - Coma
    - Respiratory:
      - Respiratory arrest
    - Cardiovascular:
      - Cardiac arrest
- Treatment:
  - Identify and treat the underlying cause
  - Reduce magnesium intake:
    - Eliminate ingestion of magnesium-containing medications.
    - Limit dietary intake of foods high in magnesium.
  - In the setting of adequate renal function:
    - Promote urinary excretion:
      - Increase fluid intake.
      - Administer diuretics.
  - In the setting of impaired renal function:
    - Hemodialysis
  - Symptomatic hypermagnesemia:
    - Administration of IV calcium gluconate will oppose effects on cardiac muscle
  - Educate patient about:
    - Plan of care
    - Signs and symptoms of hypermagnesemia
    - Avoidance of foods high in magnesium
    - Importance of taking medications as instructed
- Monitoring:
  - Patient assessment to identify changes in condition and avoid overcorrecting
  - Correct administration of ordered medications

- Serum magnesium levels
- Serum calcium levels
- Nursing diagnosis:
  - Many nursing diagnoses are appropriate for the patient experiencing hypermagnesemia. Some diagnoses include:
    - Risk for electrolyte imbalance related to excessive intake of magnesium and renal dysfunction
    - Risk for injury related to altered mental status, muscle weakness
    - Risk for activity intolerance related to muscle weakness
    - Risk for decreased cardiac output related to hypotension

ACID–BASE REGULATION

▶ Acidity or alkalinity of solutions is dependent on the amount of hydrogen (H^+) ions present, expressed as pH.

▶ The pH of a solution can range from 1 to 14, where 7 is neutral. The body is slightly alkaline with a normal arterial pH of 7.35 to 7.45.

▶ Acidosis is considered to be a pH of <7.35 and alkalosis is considered to be a pH of >7.45.

▶ Three mechanisms maintain the balance between acids and bases and regulate the pH of the body between 7.35 to 7.45. These include the buffer system, respiratory system, and renal system.

- Buffer system:
  - Primary system of regulation
  - Reacts to changes in acid–base balance immediately.
  - Converts strong acids into weaker acids or binds them so they are neutralized.
  - Can maintain normal pH only as long as respiratory and renal systems are working properly.
  - Maintains a 20:1 ratio between bicarbonate (HCO_3^-) and carbonic acid (H_2CO_3)
  - Present in all body fluids:
    - Primary buffer system in ECF is carbonic acid–bicarbonate.
    - Phosphate, protein, and hemoglobin are also buffers.
- Respiratory system:
  - Second fastest regulatory system; reacts in changes in minutes and is most effective in a matter of hours to correct acid–base imbalances.
  - Aids in maintaining normal pH through excretion of CO_2 and water by the lungs.
  - The concentration of CO_2 in the blood is directly related to the amount of carbonic acid and hydrogen.
    - An increased respiratory rate expels more CO_2, leaving less in the blood, which leads to less carbonic acid, less hydrogen, and an alkalotic state.
    - A decreased respiratory rate leads to retention of CO_2 in the blood, which leads to increased carbonic acid, increased hydrogen, and an acidotic state.
  - The respiratory center resides in the medulla and controls the rate of CO_2 excretion.
  - If a respiratory problem is the cause of an acid–base imbalance, the respiratory system cannot correct the change in pH.
- Renal system:
  - Slowest to respond to changes; reacts in hours to days after a change in pH.
  - Capable of maintaining acid–base balance for prolonged period in patients with chronic imbalances.

Clinical Consideration
Older adults have impaired abilities with regard to respiratory system compensation.

Clinical Consideration
Impaired ability of the renal system to compensate for acid load occurs in the older adult.

- Normally, the kidneys reabsorb and conserve all bicarbonate that is filtered and excrete some of the acid that results from cellular metabolism.
- The pH of urine is normally acidic (typically pH of 6), but compensatory mechanisms allow alteration of the pH through reabsorption of more bicarbonate and elimination of excess hydrogen. This will increase the blood pH and lower the pH of the urine.
- If a renal (metabolic) problem is the cause of an acid–base imbalance, the renal system cannot correct the change in pH.

▌ Disruptions in acid–base balance occur when something causes an alteration to the ratio of 20:1 base-to-acid and compensatory mechanisms are deficient or fail to restore the balance.

▌ Imbalances are classified as respiratory or metabolic in nature and as acidosis or alkalosis based on the pH.

▌ Acidosis is the result of increased carbonic acid (retention of CO_2 from hypoventilation) (respiratory) or decreased HCO_3^- (metabolic).

- Acidosis can cause hyperkalemia, as H^+ will enter the cell in exchange for potassium.

▌ Alkalosis is the result of a decrease in carbonic acid ("blowing off" CO_2 in excess from hyperventilation) (respiratory) or an increase in HCO_3^- (metabolic).

- Alkalosis can cause hypokalemia, as H^+ will exit the cell in exchange for potassium.

▌ Imbalances can be acute or chronic, and mixed imbalances can occur.

ACID–BASE IMBALANCES

▌ Respiratory acidosis (Table 6.6)

- Retention of CO_2 as the result of hypoventilation
- Compensation to correct the altered pH occurs through increased retention of bicarbonate by the renal system
- Example of uncompensated ABG: pH 7.33, $PaCO_2$ 55, HCO_3^- 24

▌ Respiratory alkalosis (Table 6.6)

- Excretion of CO_2 as the result of hyperventilation
- Compensation to correct the altered pH occurs through increased excretion of bicarbonate by the renal system
- Example of uncompensated ABG: pH 7.50, $PaCO_2$ 28, HCO_3^- 25

▌ Metabolic acidosis (Table 6.6)

- Results from increased acid production or ingestion, decreased acid excretion, or loss of base (bicarbonate)
- Compensation to correct the altered pH occurs through increased excretion of CO_2 by the respiratory system
- Example of uncompensated ABG: pH 7.31, $PaCO_2$ 39, HCO_3^- 19

▌ Metabolic alkalosis (Table 6.6)

- Results from loss of acid or retention of base (bicarbonate)
- Compensation to correct the altered pH occurs through increased retention of CO_2 by the respiratory system
- Example of uncompensated ABG: pH 7.49, $PaCO_2$ 41, HCO_3^- 32

▌ Treatment

- Treatment for acid–base imbalances is aimed at identifying and correcting the underlying cause

TABLE 6.6	ACID–BASE IMBALANCES		
Imbalance	Causes	Manifestations	Laboratory Findings
Respiratory acidosis	Chronic respiratory conditions (e.g., COPD) Overdose (e.g., barbiturates, sedatives, etc.) Chest-wall abnormality Severe pneumonia Atelectasis Weakened respiratory muscles Mechanical hypoventilation Pulmonary edema	Neurologic: lethargy, confusion, dizziness, headache, seizures, coma Cardiovascular: hypotension, warm, flushed skin, ventricular fibrillation Respiratory: hypoventilation, hypoxia	Plasma pH <7.35 $PaCO_2$ >45 HCO_3^- normal (uncompensated) HCO_3^- >26 (compensated)
Respiratory alkalosis	Hyperventilation: hypoxia, anxiety, fear, pain, fever, exercise Stimulation of the respiratory center: septicemia, stroke, brain injury, meningitis, encephalitis, salicylate poisoning Liver failure Mechanical hyperventilation	Neurologic: dizziness, light-headedness, confusion, headache, seizures Cardiovascular: tachycardia, dysrhythmias Respiratory: hyperventilation Gastrointestinal: nausea, vomiting, diarrhea Neuromuscular: tetany, numbness, hyperreflexia	Plasma pH >7.45 $PaCO_2$ <35 HCO_3^- normal (uncompensated) HCO_3^- < 22 (compensated)
Metabolic acidosis	Diabetic ketoacidosis (DKA) Lactic acidosis Starvation Diarrhea Renal tubular acidosis Renal failure GI fistulas Shock	Neurologic: lethargy, confusion, dizziness, headache, coma Cardiovascular: hypotension, dysrhythmias, cold, clammy skin Respiratory: Kussmaul breathing (deep, rapid respirations) Gastrointestinal: nausea, vomiting, diarrhea, abdominal pain Neuromuscular: muscle weakness	Plasma pH <7.35 $PaCO_2$ Normal (uncompensated) $PaCO_2$ <35 (compensated) HCO_3^- < 22
Metabolic alkalosis	Vomiting Nasogastric suctioning Diuretic therapy Hypokalemia Excess sodium bicarbonate intake Mineralocorticoid use	Neurologic: irritability, confusion, lethargy, headaches, seizures Cardiovascular: tachycardia, dysrhythmias Respiratory: hypoventilation Gastrointestinal: nausea, vomiting, anorexia Neuromuscular: tremors, tetany, paresthesias, muscle cramps	Plasma pH > 7.45 $PaCO_2$ Normal (uncompensated) $PaCO_2$ > 45 (compensated) HCO_3^- > 26

COPD = chronic obstructive pulmonary disease.

◗ Nursing diagnosis:

- Many nursing diagnoses are appropriate for the patient experiencing acid–base imbalances. Some diagnoses include:
  - Impaired gas exchange related to hyperventilation or hypoventilation
  - Risk for electrolyte imbalance related to shifts of electrolytes in and/or out of the cells
  - Risk for injury related to altered mental status, central nervous system depression
  - Risk for decreased cardiac output related to hypotension and/or dysrhythmias

Question	Rationale
A patient receiving IV hydromorphone (Dilaudid) via PCA is lethargic and noted to have shallow respirations at a rate of 7 per minute. The nurse realizes that the patient is likely experiencing which acid–base imbalance? A. Respiratory alkalosis B. Metabolic alkalosis C. Respiratory acidosis D. Metabolic acidosis	Answer: C Respiratory acidosis results from the retention of CO2 that occurs with hypoventilation, in this case from a potential overdose of opioid analgesic. The retention of CO2 leads to increased carbonic acid, increased hydrogen, and a resulting acidotic state. In addition to hypoventilation, one of the manifestations of respiratory acidosis is lethargy.

INTERPRETATION OF ABGs

▶ If all values are within normal limits (Table 6.7) then the ABGs are normal. For abnormal values, the following steps apply.

▶ Classify the pH:

- pH <7.35 indicates acidosis.
- pH >7.45 indicates alkalosis.

▶ Determine the cause:

- Assess the $PaCO_2$, which is the respiratory component:
  - $PaCO_2$ >45 mm Hg and pH <7.35 indicates respiratory acidosis.
  - $PaCO_2$ <35 mm Hg and pH >7.45 indicates respiratory alkalosis.
  - Problems that are respiratory in nature cause the pH and CO_2 to go in opposite directions (low and high or high and low).
- Assess the HCO_3^-, which is the metabolic component
  - HCO_3^- >26 mEq/L and pH >7.45 indicates metabolic alkalosis.
  - HCO_3^- <22 mEq/L and pH <7.35 indicates metabolic acidosis .
  - Problems that are metabolic in nature cause the pH and HCO_3^- to go in the same direction (both are low or both are high).

▶ Determine whether compensation is occurring (if the unaffected system is attempting to correct the acid–base ratio and normalize the pH) (Table 6.8)

- Assess the component ($PaCO_2$ or HCO_3^-) that is not causing the primary disturbance.

TABLE 6.7	NORMAL ARTERIAL BLOOD GAS (ABG) RANGES	
pH	7.35–7.45	
$PaCO_2$	45–35 mm Hg	
HCO_3^-	22–26 mEq/L	
	Acidotic ⟵ ⟶ Alkalotic	
PaO_2	80–100 mm Hg	
SaO_2	95–100%	

Note: The values for $PaCO_2$ are reversed to indicate acidosis with increased CO_2 and alkalosis with decreased CO_2.

TABLE 6.8	ABG INTERPRETATION EXAMPLES
Uncompensated	pH 7.50, PaCO₂ 28 mm Hg, HCO₃⁻ 24 mEq/L, PaO₂ 95 mm Hg (1) pH and PaCO₂ are abnormal. (2) pH is >7.45, indicating alkalosis. (3) PaCO₂ is <35 mm Hg, indicating possible respiratory alkalosis; since it is moving in the opposite direction of the pH, this is the primary problem (in respiratory problems, pH and CO₂ move in opposite directions). (4) HCO₃⁻ is within normal limits, indicating that the renal system is not yet attempting to compensate for the respiratory problem. (5) PaO₂ is within normal limits which is not indicative of hypoxemia Final interpretation: Uncompensated respiratory alkalosis
Partially compensated	pH 7.31, PaCO₂ 31 mm Hg, HCO₃⁻ 17 mEq/L, PaO₂ 97 mm Hg (1) All values are abnormal with exception of PaO₂. (2) pH is <7.35, indicating acidosis. (3) PaCO₂ is <35 mm Hg, indicating possible respiratory alkalosis but is moving in the same direction as the pH, so this is not a respiratory problem (4) HCO₃⁻ is <22 mEq/L, indicating possible metabolic acidosis; since it is moving in the same direction as the pH, this is the primary problem (in metabolic problems, pH and HCO₃⁻ move in the same direction). (5) PaCO₂ is outside normal limits, indicating that the respiratory system is attempting to compensate for the metabolic problem (6) PaO₂ is normal, which is not indicative of hypoxemia. Final interpretation: Partially compensated metabolic acidosis
Fully compensated	pH 7.43, PaCO₂ 28 mm Hg, HCO₃⁻ 18mEq/L, PaO₂ 96 mm Hg (1) PaCO₂ and HCO₃⁻ are abnormal and pH is normal, indicating full compensation. (2) pH, while in normal limits, is closer to the alkalotic side. (3) PaCO₂ is <35 mm Hg indicating possible respiratory alkalosis (headed in the opposite direction of the pH). (4) HCO₃⁻ is <22 mEq/L, indicating possible metabolic acidosis (however, it is headed in the opposite direction of the pH). (5) PaCO₂ varies most greatly from the normal parameters, which indicates that this is a respiratory problem (CO₂ of 28 is 7 points away from the lowest end of the normal parameter, 35, whereas the HCO₃⁻ is only 4 points away from the lowest end of the normal parameter, 22) (6) PaO₂ is normal, which is not indicative of hypoxemia. Final interpretation: Fully compensated respiratory alkalosis

- If that component remains within normal limits, no compensation is occurring. This is considered "uncompensated."
- If that component is outside normal limits and the pH is not within normal limits, compensation is occurring. This is considered "partially compensated."
- If upon interpreting the ABGs, the pH is within normal limits, this is considered "fully compensated."
  - To determine the cause of the imbalance in fully compensated ABGs, evaluate which component, CO_2 or HCO_3^- is furthest outside its normal parameters (Table 6.8).

▌ Assess the PaO_2, which should be between 80 and 100 mm Hg, and oxygen saturation, which should be >95%.

- Hypoxemia is indicated if these numbers are less than normal.
- Note that reference ranges may differ between laboratories, and consideration should be given to individual patient, as not all may be expected to maintain this range of oxygen saturation (e.g., patients with chronic obstructive pulmonary disease [COPD], the older adult patient, etc.).

▌ Considerations related to the collection of blood for ABGs include but may not be limited to the following:

- Ensure that arterial blood is used, not venous.
- Protect the patient from injury at the site of the radial puncture:

- An Allen test may be performed to test for collateral circulation (adequate ulnar circulation):
  - For the Allen test, pressure is applied to the radial and ulnar arteries at the same time. The patient opens and closes the hand repeatedly, during which time the hand should blanch. Pressure to the ulnar artery is released while maintaining pressure to the radial artery. Pink color should return to the hand within 6 seconds.
  - An abnormal Allen test suggests that ulnar circulation is inadequate and that the radial site should not be used. Poor radial artery perfusion could occur in patients who have had procedures performed on the radial artery.
  - Prevention of arterial hemorrhage can be achieved by holding pressure to the collection site for 3 to 5 minutes. This time may be longer for patients taking anticoagulants.
- To ensure accuracy of the ABG sample:
  - Use correct syringe for collection and label sample per institution policy.
  - Eliminate air and place sample on ice prior to sending for analysis.
  - Avoid collection of blood for ABGs immediately after a patient has been suctioned.
- It is possible that ABG results may not correlate with the patient's condition. If this occurs, it may be necessary to rule out hemolysis of the sample or the use of venous blood and/or repeat the blood draw to verify results. The patient's condition should be observed and treated accordingly using critical thinking.

Question	Rationale
The following ABG values are indicative of which acid–base imbalance? pH 7.31, $PaCO_2$ 36 mm Hg, HCO_3^- 17 mEq/L A. Uncompensated respiratory acidosis B. Partially compensated metabolic acidosis C. Uncompensated metabolic acidosis D. Partially compensated respiratory acidosis	Answer: C The pH is <7.35, indicating acidosis. The $PaCO_2$ is within normal limits. The HCO_3^- is <22, indicating acidosis. Since bicarbonate is the metabolic component, this is a metabolic problem. As the $PaCO_2$ is still normal, the respiratory system has not yet started to compensate to restore the acid–base ratio to normal. Final interpretation: Uncompensated metabolic acidosis

CASE STUDY

An 80-year-old man was admitted through the emergency department with diagnosis of fever and pneumonia. Symptoms on admission included a productive cough, dizziness, weakness, and confusion, which prompted his family to call 911. He was independent with activities of daily living (ADLs) prior to admission. His medical history includes hypertension and coronary artery disease. He has a remote history of smoking for 15 years, but quit 20 years ago. His current medications include hydrochlorothiazide 12.5 mg PO daily, spironolactone 25 mg PO daily, and aspirin 80 mg PO daily. Vital signs are assessed, revealing: temperature 100.8°F, heart rate 106 beats/min, blood pressure 90/50 mm Hg, respiratory rate

26 breaths/min, O2 saturation 90% while breathing room air. Physical assessment reveals the following abnormal findings.

-Neurologic: Lethargic, but arouses to voice. Oriented to person only. Speech intact, slow to respond.

-Skin: Poor skin turgor, with 1+ tenting.

-Head, eyes, ear, nose. and throat: Dry mucous membranes, cracked lips.

-Respiratory: Productive cough with moderate amounts of thick, yellow sputum. Crackles in right lower lobe on auscultation.

-Cardiovascular: Pulses +1 bilaterally radial, dorsalis pedis sites. Sluggish capillary refill, >3 seconds.

-Gastrointestinal: Last bowel movement 3 days ago. Normal for the patient is once daily.

-Genitourinary: Concentrated, dark yellow urine.

-Musculoskeletal: Weak muscle strength at 2/5 bilateral upper and lower extremities. Needs assistance to stand.

Abnormal lab values include: sodium 150 mEq/L, BUN 35 mg/dL, serum osmolality 310 mOsm/kg, hematocrit 60%, white-cell count 15,000 per microliter.

1. **Based on the assessment findings, what diagnosis might you expect?**

    ▶ *In addition to those that support the diagnosis of fever and pneumonia, the patient is also demonstrating symptoms of dehydration or an ECFVD, including hypotension and tachycardia, lethargy and confusion, dry mucous membranes and cracked lips, weak pulses and sluggish capillary refill, constipation, dark and concentrated urine, and muscle weakness. Lab values that indicate ECFVD includes the elevated sodium, which is also an incidental finding of hypernatremia, BUN, serum osmolality, and hematocrit. The underlying cause for the fluid and electrolyte imbalance is likely the fever and early pneumonia, which also put the patient at risk for respiratory alkalosis.*

2. **What diagnostic tests would you anticipate the provider to order?**

    ▶ *ABGs*

    ▶ *Sputum culture*

    ▶ *Blood cultures*

    ▶ *Urinalysis, followed by urine culture and sensitivity if abnormal*

    ▶ *Repeat labs for monitoring fluid and electrolyte status*

    ▶ *Repeat chest x-ray for follow-up on pneumonia*

    ▶ *Possible swallow evaluation if aspiration is suspected cause of pneumonia*

3. **What education would you want to provide to this patient?**

    ▶ *Treatment of dehydration*
    - *Fluid replacement*
      - *IV fluid hydration*
      - *Push oral fluids*
    - *Treatment of the underlying cause: fever, pneumonia*
      - *Prescribed medications*
        - *Antibiotics*
          - *Initiated after cultures are obtained*
        - *Antipyretics*
        - *Possible steroids and/or nebulizer treatments*
      - *Cough and deep breathing exercises, incentive spirometry*
      - *Possible need for supplemental oxygen*

- ***General plan of care including need to monitor daily weights, intake and output, vital signs, repeat blood draws, need for telemetry (if ordered), frequent skin care, oral hygiene care, need to change position frequently, safety, and fall prevention*

4. **What considerations would you make based on this patient's age?**

▶ *There are normal physiologic changes that occur with aging that increase the older adult's susceptibility to fluid and electrolyte imbalances. These include changes to the kidneys, decreased renal blood flow, decreased glomerular filtration, and a loss of ability to concentrate urine and conserve water. Older adults also have a lower percentage of overall body water compared to younger adults because of having less lean body mass.*

▶ *In older adults, classic signs of dehydration may not be present. For example, tissue turgor is a less reliable predictor of fluid balance because of the loss of tissue elasticity with aging. Dehydration in older adults can cause atypical manifestations, such as confusion, constipation, and less commonly, fever and falls.*

▶ *Mental status changes in the older adult can indicate problems such as dehydration or infection.*

Discussion:

What may seem like a straightforward diagnosis can put the patient at risk for many other problems, including fluid, electrolyte, and acid–base imbalances, so it is important to assess and monitor for changes that may indicate that these are occurring. It is also necessary to monitor the patient to prevent overcorrection of these problems. It is important to keep in mind that the older adult patient may have atypical signs and symptoms of these conditions.

Bibliography

Black, J.M., and Hawks, J. (2009). *Medical-Surgical Nursing: Clinical Management for Positive Outcomes,* 8th ed. (St. Louis: Saunders).

Burchum, J.R., and Rosenthal, L.D. (2016). *Lehne's Pharmacology for Nursing Care,* 9th ed. (St. Louis: Elsevier).

Faes, M.C., Spigt, M.G., and Rikkert, M.O. (2007). Dehydration in geriatrics. *Geriatrics and Aging* 10, 590–596.

Kee, J.L., Paulanka, B.J., and Polek, C. (2010). *Handbook of Fluid, Electrolyte, and Acid-Base Imbalances,* 3rd ed. (Clifton Park, NY: Delmar, Cengage Learning).

Lewis, S.L., Bucher, L., Heitkemper, M., and Harding, M.M. (2017). *Medical-Surgical Nursing: Assessment and Management of Clinical Problems,* 10th ed. (St. Louis: Elsevier).

7

Gastrointestinal System

Donna Martin, DNP, RN, CMSRN, CDE, CNE

OVERVIEW

▶ The gastrointestinal (GI) system is responsible for the digestion and absorption of nutrients, which is accomplished by producing enzymes and hormones, synthesizing and storing vitamins, as well as collecting waste products and efficiently eliminating them from the body. The smooth muscle that lines the GI tract allows food and fluid intake to move by peristalsis. These organized waves of contractions propel contents of the GI tract from the esophagus through the rectum.

▶ There are several accessory organs associated with the GI system that work collaboratively to aid in the process of digestion.

▶ Water absorption and electrolyte balance can be significantly impacted by alterations in the GI system.

ANATOMY AND PHYSIOLOGY

▶ The gastrointestinal/digestive system is comprised of the:
- Mouth:
  - Lips and oral cavity for intake of food and fluids
  - Teeth for chewing
  - Tongue for swallowing
  - Salivary glands that secrete amylase to begin starch digestion
- Pharynx:
  - Passageway between the mouth and the esophagus
- Esophagus:
  - Moves food from the pharynx to the stomach
  - Upper esophageal sphincter (UES):
    - Relaxes and opens when swallowing
  - Lower esophageal sphincter (LES):
    - Closed except during swallowing, belching, and vomiting
    - Prevents gastric acid reflux into esophagus
- Stomach:
  - Serves as a food storage reservoir during the early phases of digestion
  - Several secretions from the stomach are part of the digestive process:
    - Pepsinogen digests protein.
    - Hydrochloric (HCl) acid plays a role in converting pepsinogen to pepsin.

- Lipase aids in fat digestion.
- Intrinsic factor is essential for absorption of vitamin B_{12}.
- Small intestine:
  - Middle portion of the digestive tract; consists of three portions that are the major sites of digestion and absorption:
    - Duodenum:
      - Common bile duct and main pancreatic duct are located in this portion of the small intestine, allowing bile and pancreatic secretions to enter the small intestine.
    - Jejunum
    - Ileum
  - There are multiple digestive secretions from the small intestine:
    - Enterokinase activates the conversion of trypsinogen to trypsin.
    - Amylase breaks down carbohydrates.
    - Peptidases and aminopeptidases assist with protein digestion.
    - Maltase, sucrose, and lactase convert forms of sugar into glucose.
    - Lipase aids in fat digestion.
- Large intestine:
  - Lower portion of the digestive tract; its most important function is the absorption of water and electrolytes:
    - Cecum:
      - Pouch at the junction of the ileum and colon
      - The ileocecal valve prevents the return of feces into the small intestine.
      - The appendix is located near the ileocecal valve.
    - Colon:
      - Ascending
      - Transverse
      - Descending
      - Sigmoid
    - Rectum/anal canal:
      - Internal and external sphincter muscles control the opening of the anus.
      - When the rectum fills, the external sphincter contracts and creates the urge to defecate.
- Other structures/organs:
  - Liver:
    - Largest internal organ of the body, with multiple functions:
      - Metabolic:
        - Glycogenesis—converting glucose to glycogen
        - Glycogenolysis—breaking down glycogen to glucose
        - Gluconeogenesis—forming glucose from amino acids and fatty acids
        - Synthesis of nonessential amino acids and plasma proteins
        - Synthesis of lipoproteins
        - Breakdown of triglycerides
        - Formation of ketone bodies
        - Synthesis and breakdown of cholesterol
        - Detoxification through the inactivation of drugs and harmful substances, excreting them from the body
        - Synthesis of clotting factors prothrombin and fibrinogen

- Secretory:
  - Formation of bile:
    - Bile aids in the breakdown of fatty acids and absorption of fat-soluble vitamins.
  - Formation and secretion of bilirubin
- Vascular:
  - Rich blood supply; serves as reservoir
  - Breaks down old red and white cells
  - Removes bacteria and toxins from the blood
- Storage:
  - Glycogen for conversion to glucose
  - Vitamins A, B_1, B_2, B_{12}, D, E, and K and folic acid
  - Fatty acids
  - Minerals; iron and copper
  - Amino acids; albumin
- Biliary tract:
  - Gallbladder:
    - Concentrates and stores bile
    - Contracts and releases bile in response to fat intake
  - Biliary ducts:
    - Cystic duct:
      - Moves bile
    - Common bile duct
      - Hepatic ducts and cystic duct join
      - Moves bile to the duodenum at the ampulla of Vater
- Pancreas:
  - Has endocrine and exocrine functions:
    - Endocrine:
      - Occur in the islets of Langerhans
        - β cells secrete insulin and amylin.
        - α cells secrete glucagon.
        - δ cells secrete somatostatin.
        - F cells secrete pancreatic polypeptide.
    - Exocrine:
      - Production and secretion of digestive enzymes:
        - Amylase breaks down carbohydrates.
        - Lipase aids in fat digestion.
- Gerontologic considerations:
  - Age-related changes:
    - Decreased number of taste buds
    - Decreased sense of smell and taste
    - Periodontal disease, loss of teeth, ill-fitting dentures
    - Delayed esophageal emptying
    - Changes in the esophageal sphincters
    - Slowed GI motility
  - Other factors:
    - Medications that contribute to constipation

- Decreased activity/mobility
- Dietary changes:
  - Decreased fluid intake
  - Decreased dietary fiber
- Cognitive and neurologic disorders

DIAGNOSTIC TESTS

▶ Radiology:

- Barium swallow—upper GI
  - Visualization of transit of barium (contrast dye) to identify abnormalities in the lower esophagus, stomach and upper duodenum
- Small bowel follow-through:
  - Use of barium to visualize positioning, motility, and patency of the small intestine.
- Barium enema—lower GI
  - Visualization of transit of barium to identify abnormalities in the normal filling of the appendix, terminal ileum, and colon
- Cholangiography:
  - X-ray examination of the bile ducts, using a radiopaque dye as a contrast medium
- Ultrasound
- Nuclear imaging:
  - Gastric emptying scan
  - Gastroesophageal reflux scan
  - Gastroesophageal bleeding scan
- Gastric emptying breath test (GEBT):
  - Measures how fast food passes to the small intestine; can diagnose gastroparesis
- Computed tomography (CT)
- Magnetic resonance imaging (MRI)

▶ Endoscopy—direct visualization of various areas of the body:

- Esophagogastroduodenoscopy (EGD)
- Endoscopic retrograde cholangiopancreatography (ERCP):
  - Allows for visualization of the pancreatic, hepatic, and common bile ducts
- Video capsule endoscopy (VCE):
  - Noninvasive capsule that send images as it passes through the GI tract
- Colonoscopy
- Sigmoidoscopy

▶ Screening:

- Colonoscopy screening is recommended a minimum of every 10 years for persons over the age of 45 or as recommended by provider.

▶ Laboratory

- *Helicobacter pylori (H. pylori)*
  - Biopsy of the gastric mucosa
  - Urea breath test (byproduct of *H. pylori*)
  - Stool antigen test
  - Serum antibody test:
    - IgG anti–*H. pylori* antibody—elevated 2 months after being infected and remains elevated for more than 1 year
    - IgA anti–*H. pylori* antibody—elevated 2 months after being infected and decreases 3 to 4 weeks after treatment

Clinical Consideration
It is important that the patient evacuate all barium to prevent a fecal impaction.

Clinical Consideration
Antibody testing is considered the gold standard for diagnosing *H. pylori* infection.

- IgM anti–*H. pylori* antibody—elevated 3 to 4 weeks after being infected and is detected up to 3 months after treatment
- Liver-function tests (LFTs)
  - Alkaline phosphate (ALP)
    - Highest concentrations in liver; greatly increased with biliary disease and cirrhosis
  - Aspartate aminotransferase (AST):
    - Used to evaluate hepatocellular diseases
  - Alanine aminotransferase (ALT):
    - Predominantly found in liver; most elevations caused by the liver
  - Serum bilirubin:
    - Indicates liver and gallbladder function
  - Serum protein:
    - Measures the total amount of protein in the blood
  - Ammonia:
    - Used to support the diagnosis of severe liver diseases
  - Serum cholesterol:
    - Low levels indicate severe liver disease
  - Partial thromboplastin time (PTT):
    - With hepatocellular dysfunction and biliary obstruction, clotting factors will be altered.
  - Prothrombin time: Protime (PT) / International normalized ratio (INR):
    - With hepatocellular dysfunction and biliary obstruction, clotting factors will be altered.
  - Vitamin K:
    - Plays a vital role in the production of coagulation
- Amylase:
  - Commonly used to diagnose and monitor treatment of pancreatitis
- Lipase:
  - Acute pancreatitis is the most common cause of elevation
- Gastrin:
  - Plays a role in the release of gastric acids
- Cultures:
  - Stool
- Testing for occult blood
- Hepatitis virus studies:
  - Hepatitis A virus antibody (HAVAb)/IgM—Indicates acute HAV infection; present 4 to 6 weeks through 3 to 4 months
  - HAVAb/IgG—Indicates previous HAV exposure; present 8 to 12 weeks though 10 years
  - HAV RNA—Indicates acute HAV infection and carrier state
  - Hepatitis B early antigen (HBeAg)—Indicates acute HBV infection; present 1 to 3 weeks through 6 to 8 weeks
  - Hepatitis B early antibody (HBeAb)—Indicates acute HBV infection; present 4 to 6 weeks through 4 to 6 years
  - Hepatitis B surface antigen (HBsAg)—Indicates acute/chronic HBV infection; present 4 to 12 weeks through 1 to 3 months
  - Hepatitis B surface antibody (HBsAb) total—Indicates previous HBV infection; present 3 to 10 months through 6 to 10 years
  - Hepatitis B core antibody (HBVcAb)/IgM—Indicates acute HBV infection; present from 2-12 weeks through 3-6 months

- Hepatitis B core antibody, total—Indicates previous HBV infection; present 3 to 12 weeks for life
- Hepatitis C antibody (HCAb)/IgG—Indicates previous HCV infection; present from 3 to 4 months through 2 years
- HCV RNA—Indicates acute/chronic HCV infection; present from first day of infection
- Liver biopsy:
  - Staging fibrosis
  - Diagnosing cancer

GASTROINTESTINAL DISORDERS

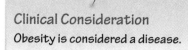

Clinical Consideration
Obesity is considered a disease.

▶ *Obesity*

- According to the U.S. Department of Health and Human Services and the Centers for Disease Control and Preventions (CDC, 2015), approximately 36% of all adults are obese. Obesity is associated with multiple health risks: heart disease, stroke, type 2 diabetes, gastroesophageal reflux disease (GERD), sleep problems, and certain types of cancer.

- *Assessment/Intervention/Education*
  - Detailed medical history:
    - History of weight loss and gain
    - Family history of being overweight
    - Previous weight loss attempts
    - Psychosocial factors
    - Barriers to weight loss
  - Risk factors:
    - Genetic link
    - Females have a higher rate of obesity
    - Higher rates of obesity in African Americans and those of Hispanic descent
    - Lower income
    - Less-educated adults
    - Overweight/obese earlier in life
  - Clinical manifestations:
    - Increased BMI
    - Waist-to-hip ratio (WHR) >0.8
    - Android body shape (apple)
  - Diagnosis:
    - Body-mass index (BMI; weight in kilograms divided by the square of the height in meters)
      - 25 to 29.9 is considered overweight
      - 30 or greater is considered obese
      - 40 or greater is considered extremely obese
  - Nursing diagnosis:
    - Imbalanced nutrition: more than body requirements
    - Disturbed body image related to weight
    - Readiness for enhanced nutrition
    - Chronic low self-esteem related to obesity
  - Treatment:
    - Nutritional therapy:
      - Restrict dietary intake.

- Include basic food groups.
- Meet minimum dietary and vitamin needs.
- Exercise:
  - Regular exercise
  - Incorporate into daily routine
  - Contributes to cardiovascular conditioning
  - Favorable effect on body-fat distribution
- Behavior modification
  - Self-monitoring—record keeping
  - Stimulus control—separate events that trigger eating
  - Rewards for meeting goals
  - Support-group participation
- Drug therapy:
  - Appetite-suppressing drugs
    - Amphetamines
      - High potential for abuse
      - Not approved for weight loss by the Food and Drug Administration
    - Nonamphetamines:
      - Potential for abuse
      - Short-term use only
- Bariatric surgical therapy:
  - Intense education and counseling is recommended prior to any bariatric procedures
  - Restrictive
    - Reduce the size of the stomach:
      - Adjustable gastric banding:
        - Inflatable band placed around the fundus
        - Delay in stomach emptying
        - Increases sense of satiety
      - Sleeve gastrectomy (gastric sleeve):
        - Removes approximately three-fourths of stomach
        - Eliminates hormone produced in the stomach that stimulate hunger
      - Gastric plication
        - Minimally invasive
        - Folds stomach wall inward, reducing size
      - Intragastric balloons
        - Minimally invasive
        - Gastric balloon inserted by endoscopy
        - Decreases appetite, reducing food intake
  - Combination of restrictive and malabsorptive:
    - Roux-en-Y gastric bypass:
      - Gastric pouch created and directly attached to small intestine
      - 90% of stomach and duodenum bypassed
      - Patient may experience *dumping syndrome*, as contents rapidly empty into the small intestine.
  - Implantable gastric stimulation:
    - Implantable device that sends electrical impulses to the vagus nerve to regulate gastric emptying
    - Stimulates a sense of fullness

- Patient teaching:
  - Lifelong lifestyle changes are part of the treatment for obesity.
  - Encourage the patient to seek support from health care providers, family, friends, and support groups.
  - Medication therapy is not a cure for obesity.
  - Surgical interventions also require lifestyle changes.

Question	Rationale
The nurse is caring for a patient who underwent gastric resection. Which of the following complications should the nurse discuss in the discharge teaching? A. Gastric spasms B. Dumping syndrome C. Weight gain D. Constipation	Answer: B Dumping syndrome occurs when food moves too quickly through the stomach to the intestine, without going through the normal digestion process. Diarrhea is a common complication due to the rapid movement of food and fluids through the gastrointestinal system. Gastric spasms and weight gain are not complications of a gastric resection.

▶ *Gastroesophageal Reflux Disease (GERD)*

- GERD is the most common GI problem. It is a syndrome in which there is mucosal damage caused by stomach acid reflux into the lower esophagus. Gastric acid and pepsin secretions reflux into the esophagus, causing irritation and inflammation.
- *Assessment/Intervention/Education*
  - Detailed medical history:
    - Frequency of heartburn/regurgitation:
    - Risk factors:
      - Obesity
      - Hiatal hernia
      - Certain foods
      - Stressors
      - Alcohol
      - Cigarette/cigar smoking
  - Clinical manifestations:
    - Pyrosis (heartburn)
    - Dyspepsia (regurgitation)
    - Respiratory symptoms:
      - Coughing
    - Otolaryngologic symptoms
    - Chest pain relieved with antacids
  - Complications:
    - Esophagitis:
      - Inflammation with possible ulcerations

- Barrett's esophagus (esophageal metaplasia):
  - Precancerous cell changes
  - Increased chance of esophageal adenocarcinoma
  - Aspiration of gastric secretions
- Diagnosis:
  - Endoscopy:
    - Assesses for scarring and/or inflammation of the esophagus
    - Assesses for change in esophageal cells
    - Assesses LES function
    - Biopsy to determine degree of dysplasia
  - Barium swallow:
    - Visualization of transit of barium to identify abnormalities in the lower esophagus, stomach, and upper duodenum
  - Manometric studies:
    - Measures pressure in esophagus
    - Assesses esophageal motility
  - Radionuclide studies:
    - Detects reflux of gastric contents
- Nursing diagnosis:
  - Acute pain related to irritation of esophagus by gastric acid
  - Ineffective airway clearance related to reflux of gastric contents into the esophagus and tracheal/bronchial tree
  - Risk for aspiration related to entry of gastric contents into the tracheal/bronchial tree
- Treatment:
  - Elevate head of bed for 2 to 3 hours after eating
  - Avoid alcohol
  - Reduce/avoid acidic foods
  - Medications: (Table 7.1)
    - Proton-pump inhibitors
    - H_2-receptor blockers
    - Prokinetic drug therapy
    - Cholinergic drugs
    - Antacids
  - Surgery if conservative treatment ineffective:
    - Antireflux surgery
    - Endoscopic mucosal resection
    - Ablation
- Patient teaching:
  - Do not lay supine for 2 to 3 hours after food/fluid intake.
  - Avoid triggers.
  - Eliminate foods that decrease LES pressure:
    - Chocolate
    - Peppermint
    - Fatty foods
    - Coffee
    - Tea
  - Take prescribed medications consistently
  - Quit smoking

TABLE 7.1	GASTROINTESTINAL MEDICATIONS
Medication	Action
Proton-pump inhibitors (PPIs) Esomeprazole (Nexium) Lansoprazole (Prevacid) Omeprazole (Prilosec) Pantoprazole (Protonix)	Decrease HCl acid secretion by inhibiting the proton pump responsible for the secretion of H^+. Decrease irritation of the esophageal and gastric mucosa.
Histamine (H2)-Receptor Blockers Cimetidine (Tagamet) Famotidine (Pepcid) Nizatidine (Axid) Ranitidine (Zantac)	Block histamine on the H_2 receptors to decrease HCl acid secretion. Reduce the conversion of pepsinogen to pepsin. Decrease irritation of the esophageal and gastric mucosa.
Prokinetic Agents Metoclopramide (Reglan)	Reduce reflux. Increase gastric motility and emptying.
Cholinergic Bethanechol (Urecholine)	Increase lower esophageal sphincter pressure. Increase esophageal and gastric emptying.
Antacids, Acid Neutralizers Aluminum hydroxide Calcium carbonate (Tums) Magnesium oxide (MagOx) Sodium bicarbonate (Alka-Seltzer) Sodium citrate Aluminum and magnesium (Maalox, Mylanta) Aluminum/magnesium trisilicate (Gaviscon)	Neutralize HCl acid.
Cytoprotective drugs Sucralfate (Carafate) Misoprostol (Cytotec)	Provide protection to the mucosa of the esophagus, stomach, and duodenum.

▶ *Hiatal Hernia*

- A portion of the stomach that protrudes into the esophagus through an opening in the diaphragm. The most common type of hernia is a *sliding hernia*, which occurs when the patient is supine and typically resolves when the patient stands upright. A *rolling (paraesophageal) hernia* occurs when the fundus and a portion of the stomach roll up through the diaphragm, forming a pocket alongside the esophagus. An acute rolling hernia is considered a medical emergency because of the strangulation of the hernia.

- *Assessment/Intervention/Education*
  - Detailed medical history:
    - Check for a history of factors that increase intraabdominal pressure:
      - Intense physical exertion
      - Repetitive heavy lifting
      - Pregnancy
      - Ascites
      - Abdominal tumors
    - Heartburn or reflux
  - Risk factors:
    - Older age
    - Obesity
    - Weakening of diaphragm
  - Clinical manifestations:
    - May be asymptomatic
    - If symptomatic, symptoms similar to those of GERD

- Diagnosis:
  - Upper GI—barium swallow
  - May be identified on a chest x-ray
- Nursing diagnosis:
  - Acute pain related to gastroesophageal reflux
  - Nausea related to gastric contents in the esophagus
- Treatment:
  - Management same as for GERD
  - Surgery:
    - Reduction of the herniation
    - Closing the defect
    - Secure the stomach to prevent it from herniating
- Patient teaching:
  - Importance of following prescribed dietary regimen
  - Treatment options, including medications

Question	Rationale
A female patient has a sliding hiatal hernia. What nursing intervention will prevent the symptoms of heartburn that she is experiencing? A. Keep the patient NPO (non per os; nothing by mouth). B. Put the bed in the Trendelenburg position. C. Have the patient eat four to six smaller meals each day. D. Encourage the patient to wear form-fitting clothes	Answer: C Eating smaller meals during the day will decrease the gastric pressure and the symptoms of hiatal hernia. Keeping the patient NPO or in a Trendelenburg position is not appropriate. The head of the bed should be elevated. Patients should be encouraged to wear loose-fitting clothes.

▶ *Esophageal Varices*

- Esophageal varices are enlarged and dilated veins in the esophagus. They are caused by portal hypertension, which is most often associated with cirrhosis. Increased pressure can cause these varices to rupture, which is considered a medical emergency.
- *Assessment/Intervention/Education*
  - Detailed medical history:
    - Cirrhosis of the liver
    - Portal hypertension
    - Previous bleeding varices
  - Risk factors:
    - Excess alcohol ingestion
    - History of liver disease
  - Clinical manifestations:
    - Hematemesis
    - Melena (black stools)
    - Abdominal pain

- May have ascites and bruits heard over the upper abdominal area
  - Tortuous epigastric vessels
- Diagnosis:
  - Endoscopy
- Treatment:
  - Endoscopic ligation of bleeding varices
  - Life-threatening emergency if varices rupture
  - Admit/transfer to intensive care unit (ICU)
  - Balloon tamponade
  - Transjugular intrahepatic portosystemic shunt (TIPS) procedure
  - Beta-blockers
- Patient teaching:
  - Teach the patient when to seek medical attention
  - Follow treatment plan to prevent rupture of varices:
    - Abstain from alcohol use.
    - Avoid aspirin (ASA) and nonsteroidal antiinflammatory drugs (NSAIDs).
    - Avoid straining that may trigger hemorrhage.

▶ **Gastritis**

- Inflammation of the gastric mucosa occurs when there is breakdown in the normal gastric barrier. Acute gastritis is self-limiting lasting a few hours to a few days and typically results in complete healing. Chronic gastritis requires a lifelong change or treatment to prevent symptoms.
- *Assessment/Intervention/Education*
  - Detailed medical history:
    - Alcohol abuse
    - GI problems:
      - Hiatal hernia
      - Crohn's disease
      - Reflux
    - Renal failure
    - Burns
    - Sepsis
  - Risk factors:
    - Drugs that contribute to gastritis:
      - ASA
      - NSAIDs
      - Corticosteroids
      - Iron supplements
    - Diet:
      - Alcohol
      - Spicy foods
    - Microorganisms:
      - *Helicobacter pylori*
      - Mycobacterium
      - Salmonella
      - Cytomegalovirus
      - Syphilis

Clinical Consideration
H. pylori is the causative organism for most cases of gastritis.

- Environmental factors:
  - Radiation
  - Smoking
- Clinical manifestations:
  - Symptomatic
  - Anorexia
  - Nausea
  - Vomiting
  - Epigastric tenderness
  - Chronic gastritis problems:
    - Loss of intrinsic factor
    - Cobalamin deficiency (vitamin B_{12})
    - Anemia
- Diagnosis:
  - Based on symptoms and alcohol abuse
  - Testing for *H. pylori*
- Nursing diagnosis:
  - Acute pain related to inflammation of gastric mucosa
  - Imbalanced nutrition: less than body requirements related to vomiting, inadequate intestinal absorption of nutrients, restricted dietary regimen
- Treatment:
  - Eliminate cause of gastritis
  - Nutrition consult
  - Eliminate alcohol ingestion
  - Treat cobalamin deficiency and anemia
  - Treat *H. pylori* infection
- Patient teaching:
  - Importance of eliminating alcohol
  - Avoid causes of gastritis symptoms

Peptic Ulcer Disease (PUD)

- Erosion along the GI tract from HCl acid and pepsin secretions that may be acute or chronic in nature. Acute ulcers involve superficial erosion of the mucosal wall with minimal inflammation that resolves when the cause is removed or eliminated. Chronic ulcers are more common than acute and are defined as a long-term exposure to inflammation with erosion through the mucosal wall that results in the formation of fibrous tissue.
- PUD can occur anywhere in the GI tract where there is an acidic environment. Gastric and duodenal ulcer presentations are different, but the treatment is similar for the various types of ulcers.
  - Gastric ulcers:
    - Less common
    - Can occur in any portion of the stomach
    - Occur more often in women over 50 years old
    - May result in an obstruction
  - Duodenal ulcers:
    - Accounts for the majority of PUD
    - Occur more often in adults 35 to 45 years old
    - *H. pylori* found in 90 to 95% of cases

- *Assessment/Intervention/Education*
  - Detailed medical history:
    - Symptoms of epigastric pain
    - Habits that increase gastric acid secretions:
      - Alcohol intake
      - Ingestion of large quantities of coffee
      - Smoking
    - History of GI disorders
    - *H. pylori*
    - Taking medications that cause gastric irritation:
      - NSAIDs
      - ASA
  - Clinical manifestations:
    - Epigastric pain
    - Referred back pain
    - May experience bloating, nausea, and vomiting
    - May be asymptomatic:
      - Older adults
      - Those taking NSAIDs
    - Gastric:
      - Epigastric pain 1 to 2 hours after eating
      - Epigastric burning
      - Excessive flatus
    - Duodenal:
      - Epigastric pain several hours (2 to 5 hours) after eating when gastric acid comes in contact with ulcerations
      - Epigastric burning
      - Abdominal cramping
  - Diagnosis:
    - Endoscopy for visualization and biopsy
    - Determine if *H. pylori* is present:
      - Invasive test:
        - Biopsy
      - Noninvasive test:
        - Urea (by-product of *H. pylori*) breath test
        - Stool antigen test
        - Serum antibody test (antibodies present for past and current infection)
    - Barium contrast study to assess for obstruction
  - Nursing diagnosis:
    - Acute pain related to irritation from gastric secretions
    - Fatigue related to loss of blood, chronic illness
    - Nausea related to gastrointestinal irritation
  - Complications:
    - Hemorrhage
    - Perforation
    - Gastric-outlet obstruction
  - Treatment:
    - Treat *H. pylori* infection
      - Antibiotics, if appropriate

Clinical Consideration

All these complications are considered an emergency and may require surgical intervention.

- Medications:
  - Proton-pump inhibitor (PPI) medications
  - H_2-receptor blockers
  - Antacids
  - Cytoprotective drugs
  - Tricyclic antidepressants:
    - Decrease acid secretion
    - May help with pain relief
- Smoking cessation
- Dietary modification:
  - Avoid/restrict alcohol
- Surgery:
  - May result in *dumping syndrome*—nutrients not able to be absorbed because the gastric contents empty too quickly into the intestine; can cause nausea, vomiting, and weakness
- Patient teaching:
  - Adherence to therapy, as ulcers tend to recur
  - Smoking, stress, and depression can delay healing
  - Long-term follow-up
    - Endoscopy every 3 to 6 months
  - Teach patient about medications
    - Use enteric coated ASA
  - Teach patient to notify provider about:
    - Recurrence of epigastric pain
    - Blood in stool
    - Blood in emesis

Gastrointestinal (GI) Bleeding

- GI bleeding is any type of bleeding that originates in the GI tract. Bleeding of the GI tract is not a disease, but rather a symptom of another disease or condition.
- **Assessment/Intervention/Education**
  - Detailed medical history:
    - History of previous bleeding
    - Alcohol intake
    - Medications:
      - ASA
      - NSAIDs
      - Corticosteroids
      - Anticoagulants
    - GI-tract disorders:
      - Cancer
      - PUD
      - Varices
      - Gastritis
      - Diverticulitis
      - Polyps
  - Clinical manifestations:
    - Acute bleed:
      - Change in vital signs

- Symptoms of hypovolemic shock
- Decreased urine output
  - Upper GI bleed:
    - Bright red blood in emesis, arterial
    - Coffee-ground emesis—old blood in stomach
    - Melena—slow GI bleed
  - Lower GI bleed:
    - Presentation typically varies based on location of bleed
    - Bright red blood—descending colon and rectal bleed
    - Maroon stools—ascending colon bleed
    - Melena—cecal bleeding
- Diagnosis:
  - Endoscopy visualization
  - Emesis and stool with frank or occult blood
  - Complete blood count decreased/decreasing
- Nursing diagnosis:
  - Deficient fluid volume related to blood loss
  - Fatigue related to blood loss
- Treatment:
  - Endoscopy:
    - Stop bleeding by thrombosing the vessel.
    - Apply clips/bands to compress the vessel.
  - Medications:
    - PPIs
    - Epinephrine injection during endoscopy
    - Decrease esophageal bleeding:
      - Octreotide (Sandostatin)
      - Vasopressin (Pitressin)
  - Surgery—if endoscopy and medications fail
  - Blood transfusion
- Patient teaching:
  - Avoid gastric irritants.
  - Take drugs that are gastric irritants with food.
  - Importance of adhering to drug therapy.

Question	Rationale
A 62-year-old patient was admitted with epigastric pain due to a gastric ulcer. Which patient assessment requires an urgent change in the plan of care? A. Chest pain relieved with eating or drinking B. Rigid abdomen and vomiting C. Back pain 3 or 4 hours after eating a meal D. Burning epigastric pain 1 hour after eating	Answer: B A rigid abdomen with vomiting may indicate a perforation of the ulcer and requires immediate attention. Chest pain that is relieved by eating or drinking and back pain 3 to 4 hours after a meal is more likely to occur with a duodenal ulcer. It is not uncommon to experience burning epigastric pain 1-2 hours after a meal with a gastric ulcer.

▶ *Appendicitis*

- Appendicitis is the inflammation of the appendix, typically caused by an obstruction of the lumen, causing an accumulation of mucus that becomes infected, potentially causing perforation and peritonitis. A delay in treatment may result in a poor outcome and may even be fatal.

- *Assessment/Intervention/Education*
  - Detailed medical history:
    - Onset of abdominal pain/discomfort—no analgesics or light analgesics until cause of pain determined
  - Clinical manifestations:
    - Pain near the umbilicus moving to right lower quadrant (McBurney's point)
    - Rebound pain/tenderness
    - Nausea/vomiting
    - Poor appetite
    - Fever and chills
  - Complications:
    - Abscess
    - Rupture of appendix
    - Sepsis
  - Diagnosis:
    - CT scan
    - White-cell count elevated to >10,000/mm^3
    - C-reactive protein
  - Nursing diagnosis:
    - Acute pain related to inflammation of appendix
    - Risk for infection related to infected appendix
  - Treatment:
    - Keep patient NPO
    - Assess for signs and symptoms of perforation (surgical emergency)
    - Appendectomy
    - Antibiotics
  - Patient teaching:
    - Postoperative care of surgical site
    - Signs and symptoms of infection

Clinical Consideration

Do not use a heating pad or administer enemas or laxatives, as doing so may cause an inflamed appendix to rupture.

Question	Rationale
The provider orders an enema for a patient with suspected appendicitis. Which of the following actions should the nurse take? A. Explain the procedure to the patient, B. Prepare the enema with 750 to1000 ml of lukewarm tap water. C. Question the provider order. D. Position the patient in left Sims position.	Answer: C An enema is contraindicated for a patient with actual or suspected appendicitis. All the other actions are correct only if enema administration is appropriate.

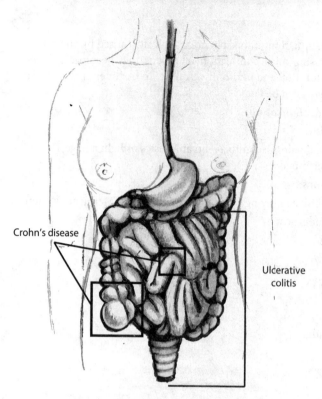

Crohn's disease

Ulcerative colitis

Figure 7.1 Location of inflammation

▶ *Inflammatory Bowel Disease (IBD)*

- IBD is an autoimmune disease that causes chronic inflammation of the GI tract, with periods of exacerbation and remission. These exacerbations of inflammation cause tissue damage and destruction. IBD is divided into two classifications: ulcerative colitis and Crohn's disease.

- In ulcerative colitis, the inflammation is limited to the colon; it starts at the rectum and spreads up the colon. The area of inflammation is continuous and involves only the mucosa.

- Crohn's disease involves inflammation at any point in the GI tract, but is most frequently found in the distal ileum. Inflammation involves the entire thickness of the bowel wall. There is cobblestoning of the mucosal wall, and patches of healthy tissue can be found between areas of inflammation. (Figure 7.1)

- *Assessment/Intervention/Education*
  - Detailed medical history:
    - Family members with IBD
    - Jewish origin
    - Genetic predispositions
    - Inflammatory disorders:
      • Multiple sclerosis
      • Psoriasis
    - Genetic syndromes:
      • Cystic fibrosis
  - Risk factors:
    - Environmental factors that can impact the normal GI flora and the immune system:
      • Diet
      • Air pollution

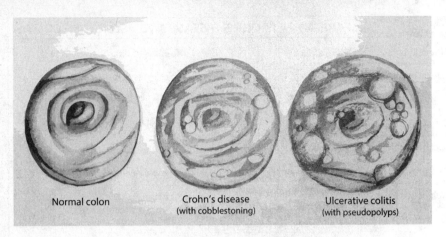

Normal colon

Crohn's disease
(with cobblestoning)

Ulcerative colitis
(with pseudopolyps)

Figure 7.2 Intestinal wall changes

- Stress
- Smoking
- Clinical manifestations: (Table 7.2 and Figure 7.2)
  - Both ulcerative colitis and Crohn's disease:
    - Diarrhea
    - Abdominal pain
    - Fatigue
  - Ulcerative colitis only:
    - Fever during exacerbations
    - Rectal bleeding
    - Tenesmus
    - Pseudopolyps—inflamed projections into the intestinal lumen
  - Crohn's disease only:
    - Fever
    - Weight loss
    - Nutritional deficits
    - Small bowel involvement
- Complications:
  - Both ulcerative colitis and Crohn's disease:
    - Hemorrhage
    - Perforation
    - Increased incidence of *Clostridium difficile* infection
  - Ulcerative colitis only:
    - Toxic megacolon
    - Increased incidence of colorectal cancer after 10 years
  - Crohn's disease only:
    - Perianal abscesses and fistulas
    - Strictures
    - Increased incidence of small bowel cancer
  - Systemic problems:
    - Peripheral arthritis
    - Ankylosing spondylosis
    - Finger clubbing
    - Gallstones

TABLE 7.2	COMPARISON OF CROHN'S DISEASE AND ULCERATIVE COLITIS	
Characteristic	Crohn's Disease	Ulcerative Colitis
Age on onset	Typically teens to 30	Typically teens to 30 and over 60
Steatorrhea	Frequent	Absent
Diarrhea	Common	Common, up to 30 stools a day
Rectal bleeding	Occasional	Common
Pain, abdominal	Common, cramping	Common, severe
Weight loss	Yes	Not typically
Fever	Common	During exacerbations
Tenesmus	Rare	Common
Malabsorption, nutritional deficits	Significant	Minimal
Location	Ileum, right colon	Starts at rectum, travels up left colon
Distribution	Interspersed among healthy tissue	Continuous segment
Depth	Entire thickness of bowel wall	Mucosal layer
Appearance	Cobblestoning due to fissures and edema	Pseudopolyps due to inflamed mucosa
Complications	Bowel abscess Fistula formation Strictures Intestinal obstruction Perforation	Hemorrhage Abscess formation Perforation Toxic megacolon Increased incidence of colon cancer

- Kidney stones
- Liver disease
- Osteoporosis
- Diagnosis:
  - Rule out other diseases
  - Diagnostic studies identify severity and complications:
    - Barium enema
    - Small bowel follow-through
    - Abdominal ultrasound
    - CT scan
    - MRI
    - Colonoscopy
    - Video capsule endoscopy
  - Laboratory
    - CBC—determine anemia
    - WBC—determine toxic megacolon or perforation
    - Serum electrolytes—levels decreased due to diarrhea
    - Stool specimens—check for blood
- Nursing diagnosis:
  - Diarrhea related to bowel inflammation

TABLE 7.3	INFLAMMATORY BOWEL DISEASE (IBD) MEDICATIONS
Medication	Action
5-Aminosalicylates (5-ASA) **Oral** Sulfasalazine (Azulfidine) Olsalazine (Dipentum) Mesalamine (Pentasa) **Topical** 5-ASA enema (Rowasa) Mesalamine suppositories (Canasa)	First-line therapy Decreases inflammation Used to achieve remission and prevent flare-ups
Antimicrobials Metronidazole (Flagyl) Ciprofloxacin (Cipro) Clarithromycin (Biaxin)	Used to treat suspected infections
Corticosteroids **Oral** Prednisone **Topical** Hydrocortisone suppository or enema **IV** Methylprednisolone	Used short term to achieve remission
Immunosuppressants 6-mercaptopurine (6-MP) Azathioprine (Imuran) Methotrexate	Used to maintain remission with corticosteroids
Biologic and target therapy **Antitumor necrosis factor agents** Infliximab (Remicade) Adalimumab (Humira) Certolizumab pegol (Cimzia) Golimumab (Simponi) **Integrin receptor antagonists** Natalizumab (Tysabri) Vedolizumab (Entyvio)	Used to achieve and maintain remission for Crohn's disease when conservative therapy has failed Patients may produce antibodies against these medications

- Treatment:
  - Induce and maintain remission
  - Medications (Table 7.3)
  - Diet:
    - High calorie
    - High protein
    - High vitamin
    - May need total parenteral nutrition (TPN) for bowel rest
  - Support group
  - Surgery:
    - Both ulcerative colitis and Crohn's disease:
      - Drainage of abscess
      - Massive hemorrhage
      - Perforation
    - Ulcerative colitis only:
      - Total proctocolectomy with ileal pouch/anal anastomosis
      - Total proctocolectomy with permanent ileostomy

- Crohn's disease only:
    - Resect diseased sections with reanastomosis.
    - Repair fistulas.
    - Relieve strictures.
    - Correct obstructions.
- Patient teaching:
    - Importance of rest and nutrition
    - Importance of following treatment plan to minimize exacerbations
    - Action and side effects of medications
    - Symptoms of recurrence
    - When to seek medical care

Question	Rationale
Crohn's disease is described as a chronic disease that causes relapses. Which of the following areas in the GI system may be involved with this disease? A. Only the mucosal layer of the sigmoid colon. B. The entire length of the large colon. C. The entire large colon through the layers of mucosa and submucosa. D. The small intestine and colon; affecting the entire thickness of the bowel.	Answer: D Crohn's disease involves inflammation at any point in the GI tract and involves the entire thickness of the bowel wall. In ulcerative colitis, the inflammation is limited to the colon; it starts at the rectum and spreads up the colon. The area of inflammation is continuous and involves only the mucosa.

▶ *Intestinal Obstruction*

- Blockage of the small intestine or colon. A complete obstruction occurs when no intestinal contents are able to pass; a partial obstruction allows small amounts of stool to pass through the intestines. Failure to correct an obstruction eventually leads to necrosis and perforation.
- *Assessment/Intervention/Education*
    - Detailed medical history:
        - Recent surgery
        - Change in bowel habits
        - Medications that cause constipation
    - Risk factors:
        - Colorectal cancer
        - Recent or past surgery:
            - Paralytic ileus
            - Postoperative adhesions
        - Hernia
        - Crohn's disease
        - Opiate usage
    - Clinical manifestations:
        - Abdominal pain
        - Vomiting

- Distention
- Constipation
- Third spacing of fluids in the bowel lumen
- Diagnosis:
  - Radiology :
    - CT scan
    - Abdominal x-rays
    - Sigmoidoscopy
    - Colonoscopy
  - Laboratory:
    - White-cell count
    - Hemoglobin/hematocrit—decrease may indicate bleeding or strangulation with necrosis
    - Electrolytes—may indicate dehydration
    - Arterial blood gases (ABGs)—vomiting may cause metabolic alkalosis.
- Nursing diagnosis:
  - Acute pain related to distended abdomen
- Treatment:
  - Varies with cause of obstruction
  - Correction of the obstruction:
    - NPO—rest the bowel
    - IV fluids
    - Colonoscopy to remove polyps, strictures, and tumors
    - Surgery to relieve obstruction:
      - Partial or total colectomy
      - Possible colostomy
      - Possible ileostomy
- Patient teaching:
  - Prevent constipation.
  - Ensure adequate fluid intact.
  - Eat a healthy, well-balanced meal.
- Ostomy surgery
  - A portion of the bowel being brought to the surface of the abdomen, in the form of a stoma. An ostomy can be temporary or permanent.
    - Ileostomy—located in the ileum:
      - Liquid to semiliquid stool
      - Indications: ulcerative colitis, Crohn's disease, trauma, and cancer
    - Colostomy—located in the colon
      - Indications: perforating diverticulitis, fistulas, tumors, and cancer
      - Stool consistency is dependent on location of stoma:
        - *Ascending*—semiliquid stool
        - *Transverse*—semiliquid to semiformed stool
        - *Sigmoid*—formed stool
  - Types of ostomies:
    - End stoma:
      - One stoma
      - Permanent if distal bowel removed
      - Temporary if Hartmann pouch created for anastomosis of the intestines in the future

- Loop stoma:
  - One stoma
  - Proximal and distal openings
  - Temporary
- Double-barreled stoma:
  - Two stomas
  - Proximal stoma functions, distal stoma is nonfunctioning
  - Temporary

▶ *Diverticulitis*

- Inflammation of one or more diverticula, most commonly found in the left sigmoid and descending colon. Diverticula are dilations or outpouchings of the colon mucosa.
- *Assessment/Intervention/Education*
  - Detailed medical history:
    - Known history of diverticula
    - Dietary intake
  - Risk factors:
    - Low-fiber diet
    - Age-related changes of the colon
    - obesity
  - Clinical manifestations:
    - May be asymptomatic
    - Pain, usually in left lower abdomen
    - Change in bowel habits
    - Acute manifestations:
      - Hemorrhage
      - Perforation
      - Peritonitis
    - Chronic manifestations:
      - Abscess
      - Strictures
      - Fistulas
      - Obstruction
  - Diagnosis:
    - Colonoscopy
    - Sigmoidoscopy
    - CT scan
  - Nursing diagnosis:
    - Acute pain related to inflammation of bowel
    - Constipation related to dietary deficiency of fiber and roughage
    - Diarrhea related to increased intestinal motility caused by inflammation
  - Treatment:
    - Diet:
      - Acute episode—NPO to allow the colon to rest
      - High-fiber diet
    - Medications:
      - Anticholinergics
      - Antispasmodics
      - Antiinflammatory
      - Bulk laxatives

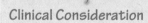

Clinical Consideration

There is no evidence to support that a diet that avoids nuts and seeds will prevent diverticulitis.

- Increase physical activity
- Antibiotics if abscess or perforation is suspected
- Surgery if conservative therapy fails
- Patient teaching:
  - Ways to prevent recurrence of symptoms:
    - Weight reduction
    - High-fiber diet
    - Regular exercise
    - Increase fluids
  - Avoid increasing intraabdominal pressure

Hepatitis

- Hepatitis involves injury to hepatocytes due to the inflammation caused by viruses, alcohol, medications, autoimmune diseases, or metabolic abnormalities, leading to liver dysfunction.
- After the acute phase, the liver cells usually regenerate, resuming normal function. On occasion acute hepatitis causes severe damage to the liver cells, ultimately leading to liver failure.
- Chronic hepatitis is the result of continual destruction of the hepatocytes, the formation of scar tissue and fibrosis as the liver cells attempt to regenerate. This may result in cirrhosis and liver failure.
- Viral hepatitis is categorized into various types with similar manifestations, while mode of transmission and the course of each disease differs.
- *Assessment/Intervention/Education*
  - Clinical manifestations:
    - Acute hepatitis:
      - Flu-like symptoms
      - Anorexia
      - Lethargy/malaise
      - Nausea/vomiting
      - May or may not have jaundice
      - Clay-colored stools
      - Rash, angioedema
      - Right-upper-quadrant tenderness
      - Weight loss
    - Chronic hepatitis:
      - Jaundice
      - Dark urine
      - Pruritus (generalized itching)
      - Spider angiomas
      - Ascites
      - Anemia
      - Coagulation abnormalities
      - Steatorrhea
  - Complications:
    - Portal hypertension
    - Cirrhosis
    - Liver cancer
  - **Hepatitis A (HAV)**
  Spread by the fecal–oral route, from contaminated food or drinking water

- *Assessment/Intervention/Education*
  - Risk factors:
    - Drug users
    - Travel to developing countries
    - Poor sanitation
    - Contaminated food or water
  - Diagnosis:
    - Laboratory testing:
      - HAVAb/IgM
      - HAVAb/IgG
      - HAV RNA
  - Treatment:
    - There are no medications for the treatment of HAV.
    - Infections is self-limiting and should resolve within several weeks.
    - Periods of rest to decrease metabolic demands.
  - Patient teaching:
    - Prevention:
      - Hepatitis A vaccine
      - Handwashing before eating and after having a bowel movement
      - Proper handling of food and food preparation
      - Postexposure prophylaxis treated with gamma globulin

> **Clinical Consideration**
> HBV is more infectious than human immunodeficiency virus.

- **Hepatitis B (HBV)**

Bloodborne pathogen that is spread by exposure to blood or blood products; HBV can live on surfaces for a minimum of 7 days.

- *Assessment/Intervention/Education*
  - Risk factors/transmission:
    - Hemodialysis
    - Sharing needles/syringes
    - Tattoos
    - Piercings
    - High-risk sexual practices:
      - Multiple partners
      - No protection
    - Health care workers
    - Perinatal
    - Transfusion recipients
  - Diagnosis:
    - Laboratory testing:
      - HBeAg
      - HBeAb
      - HBsAg
      - HBsAb total
      - HBVcAb/IgM
  - Treatment:
    - May resolve with no complications
    - Well-balanced diet, with adequate calories
    - Periods of rest to decrease metabolic demands
    - Medications: (Table 7.4)
      - Nucleoside and nucleotide analogs
      - Interferon

TABLE 7.4 HEPATITIS MEDICATIONS

Medication	Action
Nucleoside and nucleotide analogs Adefovir dipivoxil (Hepsera) Entecavir (Baraclude) Ribavirin (Ribashere)	Used for chronic HBV Prevents viral replication
Immune modulators Interferon (Pegintron)	Used for chronic HBV and HCV Stimulates a natural immune response Administered subcutaneously Not well tolerated because of numerous side effects

Direct-acting antivirals (DAAs)
NS3/4A protease inhibitors
  Simeprevir (Olysio)
NS5B Polymerase inhibitors
  Sofosbuvir (Sovaldi)
NS5A inhibitors
  Ledipasvir
Combination therapy of the various DAAs
  Sofosbuvir + ledipasvir (Harvoni)
	Used for chronic HCV
	Many medications are only used in combination therapy
	Almost all of these are teratogenic

- Abstinence from alcohol and other hepatotoxic substances
- Patient teaching:
  - Dispose of sharps properly.
  - Use condoms for sexual intercourse.
  - Potential development of chronic hepatitis B.
  - Prevention:
    - Modify high-risk behaviors
    - Avoid sharing needles, syringes, personal items
    - Hepatitis B vaccine (Heptavax B, Recombivax HB) for prevention
    - Postexposure prophylaxis: hepatitis B immune globulin (HBIg)
    - For patients with chronic hepatitis B: surveillance for cirrhosis and hepatocellular cancer
- **Hepatitis C (HCV)**
  Bloodborne pathogen that is spread by exposure to blood or blood products. Most patients with HCV are unaware that they have been infected as the symptoms are mild. Chronic infection develops in more than two-thirds of infected individuals. Based on this, the CDC recommends that all people born between 1945 and 1965 be screened for HCV.
- ***Assessment/Intervention/Education***
  - Risk factors:
    - Hemodialysis
    - Sharing needles/syringes
    - Tattoos
    - Piercings
    - High-risk sexual practices:
      - Multiple partners
      - No protection
  - Diagnosis:
    - Laboratory testing:
      - HCVAb/IgG
      - HVC RNA

> **Clinical Consideration**
> HBV and HBC account for 80% of all cases of liver cancer.

- Treatment:
  - Well-balanced diet, with adequate calories
  - Periods of rest to decrease metabolic demands
  - Medications: (Table 7.4)
    - Interferon
    - Direct-acting antivirals (DAAs)
      - NS3/4A protease inhibitors
      - NS5B polymerase inhibitors
      - NS5A inhibitors
      - Combination therapy of the various DAAs
  - Abstinence from alcohol
- Patient teaching:
  - Dispose of sharps properly.
  - Use condoms for sexual intercourse.
  - Avoid hepatotoxic substances/medications.
  - Calamine lotion for pruritus.
  - Prevention:
    - Avoid sharing needles, syringes, personal items
    - For patients with chronic hepatitis C, surveillance for development of cirrhosis and hepatocellular cancer

Cirrhosis

- Destruction of liver cells that results in fibrosis and nodules of the liver tissue found in patients with end-stage liver disease.
- **Assessment/Intervention/Education**
  - Detailed medical history:
    - Hepatitis
    - Alcohol intake
    - Right-sided heart failure
    - Chronic biliary obstruction
    - Assess for spontaneous bacterial peritonitis (SBP) if patient has ascites.
    - Medications:
      - ASA
      - Acetaminophen
      - NSAIDs
      - Anticoagulants
      - Hepatotoxic medications
  - Complications:
    - Portal hypertension
    - Esophageal and gastric varices
    - Abdominal ascites
    - Peripheral edema
    - Hepatic encephalopathy
      - Neurotoxic effects from excess ammonia—crosses the blood–brain barrier
      - Changes in mental status
      - Impaired consciousness
  - Clinical manifestations:

Clinical Consideration

Acetaminophen can cause liver failure if total daily dose is exceeded.

- Early:
  - No symptoms may be apparent
  - Fatigue
  - Liver enlargement
- Late:
  - Symptoms from liver failure and portal hypertension
  - Jaundice
  - Peripheral edema
  - Ascites
  - Skin lesions:
    - Spider angiomas
  - Hematologic disorders:
    - Thrombocytopenia
    - Leukopenia
    - Anemia
    - Coagulation disorders:
      - Bleeding
      - Petechiae
      - Bruising
  - Peripheral neuropathy
  - Spontaneous bacterial peritonitis (SBP)
- Diagnosis:
  - Abnormal liver-function tests (LFTs):
    - AST and ALT initially elevated
    - AST and ALT may be normal with end-stage liver failure
  - Other labs:
    - Decreased serum protein and albumin
    - Increased bilirubin and globulin
  - Diagnostic tests:
    - Liver biopsy—*gold standard.*
    - Ultrasound not reliable for cirrhosis diagnosis.
    - Ultrasound elastography (Fibroscan) can determine degree of liver fibrosis.
- Nursing diagnosis:
  - Excess fluid volume related to portal hypertension
  - Imbalanced nutrition: less than body requirements related to utilization and storage of nutrients
- Treatment:
  - Rest
  - Avoid alcohol intake
  - Avoid ASA, acetaminophen, NSAIDs
  - There is no specific drug therapy for cirrhosis
  - Treatment of symptoms and complications (Table 7.5)
- Patient teaching:
  - Alcohol abstinence
  - Provide information on support groups/Alcohol Anonymous (AA)
  - Avoid over-the-counter (OTC) medications that are hepatotoxic

TABLE 7.5	MEDICATIONS FOR TREATMENT FOR CIRRHOSIS COMPLICATIONS
Control bleeding of esophageal and gastric varices Octreotide (Sandostatin) Vasopressin (Pitressin)	
Reduce portal venous pressure and esophageal varices Propranolol (Inderal) Nadolol (Corgard)	
Decrease ammonia levels Lactulose Rifaximin (Xifaxan) Neomycin sulfate	
Address clotting abnormalities Vitamin K	
Decrease gastric acid Esomeprazole (Nexium) Lansoprazole (Prevacid) Omeprazole (Prilosec) Pantoprazole (Protonix)	

Question	Rationale
A patient is admitted with liver failure and cirrhosis. The patient is also noted to have ascites. The nurse understands that this has occurred because of: A. Blood accumulation in the abdomen due to decreased clotting factors. B. Portal hypertension and hypoalbuminemia causing fluid to shift into the peritoneal cavity. C. Delayed peristalsis causing distention of the bowel. D. Serum bile salts contributing to peritoneal edema.	Answer: B Portal hypertension and hypoalbuminemia are often seen with cirrhosis and contribute to the shift of fluid into the peritoneal cavity. Patients with cirrhosis will often have coagulation disorders, although these do not contribute to the development of ascites. Decreased peristalsis and bile salts are not contributing factors for ascites.

▌ *Pancreatitis*

- Pancreatitis is the inflammation of the pancreas and is defined as either acute or chronic in nature.
- Acute pancreatitis occurs suddenly and typically resolves after treatment is initiated. The most common cause of acute pancreatitis is gallbladder disease/stones that cause irritation or blockage of the common bile duct. This blockage leads to an accumulation of digestive enzymes that can cause autodigestion of the pancreas.
- Chronic pancreatitis is recurrent or ongoing inflammation of the pancreas that does not resolve, leading to fibrosis of the pancreas. An acute episode of pancreatitis can be a precursor to the chronic form of this disease, although the most common cause of chronic pancreatitis is consumption of large quantities of alcohol.
- *Assessment/Intervention/Education*
  - Detailed medical history:
    - Gallbladder disease
    - Chronic alcohol intake

- Previous ERCP procedure
- Medications:
  - Thiazide diuretics
  - Furosemide (Lasix)
- Recent viruses
- Risk factors:
  - Gallstones
  - Alcohol consumption
  - Trauma to biliary tract
  - High triglycerides
  - Smoking
- Clinical manifestations:
  - Acute:
    - Pain:
      - Sudden or gradual onset
      - Left upper quadrant
      - Midepigastric
      - Pain may radiate to back
      - Aggravated by eating
    - Nausea/vomiting
    - Low-grade fever
    - Jaundice
    - Decreased bowel sounds
    - Ecchymosis
      - Discoloration of abdominal wall
      - Grey Turner spots—discoloration in flank regions indicating a retro-peritoneal bleed
      - Cullen sign—discoloration of the umbilical area indicating bleeding in the peritoneum
  - Chronic
    - Pain
      - Abdominal pain at increasing intervals
      - Pain eventually becomes constant
    - Jaundice
    - Dark urine
    - Steatorrhea
    - Weight loss
- Complications:
  - Local:
    - Pseudocysts:
      - Inflammation due to fluid and debris accumulation
      - Usually resolves without intervention
    - Pancreatic abscess:
      - Infected pseudocyst
      - Needs to be surgically drained
  - Respiratory—due to spillage from pancreas affecting the diaphragm:
    - Atelectasis
    - Left pleural effusion
    - Pneumonia
    - Acute respiratory distress syndrome (ARDS)

- Cardiovascular
  - Activation of prothrombin due to release of trypsin
  - Risk for thrombi, emboli, disseminated intravascular coagulation (DIC)
- Pancreatic cancer
- Diabetes—due to pancreatic dysfunction
- Tetany—from hypocalcemia
- Abdominal compartment syndrome ascites
- Diagnosis:
  - ERCP
  - MRCP—determines gallstones
  - CT with contrast—determines pseudocysts, abscess, and severity
  - Laboratory tests:
    - Serum amylase elevated in acute disease
    - Serum lipase elevated in acute disease
- Nursing diagnosis:
  - Acute pain related to injury from distention and injury of pancreas.
  - Ineffective health management related to not following treatment plan, lack of follow-up care, and continued alcohol consumption.
- Treatment:
  - Acute:
    - Hydration
    - Pain management
    - Manage complications
    - Decrease pancreatic enzymes:
      - NPO
      - Suction gastric contents
    - Endoscopic or CT-guided aspiration of fluid
    - Antibiotics, if appropriate
    - ERCP to remove stones
    - Adequate nutrition
  - Chronic:
    - Pain management:
      - Analgesics
      - Tricyclic antidepressants may help to reduce neuropathic pain.
    - Medications to replace pancreas functions
      - Pancrelipase (Pancrease) replaces the pancreatic enzymes amylase, lipase, and trypsin.
      - Bile salts assist with absorption of vitamins.
      - Insulin or oral hypoglycemic agents for hyperglycemia
    - Adequate nutrition—small bland meals
    - Abstain from alcohol and caffeinated beverage consumption
    - Common-bile-duct stent placement
    - Roux-en-Y pancreatojejunostomy—surgical diversion of bile from pancreas to jejunum
- Patient teaching:
  - Prevention of attacks:
    - Abstain from alcohol
    - Take enzymes with food

- Monitor stool for steatorrhea
- Notify provider immediately if experiencing symptoms of worsening pancreatitis

▶ *Cholecystitis and Cholelithiasis*

- Cholecystitis occurs when there is inflammation of the gallbladder. This inflammation is typically associated with stones or biliary sludge.
- *Cholelithiasis* is defined as stones in the gallbladder that can cause spasms of the gallbladder and ductal system.
- Gallstones are classified based on the composition:
  - Cholesterol
  - Bile
  - Mixed
- *Assessment/Intervention/Education*
  - Detailed medical history:
    - Age, females over 40
    - Postmenopausal women
    - Estrogen replacement or oral contraceptives
    - Sedentary lifestyle
    - Obesity
  - Clinical manifestations:
    - May be asymptomatic
    - Indigestion
    - Right-upper-quadrant pain, exacerbated by fatty foods
    - Referred pain—right shoulder and scapula
    - Chronic symptoms:
      - Fat intolerance
      - Dyspepsia
      - Pyrosis
      - Excessive flatus
    - If bile duct is obstructed
      - Jaundice
      - Dark amber/brown urine
      - Clay-colored stool
      - Steatorrhea
  - Complications:
    - Common bile duct (CBD) obstruction
    - Cholangitis—inflammation of biliary ducts
    - Pancreatitis
    - Perforation/rupture of gallbladder
    - Peritonitis
    - Sepsis
    - Death
  - Diagnosis:
    - Ultrasound of the gallbladder—can identify stones
    - ERCP
    - Percutaneous transhepatic cholangiography
    - Radionucleotide imaging: hepatobiliary iminodiacetic acid (HIDA) scan, cholescintigraphy, cholangiography

- Laboratory:
  - White-cell count
  - Bilirubin levels
  - LFTs:
    - Alkaline phosphate
    - ALT
    - AST
  - Serum amylase
- Treatment:
  - Cholecystitis:
    - Pain control
    - Nasogastric tube (NGT) for severe nausea and vomiting
    - Anticholinergics to decrease gastric secretions and smooth muscle spasms
    - Small low-fat, high-fiber meals
  - Cholelithiasis—conservative treatment:
    - Cholesterol solvents:
      - Ursodeoxycholic acid (ursodiol)
      - Chenodeoxycholic acid (chenodiol)
    - Extracorporeal shock-wave lithotripsy (ESWL)
    - ERCP:
      - Stone removal
      - Dilation of biliary ducts
      - Stent placement
  - Surgery:
    - Laparoscopic cholecystectomy
    - Open cholecystectomy
    - Trans-hepatic biliary catheter
- Patient teaching:
  - Predisposing factors
  - Explain purpose and preparation for procedures
  - Conservative treatment:
    - Avoid irritants
    - Limit fat intake, take small meals
  - Postoperative teaching:
    - Watch for signs of infection
    - Referred shoulder pain due to CO_2 retention after laparoscopic cholecystectomy
    - A low-fat diet is better tolerated postoperatively
    - T-tube/drain care

CASE STUDY

A 45-year old-man with a history of cirrhosis, esophageal varices, hepatitis C, and hypertension has been admitted to a medical-surgical unit with increasing confusion, lethargy, and a blood pressure of 144/86 mm Hg. His family states that he has not been sleeping much in the past few days and that he has been much more unsteady when walking. Currently he is alert and oriented to person only. On assessment, abdominal distention is present. The provider orders a complete blood count, comprehensive metabolic profile, liver-function tests, serum ammonia level, and an abdominal ultrasound. See Table 7.6 for significant lab results. The abdominal ultrasound reveals a fatty liver and moderate amount of ascites. After reviewing the diagnostic test results, the provider orders an endoscopy.

TABLE 7.6	LABORATORY TEST RESULTS	
Test	Result	Normal
Hemoglobin (Hgb)	9.5 g/dL	14–18 g/dL (male)
Hematocrit (Hct)	28.4%	42–52% (male)
Serum glucose, fasting	192 mg/dL	74–106 mg/dL
BUN	42 mg/dL	10–20 mg/dL
Serum creatinine	1.5 mg/dL	0.6–1.2 mg/dL
Total protein	5.2 g/dL	6.4–8.3 g/dL
Albumin	3.0 g/dL	3.5–5.0 g/dL
Ammonia	119 µg/dL	10–80 µg/dL

1. **Based on assessment findings what diagnosis might you expect?**
   - *The clinical manifestations of changes in mental status, altered sleep pattern, elevated serum ammonia, abdominal distention (ascites), and fatty liver infiltrates are consistent with hepatic encephalopathy.*

2. **What nursing interventions would you include in this patient's plan of care?**
   - *Fall precautions*
   - *Seizure precautions*
   - *Daily weights*
   - *Strict intake and output*
   - *Neurologic assessment every 4 hours*
   - *Prepare the patient for a possible paracentesis*

3. **The patient is diagnosed with ascites and portal hypertension. What education would you provide to the patient and family? What complications may arise from portal hypertension? How do you assess for ascites?**
   - *Ascites refers to the accumulation of fluid in the peritoneal cavity. This occurs because of obstructed blood flow in the liver. In addition, low albumin may contribute to low oncotic pressure and third spacing of fluid.*
   - *Portal hypertension is an abnormally high blood pressure in the large vein that brings blood from the intestine to the liver.*
   - *Ascites and varices are consequences of portal hypertension.*
   - *Since the liver is unable to break down hormones such as aldosterone, which may contribute to ascites, an aldosterone-blocker such as spironolactone may be ordered.*
   - *Lasix may be part of the treatment of ascites.*
   - *Assessment findings of ascites includes:*
     - *Increased abdominal girth and weight*
     - *Dull percussion over fluid*
     - *Presence of a fluid wave*
     - *Abdominal striae and distended veins*

4. **What medication would you anticipate the provider ordering to help lower the ammonia level? Why would this medication be administered? What adverse effects might this patient experience?**

   ▶ *Lactulose is a laxative that helps to lower ammonia levels. The expected and desired effect would be multiple stools per day.*

   ▶ *It is critical to avoid an elevated ammonia level, as this can cause confusion, restlessness, loss of consciousness, seizures, and possible coma.*

   ▶ *Adverse effects of lactulose include:*
   - *Diarrhea*
   - *Intestinal bloating*
   - *Cramps*
   - *Hypokalemia*
   - *Dehydration*

5. **Why might the provider order a gastroscopy for this patient?**

   ▶ *The patient has a history of esophageal varices, a complication associated with cirrhosis. Since the patient is anemic, and his blood pressure has been elevated, there may be some varices that are bleeding that need to be cauterized or banded. The patient may be evaluated for a TIPS procedure, and the liver transplantation team may be asked to evaluate him to determine whether he is a candidate for liver transplantation. In addition, part of the workup may include a CT scan to rule out hepatocellular cancer, which can occur secondary to chronic hepatitis C.*

Discussion

Caring for patient with cirrhosis can be challenging, as for the development of clinical manifestations and complications such as spider angiomas, esophageal varices, gynecomastia, splenomegaly, abdominal ascites, mental confusion, skin hemorrhages, and edema is not uncommon. Hepatic encephalopathy is a life-threatening complication of liver failure caused by the liver being unable to metabolize ammonia; this causes the serum ammonia level to rise to toxic levels. It will be important to teach patients with cirrhosis to abstain from alcohol and to watch for signs and symptoms of problems that need to be reported to the provider. Teach the patient and family to notify the provider if they experience changes in mental status, signs of bleeding (bloody, black or tarry stools), and hematemesis.

Bibliography

Ankner, G.M. (2012). *Medical-Surgical Nursing,* (2nd ed. (Clifton Park, NY: Delmar).

Aschenbrenner, D.S., and Venable, S.J. (2012). *Drug Therapy in Nursing,* 4th ed. (Philadelphia: Wolters Kluwer).

Boynton, W., and Floch, M. (2013). New strategies for the management of diverticular disease: Insights for the clinician. *Therapeutic Advances in Gastroenterology* 6, 205–213.

Center for Disease Control and Prevention. (2015). Viral hepatitis. Accessed October 30, 2017, from https://www.cdc.gov/hepatitis/hcv/index.htm

Grossman, S., and Porth, C.M. (2013). *Pathophysiology: Concepts of Altered Health States.* 9th ed. (Philadelphia: Lippincott Williams & Wilkins).

Haq, I., & Tripathi, D. (2017). Recent advances in the management of variceal bleeding. *Gastroenterology Report* 5(2), 113–126.

Lee, W.M. (2012). Acute liver failure. *Seminars in Respiratory Critical Care Medicine* 33(1), 36-45.

Lewis, S.L., Bucher, L., Heitkemper, M., & Harding, M.M. (2017). *Medical-Surgical Nursing: Assessment and Management of Clinical Problems,* 10th ed. (St. Louis: Elsevier).

Moggia, E., Koti, R,, Belgaumkar, A.P., Fazio, F., Pereira, S.P., Davidson, B.R., and Gurusamy, K.S. (2017). Pharmacological interventions for acute pancreatitis. *Cochrane Database of Systematic Reviews* 4. DOI: 10.1002/14651858.CD011384.pub2.

National Guideline Clearinghouse (NGC). (2016). Guideline summary: cirrhosis in over 16s: assessment and management. In: National Guideline Clearinghouse (NGC) [website]. Rockville, MD: Agency for Healthcare Research and Quality (AHRQ). Accessed May 31, 2018, from https://www.guideline.gov

National Guideline Clearinghouse (NGC). (2015). Guideline summary: irritable bowel syndrome in adults: diagnosis and management of irritable bowel syndrome in primary care. In: National Guideline Clearinghouse (NGC) [website]. Rockville, MD: Agency for Healthcare Research and Quality (AHRQ). Accessed May 31, 2018, from https://www.guideline.gov

Ogden, C.L., Carroll, M.D., Fryar, C.D., and Flegal, K.M. (2015). Prevalence of obesity among adults and youth: United States, 2011-2014. NCHS data brief, no. 219. Hyattsville, MD: National Center for Health Statistics.

Pagana, K.D., Pagana, T.J., and Pagana, T.N. (2017). *Mosby's Diagnostic and Laboratory Test and Reference,* 13th ed. (St. Louis: Elsevier).

Potter, P.A., Perry, A.G., Stockert, P.A., & Hall, A.M. (2016). *Fundamentals of Nursing,* 9th ed. (St. Louis: Elsevier).

Rezapour, M., Ali, S., and Stollman, N. (2017). Diverticular disease: An update on pathogenesis and management. *Gut Liver.* Available at https://www.ncbi.nlm.nih.gov/pmc/articles/PMC5832336/

8

Respiratory System

Donna Martin, DNP, RN, CMSRN, CDE, CNE

OVERVIEW

The primary function of the respiratory system is to exchange oxygen and carbon dioxide to maintain these levels within a narrow therapeutic range. This occurs through the normal respiratory process, with inhalation to supply the body tissues with oxygen and exhalation to eliminate waste products (carbon dioxide) from the body. The exchange of oxygen (O_2) and carbon dioxide (CO_2) occurs at the aveolar and capillary levels.

▶ O_2 levels are measured as the arterial partial pressure of oxygen (PaO_2) by arterial blood gases and as oxygen saturation (SaO_2) by pulse oximetry. A PaO_2 level of 80 to 100 mm Hg and an SaO_2 reading of 90% or greater is considered normal.

▶ Carbon dioxide levels can be measured as serum carbon dioxide and as arterial partial pressure of carbon dioxide ($PaCO_2$) by arterial blood gases. The normal serum carbon dioxide is 23 to 30 mEq/L, and the normal $PaCO_2$ is 35 to 45 mm Hg.

ANATOMY

▶ The respiratory system is comprised of the:
- Upper airway:
  - Nose:
    - Warms, humidifies, and filters inhaled air
  - Sinuses:
    - Assist with warming and humidifying inhaled air
  - Pharynx:
    - Provides a passage for airflow to the lungs
  - Epiglottis:
    - Small flap behind the tongue that closes to protect the airway during swallowing
    - Prevents solids, liquids, and secretions from entering the lungs
  - Larynx:
    - Houses the vocal cords for speech
  - Trachea:
    - Moves mucous and particles away from the lungs
    - Branches into the right and left branches
    - The point of bifurcation is the carina (sensitive to stimulation, which causes coughing)

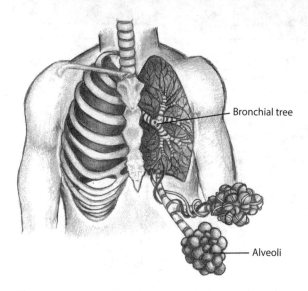

Bronchial tree

Alveoli

Figure 8.1 Lower Respiratory System

- Lower airway: (Figure 8.1)
  - Bronchi:
    - Only part of lower airway located outside the lungs
    - Lined with cilia, which move mucus from lower airway
    - Right bronchus shorter and straighter, making aspiration more likely
  - Bronchioles:
    - Constrict and dilate in response to stimuli
  - Alveoli:
    - Over 300 million small sacs in the adult lungs
    - Primary site of O_2 and CO_2 exchange
    - Surfactant secreted to prevent alveoli collapse
- Pulmonary vascular system:
  - Pulmonary veins:
    - Carry oxygenated blood from lungs to systemic circulation
  - Pulmonary arteries:
    - Carry unoxygenated blood to lungs for CO_2 excretion and exchange for O_2
- Pleura:
  - Parietal pleural layer lines inside of thoracic cavity
  - Visceral pleural layer covers lung tissue
  - Intrapleural—space between layers; provides lubrication and facilitates expansion of the lungs
- Gerontologic considerations:
  - Age-related changes:
    - Chest-wall stiffening
    - Costal cartilage calcification
    - Decreased elastic recoil of lungs
    - Decreased chest-wall compliance
    - Decreased cilia function
    - Decreased ability to forcefully cough, causing retained mucus
    - Decreased ability to fight off infection
    - Increased use of accessory muscles
    - Increased residual volume

TABLE 8.1	BREATH SOUNDS				
	Location		Pitch	Volume	Respiratory cycle
Bronchial/tracheal	Trachea and larynx		High	Loud	Inspiratory < expiratory
Bronchovesicular	Between the scapulae, near sternum, first and second intercostal spaces		Moderate	Medium	Inspiratory = expiratory
Vesicular	Peripheral lung fields		Low	Soft	Inspiratory > expiratory
Adventitious (added sounds not normally heard on auscultation)	Can be noted in any lung fields	*Crackles*	Fine—high pitched, crackling, popping Coarse—low pitched, gurgling, bubbling	Fine—soft Course—loud	Inspiratory Inspiratory and expiratory
		Wheeze	May be high pitched or low pitched, musical	Soft to loud	Inspiratory and expiratory (more prominent)
		Pleural rub	Low pitched, superficial	Soft to loud	Inspiratory
		Stridor	High pitched crowing	Loud in upper airway	Inspiratory

TABLE 8.2	RESPIRATORY DEFENSE MECHANISMS
Mechanism	Action
Filtration of air	Prevents particles from entering the lungs.
Mucus clearance	Cilia propel mucus and particles up the respiratory system.
Cough reflex	Helps clear the airway with forceful, high-pressure airflow.
Bronchoconstriction	Bronchi constrict to prevent irritants from entering the lungs.
Alveolar macrophages	Debris deep in lungs are phagocytized and then moved to the bronchioles for removal.

PHYSIOLOGY OF RESPIRATION

▶ Oxygenation:
  • The process of O_2 transport in the blood
  • O_2 and CO_2 move across the alveolar–capillary membrane by diffusion
▶ Ventilation: (Table 8.1)
  • Inspiration:
    • Movement of air in the lungs during inhalation
    • Caused by intrathoracic pressure changes due to the contraction of the diaphragm and intercostal muscles
  • Expiration:
    • Movement of air out of the lungs during exhalation
    • Passive process due to the elastic recoil and the lung's tendency to return to its original size
▶ Compliance and resistance
  • Compliance—ability of the lungs to inflate because of their elasticity
  • Resistance—due to airways impeding normal breathing process
▶ Respiratory defense mechanisms (Table 8.2)

Question	Rationale
When teaching a patient about the most important respiratory defense mechanism distal to the bronchioles, which topic would the nurse include? A. Alveolar macrophages B. Reflex bronchoconstriction C. Filtration of air D. Cough reflex	Answer: A The alveolar macrophages are distal to the bronchioles. While reflex bronchoconstriction occurs in the bronchioles, filtration of air occurs in the upper airway, and cough reflex is a defense mechanism of the large airways.

DIAGNOSTIC TESTS

▶ Radiology:
  • Chest x-ray:
    • For screening and evaluating changes
  • Computed tomography (CT) scan:
    • Used to diagnose suspicious lesions
    • Spiral CT to diagnose pulmonary embolism
  • Magnetic resonance imaging (MRI):
    • Allows for more in-depth diagnosis of lesions
  • Ventilation–perfusion (VQ) scan:
    • Assesses ventilation and perfusion of lungs
    • May be used in determination of pulmonary embolism
▶ Pulmonary angiography
  • Invasive procedure allowing for visualization of the pulmonary circulation through the use of contrast media
▶ Pulmonary-function tests (PFTs)
  • Uses spirometry to evaluate lung function
▶ Tuberculosis bacilli (TB) skin test
  • Determine if patient has been exposed to TB
▶ Bronchoscopy:
  • Invasive procedure requiring patient sedation
  • Flexible scope for diagnosis, biopsy, lavage, and removal of foreign objects from the respiratory system
▶ Thoracentesis:
  • Invasive procedure
  • Removal of pleural fluid for treatment and diagnosis
  • Monitor after procedure for pneumothorax
▶ Laboratory:
  • Hemoglobin:
    • Reflects the amount of hemoglobin available to transport O_2

Clinical Consideration

Positive TB skin test does *not* indicate that the patient has active TB, further testing must be done.

TABLE 8.3	ARTERIAL BLOOD GAS VALUES
ABG Components	Normal Value
pH	7.35–7.45
$PaCO_2$	35–45
HCO_3	21–28
PaO_2	>80

- Arterial blood gases (ABGs) (Table 8.3)
  - Steps to interpret ABGs:
    - First determine the pH value:
      - >7.45 indicates alkalosis
      - <7.35 indicates acidosis
    - Then evaluate $paCO_2$:
      - If >45 and pH <7.35—respiratory acidosis
      - If <35 and pH >7.45—respiratory alkalosis
    - Next evaluate HCO_3:
      - If >28 and pH >7.45—metabolic alkalosis
      - If <21 and pH <7.35—metabolic acidosis
    - Determine whether compensation is present; this occurs when the body's unaffected system (lungs or kidneys) acts to restore the acid–base ratio and normalize the pH:
      - No compensation: The unaffected system has not begun to restore the acid-base ratio and normalize the pH.
      - Partial compensation: The unaffected system is attempting to correct the acid–base ratio and normalize the pH but has not corrected them.
      - Full compensation: The pH has normalized through the compensation of the unaffected system.
    - Assess for hypoxemia:
      - PaO_2 <80 indicates hypoxemia
- Sputum specimens:
  - Culture and sensitivity—for diagnosis and treatment of infection
  - Gram stain—classify bacteria as gram-positive or gram-negative
  - Acid-fast bacteria (AFB) culture—used to diagnosis TB
  - Cytology—to determine presence of abnormal cells and malignancy
- Lung biopsy:
  - May be obtained by bronchoscopy, transthoracic needle aspiration (with CT guidance), or open lung biopsy during surgery
  - Allows for lung cells/tissue to be analyzed under microscopic conditions

> **Clinical Consideration**
>
> Compensation is a temporary fix and is not considered correction; correction occurs only with resolution of the underlying disorder.

NURSING DIAGNOSIS

Various nursing diagnoses are appropriate for patient experiencing respiratory disorders. Some examples include:

▸ Ineffective airway clearance related to excessive secretions, inflammation, tracheobronchial narrowing

▸ Impaired gas exchange related to decreased alveolar-capillary surface or VQ inequality

▶ Ineffective breathing pattern related to anxiety, loss of functional lung tissue, pain

▶ Activity intolerance related to imbalance between oxygen supply and demand

▶ Deficient knowledge related to medication and treatment. (Table 8.4)

TABLE 8.4 RESPIRATORY MEDICATIONS	
Medication	Action

Anticholinergics
  Ipratropium, inhaled (Atrovent)
  Tiotropium, inhaled (Spiriva)
	Dilate the airways of the trachea, bronchi, and alveoli, making respiration and gas exchange easier.

Antihistamines
  Loratadine (Claritin)
  Cetirizine (Zyrtec)
  Fexofenadine (Allegra)
  Desloratadine (Clarinex)
  Levocetirizine (Xyzal)
  Pseudoephedrine
	Block histamine; relieve allergic response of itching, sneezing, and runny nose.

Antitussives
  Codeine
  Hydrocodone
  diphenhydramine hydrochloride (Benadryl)
	Help to suppress the cough reflex by acting on the cough center receptors in the medulla.

Bronchodilators
Beta adrenergic agonists*
Oral
  Albuterol (Proventil, Volmax)
  Terbutaline (Brethine)
Inhaler
  Albuterol (Proventil)
  Levalbuterol (Xopenex)
  Pirbuterol (Maxair Autohaler)
  Salmeterol (Serevent Diskus)
	Dilate the airways of the trachea, bronchi, and alveoli making it easier for respiration and gas exchange.

Methylxanthines Theophylline	Stimulates respirations, dilates coronary and pulmonary vessels, and relaxes smooth muscles.

Corticosteroids
Oral
  Prednisone
  Prednisolone
Nasal spray
  Budesonide (Rhinocort)
  Fluticasone (Flonase)
  Mometasone (Nasonex)
Inhaled
  Beclomethasone dipropionate (Qvar)
  Budesonide (Pulmicort)
  Flunisolide (AeroBid)
  Fluticasone propionate (Flovent)
  Triamcinolone (Azmacort)
	Antiinflammatory action used to reduce edema of the airways.

Decongestants Pseudoephedrine (Sudafed)	Stimulate adrenergic receptors; nasal congestion reduced because of vasoconstriction.
Expectorants Guaifenesin (Humibid, Robitussin)	Loosen bronchial secretions and stimulate for elimination by coughing.
Mucolytics Acetylcysteine (Mucomyst)	Thins secretions to make cough more productive.
* Use with caution in patients with hypertension, diabetes, or narrow-angle glaucoma.	

RESPIRATORY DISORDERS

▶ *Airway obstruction*

- May be partial or complete
- Acute form is a medical emergency and requires immediate intervention

- Can be caused by aspiration, inflammation, infection, trauma, abscesses, or stenosis
- **Assessment/Intervention/Education**
  - Detailed medical history:
    - Allergic reactions
    - Malignancies
    - Infection
    - Trauma
  - Clinical manifestations—vary depending on location of the obstruction:
    - Coughing
    - Choking
    - Wheezing
    - Stridor
    - Accessory muscle use
    - Suprasternal and intercostal retractions
  - Treatment:
    - Immediately restore a patent airway:
      - Abdominal thrusts
      - Cricothyroidotomy
      - Endotracheal tube (ET) intubation
    - Tracheostomy for long-term airway management:
      - Cuffed tube:
        - Cuff inflated to:
          - Keep tube in place
          - Prevent aspiration
      - Uncuffed tube:
        - Primarily used for long-term tracheostomy
        - Allows patient to talk and eat
      - Fenestrated tube:
        - Has an opening on the surface of the tube
        - Allows patient to speak
      - Nonfenestrated tube
    - Suctioning:
      - Assess need for suctioning every hour, at a minimum.
      - Use sterile technique.
      - Hyperoxygenate patient prior to beginning suctioning.
      - Gently insert suction catheter, **without suction.**
      - Advance catheter until patient coughs.
      - Continuous suction should be applied for a maximum of 10 to 15 seconds while withdrawing the catheter.
      - Wall suction is set between 80 and 120 mm Hg.
      - Wait a minimum of 30 seconds before suctioning patient again.
      - Hyperoxygenate patient for 30 seconds between each suctioning.
      - Repeat until airway is clear.
      - Suction oropharynx once airway suctioning is completed.
    - Promote high Fowler's position.
    - Provide supplemental oxygen as ordered.
    - Perform tracheostomy care per hospital protocol:
      - May be a shared responsibility with nursing and respiratory therapy.
      - Explain procedure to patient.

Clinical Consideration

In order to avoid injury, do not use suction routinely.

- Place patient in a semi-Fowler's position.
- Suction tracheostomy tube.
- Remove old dressing.
- Use sterile technique.
- Use sterile normal saline or H_2O.
- Unlock, remove, and clean inner cannula for a nondisposable tracheostomy.
- Remove and discard disposable inner cannula.
- Reinsert clean inner cannula or new inner cannula.
- Clean stoma area.
- Change tracheostomy straps/ties; use two people to prevent accidental tube removal.
- Use a precut dry 4 x 4 gauze dressing if there is drainage from stoma site noted.
  - Assess tracheostomy site a minimum of once a shift:
    - Monitor for complications:
      - Infection
      - Stoma drainage or bleeding
      - Air leak
      - Aspiration
      - Impaired cough
      - Tracheal necrosis
      - Tube displacement
- Patient teaching:
  - Explain the purpose of procedures:
    - Suctioning
    - Tracheostomy care
  - Instruct patient to notify provider of any shortness of breath, displacement of tube, or increase/change in secretions.

Asthma

- A *reversible* bronchospasm
- According to the Centers for Disease Control and Prevention (CDC; 2017), over 26.5 million Americans (both adults and children) suffer from this respiratory disease. *Asthma* is defined as a chronic inflammation of the airways and is characterized by episodes of wheezing, coughing, chest tightness, and breathlessness. (Figure 8.2) Recurrent episodes occur because of changes in the respiratory system from bronchoconstriction, airway edema, airway hyperresponsiveness, and airway remodeling.
- A stepwise approach to treatment is dependent on the severity and control:
  - Severity—Take into account the current impact it has on daily activities and the risk for future exacerbations. Classifications include: (Table 8.5)
    - Intermittent
    - Persistent mild
    - Persistent moderate
    - Persistent severe
  - Classifications of control include: (Table 8.6)
    - Well controlled
    - Not well controlled
    - Very poorly controlled

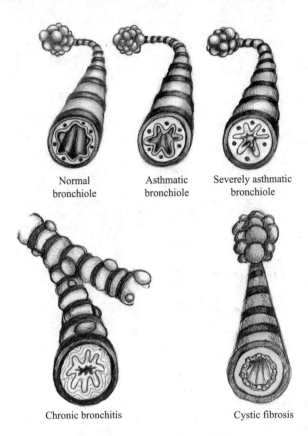

Normal
bronchiole

Asthmatic
bronchiole

Severely asthmatic
bronchiole

Chronic bronchitis

Cystic fibrosis

Figure 8.2 Disease impact on bronchioles

TABLE 8.5	ASTHMA SEVERITY CLASSIFICATIONS			
	Intermittent	Persistent Mild	Persistent Moderate	Persistent Severe
Impairment				
Frequency of symptoms	≤2 days a week	> 2 days a week, not daily	Daily	Much of the day
Effect on nighttime awakening	≤2 times a month	3–4 times a month	More than once a week	Nightly
Use of short-acting beta-agonist for control	≤2 days a week	>2 days a week, not more than once a day	Daily	Several times a day
Impact on daily activities	No limitation	Minor limitation	Some limitation	Extreme limitation
Lung function	Normal FEV_1 between exacerbations FEV_1 80% of predicted FEV_1/FVC normal	FEV_1 80% of predicted FEV_1/FVC normal	FEV_1 >60% but <80% of predicted FEV_1/FVC reduced by 5%	FEV_1 <60% of predicted FEV_1/FVC reduced > 5%
Risk				
Exacerbations requiring the use of steroids	0–1 times a year	≥2 times a year*	≥2 times a year*	≥2 times a year*

*Frequency and severity of exacerbations should be taken into consideration.
FEV_1 = forced expiratory volume in 1 second; FVC = forced vital capacity.
Adapted from the National Heart, Lung, and Blood Institute National Asthma Education and Prevention Program. Expert Panel Report 3: Guidelines for the diagnosis and management of asthma. Accessed June 3, 2018, from https://www.nhlbi.nih.gov/files/docs/guidelines/asthgdln.pdf

TABLE 8.6   ASTHMA CONTROL

	Well Controlled	Not Well Controlled	Very Poorly Controlled
Impairment			
Frequency of symptoms	<2 days a week	>2 days a week	Throughout day
Effect on night time awakening	<2 times a month	1–3 times a week	>4 times a week
Use of short-acting beta-agonist for control	<2 days a week	>2 days a week	Several times a day
Impact on daily activities	No limitation	Some limitation	Extreme limitation
Lung function: FEV_1	80% of predicted	60–80% of predicted	<60% of predicted
Peak flow	80% of personal best	60–80% of personal best	<60% of personal best
Risk			
Exacerbations requiring the use of steroids	0–1 times a year	>2 times a year*	>2 times a year*

Frequency and severity of exacerbations should be taken into consideration.
Adapted from the National Heart, Lung, and Blood Institute National Asthma Education and Prevention Program. Expert Panel Report 3: Guidelines for the diagnosis and management of asthma. Accessed June 3, 2018, from https://www.nhlbi.nih.gov/files/docs/guidelines/asthgdln.pdf

- ***Assessment/Intervention/Education***
  - Detailed medical history:
    - Recurrent respiratory infections
    - Frequency of symptoms/episodes:
      - Cough
      - Wheeze
      - Difficulty breathing
      - Chest tightness
    - Triggers:
      - Exercise/activity
      - Changes in weather:
        - Cold air
        - Dry air
      - Allergens:
        - Animals
        - Cockroach droppings
        - Dust
        - Mold
        - Pollen
        - Food
      - Illness:
        - Upper respiratory infections
        - Sinusitis/rhinitis
        - Nasal polyps
      - Air pollutants:
        - Smoke
        - Exhaust fumes
        - Perfumes
        - Aerosol sprays

- Drugs:
  - Aspirin
  - Nonsteroidal antiinflammatory drugs (NSAIDs)
  - Beta-blockers
- Other:
  - Reflux/gastroesophageal reflux disease (GERD)
  - Emotions
- Clinical manifestations:
  - Dyspnea
  - Tachypnea
  - Wheezing—most notably on expiration:
    - Note: a "silent chest," with no breath sounds on auscultation, may be an ominous sign of decreased air movement in and out of the lungs. Hearing some wheezes may indicate that air is actually getting in/out of lungs.
  - Accessory-muscle use/intercostal retractions
    - Pursed lip breathing
    - Nasal flaring
    - Difficulty speaking
    - Coughing/ineffective cough
    - Decreased pulse oximetry
    - Cyanosis
    - Peak flow/incentive spirometer:
      - Decreased expiratory peak flow
- Diagnosis (refer to Tables 8.2 and 8.3)
- Treatment:
  - Metered-dose inhaler (MDI)
  - Medications (Table 8.5)
    - Rescue/quick relief
      - Bronchodilators
      - Anticholinergics
    - Long-acting
    - Corticosteroids:
      - Inhaled
      - Oral
  - Nebulizer
  - High Fowler's position
  - Supplemental oxygen
  - Eliminate exposure to triggers
- Patient teaching:
  - Have an asthma action plan
  - Peak flow assessment daily
  - Smoking cessation
  - Prevention:
    - Avoid triggers
    - Reduce stress, teach coping mechanisms
  - Medications:
    - Correct use of metered dose inhaler (MDI)—assess correct use at each interaction
    - Long-term control medications
    - Rescue medications

Question	Rationale
The provider prescribes albuterol sulfate (Proventil) for a patient with newly diagnosed asthma. When teaching the patient about this drug, the nurse should explain that it may cause: A. Nasal congestion B. Nervousness C. Lethargy D. Hypotension	Answer: B Albuterol may cause nervousness. The inhaled form of the drug may cause dryness and irritation of the nose and throat, insomnia, and hypertension. Other adverse effects of albuterol include tremor, dizziness, tachycardia, palpitations, and muscle cramps. Nasal congestion, lethargy, and hypotension are not noted to be secondary symptoms with this drug.

▶ *COPD*

- Chronic obstructive pulmonary disease (COPD) is a progressive disease that affects more than 16 million adults and is the third leading cause of death in the United States (NIH, 2017).
- In the past the term *COPD* included both emphysema and chronic bronchitis, with many patients having both of these conditions.
  - Emphysema involves loss of elasticity or damage to the alveoli, causing the alveoli to become enlarged and decreasing the amount of gas exchange that can occur.
  - In bronchitis, the linings of the airway are irritated, inflamed, and swollen, contributing to an increased production of mucus, which blocks the airway.
- The Global Initiative for Chronic Obstructive Lung Disease (GOLD) defines COPD as "a common, preventable and treatable disease that is characterized by persistent respiratory symptoms and airflow limitation that is due to airway and/or alveolar abnormalities" (GOLD, 2017). The airflow limitation is caused by small-airway disease and parenchymal destruction. Chronic inflammation causes structural changes in the lung and ultimately contributes to the alveolar abnormalities (Table 8.7).
- *Assessment/Intervention/Education*
  - Detailed medical history:
    - Long-term exposure to lung irritants
    - History of smoking
    - Symptoms:
      - Ongoing cough with or without mucus
      - Shortness of breath, especially with activity
      - Chest tightness

Clinical Consideration

The terms *chronic bronchitis* and *emphysema* are not used in the GOLD definition of COPD.

Clinical Consideration

Primary risk factors are smoking and exposure to secondhand smoke.

TABLE 8.7	GOLD COPD CLASSIFICATIONS
Mild	$FEV_1 \geq 80\%$ of predicted
Moderate	$50\% \leq FEV_1 < 80\%$ of predicted
Severe	$30\% \leq FEV_1 < 50\%$ of predicted
Very severe	$FEV_1 < 30\%$ of predicted

- Common triggers of exacerbations:
  - Illness:
    - Colds
    - Respiratory infections
  - Exposure to lung irritants:
    - Smoking
    - Air pollution
    - Temperature extremes:
      - Heat
      - Cold
- Clinical manifestations:
  - Barrel chest due to increased anterior–posterior diameter
  - Dyspnea
  - Tachypnea
  - Wheezing
  - Difficulty speaking
  - Ineffective cough
  - Pulse oximetry
  - Finger clubbing
  - Decreased peak flow/incentive spirometer
- Diagnosis:
  - Pulmonary-function test (FEV_1/FVC <70% of predicted)
  - Bronchoscopy
- Treatment:
  - Symptom management:
    - Oxygen:
      - Avoid high concentrations of O_2, which can cause an increased mismatch between ventilation and perfusion within the lung:
        - Decreased respirations
        - Increased buildup of CO_2
        - Decreased responsiveness
        - Breathing ceases
    - Pursed lip breathing:
      - To promote positive end-expiratory pressure, which distends the aveoli and creates a greater surface for O_2 and CO_2 exchange
    - Anxiety can make dyspnea worse—vicious cycle
    - Depression:
      - Consider antidepressants
    - Lung transplantation:
      - Single-lung
      - Bilateral lung
    - Hospice for end-stage COPD
  - Slow progression of disease process:
    - Smoking cessation
    - Avoid lung irritants
  - Improve activity/exercise tolerance:
    - Pulmonary rehabilitation

Clinical Consideration
There is no cure for COPD; the goal is symptom management.

Clinical Consideration
Administer O_2 with caution in patients with COPD.

> **Clinical Consideration**
>
> Two separate pneumococcal vaccines are recommended (PCV13 pneumococcal conjugate and PPSV23 pneumococcal polysaccharide vaccine).

> **Clinical Consideration**
>
> There is a significant increase of oral candidiasis in patients taking ICS; teach patient to rinse mouth after inhalation and notify provider of any changes in oral cavity.

- Preventing complications:
    - Immunizations:
        - Pneumonia vaccines
        - Influenza vaccine yearly
    - Eliminate exposure to illness.
    - Avoid respiratory stressors.
- Medications:
    - Bronchodilators
    - Antimuscarinics
    - Antiinflammatory agents
    - Inhaled corticosteroids (ICS)
- Decrease exposure to illness:
    - Avoid crowds.
    - Avoid others who are sick.
- Patient teaching:
    - Smoking cessation
    - Oxygen safety
    - Pursed lip breathing
    - Balance activity and rest
    - Notify provider of worsening symptoms,
    - Take medications as prescribed,
    - Review inhaler technique at each visit,
    - Rinse out mouth after using ICS.

Question	Rationale
Which nursing action would best promote adequate gas exchange for a patient with advanced COPD? A. Encouraging the patient to drink three glasses of fluid a day B. Keeping the patient in semi-Fowler's position C. Obtaining an order for a sedative D. Administering oxygen using a high-flow Venturi mask	Answer: D To promote adequate gas exchange, the nurse should use a Venturi mask to deliver a specified, controlled amount of oxygen consistently and accurately. Drinking three glasses of fluid daily would not be sufficient to liquefy secretions. Patients with COPD should be placed in high Fowler's position and should not receive sedatives that may further depress the respiratory center.

▶ *Pneumonia*
- Infection of the lungs that may be viral, bacterial, or fungal; typically more serious in patients who:
    - Are over the age of 65
    - Have chronic conditions such as heart failure and COPD
    - Have immune system compromise due to conditions such as HIV or receiving chemotherapy
    - Have undergone organ transplantation
- Types of pneumonia
    - Community-acquired pneumonia (CAP)—most common form
        - *Streptococcus pneumoniae*—most common organism

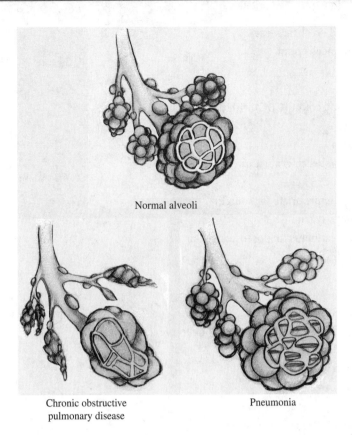

Figure 8.3 Disease effect on alveoli

- Hospital–acquired pneumonia (HAP)—develops during hospitalization, usually more serious since the person is already ill
  - Most common organisms—*Pseudomonas aeruginosa, Escherichia coli, Klebsiella pneumoniae*
- Ventilator-associated pneumonia (VAP)
- Aspiration pneumonia—due to aspiration of gastric contents, vomit, or saliva into the respiratory tract
- ***Assessment/Intervention/Education***
  - Detailed medical history:
    - Recent illness (cold, upper respiratory infection)
    - Pneumonia vaccine status
    - Swallowing problems/aspiration
    - GERD
    - Symptoms:
      - High fever
      - Shaking/chills
      - A cough, with or without mucus, that doesn't improve or worsens
      - Shortness of breath with normal daily activities
      - Chest pain with breathing or coughing
      - Feeling worse after a recent illness (cold, flu)
  - Clinical manifestations:
    - Dyspnea
    - Ineffective cough
    - Oxygen saturation decreased
    - Fine or coarse crackles on auscultation

Clinical Consideration

Older adults may be afebrile and present with atypical symptoms, such as changes in mental status.

- Infiltrate noted on chest x-ray
- Elevated white-cell count
- Diagnosis:
  - Chest x-ray
  - Complete blood count (CBC) with differential
  - Sputum culture
  - Blood cultures
  - Swallow study/speech evaluation
- Treatment:
  - Antibiotics (if appropriate for source)
  - Supplemental oxygen
  - Respiratory treatments to loosen secretions
  - Adequate hydration
- Patient teaching:
  - Prevention:
    - Receive pneumonia vaccines
    - Elevate head of bed and turn to left side to prevent aspiration
  - Adequate fluid intake
  - Complete course of antibiotics
  - Frequent oral care

▶ *Atelectasis*

- Partial or complete collapse of the aveoli.
  - Risk factors:
    - Lung disease:
      - Infection
      - Airway obstruction
      - COPD
    - General anesthesia (24 to 48 hours postoperatively)
    - Pain
    - Opioid use
    - Smoking
- *Assessment/Intervention/Education*
  - Detailed medical history:
    - Recent surgery with general anesthesia
    - History of smoking
    - History of lung disease
    - Symptoms:
      - Increased sputum production
      - Dyspnea
  - Physical assessment:
    - Diminished lung sounds
    - Inspiratory crackles
    - Low-grade fever
    - Decreased pulse oximetry
  - Diagnosis:
    - Chest x-ray
    - Basilar crackles on auscultation

- Treatment:
  - Oxygen to maintain oxygen saturation ≥90%
  - Head of bed elevated
  - Encourage patient to do coughing and deep breathing exercises
  - Incentive spirometry—use every hour
  - Encourage fluids/adequate hydration
  - Address pain, if needed, so patient will take deep breaths
  - Antibiotics (if appropriate)
- Patient teaching:
  - Prevention of alveoli collapse postoperatively or when immobile
    - Early ambulation
    - Correct use of incentive spirometer
    - How to perform coughing and deep breathing exercises
  - Notify provider of worsening symptoms

▶ *Acute Respiratory Distress Syndrome (ARDS)*

- A sudden and acute form of respiratory failure that causes significant lung injury and tissue damage, including fluid accumulation and decreased lung compliance. Referred to as noncardiogenic or increased permeability pulmonary edema. The 50% mortality rate is due to tendency toward multisystem organ failure. This is the pulmonary manifestation of a systemic disorder that triggers an uncontrolled inflammatory response. A majority of patients with ARDS require critical care because of the severity of illness and need for mechanical ventilation.
- *Assessment/Intervention/Education*
  - Detailed medical history:
    - History of aspiration, pneumonia, sepsis, injury to the lungs, surgery, fractures, transfusion therapy, or trauma
    - Use of drugs that can cause ARDS:
      - Heroin
      - Aspirin
  - Clinical manifestations:
    - Presentation of symptoms may be subtle
    - Early signs:
      - Tachypnea
      - Dyspnea
      - Cough
      - Restlessness
      - Hypoxemia
      - Fine scattered crackles on auscultation
    - Late signs:
      - Tachycardia
      - Diaphoresis
      - Mental status changes
      - Cyanosis
      - Coarse and diffuse crackles on auscultation
  - Diagnosis:
    - Hypoxemia despite increased O_2 administration
    - Profound respiratory distress
    - Chest x-ray with extensive consolidation and infiltrates

- Treatment:
  - Oxygen administration
  - Respiratory support:
    - Mechanical ventilation with positive end-expiratory pressure (PEEP)
    - Prone and lateral positioning
    - Chest physiotherapy (CPT)
  - Maintain cardiac output and tissue perfusion to prevent multisystem organ failure.
  - Maintain nutrition and fluid balance.
  - Meticulous supportive care and avoidance of secondary infections
  - Medications:
    - Bronchodilators:
      - Increase alveolar ventilation
    - Diuretics:
      - Reduce pulmonary congestion
    - Antibiotics:
      - Treat pulmonary infections
    - Sedation and analgesia:
      - Reduce O_2 consumption
- Patient teaching:
  - Treatment plan
  - Importance of increasing activity as tolerated
  - Prevention of complications of immobility

Question	Rationale
When assessing a patient for early signs or symptoms of inadequate oxygenation, the nurse would anticipate that the patient would present with: A. Dyspnea and hypotension B. Apprehension and restlessness C. Cyanosis and cool, clammy skin D. Increased urine output and diaphoresis	Answer: B Apprehension and restlessness are early signs and symptoms of inadequate oxygenation. Increased urine output does not indicate oxygenation status. The other symptoms are indicative of late signs of decreased oxygenation.

▶ *Cystic Fibrosis*

- An autosomal recessive disorder that is characterized as a defect in the transport of sodium and chloride in and out of the epithelial cells. This defect primarily affects the lungs, as well as the gastrointestinal tract and reproductive system. It is most well known for the progressive effect it has on the airways—starting with the small airways, migrating to the large airways, and finally resulting in lung tissue destruction. It causes production of abnormally thick mucous secretions and dysfunction of the exocrine glands.

- *Assessment/Intervention/Education*
  - Detailed medical history:
    - Recurrent lung infections; bronchitis, pneumonia
    - History of pancreatic insufficiency and/or diabetes
    - Biliary disorders
    - Malnutrition and weight loss
  - Clinical manifestations:
    - Thick, sticky mucous
    - Frequent cough
    - Increased yellow/green sputum
    - More frequent exacerbations
    - Worsening bronchiectasis
    - May lead to respiratory failure
  - Diagnosis:
    - Often diagnosed during first year of life
    - Clinical presentation
    - Family history
    - Genetic testing
    - Laboratory testing—sweat chloride test, gastrointestinal (GI) enzyme evaluation
  - Treatment:
    - Treat symptoms as they occur:
      - Relief of bronchoconstriction and airway obstruction
    - Aggressive CPT
    - Bronchodilators
    - Mucolytics
    - Nutritional support, including pancreatic-enzyme replacement
    - Influenza/pneumococcal vaccines
    - Antibiotics
    - Corticosteroids
    - Supplemental oxygen
    - Lung transplantation
    - Patient and family support from interdisciplinary team—physicians, nurses, respiratory therapists, physical therapists, social service workers, and dietitians
  - Patient teaching:
    - Notify provider immediately of worsening symptoms
    - Reduction of exacerbations:
      - CPT with postural drainage, percussion, and vibration
      - Regular (daily) clearance of mucus
        - Positive end-expiratory pressure (PEEP) devices (Acapella, Flutter)
        - Breathing exercises
        - Huff coughing
        - Pursed lip breathing
    - Referral to Cystic Fibrosis Foundation

Influenza

- Commonly referred to as "the flu," this is a highly contagious viral illness of the nose, mouth, and lungs. Influenza affects up to 20% of the U.S. population each year and can contribute significantly to death from flu-related complications (CDC, 2017).

- Strains of the influenza virus vary from year to year, making it challenging to forecast the vaccine composition.
- *Assessment/Intervention/Education*
  - Detailed medical history:
    - Chronic medical conditions
    - Yearly flu vaccine?
  - Clinical manifestations:
    - Comes on suddenly
    - Fever, chills
    - Cough
    - Fatigue
    - Body aches
    - Headache
  - Diagnosis:
    - Symptoms and clinical judgment
    - Rapid influenza tests
  - Treatment:
    - Rest
    - Antiviral medications within 24 to 48 hours of onset
    - Hydration
    - Acetaminophen/NSAIDs
    - Droplet precautions implemented for patients with suspected or confirmed influenza for 7 days after illness onset or until 24 hours after the resolution of fever and respiratory symptoms, whichever is longer, while a patient is in a health care facility (CDC, 2017).
  - Patient teaching:
    - Prevention:
      - Receive the yearly influenza vaccine:
        - Exclusions include patients with:
          - Egg allergy
          - History of Guillain–Barré syndrome
      - Take measures to reduce spread:
        - Proper and frequent handwashing.
        - Cover mouth when coughing or sneezing.
        - Avoid close contact with others who are ill.
        - Clean and disinfect potentially contaminated surfaces and objects.
    - Notify provider if influenza is suspected:
      - Take antiviral drugs (if prescribed)
    - Notify provider of worsening symptoms

> **Clinical Consideration**
> The rapid influenza test results may vary and may produce false negative results in adults.

Pleural Effusion

- Accumulation of fluid in the pleural space, secondary to other disease processes. Effusions are characterized by their etiology. An empyema is purulent fluid in the plural space, typically caused by pneumonia, TB, or other lung infections.
- *Assessment/Intervention/Education*
  - Detailed medical history:
    - Assess for chronic conditions
      - Congestive heart failure (CHF)
      - Chronic kidney disease
      - Cirrhosis
      - Cancer/malignancy

- Recent conditions may include:
  - Pneumonia
  - TB
  - Infection/surgical wounds of the chest
- Clinical manifestations:
  - Fever
  - Dyspnea
  - Chest pain that is worse on inspiration
  - Decreased chest movement on affected side
  - Diminished breath sounds on auscultation
  - Empyema may also cause:
    - Fever
    - Cough
    - Weight loss
    - Elevated white cell counts
- Diagnosis:
  - Chest x-ray
  - CT scan
- Treatment:
  - Identify and treat underlying cause.
  - Small effusions may not require drainage.
  - Thoracentesis:
    - Chest x-ray postprocedure to assess for pneumothorax
    - Monitor for signs and symptoms of respiratory distress
  - Antibiotics for empyema
  - Diuretics if related to heart failure/cirrhosis
- Patient teaching:
  - Prevention:
    - Take medications as ordered for chronic diseases.
  - Notify provider of recurrent symptoms.

▶ ***Pulmonary Embolism (PE)***

- A blockage of the pulmonary artery, most often caused by a deep vein thrombosis (DVT). Other sources of emboli include fat, air, bone marrow, or tumor tissue. The embolism travels through the circulatory system until it becomes lodged in a smaller blood vessel in the pulmonary vasculature.
- The term *venous thromboembolism* (VTE) can be used to describe both PE and DVT.
- ***Assessment/Intervention/Education***
  - Detailed medical history:
    - Chronic medical conditions
    - History of clotting disorders, VTE
    - Recent long-bone fracture
    - Risk factors:
      - History of any VTE
      - Obesity
      - Recent surgery
      - Periods of immobility
      - Smoking
      - Birth control pills/hormone-replacement therapy (HRT)
      - Pregnancy
      - Trauma

- Clinical manifestations:
  - Small emboli may go undetected, or patient may report vague symptoms
  - Symptoms may be sudden in onset
  - Dyspnea
  - Tachypnea
  - Hypoxemia
  - Chest pain, especially on inspiration
  - Cough
  - Crackles or wheezing on auscultation
  - Hemoptysis
  - Tachycardia
  - Hypotension
  - Fever
  - Syncope
  - Change in mental status
- Diagnosis:
  - Elevated d-dimer
  - Positive VQ scan
  - Positive spiral CT scan
  - Pulmonary angiography
- Treatment:
  - Bed rest
  - Oxygen
  - Anticoagulant therapy—see Chapter 9
    - Heparin infusion
    - Low-molecular-weight heparin (Lovenox)
    - Coumadin
  - Cardiac monitoring
  - Monitor labs:
    - Partial thromboplastin time (PTT)
    - Prothrombin time (PT)
    - International normalized ratio (INR)
- Prevention:
  - Early ambulation
  - Leg exercises
  - Sequential compression stockings
  - Anticoagulant prophylaxis
  - Inferior vena cava (IVC) filter for high-risk patients
- Patient teaching:
  - Prevention and VTE prophylaxis
  - Anticoagulant management and side effects

▶ *Obstructive Sleep Apnea (OSA)*

- Partial or complete upper-airway obstruction that occurs during sleep, resulting in a cessation of respiratory airflow for greater than 10 seconds. This obstruction can be due to the tongue and soft palate falling backward during sleep, causing an obstruction of the pharynx and/or the narrowing of the airway passages due to relaxation of the muscles during sleep.
- The cessation of breathing causes periods of arousal as the patient snorts or gasps to open the airway, resulting in frequent sleep disruptions.

- The long-term effects of untreated OSA include hypertension, cardiac dysrhythmias, atherosclerosis, and heart failure.
- *Assessment/Intervention/Education*
  - Detailed medical history:
    - Daytime sleepiness
    - Frequent awakening during sleep
    - Snoring
    - Risk factors:
      - body-mass index (BMI; weight in kilograms divided by the square of the height in meters) >30
      - >65 years of age
      - Neck circumference >17 inches
      - Abnormalities of the upper airway
      - Acromegaly (refer to Chapter 11)
      - Smoking
  - Clinical manifestations:
    - Frequent awakening/arousals during sleep
    - Insomnia
    - Daytime sleepiness
    - Witnessed episodes of apnea during sleep
    - Snoring
  - Diagnosis:
    - Positive OSA sleep screen indicates need for further follow-up.
    - Positive sleep study:
      - Periods of apnea lasting at least 10 seconds.
      - Five or more episodes of apnea per hour, with a 3 to 4% reduction in oxygen saturation.
      - *Severe apnea* is defined as more than 30 apnea events in an hour.
  - Treatment:
    - Weight loss; bariatric surgery may be an option
    - Wearing an oral appliance (mouth guard) at night to shift mandible and tongue forward, keeping the airway open
    - Continuous positive airway pressure (CPAP) mask
    - Bilevel positive airway pressure (BiPAP) mask
    - Surgical procedure, as a last option, if other treatments fail
  - Prevention:
    - Side sleeping
    - Avoid sedatives and alcohol prior to sleep
    - Maintain target BMI and weight
  - Patient teaching:
    - Proper use of equipment
    - Avoid driving when experiencing excessive daytime sleepiness
    - Importance of treatment to decrease risk of cardiovascular complications, impaired memory, and possible interpersonal and employment difficulties

> **Clinical Consideration**
> CPAP is the treatment of choice for patients with >15 apnea episodes per hour.

- **Pulmonary Edema**
  - Extravascular (third spacing) collection of fluid in the lung tissues, most often a complication of heart failure. Other causes include overhydration of IV fluids, nephrotic syndrome, altered capillary permeability of the lungs, O_2 toxicity, ARDS, and malignancies of the lymphatic system.
  - Refer to "Heart Failure" section in Chapter 9.

▶ *Cor Pulmonale*

- An enlarged right ventricle caused by a disorder of the respiratory system, with COPD being the most common cause. These patients typically present with pulmonary hypertension, with or without cardiac failure.
- Refer to "Heart Failure" section in Chapter 9.

▶ *Pneumothorax*

- Due to accumulation of air in the pleural space. The air changes the negative pressure between the visceral and parietal pleura, causing a collapse of the lung. The size and type of pneumothorax will determine the interventions and urgency of treatment.
- Types:
  - Spontaneous:
    - Occurs suddenly without injury, usually due to rupture of small air-filled sac defects (blebs) usually in healthy, young individuals or those with a history of lung disease
    - Risk factors:
      - Male gender
      - Tall, slender stature
      - Smoking
      - Previous history of spontaneous pneumothorax
      - Rapid decompression with scuba diving
      - COPD
      - Asthma
      - Cystic fibrosis
      - History of pneumonia
  - Iatrogenic pneumothorax:
    - A laceration or puncture of the lung occurs during a medical or surgical procedure.
  - Tension pneumothorax:
    - Occurs when air enters the pleural space and is trapped, causing compression on the affected side
    - Continued accumulation of air causes a mediastinal shift toward the unaffected side, as seen by a tracheal deviation
    - Can be caused by an open or closed pneumothorax
    - If the tension is not relieved, the respiratory and/or cardiovascular system will be ineffective, causing death
  - Hemothorax:
    - Accumulation of blood in the pleural space due to an injury to the chest, lung, or mediastinum
    - A traumatic hemothorax requires that a chest tube be inserted immediately to remove the blood.
- *Assessment/Intervention/Education*
  - Detailed medical history:
    - History of pneumothorax
    - Chest trauma; blunt or penetrating
    - Motor vehicle accident
    - Recent scuba diving
  - Clinical manifestations:
    - Shortness of breath
    - Dyspnea
    - Diminished or absent breath sounds on affected side

Clinical Consideration

Tension pneumothorax is *always* a medical emergency!

- Hyperresonance on percussion
- Flail chest
- Tracheal deviation
- Subcutaneous emphysema
- Diagnosis:
  - Chest x-ray
- Treatment:
  - Depends on type and severity of pneumothorax
  - Needle decompression in emergency situations
  - Chest-tube insertion (Table 8.8)
  - Oxygen
- Patient teaching:
  - Explain pneumothorax and treatment.
  - Importance of sitting up, coughing and deep breathing, and using incentive spirometer
  - Use of pain medications as needed
  - Notify provider of worsening symptoms

Question	Rationale
What clinical manifestation might a patient with a moderate-to-severe pneumothorax exhibit? A. Bradypnea B. Dyspnea C. Dull pain on the affected side D. Tracheal deviation	Answer: D A small pneumothorax can cause dyspnea, mild tachycardia, and mild tachypnea. A moderate-to-severe pneumothorax can cause respiratory distress, shallow rapid respirations, absent breath sounds over affected area, and tracheal deviation.

Pulmonary Tuberculosis (TB)

- Infectious disease caused by the *Mycobacterium tuberculosis* organism. It is usually in the lungs, but any organ can be infected. Transmission of the *Mycobacterium tuberculosis* bacilli occurs by inhalation of the microscopic airborne particles.
- Leading cause of death in patients with human immunodeficiency virus (HIV) infection.
- Latent TB infection occurs when a person has a positive TB skin test or a positive QuantiFERON-TB Gold test and is asymptomatic, with no signs of active disease. Active TB disease develops in less than 10% of individuals who are infected. Disease may be dormant for many years and be reactivated during periods of stress.
- There is an increasing number of multidrug-resistant strains of TB (MDR-TB).
- *Assessment/Intervention/Education*
  - Detailed medical history:
    - Chronic medical conditions:
      - HIV infection
      - Malignancy
      - Long-term corticosteroid use

TABLE 8.8	NURSING RESPONSIBILITIES FOR CHEST-TUBE CARE, MAINTENANCE, AND REMOVAL

Chest-tube insertion
Procedure may be done bedside
Gather supplies
    Antiseptic solution
    Pleural drainage system
    Occlusive dressing
Make sure consent was obtained
Position patient
Pain management
Postprocedure chest x-ray ordered
	Nursing interventions
	Explain procedure to patient/family
	Set up pleural drainage system with sterile water
	    Fill water seal chamber to 2-cm mark
	    Fill suction control chamber to 20-cm mark
	Patient positioning
	    Head of bed elevated 30–60 degrees
	    Position upright or side-lying
	    Arm raised above the head on affected side
	Assist provider with chest-tube insertion
	Assess patient for pain; administer pain medications as needed

Chest-tube maintenance
Assessment
    Patient status
    Pleural drainage system
Pain management
Patient activity
Documentation
	Nursing interventions
	Patient assessment
	    Assess respiratory status a minimum of every 4 hours
	    Monitor for subcutaneous emphysema at chest-tube site
	Pleural drainage system
	Tubing
	    Keep tubing below chest level.
	    Do not compress or occlude tubing.
	    Do not clamp drainage system tubing.
	    Do not milk or strip drainage system tubing.
	    Keep connections tight, and tape all connections.
	Water seal chamber
	    Keep the chamber filled to the fill line.
	    Observe for fluctuations and bubbling.
	Chest drainage chamber
	    Do not raise drainage container to the level of chest.
	    Secure the drainage system to prevent tipping.
	    Mark the drainage according to hospital policy.
	    Change the unit if the collection chamber is full.
	Suction control
	    Keep the suction control chamber at the ordered level.
	    Dial wall suction until continuous bubbling is seen.
	    Evaluate for a leak if there is no bubbling.
	Chest-tube dressings
	    Change per hospital protocol
	    Use an occlusive dressing
	    Maintain strict sterile asepsis
	Pain management
	    Administer pain medications as needed
	Activity
	    Encourage coughing, deep breathing, and use of incentive spirometer to assist with lung expansion.
	Document above interventions

Chest-tube removal Gather supplies Occlusive dressing Pain medication	**Nursing interventions** Explain procedure to patient/family Administer pain medications 30–60 minutes prior to chest-tube removal. Have patient perform Valsalva maneuver while tube is being removed. Immediately cover chest tube site with an airtight dressing.

- Risk factors:
  - Homeless
  - Foreign-born
  - Living or working in institutions such as:
    - Long-term–care facilities
    - Prisons
    - Shelters
    - Hospitals

- IV drug users
- Poor access to health care/lower socioeconomic group
- Close contact with someone who has active TB
- Clinical manifestations:
  - Latent TB infection—not contagious
    - No symptoms
  - Active TB infection—contagious
  - Symptoms of active TB typically develop 2 to 3 weeks after infection
    - Bad cough that lasts 3 weeks or longer
    - Pain in the chest
    - Coughing up blood or sputum
    - Weakness or fatigue
    - Weight loss
    - No appetite
    - Night sweats
    - Fever/chills
- Diagnosis:
  - Tuberculin skin test:
    - Mantoux purified protein derivative (PPD) administered intradermally
    - Read 48 to 72 hours after administration
    - Induration >10 mm indicates infection (*Note:* Interpretation of induration may be different in individuals who are immunocompromised.)
    - Does not confirm active disease
  - QuantiFERON-TB Gold test:
    - Blood test
    - Positive result indicates infection.
    - Does not confirm active disease
  - Chest x-ray may indicate active TB infiltrates.
  - AFB smear and culture
    - Most definitive diagnostic test for active TB infection
    - Three specimens collected on three different days
- Treatment:
  - Latent TB infection:
    - Isoniazid treatment recommended for 6 to 9 months
    - Monitor periodically to assess for active disease
  - Active TB infection:
    - Need to treat aggressively
    - Recommended treatment for 6 to 9 months
      - Isoniazid
      - Rifampin
      - Pyrazinamide
      - Ethambutol
    - It is critical that patients complete treatment to prevent development of MDR-TB.
    - Need for follow-up with possible contacts/family
  - Monitor vitamin B_9 level and administer supplements as needed.
  - Isolation for inpatient setting:
    - Airborne:
      - Staff must wear N95 or high-efficiency particulate air (HEPA) respirator
      - Negative pressure room

Clinical Consideration

A positive TB skin test and/or QuantiFERON-TB does not confirm active disease.

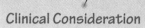

Clinical Consideration

Noncompliance with TB medication regimen significantly contributes to MDR-TB.

- Patient teaching:
    - Airborne isolation precautions during hospitalization
    - Importance of compliance with long-term medication treatment, taking medications *exactly* as prescribed
    - Adverse side effects of drugs (major side effect is nonviral hepatitis) and when to seek medical treatment
    - Need for follow up AFB smears, cultures, and chest x-rays
    - Cough and secretion hygiene
    - Use of masks and need for teaching with family and contacts

CASE STUDY

A 79-year-old woman was admitted directly from the primary care physician's office. Symptoms included increasing cough, shortness of breath, activity intolerance, and fatigue. Her medical history includes COPD, hypertension, hypercholesterolemia, a stable abdominal aortic aneurysm, and she reports increasing memory loss. She smoked for over 40 years, quitting approximately 15 years ago. She has not had an exacerbation of her COPD in over a year. Current medications include:

Atorvastatin (Lipitor) 40 mg daily

Hydrochlorothiazide 25 mg daily

Venlafaxine (Effexor) 37.5 mg daily

Vitamin D capsule daily

Tiotropium bromide (Spiriva HandiHaler) inhaler twice daily

Formoterol/mometasone (Dulera) inhaler twice daily

Ipratropium bromide (Atrovent) nasal spray twice daily

Temazepam (Restoril) capsule at bedtime

Docusate (Colace) 1 to 2 capsules daily

Ipratropium bromide (Atrovent) inhaler 2 puffs *as needed for shortness of breath*

Azithromycin (Zithromax) 250 mg daily for 5 days *for beginning COPD exacerbation*

Prednisone 40 mg oral for 5 days *for beginning COPD exacerbation*

She uses 3 L continuous O_2 at home and 3 L intermittent O_2 when out. Her activity has been decreased over the past 5 days. She contacted her provider and was instructed to begin her azithromycin and prednisone regimen. After 24 hours, she was not feeling any better, was seen by the provider in the office, and was subsequently admitted to the hospital. Upon admission to the acute care unit, her assessment reveals that the she is afebrile, blood pressure 98/66 mm Hg, heart rate 120 beats/min, respiratory rate 24 breaths /min, and O_2 saturation 86 to 90% while breathing room air. She also has a frequent nonproductive cough, and diminished breath sounds noted in the right lower lung field.

1. Based on assessment findings what diagnosis might you expect?

▶ *The patient is demonstrating symptoms of several possible respiratory disorders. It is apparent that the patient is experiencing an exacerbation of her COPD, although the trigger most likely is another respiratory problem.*

▶ *The diminished breath sounds, nonproductive cough, hypoxemia, and ineffective antibiotic and steroid regimen should cause the provider to suspect possible pneumonia.*

2. **What other information would be important to know?**
   - ▶ *Has the patient had her flu shot this season?*
   - ▶ *Has the patient had the recommended pneumonia vaccines?*
   - ▶ *Has the patient recently been exposed to others who are ill?*

3. **What diagnostic tests would you anticipate the provider to order?**
   - ▶ Chest x-ray
   - ▶ ABGs
   - ▶ White-cell count with differential
   - ▶ Nasal swab for influenza

4. **What education would you provide to this patient?**
   - ▶ *Treatment of pneumonia:*
     - • *Antibiotics*
     - • *Fluid hydration*
     - • *Cough and deep breathing exercises*
     - • *Possible need for IV steroids and nebulizer treatments*
   - ▶ *Prevention:*
     - • *Avoid crowds and other who are ill.*
     - • *Get the yearly flu shot.*
     - • *Get the pneumonia vaccines (if patient has not already received).*

5. **What should you consider based on this patient's age?**
   - ▶ *The older adult may be afebrile even when experiencing an infection.*
   - ▶ *Respiratory infections may last longer and be more severe because of a decreased immune response, decreased cough, and decreased cilia and alveolar macrophage function.*

Discussion

Patients with COPD are at greater risk for other respiratory disorders, especially as they age; therefore, it is critical to ensure that these patients prevent exposure to other illnesses. Be sure to check whether these patients have received the pneumonia vaccines and the yearly flu vaccine. Education should include avoiding crowds and others who are known to be ill, avoiding going outdoors in weather conditions that can predispose the patient to illness, and notifying the provider early if not feeling well.

Bibliography

Aschenbrenner, D.S., and Venable, S.J. (2012). *Drug Therapy in Nursing*, 4th ed. (Philadelphia: Wolters Kluwer).

Black, J.M., and Hawks, J. (2009). *Medical-Surgical Nursing: Clinical Management for Positive Outcomes*, 8th ed. (St. Louis: Saunders).

Centers for Disease Control and Prevention. (2018). Asthma Data. Accessed July 1, 2018, from https://www.cdc.gov/asthma/most_recent_data.htm

Centers for Disease Control and Prevention. (2017). Influenza (flu). Accessed September 12, 2017, from https://www.cdc.gov/flu/about/index.html

Cho, Y.J., Moon, J.Y., Shin, E.-S., Kim, J.H., Jung, H., Park, S.Y., … Choi, W.I. The Korean Academy of Tuberculosis and Respiratory Diseases Consensus Group. (2016). Clinical practice guideline of acute respiratory distress syndrome. *Tuberc Respir Dis* 79, 214–233.

Global Initiative for Chronic Obstructive Lung Disease (GOLD). (2017). Global strategy for the diagnosis, management and prevention of COPD, 2017 report. Accessed June 3, 2018, from http://goldcopd.org

Jarvis, C. (2015). *Physical Examination and Health Assessment*, 7th ed. (St. Louis: Elsevier).

Lewis, S.L., Bucher, L., Heitkemper, M., and Harding, M.M. (2017). *Medical-Surgical Nursing: Assessment and Management of Clinical Problems,* 10th ed. (St. Louis: Elsevier).

NIH National Heart, Lung, and Blood Institute. (2016). Pneumonia. U.S. Department of Health and Human Services. Accessed September 1, 2017, from https://www.nhlbi.nih.gov/health/health-topics/topics/pnu

NIH National Heart, Lung, and Blood Institute. (2017). What is COPD? U.S. Department of Health and Human Services. Accessed September 1, 2017, from https://www.nhlbi.nih.gov/health/health-topics/topics/copd/

O'Driscoll, B.R. (2008). Overdose on oxygen? AHRQ Patient Safety Network. Accessed June 3, 2018, from https://psnet.ahrq.gov/webmm/case/172#

Pagana, K.D., Pagana, T.J., & Pagana, T.N. (2017). *Mosby's Diagnostic & Laboratory Test Reference,* 13th ed. (St. Louis: Elsevier).

9

Cardiovascular System

Patricia Braida MSN, RN, AGPCNP-BC

The cardiovascular system includes the heart and the blood vessels throughout the body. It is responsible for supplying oxygenated blood to organs and tissues. According to Benjamin et al., (2018), there has been a decline in heart disease in the United States due to increased awareness and improved treatment strategies for hyperlipidemia, hypertension, heart failure, and heart attack. Cardiovascular disease (CVD) is responsible for more deaths in the United States each year than cancer and chronic lower respiratory diseases combined. Coronary heart disease is the most common cause of cardiovascular death; it accounts for 1 of every 7 deaths in the United States. Stroke, heart failure, high blood pressure, diseases of the arteries, and other CVDs also contribute to CVD death rates.

OVERVIEW: STRUCTURES AND FUNCTIONS

Structures of the Heart

- Normally the size of an adult fist, located to the left of the mediastinum.
- Four chambers: right and left atria and right and left ventricles, divided vertically by a fibrous septum.
- Muscular, hollow organ consisting of three layers: epicardium (outer layer), myocardium (middle layer responsible for contraction), and endocardium (innermost layer lining the chambers and the heart valves).
- The heart is protected by pericardium consisting of an inner visceral layer and an outer, fibrous, parietal layer. Normally only 5 to 15 ml of serous fluid is in this space and allows for smooth movement as the heart contracts.
- Four heart valves keep the blood moving forward through the heart—heart sounds are generated by closure of the heart valves; in adults:
  - Auscultate normal heart sounds with the diaphragm of the stethoscope
  - Auscultate extra/abnormal heart sounds with the bell of the stethoscope
    Across the precordium:
    - Aortic area—second right intercostal space (ICS), next to sternum
    - Pulmonic—second left ICS, next to sternum
    - Erb's point—third left ICS, next to sternum
    - Tricuspid—fifth left ICS next to sternum
    - Mitral—fifth ICS, left midclavicular line (MCL)

- S1—lub—beginning of systole (ejection)—closure of tricuspid and mitral valves
- S2—dub—beginning of diastole (filling)—closure of aortic and pulmonic valves
- If there are valve abnormalities, there may be extra sounds between S1 and S2 or after S2.
- Note whether the extra/abnormal sound was heard during systole or during diastole.
- Note where the sound was heard best/loudest on the chest wall, as this can give you a clue as to which heart valve is affected (may be related to valvular regurgitation or stenosis).
- Split S2 with inspiration and an S4 may be normal in healthy adults

> **Clinical Consideration**
> While auscultating the "lub" heart sound and simultaneously palpating the radial pulse, the nurse is assessing systole.

> **Clinical Consideration**
> The coronary arteries fill during diastole.

Question	Rationale
If a patient has mitral regurgitation, where would the nurse best auscultate the abnormal heart sound? A. At the fifth intercostal space, left midclavicular line B. At the right sternal border C. At the second intercostal space to the right of the sternum D. At the second intercostal space to the left of the sternum	Answer: A Sounds referred from the mitral valve are best heard at the fifth intercostal space, left midclavicular line. This particular abnormal heart sound would be heard during systole because some blood is regurgitating back up into the left atrium (LA) when the left ventricle (LV) is contracting (systole) and trying to eject the blood forward.

Coronary Artery Perfusion of the Myocardium

▶ The myocardium has its own circulation from the aorta to the coronary arteries to the myocardium. This occurs during diastole (ventricular filling, relaxation phase).

▶ Right main coronary artery (RCA):

- Perfuses right atrium (RA), right ventricle (RV), inferior part of LV, posterior septal wall, and sinoatrial (SA) and atrioventricular (AV) nodes
- Decreased perfusion may cause conduction system disturbances, hypotension, posterior wall infarct or RV infarct.

▶ Left main coronary artery that divides into the left anterior descending (LAD) and circumflex arteries

- LAD artery:
  - Perfuses the anterior wall of LV, anterior ventricular septum, LV apex.
  - Decreased perfusion may cause ACS, myocardial infarction, decreased LV contractility, heart failure, conduction system disturbances/heart block, and dysrhythmias.
- Left circumflex artery:
  - Perfuses the LA, lateral and posterior surfaces of the LV.
  - Decreased perfusion problems same as for LAD artery.

> **Clinical Consideration**
> Patients with an anterior-wall myocardial infarction (MI) often have disease in the LAD coronary artery.

Conduction System of the Heart

▶ System creates and transports electrical impulses and action potentials throughout the heart.

▶ Action potential causes heart cells to depolarize and heart muscle to contract.

▶ Normally, electrical impulse starts in main pacemaker of the heart (SA node), located in RA:

- Impulses generated at rate of 60 to 100 times per minute
- Under control of sympathetic and parasympathetic nervous systems
- Atria are depolarized and contract to empty in diastole
- Represented by the P wave on the electrocardiogram (ECG)

▶ Impulses go to the AV node in lower septum via internodal pathways:

- If SA does not generate an impulse, the AV node is capable of generating impulses at 40 to 60 times per minute, which may not be enough to sustain cardiac output for very long.

▶ Impulse then travels to bundle of His in the interventricular septum, to the right and left bundle branches, and finally to the Purkinje fibers (represented by PR interval on ECG; normal time <0.20 second).

- Purkinje fibers conduct impulses through the ventricles within 0.12 second and the right and left ventricles contract, or depolarize; this corresponds to systole.
- If the SA and AV nodes fail, the Purkinje fibers can take over as the pacemaker of the heart, generating a rate of 20 to 40 times per minute; this is very slow and would not sustain life for long if the other pacemakers did not take over.
- QRS complex on the ECG represents depolarization of the ventricles; normal is 0.12 second.

▶ Final phase is repolarization, when contractile cells and electrical conduction cells start to return to the resting potential; the absolute refractory period is when the myocardium is not responsive to stimuli; the relative refractory period is when the heart starts to become responsive to stimuli:

- Represented by the T wave on the ECG
- May see U wave right after T wave; represents repolarization of Purkinje fibers or can be associated with hypokalemia (see Chapter 6)

Cardiac Output

- Systole—depolarization of the ventricles, ejection of blood from RV to lungs and LV to aorta
- Diastole—relaxation, filling of the ventricles (coronary artery perfusion during diastole)
- Cardiac output (CO)—amount of blood ejected by each ventricle in 1 minute; normal is 4 to 8 L/min
- Cardiac index (CI)—CO divided by body-surface area (BSA), adjusting the CO to the patient's size
- Cardiac reserve—In health, the body has the ability to respond to demands to increase cardiac output to tissues as needed.
- Stroke volume × heart rate (HR) = CO
- Increasing HR, preload, contractility, and afterload increase oxygen demand on the heart, affecting CO.
  - Heart rate—if too high or too low can cause decreased cardiac output
  - Preload—amount of blood in the ventricle at end of diastole, just before the next contraction:
    - Starling law—up to a certain point, the greater the myocardial stretch from blood in the ventricle, the greater the force of ventricular contraction
    - Increased by hypertension, aortic-valve disease, fluid overload
    - Decreased by venodilators, diuretics, sitting in high Fowler's position

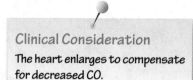

- Afterload—resistance against which the ventricle has to pump:
  - Hypertension, aortic stenosis increase afterload
  - LV hypertrophy (enlargement of heart muscle) occurs after longstanding ejection against high resistance
- Contractility—the force of myocardial contraction; can affect CO; increased by sympathetic nervous system (SNS) stimulation and positive inotropic drugs; can be decreased by hypoxia and acidosis

Vascular System

▶ Arteries/arterioles—carry blood from left side of heart to body; arterioles major control of arterial blood pressure (BP) and distribution of blood flow:

- Blood pressure:
  - Determined by cardiac output (blood going out of the heart) and arteriole resistance
  - Blood pressure = CO × peripheral vascular resistance (see section on "Hypertension")
  - Mean arterial pressure (MAP)
    - MAP = [SBP + 2(DBP)] divided by 3
    - Used to determine adequate tissue and organ perfusion
    - Pressure greater than 60 mm Hg is needed to perfuse the tissues and organs
  - Regulation of blood pressure:
    - Autonomic nervous system (ANS) responding to chemoreceptors (e.g., vasoconstrict if hypoxemia is present and will increase blood pressure; SNS will increase HR and constrict peripheral blood vessels if hypovolemia is sensed).
    - Kidneys activate renin–angiotensin–aldosterone system (RAAS) when they recognize decreased perfusion.
    - The endocrine system stimulates SNS at the cellular level, releasing catecholamines, histamines, kinins, etc.

▶ Capillaries—exchange location for nutrients and metabolic processes; connect arterioles and venules

▶ Veins/venules—return blood to right atrium; low pressure, capacitance vessels

Autonomic Nervous System

▶ Regulates cardiovascular system

▶ Sympathetic and parasympathetic receptors and fibers throughout body

▶ Heart:

- β_1-adrenergic receptors (sympathetic) in SA node and in ventricles—stimulation of β_1 increases heart rate and contraction.
- Parasympathetic stimulation of the heart slows HR.

▶ Blood vessels—SNS controls:

- α_1-adrenergic receptors—in vascular smooth muscle
  - Stimulation—vasoconstriction
  - Decreased or blocked stimulation—vasodilation
  - Some parasympathetic nerves in blood vessels

▶ Baroreceptors:

- Sense hypoxemia, hypercapnia (chemoreceptors), volume (stretch receptors)
- ANS responds with inhibition or stimulation of either the sympathetic or parasympathetic nervous system as needed to maintain homeostasis.

- Example: if the stretch receptors in aortic arch and carotid sinus sense fluid over-load, SNS is inhibited and the parasympathetic nervous system (PNS) is stimu-lated to decrease HR and vasodilate to lower blood pressure.

Question	Rationale
The nurse is aware that if a β_1 selective adrenergic blocker, such as metoprolol (Lopressor), is administered, sympathetic stimulation of the heart will: A. Be enhanced, and the heart rate and strength of contraction will increase. B. Be decreased, and the heart rate and strength of contraction will decrease. C. Not be affected, but the angiotensin-converting enzyme (ACE) will be inhibited. D. Decrease heart rate and increase oxygen demand in the heart.	Answer: B β_1-adrenergic receptor blockers decrease the SNS response. Metoprolol blocks β_1-receptors in the heart and decreases heart rate, thereby decreasing oxygen demand and consumption. β_1-adrenergic receptor blockers also reduce force of contraction of the ventricle, which also reduces oxygen demand. In addition, AV node (AVN) impulse conduction is decreased. ACE is inhibited by medications such as enalapril (Vasotec).

ASSESSMENT OF THE CARDIOVASCULAR SYSTEM

Patient History:
- History of present illness
- Risk factor assessment—modifiable and nonmodifiable
- Medical and surgical history
- Use of alcohol, cigarettes, illicit drugs
- Medications
- Diet/nutrition history
- Weight patterns
- Psychosocial history
- Employment, functional status
- Family history and genetic risk
- Review of systems

Physical Assessment Using Inspection, Palpation, and Auscultation
- Vital signs, heart rhythm
- Appearance
- Skin
- Peripheral vascular assessment
- Precordium
- Lung sounds
- Other as dictated by history (e.g., reports of abdominal bloating, scrotal edema with heart failure)

Question	Rationale
The nurse is explaining to a new graduate nurse that the elderly are more likely to have systolic hypertension because of: A. Increased viscosity of the blood in the elderly on diuretics B. Increased ability of the kidneys to retain salt C. Increased stiffness of the aorta and blood vessels D. Hypersensitivity of the baroreceptors to changes in position	Answer: C The aorta and other large arteries become thicker, less distensible, and stiffen with aging. The systolic blood pressure increases to compensate for this. The kidneys are less able to retain salt. In the elderly, baroreceptors are less sensitive to changes in position, making them more susceptible to dizziness and falls.

> **Clinical Consideration**
>
> Troponin levels can mirror the degree of myocardial damage.

Diagnostic Studies

- Troponin—marker of myocardial damage from acute coronary syndrome (ACS)
  - Troponins T and I are the earliest markers of myocardial necrosis or acute myocardial infarction (AMI)
  - Any increase indicates risk of CVD
  - Serial values checked to observe for peak and downward trend
  - Troponin T reference value <0.1 ng/mL
  - Troponin I reference value <0.03 ng/mL
- Creatine kinase myocardial band (CKMB) can support diagnosis of myocardial infarction (MI):
  - Released within 6 hours after myocardial muscle injury; can quantify degree of injury
  - May be drawn serially to assess myocardial damage
  - Reference value would be 0%
- Myoglobin—found in cardiac and skeletal muscle:
  - Indicates cardiac muscle injury or death and rises within 3 hours after death
  - Trauma to skeletal muscles can also cause elevations
  - Reference range: <90 µg/L
- Serum lipids—a risk for CAD and peripheral arterial disease (PAD)
  - Requires a 12-hour fast
  - Recommendation values for lipid values (Stone et al., 2014)
    - Total cholesterol <200 mg/dL
    - High-density lipoprotein (HDL) (protectant) >40 mg/dL (men)
    - HDL (protectant) >50 mg/dL (women)
    - Low-density lipoprotein (LDL) (associated with increased risk of CAD) <100 mg/dl; <70 mg/dL may be recommended for those with diabetes, ASCVD (atherosclerotic cardiovascular disease), or with increased risk of ASCVD
    - Triglycerides <150 mg/dL
    - Other lipid studies may be ordered for patients with familial hypercholesterolemia (FH)
- Homocysteine—risk factor for CVD; may contribute to damaged endothelium
  - Reference range: 4–14 µmol/L
- B-type natriuretic peptide (BNP)—released by the ventricles, in response to heart failure, to oppose action of RAAS and increase excretion of sodium in the urine

- Helps differentiate cardiac (heart failure [HF]) from a respiratory cause of dyspnea
    - Reference value: >100 μg/mL indicates heart failure
- N-terminal pro B-type natriuretic peptide (NT-proBNP)—same action as BNP; clinically used interchangeably with BNP
    - Same clinical significance as BNP
    - Reference value: <125 pg/mL (for those <74 years old)
    - Reference value: <450 pg/mL (for those >75 years old)
- Chest x-ray
- 12-lead ECG provides information about rate, rhythm, interval measurements, hypertrophy, electrolyte imbalances, and effectiveness of drugs:
    - Presence of ST- or T-wave changes indicative of possible ischemia
    - The leads of ECG affected by ST/T-wave changes can guide location/extent of myocardial ischemia and/or infarction.
    - Can be obtained at rest or with exercise testing
- Holter monitoring—24 to 48 hours of heart rhythm monitoring; patient keeps diary and documents signs and symptoms
- Event monitor—patient keeps for 30 days; attaches electrodes as needed to transmit ECG to provider or when patient has specific symptoms
- Exercise stress test—assesses cardiovascular response to exercise; 12-lead ECG to observe for any ST/T-wave depression, elevation, or inversion indicative of ischemia:
    - No cigarettes, alcohol, or caffeine the day of the test
    - Patient usually told to withhold rate-controlling medications (beta-blockers; calcium-channel blockers)
    - Light meal 2 hours before test may be allowed
    - Patient reports chest pain, dyspnea, dizziness, palpitations
- Echocardiography—noninvasive; assesses LV function, size of heart, valvular function, presence of thrombi, or vegetation
- Pharmacologic stress echocardiography—used for patients who cannot exercise; dobutamine or other drug is used to increase contractility of the heart; 12-lead ECG is observed for any changes.
- Transesophageal echocardiography (TEE)—uses an endoscope to evaluate cardiac structures and function; patient must be NPO (nothing by mouth) before the procedure; monitored anesthesia care for procedure
- Arteriography—invasive procedure that uses contrast media and fluoroscopy to evaluate peripheral arteries and/or coronary arteries
- Cardiac catheterization—invasive test that may look at left- and/or right-sided heart function and the coronary arteries:
    - NPO for prescribed time before procedure
    - Patient may receive contrast media; fluoroscopy is used; patient usually receives some sedation.
    - If disease is found, patient may have percutaneous coronary intervention (PCI) which may include balloon angioplasty and stent placement.
    - Recovery occurs in monitored setting.
    - Insertion-site extremity is kept straight for period of time per provider protocol.
    - The insertion site and circulation in the extremity are carefully assessed.
- Multigated acquisition (MUGA) scan—nuclear scan that uses radioactive isotope and ECG monitoring to evaluate LV function.
- Single-photon-emission computed tomography (SPECT)—use of radioactive isotope to determine risk of infarction, size of infarction by looking at

Clinical Consideration

BNP is elevated with atrial and/or ventricular stretching; it will not be produced with a primary respiratory problem.

Clinical Consideration

Beta-blockers and calcium-channel blockers can affect the normal cardiovascular response to exercise.

coronary artery blood flow, motion of ventricles, ejection fraction (EF), and chamber sizes.

- Exercise (stress) nuclear imaging—nuclear images at rest and with exercise to evaluate wall function and myocardial perfusion:
    - If patient cannot exercise, regadenoson (Lexiscan) or adenosine (Adenocard) can be given IV to simulate the effects of exercise.
    - Patient must refrain from caffeine and tobacco for 12 hours before test.
    - If adenosine used, no aminophylline for 12 hours before test.
    - No beta-blockers or calcium-channel blockers for 24 hours before test.
- Cardiac computed tomography (CT), with or without contrast material:
    - Heart, coronary anatomy, circulation, and blood vessels are assessed.
- Coronary CT angiography (CTA), with contrast material:
    - CT used to look at blood vessels and diagnose CAD.
- Cardiovascular magnetic resonance imaging (CMRI):
    - Noninvasive—evaluates proximal coronary arteries, ejection fraction (EF), CO
- Magnetic resonance angiography (MRA):
    - Uses IV contrast material to evaluate abdominal aortic aneurysms (AAAs) and vascular disease
- Calcium-scoring CT scan:
    - Noninvasive, quantifies calcification (calcium score) in coronary arteries and valves
    - Often used in asymptomatic patients to evaluate risk of heart disease; follow-up evaluation needed if score is high
- Electrophysiology study (EPS):
    - Invasive study used to evaluate and/or treat patients with dysrhythmias
    - Antiarrhythmic drugs withheld prior to procedure
    - NPO before the procedure
    - Monitor vital signs, insertion site, and heart rhythm after procedure

Clinical Consideration

The goal of EPS is to induce the dysrhythmia while off medication to determine the appropriate treatment.

Question	Rationale
The nurse is caring for a patient who is having an exercise stress test at 1 p.m. The patient states that he had a bagel and orange juice at 6 a.m. He reports that he took all his morning medications as directed, including metoprolol (Lopressor) 50 mg. Which is the priority nursing action? A. Shave the patient's chest in order to apply the ECG electrodes. B. Explain what the patient should expect during the test. C. Inform the cardiologist that the patient did take his beta-blocker this morning. D. Inform the cardiologist that the patient ate a bagel and orange juice.	Answer: C The patient is allowed to have an early, light breakfast if he is having a stress test in the afternoon. Taking beta-blockers can blunt the heart rate response to exercise. The rationale for the treadmill test is to observe the response to exercise and physical stress. Patient signs and symptoms, blood pressure, and heart rate response to exercise are assessed. Beta-blockers decrease heart rate, conduction through the AV node, and ventricular contractility. Typically, the patient is instructed not to take the beta-blocker the day before and the day of the test. The patient is asked to bring the medication to take after the treadmill test.

DYSRHYTHMIAS

Electrocardiogram

▶ Electrical activity of the heart can be detected by placing electrodes on the patient's body and recording an electrocardiogram. The electrical activity represents depolarization and repolarization of the heart, including the action potential. The 12-lead electrocardiogram records electrical forces in the front, side, and back of the heart. It can give valuable information about:

- Rate, rhythm (e.g., bradycardia, tachycardia, atrial fibrillation)
- Measured intervals on the ECG tracing
- Structural changes (e.g., atrial enlargement, ventricular hypertrophy)
- Conduction disturbances (e.g., heart blocks)
- Effects from drugs (e.g., digoxin)
- Ischemia, infarction (e.g., ACS)
- Acid–base or electrolyte disturbances (e.g., hyperkalemia, hypokalemia)

▶ Patient can also be monitored with telemetry (one or more leads) continuously if indicated in acute care or perhaps at home to correlate symptoms (e.g., palpitations) with rhythm changes.

▶ Interpretation of rhythm strips (Table 9.1)

- Measuring waveforms and intervals and rate. (Figure 9.1)

TABLE 9.1	EVALUATING HEART RHYTHM
Steps	Clinical Considerations
Step 1: Evaluate the P waves and the atrial rhythm • Are they present? • Is there one for every QRS complex? • Are there more P waves than QRS complexes? • Do they all look the same? Upright or inverted? • Are there fibrillatory waves instead of defined P waves? • What is the P-to-P interval? • Is the atrial rhythm regular? • If the rhythm is irregular, is there a pattern?	• If there are no discernible P waves, and the QRS complexes are irregularly irregular, the patient may be in atrial fibrillation. • If the P waves are very tall, this could indicate atrial enlargement. • If some of the P waves occur earlier/out of sequence, this could indicate premature atrial contractions. • If the P-to-P-wave interval remains regular and there are some P waves without QRS complexes, this could indicate second- or third-degree heart block. • Heart blocks can occur secondary to ischemia or other diseases that may slow conduction. Beta-blockers, digoxin, and calcium-channel blockers can also slow conduction. • Must evaluate the patient for any associated symptoms and possibly hold medications that can cause heart block. • Patients with symptomatic second- or third-degree AV block may need any/or a combination of the following: drugs, a transcutaneous pacemaker, a temporary transvenous pacemaker, or a permanent pacemaker.
Step 2: Calculate the atrial rate • Can determine rate by using the ECG paper. Paper is marked in 3-second increments, which is 15 large boxes. Obtain a 6-second rhythm strip (30 large boxes) and count the number of P waves in the 6-second strip. Multiply this number by 10 to give you the atrial rate in 1 minute. (Figure 9.1)	• Normal is between 60 and 100 beats/min • PSVT can produce atrial rate between 150 and 250 beats/min • The longer the patient is in PSVT and the higher the ventricular response, the more likely the patient is to experience signs/symptoms of decreased CO. (See entry for PSVT in section on "Common Dysrhythmias in Medical-Surgical Nursing.")

(continued)

TABLE 9.1   *(Continued)*

Steps	Clinical Considerations
Step 3: Determine the PR interval • Count the number of small squares from the beginning of the P wave to the beginning of the QRS complex. Multiply this by 0.04 second. Each small square is 0.04 second. • Is the PR interval within the normal duration of 0.12 (3 small squares) to 0.20 second (5 small squares)? • Is the PR interval constant for each QRS complex?	• If the PR interval is greater than 0.20 second, the patient could have a first-degree AV block. • First-degree AV block is usually asymptomatic. The heart rate and heart rhythm are regular. The QRS complex usually has normal configuration and duration. • It can be secondary to MI, CAD, RF, and hyperthyroidism and use of digoxin, beta-blockers, calcium-channel blockers, and flecainide. • Monitor patient with first-degree AV block for any changes in rhythm or condition. May need to reevaluate medications that can be associated with heart block. • If the PR interval is gradually lengthening until there is a P wave that is not conducted and the QRS complex is missing, this can be second-degree heart block type 1. Patients are often asymptomatic with this heart block. • In third-degree AV block, there are the normal and regular atrial contractions of 60–100 beats/min, but they are not conducted to the ventricles. The ventricular rate is regular and may be 20–60 beats/min, depending on the site of the conduction block. PR intervals are not measurable or are inconsistent. The atria and ventricles are beating independently. • Third-degree AV block usually causes symptoms related to low cardiac output; it can be associated with CAD, MI, cardiomyopathy, and systemic diseases and use of beta-blockers, calcium-channel blockers, and digoxin. • Always evaluate the patient for any symptoms associated with a change in rhythm. • See above for possible treatment of symptomatic second- and third-degree block.
Step 4: Evaluate the ventricular rhythm • Is the distance between each R wave (R-to-R-wave interval) regular? • Is it irregular? • If irregular, is there a pattern to the irregularity?	If a QRS complex occurs early and has a wide distorted shape, this can be a premature ventricular contraction PVC. • Three or more PVCs in a row is called "ventricular tachycardia (VT)." • (See "premature ventricular contractions" in the section on "Common Dysrhythmias in Medical-Surgical Nursing.")
Step 5: Calculate the ventricular rate • How many R waves are noted in a 6-second strip? (Multiply this number by 10 to determine the ventricular rate).	• Normal rate is between 60 and 100 beats/min.
Step 6: Determine the QRS duration • Is the QRS complex duration within the normal limits of 0.06 to 0.11 second? • Measure the number of small boxes from the beginning of the QRS complex to the end of the S wave and multiply by 0.04 second.	• If it is greater than 0.11 second, there may be slowed conduction in the bundle branches or ventricles.
Step 7: Assess the ST segment and T waves Are T waves present? • Are the T waves upright or inverted? • Do all the T waves have a normal shape and size? • Does it appear that P waves might be superimposed on T waves? • Are the ST segments flat (even with the isoelectric line [baseline]), elevated above the isoelectric line, or depressed below the isoelectric line? If so, how many millimeters above or below isoelectric line?	• Tall peaked T waves can be secondary to hyperkalemia. • Changes in the ST/T waves can be signs of ischemia—must always correlate with patient signs and symptoms. • Evaluate for ST/T-wave changes in all 12 leads of ECG (not just in 1 or 2 leads on telemetry strip). • Always compare ECG changes to patient's baseline. • Acute ST-segment elevation can possibly indicate an acute injury pattern, STEMI; always correlate with patient assessment.

(continued)

TABLE 9. 1	(Continued)
Steps	Clinical Considerations
Step 8: Determine the QT duration • Count the number of small boxes from the beginning of the QRS complex to the end of the T wave, multiply by 0.04 second.	• Normal QT interval (QTc) is within 0.34 to 0.43 second. • May change with heart rate, certain drugs, and electrolyte disturbances. • QT interval is monitored periodically in patients receiving certain medications. • QTc prolongation can predispose to torsades de pointes, a life-threatening dysrhythmia.
Step 9: Put it together • Where is the rhythm originating from? • What is the rate? • What kind of rhythm? Abnormal/normal? • Are there extra or ectopic beats on the rhythm strip as well?	• Always evaluate your patient if there are any changes in the heart rhythm and assess for related symptoms. • Notify health care provider as appropriate. • What will the treatment be, if any?

(Elmoselhi, 2018; Fuster, Harrington, Narula, and Eapen, 2017)

AV = atrioventricular; CAD = coronary artery disease; CO = cardiac output; ECG = electrocardiogram; MI = myocardial infarction; PSVT = Paroxysmal supraventricular tachycardia; PVC = premature ventricular contraction; RF = rheumatic fever; EF = Ejection Fraction; STEMI = ST-segment elevation myocardial infarction.

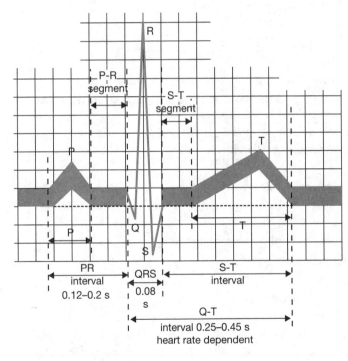

Figure 9.1 Normal ECG Complex

Fuster et al., 2017

Common Rhythms/Dysrhythmias in Medical-Surgical Nursing

- Normal sinus rhythm (Figure 9.2):
  - Ventricular and atrial rates 60 to 100 beats/min
  - QRS complexes and P waves regular and uniform
  - PR interval 0.12 to 0.20 second, constant
  - QRS interval <0.12 second
  - Ventricular and atrial rates the same

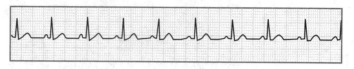

Figure 9.2 Normal Sinus Rhythm

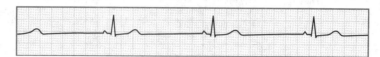

Figure 9.3 Sinus Bradycardia

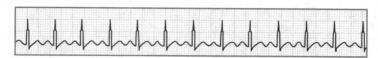

Figure 9.4 Sinus Tachycardia

- Sinus bradycardia (Figure 9.3):
  - Ventricular and atrial rates <60 beats/min
  - QRS complex for every P wave
  - See "Sinus rhythm," for the other criteria.
  - Clinical significance:
    - Normal for patient if sleeping or in aerobically trained athletes.
    - Assess for underlying causes; acute myocardial infarction (AMI), increased intracranial pressure (ICP), hypothyroid.
    - Treat if signs and symptoms of low cardiac output: hypotension; dizziness; confusion; weakness; cool, pale, clammy skin.
  - Treatment:
    - Withhold beta-blockers, calcium-channel blockers, and digoxin.
    - Give atropine if symptomatic; evaluate need for intravenous fluids (IVF); may also need dopamine, epinephrine, or transcutaneous pacemaker.
- Sinus tachycardia—originates in sinus node (Figure 9.4):
  - Rate can be from 101 to 200 beats/min
  - One QRS complex for every P wave
  - See "Sinus rhythm," for other criteria.
  - Clinical significance:
    - Assess for underlying causes, such as dehydration, bleeding, pain, anxiety, fever, exercise, anemia, hyperthyroidism, fear, decreased cardiac output, and stress.
    - Is the patient symptomatic? Is there chest pain/angina due to increased myocardial oxygen demand?
  - Treatment:
    - Treat cause
    - Beta-blocker or calcium-channel blocker (Use caution when giving calcium-channel blocker to patients with HF.)
- Atrial fibrillation—disorganization of atrial electrical activity, resulting in loss of atrial contraction, or "atrial kick" at end of diastole; atrial contraction can contribute significantly to cardiac output and this is why patients can become symptomatic when they are in atrial fibrillation (Figure 9.5):
  - Atrial rate >400 beats/min; ventricular rate irregularly irregular.
    - QRS complexes are the same, but the R to R interval is irregular.

Clinical Consideration

When the heart rate increases, coronary artery diastolic filling times are decreased, predisposing to myocardial ischemia and chest pain in those with CAD.

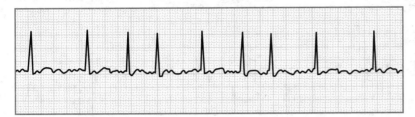

Figure 9.5 Atrial Fibrillation

- No measurable PR interval
- P waves are not discernible; they appear as wavy baseline
- Clinical significance:
  - Is this rhythm persistent (baseline rhythm for >7 days)? Or is it paroxysmal (does it come and go)?
  - Is the ventricular response controlled (between 60 and 100 beats/min)? Is there a rapid ventricular response (RVR) (>100 beats/min)?
  - Is the patient symptomatic? Are there signs/symptoms of decreased cardiac output (e.g., hypotension; HF; syncope; altered mental status; chest pain; thready peripheral pulses; skin pale/dusky, cool, and/or diaphoretic?)
  - Occurs in patients with valvular disease, CAD, cardiomyopathy, thyrotoxicosis, alcohol consumption, caffeine, stress, and heart surgery.
- Treatment:
  - Goal:
    - Control ventricular response to between 60 and 100 beats/min
    - Prevent stroke—anticoagulation
    - Convert to sinus rhythm, if possible—amiodarone (Cordarone) or ibutilide (Corvert)
    - If the patient is not symptomatic, a beta-blocker, calcium-channel blocker, digoxin, or dronedarone (Multaq) may be administered.
  - Perhaps synchronous cardioversion
  - Anticoagulation—(see section on "Venous Thromboembolism")
    - Warfarin (Coumadin)
    - Dabigatran (Pradaxa)
    - Apixaban (Eliquis)
    - Rivaroxaban (Xarelto)
  - Warfarin (Coumadin) preferred for patients with chronic kidney disease (CKD) 5 or who are undergoing hemodialysis.
  - Ablation
  - Maze procedure (See section on "Valvular Heart Disease")
  - Pacemaker
  - Left atrial appendage (LAA) devices used to occlude or remove area in LAA that produces clots and is a source of the atrial fibrillation.
- Premature atrial contractions (PAC)—ectopic focus that starts in atrium (Figure 9.6):
  - Premature beats that usually have same QRS complex as underlying rhythm; underlying rhythm is irregular.
  - P waves are distorted, may be hidden in the in previous T wave or have different shape than those in underlying rhythm.
  - Underlying rhythm can be any rate or rhythm.
  - May be a forewarning that patient will go into supraventricular tachycardia (SVT).

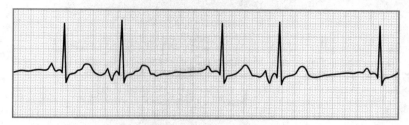

Figure 9.6 Premature Atrial Contractions

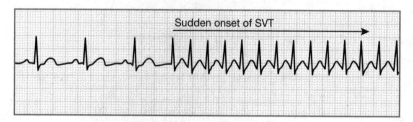

Figure 9.7 Supraventricular Tachycardia

- Normal in healthy hearts
- Clinical significance:
    - Fatigue; emotional stress; tobacco; alcohol; caffeine
    - Hyperthyroidism; hypoxia; electrolyte imbalances; chronic obstructive pulmonary disease (COPD); valvular disease; CAD
- Treatment:
    - Treat the cause; patient should not use caffeine, tobacco, or alcohol
    - Beta-blocker
- Paroxysmal atrial tachycardia (PAT) or paroxysmal supraventricular tachycardia (PSVT) or supraventricular tachycardia (SVT)—rhythm originates in ectopic focus somewhere above the bundle of His (Figure 9.7).
    - Ventricular and atrial rates are usually the same; heart rate ranges from 150 to 250 beats/min; rhythm is regular.
    - P wave present; might be hidden in previous T wave.
    - PR interval normal or shortened slightly; may be difficult to discern.
    - QRS complex is usually normal.
    - Clinical significance—associated with hyperthyroidism, stress, caffeine, tobacco, CAD, or pulmonale.
    - Treatment:
        - Vagal simulation
        - Intravenous (IV) adenosine (Adenocard) will cause conversion back to sinus rhythm.
        - IV beta-blockers or calcium-channel blockers
        - If drugs did not convert back to sinus rhythm and patient becomes unstable, may need synchronized cardioversion.
- Premature ventricular contractions (PVC) (Figure 9.8):
    - Wide, premature beats
    - Underlying rhythm can be any rate; regular or irregular

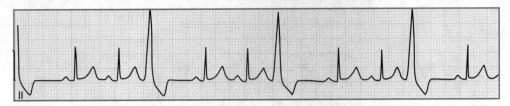

Figure 9.8 Premature Ventricular Contractions

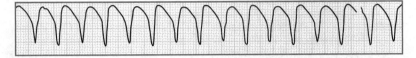

Figure 9.9 Ventricular Tachycardia

- Clinical significance:
  - Can be associated with stimulants, HF, acute MI, hypoxia, electrolyte disturbances, mitral-valve prolapse, and anxiety.
- Treatment:
  - Treat cause: administer oxygen; replace potassium and magnesium as necessary; treat acute MI; withdraw caffeine, alcohol.
  - Beta-blockers; amiodarone. Figure 9.8 Ventricular Trigemeny (every third beat is a PVC).
- Ventricular tachycardia (VT)—Three or more premature ventricular contractions (PVCs) in a row; ectopic focus fires repeatedly and the ventricle is the heart's primary pacemaker (Figure 9.9).
  - Ventricular rate is 150 to 250 beats/min; may be regular, or irregular.
  - P waves usually not visible; no PR interval.
  - QRS is wide and distorted, >0.12 second.
  - Monomorphic VT—QRSs are all the same size and shape.
  - Polymorphic VT—QRS complexes change from one size and shape to another.
  - Torsades de pointes—type of polymorphic VT that can occur secondary to prolonged QT interval in underlying rhythm.
  - Can develop into ventricular fibrillation (vfib or VF).
- Ventricular fibrillation (VF)—unorganized, chaotic foci from ventricles; lethal rhythm that does not generate any cardiac output (Figure 9.10):
  - No measurable QRS complexes or PR interval; rhythm irregular and not measurable
  - Clinical significance
    - Patient is unresponsive and has no palpable pulse or respirations.
    - Occurs with acute MI, myocardial ischemia, electrolyte abnormalities, heart defects, acidosis, drug toxicity, and cardiomyopathy.
  - Treatment:
    - Immediate cardiopulmonary resuscitation (CPR), defibrillation; drug therapy per Advanced Cardiac Life Support (ACLS)

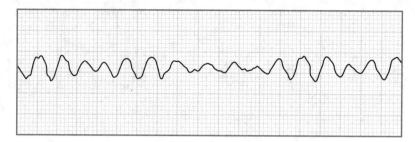

Figure 9.10 Ventricular Fibrillation

Question	Rationale
Which of the following assessment findings would alert the new graduate nurse that the patient may have atrial fibrillation? A. The pulse is 54 beats/min and regular B. The pulse is very irregular and the rate is 102 beats/min C. The pulse is bounding and regular D. There are three regular beats in a row, followed by an irregular beat	Answer: B Atrial fibrillation is an irregularly, irregular rhythm. The heart rate is often fast unless the patient is on a medication to lower the heart rate and control the ventricular response. The rhythm strip reveals no definite P waves, and the QRS complexes are present at irregular intervals.

HYPERTENSION

Hypertension is the force exerted by blood against the wall of a blood vessel. Blood pressure is critical for tissue perfusion and to meet the body's needs during rest and activity. Hypertension is defined as a systolic blood pressure (SBP) ≥130 mm Hg and/or a DBP ≥80 mm Hg (Whelton et al., 2018).

About one in three adults in the United States has high blood pressure. Only about half of people with high blood pressure have their disease under control (Merai et al., 2016).

Predisposing Factors

- Primary (essential)—90 to 95% of all cases of hypertension; cause may be unknown
- Secondary hypertension—identifiable cause (5 to 10% of hypertension in adults)
- Risk factors (Table 9.2)
- Isolated systolic hypertension (ISH):
  - An average SBP of >140 mm Hg, with an average DBP of <90 mm Hg
  - Increased incidence with aging
  - Contributes to stroke, heart failure and death
- Hypertensive crisis—hypertensive urgency or emergency
  - Causes
    - Exacerbation of chronic hypertension; preeclampsia; pheochromocytoma; cocaine; methamphetamines; monoamine oxidase (MAO) inhibitors taken with tyramine-containing foods; rebound hypertension from abrupt withdrawal of beta-blockers or clonidine; aortic dissection
  - SBP >180 mm Hg and/or DBP >110 mm Hg

TABLE 9.2	ETIOLOGY OF HYPERTENSION
Essential (Primary)	**Secondary**

Family history
African American race
Hyperlipidemia
Diabetes
Smoking
Postmenopausal
Over age 60
Excessive sodium and/or caffeine intake
Overweight/obesity
Sedentary lifestyle
Excessive alcohol intake
Low potassium, calcium, or magnesium intake
Stress
	Obstructive sleep apnea
	Kidney disease
	Acromegaly
	Hypo/hyperthyroid
	Hyperparathyroidism
	Primary aldosteronism
	Pheochromocytoma
	Cushing's disease
	Coarctation of aorta
	Brain tumors
	Encephalitis
	Pregnancy
	Low socioeconomic status
	Drugs
	   Mineralocorticoids
	   Glucocorticoids
	   Sympathomimetics

(Lewis et al., 2017; Whelton et al., 2018.)

- Hypertensive urgency—develops over hours to days, with no evidence of target organ disease
- Hypertensive emergency:
  - Signs and symptoms—target organ disease
  - Requires hospitalization if presenting with significant symptoms (encephalopathy, heart failure, bleeding in the brain, retinopathy, dissecting aortic aneurysm)
  - Don't lower blood pressure quickly (except in patient with aortic aneurysm)
- Genetics:
  - Up to age 45 years old, more men than women have hypertension.
  - After age 45, more women than men have hypertension.
  - Prevalence of hypertension among African Americans in the United States is among the highest in the world.
  - Hypertension in African Americans seems to respond better to diuretics and calcium-channel blockers (CCBs), rather than monotherapy with beta blocker or ACE inhibitors (ACEIs).
  - Chance of having hypertension increases if parent or sibling has the disease (Lewis et al., 2017; Whelton et al., 2018)

Assessment/Interventions/Education

- Clinical manifestations:
  - Silent killer—no symptoms until target organ damage
  - Dizziness, chest pain, fatigue, dyspnea
  - Hypertensive crisis (see above)
  - Target organ damage (Table 9.3)
- Diagnosis:
  - Criteria from American College of Cardiology (ACC)/American Heart Association (AHA) 2017 Guidelines, (Whelton et al., 2018) (Table 9.4)
    - Correct technique (correct cuff; sitting; no smoking, caffeine, or exercise within 30 minutes of measurement)
    - Need more than two elevated readings on more than two occasions for diagnosis
  - Rule out secondary causes

TABLE 9.3	TARGET ORGAN DAMAGE IN HYPERTENSION
Hypertensive heart disease	• Contributes to development of atherosclerosis (narrowed lumen and decreased compliance of arteries) • CAD, MI • LV hypertrophy develops because of ejecting blood against high resistance; increases oxygen demand and myocardial workload • LV dysfunction: heart failure (HF) due to decreased stroke volume and CO, and increased workload • Treatment of hypertension recommended as primary prevention in adults with no history of CVD and as secondary prevention of recurrent CVD events in those with clinical CVD (Whelton et al., 2017).
Kidney disease	• Hypertension is the leading cause of chronic kidney disease, especially in African Americans. • Almost all patients with hypertension have some evidence of kidney involvement. • Vasoconstriction of blood vessels and decreased perfusion cause nephrons to be destroyed. • Albuminuria, proteinuria, and microscopic hematuria may be present. • Increased BUN and creatinine and decreased GFR are indications of renal disease.
Cerebrovascular disease	• Atherosclerosis is the most common cause • TIA, stroke • Hypertension major risk for stroke—4 times higher than for those with normal BP • Hypertensive encephalopathy
Peripheral vascular disease	• Hypertension speeds up atherosclerosis in peripheral blood vessels. • Decreased pulses • Intermittent claudication • Decreased perfusion • Susceptibility to nonhealing wounds • Aortic aneurysm, dissection
Retinal damage	• The degree of retinal blood vessel damage often corresponds with the vessel damage in the heart, kidneys, and brain. • Blurred vision, blindness, and hemorrhage can result.

BP = blood pressure; BUN = blood urea nitrogen; CAD = coronary artery disease; CVD= cardiovascular disease; GFR = glomerular filtration rate; HF = heart failure; LV = left ventricular; MI = myocardial infarction; TIA = transient ischemic attack.

TABLE 9.4	CATEGORIES OF BLOOD PRESSURE (BP) IN ADULTS*		
BP Category	Systolic BP		Diastolic BP
Normal BP	<120 mm Hg	and	<80 mm Hg
Elevated BP	120–129 mm Hg	and	<80 mm Hg
Hypertension			
Stage 1	130–139 mm Hg	or	80–89 mm Hg
Stage 2	≥140 mm Hg	or	≥90 mm Hg

* Patients with systolic blood pressure and diastolic blood pressure in two different categories should be designated as the higher BP category.
(Whelton, et al., 2018)

- Nursing diagnosis:
  - Risk for decreased cardiac output related to decreased contractility
  - Ineffective health maintenance related to deficient knowledge regarding self-care and treatment of disease
- Treatment:
  - Lifestyle modifications first (Whelton et al., 2018)

- Weight loss—1-kg weight reduction results in 1 mm Hg reduction on SBP
- Dietary Approaches to Stop Hypertension (DASH) diet—increased fruits, vegetables, whole grains; decreased total and saturated fats
- Sodium reduction—goal of <1500 mg/day
- Physical activity—aerobic and resistance exercises 90 to 150 minutes/week
- Moderate alcohol consumption—men <2 drinks per day, women <1 drink per day
- Management of psychosocial risk factors:
  - Low socioeconomic status, stress at work, social isolation depression
  - Counseling, exercise, support groups, relaxation, stress management
- Medications (Table 9.5)
- Specific treatment goals:
  - CKD goal BP <130/80 mm Hg
  - CVD goal BP <130/80 mm Hg
  - Diabetes and hypertension: keep <130/80 mm Hg
  - Adults >65 years old with hypertension, multiple comorbidities, limited life expectancy: clinical judgment is reasonable based on concern for fall, orthostatic hypotension, and change in cognition with lowering BP aggressively
- Patient teaching:
  - Monitor BP on a regular basis and notify provider of persistent elevation.
  - Risk-factor reduction:
    - Reduce fat intake, sodium intake
    - Maintain goal weight
    - Smoking cessation
    - Increase physical activity
    - If diabetic, monitor blood glucose
    - Stress management
- Medication teaching:
  - Take medications as prescribed; do not suddenly stop taking medications.
  - Potential side effects.
  - Change position slowly to prevent dizziness, light-headedness, and transient nausea.
- Reasons for poor adherence to treatment plan:
  - Side effects
  - Patient may not have symptoms and BP may be normal, so they see no need to take medication.
  - Financial
  - Health literacy
- Strategies to improve adherence to treatment plan:
  - Determine why patient is not following recommendations.
  - Review the implications and consequences of not following the recommended treatment plan.
  - Involve patient and caregiver in decision making about drugs; plan must be compatible with patient's financial situation, culture, needs, habits, lifestyle, and wishes.
  - Long-acting or combination drugs will decrease pill burden.

Geriatric Considerations and Cardiovascular Changes

- Mitral- and tricuspid-valve calcification may occur.
- Conduction system cells can decrease in number and function, leading to slow heart rate, atrial dysrhythmias, and premature ventricular contractions.

TABLE 9.5   DRUGS FOR TREATING HYPERTENSION

Drug Name	Drug Type and Use	Mode of Action	Dosage	Adverse Effects	Clinical Considerations/Patient Teaching
Thiazide diuretics Hydrochlorothiazide Chlorothiazide (Diuril) Chlorthalidone Metolazone (Zaroxolym)	Thiazide diuretics used for essential HTN, edema, DI	Inhibit sodium and chloride reabsorption in distal convoluted tubules	**Hydrochlorothiazide** Oral: 12.5–50 mg daily	Hyponatremia, hypochloremia, dehydration, hypokalemia, hyperglycemia, hyperuricemia, orthostatic hypotension	• Check BP and potassium; monitor for orthostatic hypotension • Add foods containing potassium to diet • NSAIDs can block the diuretic effects • Can't be used if GFR <15–20 ml/min
Loop diuretics Furosemide (Lasix) Bumetanide (Bumex) Torsemide (Demadex)	Used for HTN, edema associated with HF, renal failure, cirrhosis, hypercalcemia, pulmonary edema	Inhibits sodium and chloride reabsorption in the loop of Henle and blocks reabsorption of water	**Furosemide (Lasix)** Oral: 20–120 mg daily in one dose, or divided doses IV: 20–80 mg in one dose or divided doses; can also use continuous drip	Hyponatremia, hypochloremia, dehydration, hypotension, hypokalemia, ototoxicity, hyperglycemia, hyperuricemia, hypomagnesemia	• Can be used if GFR is low • Can be combined with a thiazide diuretic • Check BP and potassium and monitor for orthostatic hypotension • Supplement diet with potassium-rich foods • If patient is receiving digoxin, hypokalemia can predispose to digoxin toxicity • Best to give diuretics in morning and early afternoon to avoid waking up in middle of night to urinate • Monitor BUN and creatinine to avoid overdiuresis.
Potassium-sparing diuretics (nonaldosterone antagonists) Amiloride (Midamor) Triamterene (Dyrenium)	Used for HTN, edema	Inhibit sodium reabsorption at the distal convoluted tubule, decreasing water reabsorption and increasing potassium retention	**Triamterene (Dyrenium)** Oral: 100 mg twice daily	Hyperkalemia, nausea, vomiting, leg cramps, dizziness, weakness, rash, orthostatic hypotension	• Monitor for orthostatic hypotension and hyperkalemia • Use carefully and follow potassium levels if patient is also on ACEI or ARB
Potassium sparing diuretics (aldosterone antagonists) Spironaldactone (Aldactone)	Used for HTN, edema, HF, premenstrual syndrome, acne in women, PCOS, hyperaldosteronism (also classified as potassium-sparing diuretic)	Block the aldosterone-specific mineralocorticoid receptors primarily in the distal convoluted tubule; decrease sodium and water reabsorption and increases potassium retention	**Spironaldactone (Aldactone)** Oral: 25–200 mg once or in divided doses (for HTN)	Hyperkalemia, orthostatic hypotension, gynecomastia, menstrual irregularities	• Frequently combined with loop or thiazide diuretics (e.g., hydrochlorothiazide/spironolactone (Aldactazide) • Monitor for orthostatic hypotension and hyperkalemia • Use with caution with patients who are taking ARBs or ACEIs • Should not be given with potassium supplements or other potassium-sparing diuretics
Adrenergic inhibitors, central-acting alpha adrenergic agonist Clonidine (Catapres)	Used for HTN, relief of severe pain, and ADHD	Selectively activates α₂ receptors in brain stem and reduces sympathetic outflow to blood vessels and the heart	**Clonidine (Catapres)** Oral: 0.1–0.3 mg daily (dose for hypertension)	Drowsiness, xerostomia, rebound HTN, constipation, impotence, gynecomastia, vivid dreams, nightmares, anxiety, depression, headache, hypotension	• Stopping medication abruptly can lead to rebound HTN, tachycardia, headache, tremors, and sweating. • Transdermal patch can be associated with skin irritation. • Gum or hard candy for xerostomia • Increased somnolence if combined with sedatives or alcohol.

Drug	Use	Action	Dose	Adverse Effects	Nursing Considerations
α₁-Adrenergic blockers Doxazosin (Cardura) Terazosin (Hytrin)	Used to treat HTN and BPH	Nonselective alpha blockers block α_1 receptors in blood vessels, cause vasodilation and lower BP; block α receptors in bladder neck and prostate, and decrease obstruction of the urethra, increasing urine flow	**Doxazosin (Cardura)** Oral: 1–4 mg daily	Hypotension, fainting, dizziness, somnolence, nasal congestion, intraoperative floppy iris syndrome, headache, xerostomia, blurred vision, polyuria	• If patient reports orthostatic hypotension and dizziness, may want to give drug at bedtime. • Change positions slowly. • Floppy iris syndrome is a complication in men undergoing cataract surgery who are taking alpha-blockers; notify ophthalmologist if taking this medication and planning surgery. • These two drugs have greater effects on BP than tamsulosin. • These two drugs are useful in men who have HTN and BPH. • Be aware of excessive hypotension that can develop from taking these drugs with nitrates, other antihypertensive drugs, and phosphodiesterase type 5 (PDE5) inhibitors (sildenafil [Viagra]).
β₁-Adrenergic blockers, cardioselective Atenolol (Tenormin) Metoprolol (Lopressor)	Used for HTN, angina, acute MI, post-MI, HF, migraine headache prophylaxis	Selectively antagonize β_1-adrenergic receptors; block contractility in ventricles and decreases CO and oxygen demand; reduce sympathetic vasoconstrictor tone; block renin secretion	**Metoprolol (Lopressor)** Oral: 12.5–200 mg twice daily, titrate to control BP and heart rate	Bradycardia, reduced CO, AV heart block, rebound excitation if abrupt withdrawal (tachycardia and dysrhythmias), fatigue, dizziness, depression	• Check BP and pulse before administering • Tell patient to never stop abruptly; must taper dose to prevent rebound cardiac excitation • Use with caution in patients with DM; can block normal sympathetic response to hypoglycemia (tachycardia, tremors, diaphoresis) • In higher doses, can cause bronchospasm; assess patients with COPD and asthma carefully • Although these drugs are not first-line treatment for HTN, they are the drug of choice for a patient who has HTN and a history of MI and/or HF • Less effective BP reduction in African Americans;
β-Adrenergic blockers, nonselective Propranolol (Inderal) Nadolol (Corgard)	Used for HTN, angina, to prevent CV event post-MI; atrial fibrillation/flutter, SVT, migraine prophylaxis, pheochromocytoma, portal HTN, Graves' disease	Block β_1- and β_2-adrenergic receptors to decrease heart rate; block impulses through AV node; decrease ventricular contractility, so decreased CO and oxygen demand; decrease renin secretion from kidney	**Propranolol (Inderal)** Oral: 40–240 mg, two to three times daily, (maximum, 640 mg/day for HTN)	Fatigue, dizziness, bradycardia, hypotension, depression, bronchoconstriction; inhibition of glycogenolysis (by blocking β_2 receptors in liver; diabetic patient can become hypoglycemic); also blocks β_1 receptors, so normal responses to hypoglycemia—tachycardia, shakiness, and diaphoresis—are blocked and patient may be unaware of hypoglycemia	• Check HR; may need to withhold if HR and/or BP become too low • Teach diabetic patients that normal signs/symptoms of hypoglycemia (activated from the sympathetic nervous system) may be blocked • Monitor for bronchospasm in patients with COPD or asthma; may need to be switched to β_1 agent such as metoprolol (Lopressor) • Monitor for AV block • Monitor for signs/symptoms of heart failure • Taper dose to discontinue

(continued)

TABLE 9.5   (Continued)

Drug Name	Drug Type and Use	Mode of Action	Dosage	Adverse Effects	Clinical Considerations/Patient Teaching
Mixed α- and β-Blockers Carvedilol (Coreg) Labetalol (Trandate)	Mixed α₁-receptor blocker and nonselective beta-blocker used for HTN, HF, cardiovascular event prevention post-MI	Block α₁-receptors to dilate arterioles and veins and decreases SVR; block β₁-receptors to reduce heart rate and contractility (cardiac output); blocks β₁-receptors on juxta-glomerular cells to block renin release from kidneys; reduce peripheral vascular resistance	**Carvedilol (Coreg):** Oral immediate release: 6.25–25 mg twice daily Oral extended release: 20–80 mg once daily	Bradycardia, postural hypotension, AV block, depression, insomnia, sexual dysfunction, fatigue, diarrhea, weight gain, dyspnea, nausea, bronchoconstriction, masked signs of hypoglycemia, depression	• Check HR and BP before giving • Observe for AV block • Be aware that orthostatic hypotension can occur; change positions slowly • Can mask signs of hypoglycemia • Can cause bronchospasm in patients with asthma or COPD
Direct vasodilators Hydralazine (Apresoline) Nitroglycerin (Nitro-Bid)	Used for essential HTN, hypertensive crisis, angina, HF, MI	Selective dilation of arterioles; decrease peripheral resistance and BP; HR and myocardial contractility increase	**Hydralazine** Oral: 10–50 mg three or four times daily for HTN IV: 10–20 mg every 2–4 hours as needed for hypertensive crisis	Reflex tachycardia, hypotension, increased blood volume, systemic lupus erythematosus–like syndrome, headache, dizziness, weakness, fatigue	• Observe for reflex tachycardia; patient often also taking beta-blocker to prevent this • Monitor BP and HR carefully, especially if patient taking other antihypertensives • Start on low dose and titrate upward slowly • Nitroglycerin relaxes arteriole and venous smooth muscle, reduces preload and SVR
ACEIs Enalapril (Vasotec) Lisinopril (Zestril) Benazepril (Lotensin) Captopril	Used for HTN, HF, acute MI, and LV dysfunction; prevention of diabetic and nondiabetic nephropathy; prevention of MI, stroke, and death in patients at high risk of CV events	Reduce levels of angiotensin II by blocking ACE; dilates arterioles, reduces vascular resistance, reduces blood volume, and prevents damage to heart and blood vessels from angiotensin II and aldosterone	**Enalapril (Vasotec)** Oral: 10–40 mg once or twice daily (maximum, 40 mg/day for HTN	First-dose hypotension, cough, hyperkalemia, renal insufficiency in patients with renal artery stenosis, angioedema, fetal injury, dizziness, hypotension, headache, fatigue, BUN/creatinine increased	• Check BP before administering • Decreased dosage for patients with kidney disease • Not to be used in pregnancy • Aspirin and NSAIDs can reduce antihypertensive effects • Angioedema is life-threatening reaction: swelling of eyes, lips, tongue, glottis, pharynx; must seek emergency treatment and discontinue drug • Monitor for hyperkalemia and be aware of other drugs that can also increase the potassium level, such as potassium-sparing diuretics and potassium supplements
ARBs Losartan (Cozaar) Valsartan (Diovan) Candesartan (Atacand)	Used for HTN, MI, HTN, diabetic nephropathy; prevention of MI, stroke, and death in people at high risk for CV events	Block angiotensin II receptors in blood vessels, the adrenals and other tissues; promote dilation of arterioles and veins; prevent damage to the heart; decrease release of aldosterone; increase excretion of sodium and water	**Losartan (Cozaar)** Oral: 25–100 mg/day; once or divided twice daily	Angioedema, renal failure in renal artery stenosis, fetal injury, fatigue, hyperkalemia, cough	• Incidence of cough and hyperkalemia is less than with ACEIs • Check BP and potassium level before administering • Assess for angioedema • If taking with other antihypertensives may cause additive effect • Not to be used in pregnancy

Renin inhibitors Aliskiren (Tekturna)	Direct renin inhibitor used for HTN	Oral: 150–300 mg/day	Fetal harm, angioedema, cough, hypotension, hyperkalemia, elevated BUN, creatinine, diarrhea	• Not to be used in pregnancy • Assess BP, serum potassium, BUN, creatinine • Assess for angioedema and cough, although incidence is low
CCBs, non-dihydropyridines Diltiazem (Cardizem) Verapamil (Calan)	**Non-dihydropyridines** Block entry of calcium into smooth muscles of peripheral arterioles, arteries, and arterioles of the heart, resulting in vasodilation and blockade of the SA node, AV node, and decreased myocardial contractility	**Diltiazem (Cardizem)** Oral: 30–60 mg four times daily for (angina)	Hypotension, dizziness, flushing, headache, edema, HF, bradycardia, AV block, rash	• Grapefruit juice can increase level of diltiazem and verapamil • Verapamil can cause constipation. • Check HR, rhythm (if on a monitor) and BP before administering • Use with caution in patients who have HF; observe for signs and symptoms of HF • If patient is also receiving digoxin, be aware of additive effects of decreasing HR and AVN conduction. Verapamil can pre-dispose to digoxin toxicity • If a non-dihydropyridine CCB and a beta blocker are used together, there may be additive effects of decreased HR and AVN conduction
Dihydropyridines Amlodipine (Norvasc) Nifedipine (Procardia)	**Dihydropyridines** Block entry of calcium into smooth muscles of peripheral arterioles and arteries, resulting in vasodilation and decreased SVR; minimal blockade of calcium channels in the heart	**Amlodipine (Norvasc)** Oral: 5–10 mg daily; start at 2.5 mg if elderly or if this is second drug for HTN	Hypotension, dizziness, edema, HF, rash, headache, gingival hyperplasia, fatigue, nausea, vomiting	• Check BP and rhythm (if on monitor) • Monitor for peripheral edema • Monitor for relex tachycardia if taking Nifedipine

(Burchum & Rosenthal, 2016; Epocrates, 2018)

ACEI = angiotensin-converting–enzyme inhibitor; ADHD = attention-deficit/hyperactivity disorder; ARB = angiotensin-receptor blocker; BP = blood pressure; BPH = benign prostatic hyperplasia; CCB = calcium-channel blocker; CV = cardiovascular; DI = diabetes insipidus; DM = diabetes mellitus; GFR = glomerular filtration rate; HF = heart failure; HR = heart rate; HTN = hypertension; LV = left ventricular; MI = myocardial infarction; NSAIDs = nonsteroidal antiinflammatory drugs; PCOS = polycystic ovary syndrome; PDE5 = phosphodiesterase type 5; RAAS = renin–angiotensin–aldosterone system; SA = sinoatrial; SVR = systemic vascular resistance; SVT = supraventricular tachycardia.

- Left ventricle increases in size, is less compliant and can't increase cardiac output and stroke volume during exercise to meet oxygen demands.
- During exercise, maximum heart rate is decreased and patient is unable to meet oxygen demands; may have dizziness, hypotension, syncope, chest pain with exercise.
- Older adults have stiff, less-distensible arteries and aorta, so systolic blood pressure increases to compensate.
- As a result of the stiff arteries, some older adults have an auscultatory gap, noted when assessing their BP. There may be a wide gap between the first Korotkoff sound heard and subsequent sounds. If the blood pressure cuff is not sufficiently inflated, the reading may not be accurate.
- Increased blood pressure leads to increased vascular resistance and left ventricle can hypertrophy trying to empty against high resistance.
- Renal function is decreased, so excretion of drugs may be altered.
- Renin response decreases in response to hyponatremia and/or hypovolemia, so patient can become hypovolemic easily.
- Baroreceptors change with age, and the patient can't adjust blood flow/heart rate quickly with position changes; orthostatic hypotension, dizziness, and fainting may contribute to fall risk, hip fractures, and head injuries.
- Orthostatic blood pressure readings should be monitored closely.
- In elderly patients, antihypertensive medications should be started at low doses and increased slowly.
- Decreased absorption of some drugs can occur secondary to decreased blood flow to the gut.

CORONARY ARTERY DISEASE AND ACUTE CORONARY SYNDROME

Cardiovascular disease (CVD) is the major cause of death in the United States. Coronary artery disease (CAD), also referred to as coronary heart disease (CHD), is the most common type of CVD. Injury, inflammation, and lipid deposits to the endothelium contribute to the development of atherosclerosis. Without treatment, or modification of risk factors, atherosclerosis may lead to partial or complete occlusion of the coronary arteries. This can result in ischemia (decreased myocardial perfusion) or infarction (necrosis or cell death) of the myocardium. Patients may have chronic stable angina, or may experience acute coronary syndrome (ACS). ACS is caused by a rupture of an atherosclerotic lesion, which can cause unstable angina or acute myocardial infarction (AMI).

CAD/Chronic Stable Angina

▌ Risk factors/etiology:
- Nonmodifiable:
  - Age
  - Gender—more common in men before age 75
  - Ethnicity—more common in white men
  - Family history/genetics
- Modifiable:
  - Elevated serum lipids
  - Hypertension
  - Tobacco
  - Physical inactivity
  - Obesity
  - Diabetes
  - Metabolic syndrome
  - Psychologic state

- Substance abuse
- Homocysteine—high levels associated with risk for CAD and CVD

Assessment/Interventions/Education

▶ Clinical manifestations:

- Angina—caused by atherosclerosis and myocardial ischemia; usually caused by >70% stenosis of coronary artery:
  - Chronic stable angina:
    - Pain, heaviness, pressure, discomfort in the chest
    - Radiation
    - Back pain
    - Burning/epigastric pain or discomfort
    - Similar, predictable pattern of onset, duration, intensity
    - Lasts for few minutes
    - Goes away when cause is removed (e.g., patient stops walking up the stairs)
    - Responds to nitroglycerin or rest
    - Controlled with medications, risk factor modification, and outpatient care
  - Prinzmetal angina—variant angina:
    - Occurs at rest
    - Due to coronary artery spasm—ST/T-wave changes with the pain
    - Increased demand or tobacco, smoke, alcohol, or cocaine use
    - Pain relieved with moderate exercise, with nitroglycerin, or spontaneously
    - Avoid precipitating factors, use CCBs and/or nitrates to control pain
  - Microvascular angina:
    - Common in postmenopausal women
    - No significant CAD or spasm of major coronary arteries
    - Ischemia from atherosclerosis or spasm of the small blood vessels in the microcirculation of the myocardium
    - Brought on by physical exertion and may have positive stress tests
    - Treatment is risk-factor modification and same as for CAD
  - Silent angina:
    - No symptoms
    - Often in diabetics secondary to neuropathy
    - ECG evidence of ischemia
  - Atypical angina:
    - Women, older adults, diabetics
    - Dyspnea, nausea, fatigue, epigastric discomfort, back pain, weakness

Question	Rationale
A patient is admitted with a diagnosis of acute MI. The nurse is aware that the following signs and symptoms indicate that the patient may be having an acute MI: A. Pain in the chest that worsens with deep breaths and movement. B. Discomfort in the epigastric area that is relieved with an antacid and belching. C. Severe, crushing chest pain that does not change and has been present for 30 minutes. D. Pain in the distal left arm with tingling in the hand that began when the patient awoke from sleeping.	Answer: C This is the classic presentation of chest pain that may occur with acute MI. Pain that worsens with deep breaths is probably pleuritic in origin. If the patient was able to obtain relief with antacid therapy and belching, the problem is probably gastrointestinal. Pain in the arm on awakening is likely related to positioning during sleep. A thorough assessment of the pain and associated symptoms would be critical.

▶ Diagnosis—establish diagnosis and rule out ACS:

- History and physical exam
- ECG
- Chest x-ray
- Stress test
- Coronary angiography
- Echocardiogram
- Cardiac troponin
- Lipid panel
- Basic metabolic panel (BMP)
- Homocysteine/C-reactive protein (CRP)

▶ Nursing diagnosis:

- Activity intolerance related to chest pain
- Anxiety related to situational crisis
- Ineffective denial related to deficient knowledge of need to seek help with symptoms

▶ Treatment (Table 9.5):

- Short-acting nitrates—Sublingual nitroglycerin (SL NTG) or translingual spray to prevent or treat angina:
  - Venodilation; decreases venous return to the heart and preload and oxygen demand; dilation of coronary arteries and collateral vessels
  - Check vital signs before and after administration of SL NTG
  - Can cause headache, hypotension, reflex tachycardia
  - SL NTG can be given every 5 minutes for maximum of three doses; if symptoms persist, contact provider/emergency medical services (EMS)
- Long-acting nitrates—isosorbide dinitrate (Isordil) (oral); Nitropaste; transdermal NTG patch
  - Same action as short-acting nitrates
  - Can cause headache, hypotension, reflex tachycardia
  - Do not withdraw abruptly
- Beta-adrenergic blockers—metoprolol (Lopressor), carvedilol (Coreg) used to prevent angina
- Calcium-channel blockers—dihydropyridines such as amlodipine (Norvasc) or non-dihydropyridines such as diltiazem (Cardizem) and verapamil (Calan):
  - Can be used to treat stable and variant angina (coronary artery spasm)
- Sodium current inhibitor—ranolazine (Ranexa); approved as first-line drug for chronic angina; can be combined with nitrates, beta-blockers, amlodipine:
  - Reduces accumulation of sodium and calcium in myocardial cells
  - Side effects include constipation, dizziness, nausea, headache, renal failure, prolonged QT interval
  - Contraindicated in hepatic impairment and in patients with prolonged QT interval
- Lipid-lowering drugs—starting at age 20, lipid profile should be assessed every 5 years; starting at age 40, formal estimation of the absolute 10-year risk for atherosclerotic CVD is to be initiated and evaluated every 4 to 6 years (Goff et al., 2013)
  - Drug therapy for hyperlipidemia (Table 9.6)

Clinical Consideration

NTG tablets must be stored at room temperature and in the original bottle to maintain potency.

TABLE 9.6	DRUGS USED TO TREAT HYPERLIPIDEMIA

Drug	Action		Side Effects	Patient teaching-Critical thinking
Statins: HMG-CoA Reductase Inhibitors (first line in lipid management)				
Atorvastatin (Lipitor) Lovastatin (Mevacor) Pravastatin (Pravachol) Simvastatin (Zocor) Rosuvastatin (Crestor)	• Increases number of liver receptors to remove LDL from blood • Decreases HMG-CoA reductase to decrease production of cholesterol • Decreases production of VLDL and TGs • Increases HDL • Slows progression of atherosclerotic CVD and decreases risk of stroke, cardiac disease, PAD, and death		• Myopathy • Rhabdomyolysis • Hepatotoxicity • Rash • GI disturbances	• Takes 4–6 weeks for maximal effect • Lifelong treatment • Not used in pregnancy • Cholesterol synthesis increases during the night, most effective if given in the evening • Avoid grapefruit/grapefruit juice • Usually will check CK and LFTs before starting drug. • If muscle pain or clinical signs or symptoms of liver disease occur, health care provider will reassess CPK and LFT levels • If combined with other cholesterol lowering drugs (not bile acid sequestrants), may develop more side effects
Nicotinic Acid				
Niacin	• Increases HDL • Inhibits synthesis of TG • Decreases LDL and VLDL	• Flushing • GI upset • Liver injury • Can elevate uric acid		• Flushing and liver injury are decreased with Niaspan (extended release) • Flushing can be decreased by taking aspirin 325 mg or NSAID 30 minutes before each dose • Take with food • Can be used with statin and bile acid sequestrant if necessary to lower cholesterol further • Assess liver enzymes before and during treatment
Folic Acid Derivatives (Fibrates)				
Gemfibrozil (Lopid) Fenofibrate (Tricor)	• Decreases TG • Increases HDL • Little to no effect on HDL	• Rashes • GI disturbances • Gallstones • Liver toxicity		• Increases risk of rhabdomyolysis in those taking statins • Must report signs of muscle injury, weakness, pain • Increases risk of bleeding in those taking warfarin (Coumadin) • Third-line drugs for managing lipid disorders
Omega-3 Fatty Acids				
Omega-3 acid ethyl esters (Lovaza) Icosapent ethyl (Vascepa)	• Decreases TG	• GI disturbances • Taste changes • Pruritus, rash • Arthralgia • Bleeding		• Can prolong bleeding time and cause bleeding: caution if taking antiplatelet or anticoagulant drugs • No evidence that these will decrease CVD • May contain fish oil with environmental contaminants (mercury, etc.)
Bile-Acid Sequestrants				
Cholestyramine (Prevalite) Colesevelam (Welchol)	• Promotes bile-acid absorption and then increases LDL receptors • Decreases LDL • Can control hyperglycemia in type 2 diabetes	• GI disturbances (bloating, constipation)		• Used as adjuncts to statins • Can interfere with absorption of some drugs such as warfarin, some antibiotics, digoxin, thiazide diuretics; give 1 hour before or 4 hours after the sequestrant • Maximal effect in 1 month
PCSK9 Inhibitors				
Alirocumab (Praluent) Evolocumab (Repatha)	• Monoclonal antibody • Inhibits PCSK9 from binding to LDL receptor and lowers LDL levels	• Injection-site reactions • Nasopharyngitis • Musculoskeletal pain • Myalgia • Increased ALT/AST • Flu-like symptoms		• Used by those with familial hypercholesterolemia and those who are intolerant to statins • Can be used by those who are not responding to statins alone • Subcutaneous injection every 2 weeks

(continued)

TABLE 9.6 *(Continued)*

Drug	Action	Side Effects	Patient teaching-Critical thinking
Cholesterol Absorption Inhibitor			
Ezetimibe (Zetia)	• Inhibits absorption of cholesterol • Lowers LDL and TG and has small effect on HDL	• Myopathy • Rhabdomyolysis • Hepatitis • Thrombocytopenia • Increased risk of gallstones	• Can be used with statin, but may increase risk of liver injury • Patients with moderate to severe liver impairment should not be given this drug.
(Burcham & Rosenthal, 2016; Epocrates, 2018)			

ALT = alanine aminotransferase; AST = aspartate aminotransferase; CK = creatine kinase; CVD = cardiovascular disease; GI = gastrointestinal; HDL = high-density lipoprotein; HMG-CoA = 3-hydroxy-3-methylglutaryl coenzyme A; LDL = low-density lipoprotein; LFT = liver-function test; PAD = peripheral arterial disease; PCSK9 = proprotein convertase subtilisin/keksin type 9; TG = triglyceride; VLDL = very-low-density lipoprotein.

- Antiplatelet therapy—aspirin, clopidogrel (Plavix):
  - Recommended for most people who are at risk for CVD, those with chronic and unstable angina, and those who have had an MI or undergone stent placement
  - Risk for bleeding; discuss with provider the risks/benefits of taking aspirin
  - Currently no evidence to support low-dose aspirin use in those less than 50 years old or older than 70 (Bibbins-Domingo, 2016)
- ACEIs—Lisinopril (Zestril) (Table 9.5)
- Cardiac catheterization—determine whether patient is a candidate for revascularization:
  - Balloon angioplasty with stent (expandable mesh-like device placed in the vessel to keep it open after the angioplasty); can be bare stent or drug-eluting stent (DES) (coated with a drug)
  - Drugs used during procedure to prevent platelet aggregation and thrombosis of the stent:
    - Unfractionated heparin (UH), heparin:
      - Acts at multiple sites in coagulation process; binds to antithrombin III, inactivating thrombin and other clotting factors
    - Low-molecular-weight heparin (LMWH); enoxaparin (Lovenox):
      - Binds to antithrombin III and selectively inhibits factor Xa, prevents conversion of fibrinogen to fibrin
    - Direct thrombin inhibitor: bivalirudin (Angiomax); argatroban:
      - Inhibits thrombin formation
    - Glycoprotein IIb/IIIa inhibitors: abciximab (ReoPro); eptifibatide (Integrilin); tirofiban (Aggrastat):
      - Binds to platelet glycoprotein IIb/IIIa receptors to reduce platelet aggregation
  - Single or dual antiplatelet therapy with aspirin and/or clopidogrel (Plavix) to prevent restenosis for a year or longer
  - Potential complications during/after coronary catheterization and PCI:
    - Acute stent thrombosis
    - Coronary artery dissection
    - Femoral or radial artery injury
    - Extension of acute MI

- - Stent embolization
  - Coronary artery spasm
  - Retroperitoneal bleeding
  - Stroke
  - Reaction to dye
  - Acute kidney injury
- Monitoring patient post-PCI:
  - Maintain bed rest with straight extremity per agency protocol
  - Assess insertion site, neurovascular assessment of involved extremity, vital signs, heart rhythm, urine output
  - Monitor for signs/symptoms of stent thrombosis—chest pain, change in vital signs, dysrhythmias
  - Monitor IV infusions of antiplatelet and anticoagulant medications
  - Patient must understand importance of taking antiplatelet medications as directed
- Coronary surgical revascularization:
  - If medical treatment has not worked
  - Patients who are not candidates for PCI:
    - Complicated lesions
    - More than three different coronary artery occlusions
    - Left main coronary artery lesion
  - May have minimally invasive procedures that avoid sternotomy and generally have faster recovery time:
    - Not everyone is a candidate for these procedures
    - MidCab (minimally invasive direct coronary artery bypass) beating heart surgery; a mini-thoracotomy is performed
    - OPCAB (off-pump coronary bypass) using median sternotomy
    - TECAB (totally endoscopic coronary bypass) surgery with smaller incisions, decreased blood loss, less pain, shorter recovery time
    - Laser revascularization
  - Traditional coronary artery bypass surgery
  - Go to intensive-care unit (ICU) after surgery
  - Assess for and prevent complications:
    - Bleeding:
      - Observe and care for all incisions
    - Venous thromboembolism (VTE):
      - Sequential compression devices
      - Manage pain to allow for early ambulation
    - Dysrhythmias—especially atrial fibrillation:
      - Beta-blockers, calcium channel blockers
      - Patient may need anticoagulation
    - Fluid and electrolyte shifts
    - Postoperative cognitive dysfunction
    - Respiratory complications:
      - Ensure adequate pain management
      - Early ambulation
      - Incentive spirometer
      - Splinting, coughing, deep breathing

Clinical Consideration

Antiplatelet medication(s) are necessary to prevent stent thrombosis.

ACUTE CORONARY SYNDROME (ACS)

Predisposing Factors/Etiology

- Risk factors for CAD
- Most MIs occur in setting of preexisting CAD
- Caused by previously stable atherosclerotic plaque rupture, which causes platelet aggregation and thrombus with partial or complete obstruction of the coronary artery
- Prolonged and not immediately reversible—ACS develops
- Can be one of these three:
  - Unstable angina (UA)—partial obstruction of coronary artery
    - Pain is new, occurs at rest, lasts longer, occurs more often, and/or is not relieved with usual measures.
  - Non-ST-segment elevation myocardial infarction (NSTEMI); sometimes called non-ST-segment elevation ACS—partial obstruction of coronary artery
  - ST-segment-elevation myocardial infarction (STEMI), or ST-segment-elevation ACS—complete obstruction of coronary artery:
    - Irreversible heart damage and necrosis after 20 minutes of ischemia and if reperfusion does not occur
    - New ECG changes when compared to previous ECG

Assessment/Interventions/Education

- ▶ Clinical manifestations:
  - MIs:
    - Chest pain comes on at rest, with activity, or while asleep; not relieved by rest, position change, nitrate administration
    - Heavy, pressure, tight, burning, crushing substernal with radiation
    - Discomfort, weakness, fatigue, indigestion
    - Ashen clammy, cool to touch, increased HR
    - Observe for signs/symptoms of HF or pulmonary edema
    - New murmur can be from papillary muscle rupture or valvular dysfunction
    - Nausea/vomiting
    - Low-grade fever
    - Denial
    - Most MIs located in LV and described by the location of the heart damage (e.g., posterior, lateral, inferior, anterior)
    - ECG changes indicate the location of the MI and which coronary artery is affected:
      - Possible complications of MI:
        - Depend on the area of the heart involved, size of the infarction, and amount of collateral circulation
        - Dysrhythmias; ventricular tachycardia and/or fibrillation most common cause of death in pre-hospital period
        - Heart failure
        - Cardiogenic shock
        - Papillary muscle dysfunction or rupture
        - Septal or LV free-wall rupture
        - Pericarditis; Dressler syndrome
  - Unstable angina (UA):
    - Pain is new, occurs at rest, lasts longer, occurs more often, is unpredictable, and/or is not relieved with usual measures.
    - May be first sign of CAD

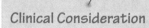

Clinical Consideration

Teach patients to call EMS when having chest pain or sign/symptoms of MI in case of dysrhythmias and hemodynamic instability.

- Lasts longer than 10 minutes
- May/may not have ECG changes
- Troponins will be negative
- Women often present with symptoms of UA: fatigue, shortness of breath, indigestion, anxiety
  - Underrecognized
  - Attributed to other things
- NSTEMI:
  - See "Clinical manifestations" of MI
  - No ST-segment elevation
  - May/may not have ST/T-wave changes on 12-lead ECG
  - Patient reports chest pain that has lasted for more than 10 minutes
  - Hard to distinguish between UA and NSTEMI until troponins are measured
  - Troponins positive for myocardial injury
  - Thrombolytic therapy not indicated
  - Patient should be brought to the catheterization lab within 12 to 72 hours after presentation; no need for emergency catheterization
- STEMI:
  - See "Clinical manifestations" of MI
  - ST-segment elevation on ECG in leads facing the damaged wall
  - Complete obstruction of coronary artery with thrombus and necrosis will occur if perfusion is not restored
  - Medical emergency
  - To limit infarct size and tissue death, the artery must be opened within 90 minutes after presentation:
    - PCI
    - Fibrinolytic (thrombolytic) therapy
- Diagnosis:
  - ECG changes (see above)—obtain serial ECGs to track changes
  - Serial cardiac troponins I and T (biomarkers)—three times, every 6 hours
  - Cardiac catheterization:
    - STEMI—within 90 minutes after presentation
    - NSTEMI—within 12 to 72 hours after presentation
    - UA—may or may not go to catheterization lab
  - Pharmacologic stress testing perhaps for UA patient
- Nursing diagnosis:
  - Activity intolerance related to imbalance between oxygen supply and demand
  - Denial related to fear, deficient knowledge about heart disease
- Treatment:
  - STEMI/NSTEMI/UA:
    - Time is critical when treating patient with STEMI.
    - Patient with STEMI/NSTEMI/UA should seek emergency treatment—call 911.
    - Assess circulation, airway, breathing.
    - Oxygen, 12-lead ECG, aspirin (unless contraindicated), NTG SL, morphine.
    - Patient/family teaching; offer reassurance, emotional support.
    - PCI with bare stent or DES:
      - Started on antiplatelet, anticoagulant therapy
    - If not at PCI-capable hospital, patient with STEMI may receive thrombolytic therapy (tissue plasminogen activator [t-PA, alteplase]) to lyse the clot and reduce infarct size

- ECG has to show acute STEMI.
- Onset of chest pain less than 12 hours ago
- Patient must not have any absolute contraindications for thrombolytic therapy
- Oral beta-blocker will be added within first 24 hours unless contraindicated
- ACEI may be added for patients with ejection fraction (EF) <40%; ARB can be used if can't tolerate ACEI
- Antidysrhythmia medication, if needed
- Lipid-lowering medications, if appropriate
- Stool softeners
- Cardiac rehabilitation
- Be aware of possible psychosocial responses to ACS:
  - Denial, depression anger, hostility, anxiety, fear, dependency, acceptance
  - Support patient and family coping strategies
- Ongoing monitoring for repeat episodes of chest pain

Geriatric Considerations: Coronary Artery Disease

▶ Older adults may have "atypical" signs and symptoms of ACS. They may report dyspnea, fatigue, indigestion, dizziness, and weakness. They may have experienced a fall or mental status changes.

▶ Don't give up on the elderly—risk-factor modification is possible.

▶ The older adult is more sensitive to salt, so suggesting salt reduction may help decrease blood pressure and fluid retention.

▶ Older adults typically need longer warm-up periods, longer rest periods, and paced activities.

▶ Activity, and the socialization that comes with some kinds of activities, increases sense of well-being, self-esteem, and self-image.

▶ Older adults should be taught how to check their heart rate and what their limits and maximum HR should be with exercise.

▶ Older adults should be reminded that they may overheat more easily because of a decreased ability to sweat.

▶ Older adults generally tolerate elective coronary-artery bypass graft (CABG) surgery well, but they have more postoperative complications such as infection, stroke, dysrhythmias, and postoperative cognitive dysfunction.

▶ Older adults may have a longer recovery post-MI or postsurgery, requiring care in a rehabilitation setting before being able to return home.

HEART FAILURE

Heart failure (HF) is the leading cause of hospital admissions in adults over age 65. As the population ages, the prevalence of heart failure continues to rise, even though the prevalence of other CVDs has decreased (Benjamin et al., 2018). It is a complex chronic illness that results from the inability of the heart to eject enough oxygenated blood to meet the needs of organs and tissues.

Ejection fraction (EF) refers to the amount of blood that is ejected (measured as a percentage) by the left ventricle with each beat. Heart failure with reduced EF (HFrEF) refers to systolic heart failure. Heart failure with preserved EF (HFpEF) refers to diastolic heart failure (Yancey et al., 2013).

▶ Pathophysiology
  - Left-sided HF—most common form:
    - Systolic HF or HF with reduced ejection fraction (HFrEF)—heart can't pump blood effectively possibly due to: increased afterload (HTN); valve abnormalities; and/or decreased contractility (MI)

- Normal EF: 55 to 60%
- Systolic HF–EF <45%
- Heart dilates and hypertrophies because of decreased stroke volume, and blood backs up
- Increased LV volume and LV end diastolic pressure (preload)
- Leads to increased pressure in LA and blood backs up in lungs
- Increased pulmonary hydrostatic pressure pushes fluid into the interstitium and alveoli
- Diastolic failure or HFpEF—stiff ventricles cannot relax during diastole and cannot fill
  - Common in women, diabetics, elderly and obese individuals.
  - Ventricle can't fill during diastole due to inability to stretch, so there is decreased SV (amount of blood that the heart ejects with each beat, in milliliters) and decreased CO.
  - EF remains normal because the percentage of total amount of blood ejected from ventricle remains the same.
  - Patient exhibits signs and symptoms of heart failure.
- Mixed diastolic and systolic heart failure—as in dilated cardiomyopathy (DCM):
  - Low EF—ventricle can't eject blood (systolic HF)
  - Ventricle is dilated and unable to fill (diastolic HF)
- Right-sided heart failure
  - RV fails due to left-sided heart failure—fluid from LV backs up into pulmonary circuit, increases pressures in the lungs and RV fails from trying to push blood into high-pressure pulmonary circuit; increased workload and RV fails:
    - COPD is another common cause of right-sided HF.
- Compensation:
  - HF can be acute or chronic
  - Heart tries to compensate for chronic decreased CO through dilation and hypertrophy and activation of the RAAS and the sympathetic nervous system.
  - CO = SV × HR
  - Heart failure can be made worse by anything that alters mechanisms that control cardiac output (e.g., increased preload, increased afterload, tachycardia, bradycardia)
  - When CO drops, heart uses compensatory mechanisms to try to maintain adequate SV
  - These compensatory mechanisms help for a while, but then become maladaptive and eventually fail:
    - RAAS:
      - Aldosterone—sodium and water retention
      - Antidiuretic hormone (ADH)—water retention
      - Endothelin—vasoconstriction and hypertrophy (remodeling) of myocardial cells
      - Proinflammatory cytokines—hypertrophy and cell death
    - SNS:
      - Epinephrine—increased HR
      - Norepinephrine—vasoconstriction
      - Increase contractility and CO initially, eventually become maladaptive and increase O_2 demand
    - Remodeling—increased ventricular muscle size:
      - RAAS and SNS increase LV workload and cause the ventricle to enlarge; its ineffective pumping leads to increased O_2 demand:

- Can contribute to development of life-threatening dysrhythmias
- Stasis of blood
- Dilation—enlargement of the chambers of the heart

▶ Risk factors/etiology:
- Primary causes:
  - CAD and HTN most common
  - Rheumatic heart disease
  - Valvular heart disease
  - Congenital heart defects (ventricular septal defect [VSD])
  - Pulmonary hypertension (PH)
  - Cardiomyopathy (e.g., viral, substance abuse)
  - Hyperthyroidism
  - Myocarditis
- Conditions that can increase the workload of the heart:
  - Anemia
  - Hypothyroidism/hyperthyroidism
  - Infection
  - Dysrhythmias
  - Endocarditis
  - Obstructive sleep apnea (OSA)
  - Pulmonary embolism
  - Paget disease
  - Nutritional deficiencies
  - Hypervolemia

(Yancey et al., 2013)

Assessment/Interventions/Education

▶ Clinical manifestations
- Acute decompensated HF—signs and symptoms of systemic and pulmonary congestion requiring hospitalization; patient may display:
  - Tachypnea
  - Hypoxemia, perhaps respiratory acidosis
  - Pulmonary edema
    - Orthopnea
    - Jugular venous distention (JVD)
    - Anxious
    - Pale, cool, clammy skin
    - Wheezing, coughing, blood tinged sputum
    - Tachycardia
    - Can show signs of decreased perfusion to other organs: altered mental status, decreased urine output, hypotension; can progress to shock
- Chronic HF:
  - Ventricular remodeling:
    - Right-sided heart failure:
      - Symptoms:
        - Fatigue
        - Right-upper-quadrant pain
        - Fullness, loss of appetite

Clinical Consideration

Increased pulmonary hydrostatic pressure causes capillaries to break and stain the sputum red, orange, or pink.

- Nausea
- Palpitations (dysrhythmias)
  - Physical assessment findings:
    - Weakness, fatigue
    - Edema
    - Chronic changes in legs: thick brown, dry skin; ulcers
    - Weight gain
    - Ascites
    - JVD
    - Anasarca
    - Hepatomegaly
- Left-sided heart failure:
  - Symptoms:
    - Weakness, fatigue
    - Dyspnea
    - Shallow respirations, tachypnea
    - Paroxysmal nocturnal dyspnea
    - Orthopnea
    - Nocturia
  - Physical assessment findings:
    - Tachypnea
    - Tachycardia
    - Point of maximal impulse (PMI) displaced to the left of the midclavicular line due to hypertrophy of ventricle, heart
    - S3 and/or S4 heart sounds
    - Altered mental status
    - Crackles
    - Pleural effusion
    - Hypoxemia
- Complications of HF:
  - Pleural effusion
  - Dysrhythmias:
    - Atrial fibrillation—prevalence increases with severity of heart failure
    - Ventricular dysrhythmias—ventricular tachycardia, ventricular fibrillation; cause of sudden cardiac death (SCD)
  - LV thrombus—due to dilated LV and/or presence of atrial fibrillation; stroke risk increased
  - Hepatomegaly—due to RV failure and backup to liver
  - Renal failure—decreased CO to kidneys

▶ Diagnosis:
- Patient history and physical exam
- Patient placed in New York Heart Association (NYHA) functional guideline class I to IV, based on tolerance of activity (e.g., NYHA III)
- ACC/AHA also developed a staging system that also suggests treatment strategies based on the stage of disease (Yancy et al., 2013) (Table 9.7)
- Complete blood count (CBC)
- CMP
- Albumin
- Thyroid-stimulating hormone (TSH; thyrotropin)

TABLE 9.7	COMPARISON OF ACCF/AHA STAGES OF HEART FAILURE AND NYHA FUNCTIONAL CLASSIFICATION
ACCF/AHA Stages of Heart Failure (HF)	**NYHA Functional Classifications**
A. At high risk for HF, but without structural heart disease or symptoms of heart failure	No equivalent
B. Structural heart disease but without signs or symptoms of HF	I. No limitation of physical activity; ordinary physical activity does not cause symptoms of HF
C. Structural heart disease with prior or current symptoms of HF	I. No limitation of physical activity; ordinary physical activity does not cause symptoms of HF
	II. Slight limitation of physical activity. Comfortable at rest, but ordinary physical activity results in symptoms of HF
	III. Marked limitation of physical activity; comfortable at rest, but less than ordinary activity causes symptoms of HF
	IV. Unable to carry on any physical activity without symptoms of HF or experiences symptoms of HF at rest
D. Refractory HF requiring specialized interventions	IV. Unable to carry on any physical activity without symptoms of HF or experiences symptoms of HF at rest
	(Yancy et al., 2013)

ACCF = American College of Cardiology Foundation; AHA = American Heart Association; HF = heart failure; NYHA = New York Heart Association.

- Liver-function test (LFT)
- ECG
- Echocardiogram:
  - EF
  - To determine if HFpEF or HFrEF
- Chest x-ray
- BNP
- Troponins
- May order the following to further assess underlying cause for HF:
  - MUGA scan
  - Stress test
  - Cardiac catheterization
  - Testing for OSA

▶ Nursing diagnosis:
- Decreased cardiac output related to impaired cardiac function, increased preload, decreased contractility, and increased afterload
- Fatigue related to disease process with decreased cardiac output

▶ Treatment:
- Patients with acute decompensated HF (ADHF) may be admitted to ICU.
- Patients with compensated HF admitted to telemetry floor.
  - Oxygen as needed
  - Intake and output, daily weights
  - Frequent vital signs, pulse oximetry
  - Frequent assessment
  - Assessment for signs/symptoms of chest pain
  - Ultrafiltration or hemodialysis to remove extra fluid

Clinical Consideration

It is important to rule out myocardial ischemia as possible cause for worsening heart failure.

- Fluid restriction
- Low-sodium diet
- VTE prophylaxis
- Assist patient in reducing anxiety
- Diuretics, ACEIs, beta-blockers, antiplatelet or anticoagulant therapy as guided by specific patient comorbidities

▶ Goals for treatment of chronic HF:

- Treat underlying cause
- Maximize CO and improve ventricular function
- Reduce symptoms
- Improve quality of life
- Reduce morbidity and mortality

- Drug therapy for chronic heart failure (Table 9.5)

  - Diuretics—furosemide (Lasix), bumetanide (Bumex)—loop diuretics; hydrochlorothiazide—thiazide diuretic
  - ACEIs—lisinopril (Zestril)
  - ARBs—losartan (Cozaar); valsartan (Diovan)
  - Beta-adrenergic blockers—metoprolol succinate (Toprol XL)—β_1-adrenergic blocker; carvedilol (Coreg)—nonselective beta-adrenergic blocker and vasodilator
  - Aldosterone antagonists—eplerenone (Inspra); spironolactone (Aldactone)
  - Vasodilators—nitrates: isosorbide dinitrate (Isordil); nitroglycerin transdermal (Nitrodur)
  - Positive inotropes—digoxin (Lanoxin); milrinone (Primacor); dobutamine (Dobutrex):
    - Digoxin increases contractility and increases O_2 consumption; blocks at the AVN and decreases HR. May be used in patients with atrial fibrillation for rate control.
    - Assess rhythm, HR, serum potassium, calcium, magnesium, renal and liver function, and digoxin level before administering. Must withhold if patient has AV block or bradycardia. Patients with liver and kidney disease may not be able to metabolize and eliminate digoxin. Observe for possible signs/symptoms of digoxin toxicity: nausea, vomiting, dysrhythmias, visual disturbances, abdominal pain, anorexia, diarrhea.
    - Milrinone or dobutamine can be given only via IV infusion and are to be used for a short time for treatment of ADHF. They are administered in step-down ICU or in ICU:
      - Milrinone increases CO and reduces afterload.
      - Dobutamine is a selective beta agonist and increases LV contractility; can cause dysrhythmias, tachycardia.
  - Cardiac sinus node inhibitor—ivabradine (Corlanor)
    - Inhibits sinus node and reduces heart rate; must be in sinus rhythm with resting HR of at least 70 beats/min and taking maximally tolerated doses of beta blockers.
    - Check HR, rhythm, BP before taking; bradycardia, hypertension, atrial fibrillation, vision disturbances are common. Notify health care provider (HCP) if dyspnea, palpitations, chest pressure.
  - Angiotensin II receptor blocker/neprilysin inhibitor—sacubitril/valsartan (Entresto):
    - Sacubitril inhibits neprilysin, decreasing atrial and brain natriuretic peptide (ANP and BNP) breakdown; this allows more ANP and BNP to be available to lower the BP and decrease sodium and water retention; valsartan blocks angiotensin II receptors, decreasing afterload and aldosterone secretion
    - Assess BP, serum potassium, BUN/creatinine. Side effects are hyperkalemia, hypotension, dizziness, cough, increasing BUN/creatinine

Clinical Consideration

Nitrates should not be used by patients who also take phosphodiesterase inhibitors [sildenafil (Viagra), and tadalafil (Cialis)] due to additive effects and severe hypotension

▶ Other treatments for chronic HF:
- Supplemental oxygen
- Low-sodium diet, maybe fluid restriction
- Rest and energy conservation
- Cardiac rehabilitation program
- Cardio Mems—device implanted to measure pulmonary pressures; wirelessly notifies HCP of worsening HF (Abraham et al., 2011)
- Implantable cardioverter–defibrillator (ICD) therapy for those with EF <35% (at risk for sudden cardiac arrest [SCA] and/or SCD); or external defibrillator vest
- Cardiac resynchronization therapy (CRT)—biventricular pacing to coordinate contractions and improve CO (Yancy et al., 2013)
- Ventricular assist device (VAD)—may be bridge to transplantation or may be destination therapy
- Heart transplantation
- Palliative care for management of symptoms and to increase quality of life
- Hospice care if death is expected within 6 months

▶ Patient teaching:
- Keep schedule as to when device (pacemakers, etc.) appointments and all health assessments are necessary
- Balance rest with activity
- Increase activity gradually, monitoring for excessive fatigue and dyspnea
- Avoid extremes of temperature
- Low-salt diet
- Small, frequent meals
- Daily weight; notify HCP if gain of 3 lb in 2 days or 3 to 5 lb in a week
- Cardiac rehabilitation program
- Notify if excessive fatigue, limitation of activities, cough, edema, dyspnea, chest pain
- Risk-factor reduction: weight, BP, lipid, management; tobacco cessation
- Medication management:
  - Take drugs per HCP instructions
  - Know actions and side effects of medications
  - Know what side effects to report to HCP
  - Learn to take BP and pulse and know target ranges for both
  - Recognize signs and symptoms of orthostatic hypotension and how to prevent
  - If taking anticoagulants, know signs/symptoms of bleeding and when to notify HCP. If taking warfarin (Coumadin), know the target range for your international normalized ratio (INR) and how often to have blood drawn.

Question	Rationale
The nurse is assessing a patient admitted with pulmonary hypertension. The patient would likely demonstrate which of the following physical assessment findings of right-sided heart failure? A. Cyanosis, frothy sputum B. Edema of the extremities and JVD C. Paroxysmal nocturnal dyspnea and tachycardia D. A systolic aortic murmur and tachycardia	Answer: B The right side of the heart is trying to empty against high resistance in the pulmonary circuit. The right ventricle may hypertrophy and become an ineffective pump. The pressure is reflected backward. Signs of backup of blood to the periphery, edema, and JVD can develop. Cyanosis, frothy sputum, paroxysmal nocturnal dyspnea and tachycardia are signs/symptoms of left-sided heart failure. A systolic aortic murmur may occur in aortic stenosis.

INFLAMMATORY CONDITIONS OF THE HEART

Infective Endocarditis (IE)

▶ Infection of the endocardial (innermost) layer of the heart and heart valves:

- Classification based on the cause (e.g., bacterial) or site of infection
- Aortic and mitral are most common valves infected
- Vegetations on the valves can embolize:
  - Aortic- or mitral-valve vegetation can embolize to brain, kidneys, spleen, extremities.
  - Pulmonic or tricuspid-valve vegetation can embolize to lungs.

▶ Risk factors/etiology:

- Most common causative organisms: *Staphylococcus aureus* and *Streptococcus viridans*—bacteria
- Most common causes:
  - Aging and calcified aortic stenosis
  - IVDA (IV drug abuse)
  - Prosthetic valves
  - Intravascular devices—(e.g., hospital-acquired infection [HAI]; methicillin-resistant *Staphylococcus aureus* [MRSA] bacteremia)
  - Renal dialysis
- Other causes:
  - Dental, urologic, surgical, gynecologic procedures
  - Funguses, viruses
  - History of endocarditis
  - Acquired valve disease (e.g., mitral-valve prolapse)
  - Pacemakers
  - Marfan syndrome
  - Cardiomyopathy
  - Heart abnormalities (e.g., atrial septal defect [ASD])
  - Congenital heart disease

Assessment/Interventions/Education

▶ Medical history:

- See Causes above
- Fever, chills, fatigue, weakness, anorexia, joint/muscle aches, headache

▶ Clinical manifestations:

- Splinter hemorrhages in nail beds (black streaks)
- Petechiae on lips, conjunctivae, buccal mucosa, ankles, feet, antecubital areas
- Osler's nodes—red, purple, painful, pea-sized lesions may be seen on fingertips or toes
- Janeway lesions—flat, painless small, red spots perhaps on fingertips, palms, soles of feet, and toes
- Roth spots—retinal hemorrhages noted in eye exam
- Aortic or mitral systolic murmur
- Perhaps HF
- Left-upper-quadrant (LUQ) pain secondary to splenomegaly and pain in flank secondary to embolization to kidney
- Ischemia and gangrene in extremities due to embolization
- Embolization to brain can cause signs/symptoms of a stroke
- Embolization to lungs can cause pulmonary embolus

▶ Diagnosis:
- History and physical exam
- Blood cultures—identify causative organism
- Echocardiogram/TEE—may show chamber enlargement, valvular dysfunction, and vegetations
- ECG
- Possibly cardiac catheterization to assess valve function

▶ Nursing diagnosis:
- Decreased cardiac output related to inflammation of lining of heart and valve leaflets and change in structure and function of valve leaflets

▶ Treatment:
- IV antibiotics guided by results of blood cultures—often for 4 to 6 weeks
- Repeat blood cultures to ensure appropriateness of antibiotics
- If valve damage is severe/life-threatening, the patient may have to undergo valve replacement
- Balance rest with activity
- Treat signs/symptoms of HF
- May need anticoagulation

▶ Patient teaching:
- Treatment of fever
- Reduce risk of reinfection—avoid sick contacts
- Early treatment of other infections
- Notify HCP of signs/symptoms of infection
- Oral hygiene and regular dental visits
- Prophylactic antibiotic therapy before certain invasive procedures:
  - Dental procedures and other select procedures/some surgeries

Acute pericarditis

▶ Inflammation of the pericardial sac:
- Risk factors/etiology:
  - Infections—viral, bacterial, fungal, toxoplasmosis, Lyme disease:
    - Most often viral related to coxsackievirus B
  - Noninfectious—renal failure, MI, lung/breast cancer, lymphoma, leukemia, radiation treatment, myxedema
  - Autoimmune—Dressler syndrome post-MI; rheumatic fever; rheumatoid arthritis, systemic lupus erythematosus, ankylosing spondylitis, postpericardiotomy syndrome (PPS)

Assessment/Interventions/Education

- Medical history/clinical manifestations:
  - See above.
  - Frequent severe chest pain that is worse with inspiration and gets better when sitting up and leaning forward
  - Pain can radiate to upper back, neck, arms, left shoulder
  - Dyspnea
  - Distant heart sounds if pericardial effusion
  - Pericardial friction rub at lower left sternal border with patient sitting forward:
    - Can be intermittent; may need to listen several times

Clinical Consideration

If the pain is pleuritic in nature (worsening with movement/deep breaths), it may respond better to NSAIDs and/or steroids.

Clinical Consideration

Sometimes pericardial friction rubs are very soft, "distant," and high-pitched and you must listen carefully.

- Possible complications
  - Pericardial effusion—fluid can accumulate quickly or slowly.
  - Cardiac tamponade—large effusion affects venous return and cardiac output:
    - If tamponade occurs acutely, the patient has greater hemodynamic compromise (trauma).
    - This is an emergency!
      - Anxious, confused, restless, chest pain
      - Muffled heart sounds, signs/symptoms of decreased cardiac output, narrow pulse pressure
      - JVD
      - Pulsus paradoxus—drop of 10 mm Hg or more in systolic blood pressure during inspiration
      - Can be life-threatening emergency—emergency pericardiocentesis
    - If tamponade has a longer onset because of chronic issue (e.g., chronic kidney disease):
      - No symptoms
      - Dyspnea
- ▶ Diagnosis:
  - ECG—diffuse ST-segment elevation
  - Echocardiogram—most helpful in diagnosis
  - CBC—leukocytosis
  - Elevated CRP and erythrocyte sedimentation rate (ESR) (markers for inflammation)
  - Troponins may be positive because of pericarditis
  - HIV antibody or antinuclear antibody (ANA)—to help determine cause if unknown
  - Fluid from pericardiocentesis is sent for evaluation to determine etiology of effusion.
- ▶ Nursing diagnosis:
  - Acute pain related to inflammation, effusion
  - Risk for decreased cardiac output related to fluid accumulation in pericardium
- ▶ Treatment:
  - Treat underlying cause
  - Pericardiocentesis—emergent with acute tamponade to relieve the pressure around the heart and/or to analyze fluid:
    - May need to go to ICU to support hemodynamic stability
  - Pericardial drain may be placed
  - NSAIDs and/or corticosteroids
  - Pericardial window surgery (if tamponade is present or to treat chronic effusion) to prevent future buildup of fluid
- ▶ Patient teaching:
  - Offer support and explanations of all procedures.
  - Explain etiology of the condition.
  - Postoperative/postprocedure care.

Clinical Consideration

ST-segment elevation can be present with generalized inflammation in the pericardium.

Myocarditis

- ▶ Diffuse or focal inflammatory process involving the myocardium that may be acute or chronic; autoimmune response that causes myocyte destruction; contractility decreases and the conduction system can be affected also.

◗ Risk factors/etiology:

- Viruses, bacteria, fungi, radiation therapy, pharmacologic, chemical
  - Coxsackie A and B viruses most common causes
- Autoimmune
- Can cause dilated cardiomyopathy

Assessment/Interventions/Education

◗ Medical history:

- Flu-like symptoms—fever, fatigue, malaise, myalgia, dyspnea, lymphadenopathy, nausea, vomiting
- May report minimal symptoms, infection may resolve on its own
- May report early cardiac symptoms: pleuritic chest pain 7 to 10 days after viral illness

◗ Clinical manifestations:

- May develop severe HF, pericardial friction rub, JVD, edema, angina, S3 heart sound

◗ Diagnosis:

- ECG—diffuse ST-segment elevation due to pericarditis
- Echocardiogram
- CBC
- Throat, blood, and stool cultures to assess for possible causative infectious agent
- CRP and ESR—elevated from inflammation
- Viral titers
- Endomyocardial biopsy to confirm damage to myocytes
- Elevated troponins

◗ Nursing diagnosis:

- Decreased CO related to altered preload and afterload
- Activity intolerance related to decreased cardiac output

◗ Treatment:

- Treatment of HF (see section on "HF treatment")
- Immunosuppressant agent if autoimmune cause
- Treat organism as indicated if acute viral or bacterial cause
- Use digoxin cautiously because of concern for sensitivity to digoxin; monitor for signs/symptoms of toxicity and possibly dysrhythmias
- Anticoagulation if low EF
- Continuous cardiac monitoring for dysrhythmias
- May need intraaortic balloon pump or VAD if condition deteriorates
- If the patient's condition continues to deteriorate despite medical therapy, heart transplantation may be required

◗ Patient teaching:

- Most patients recover spontaneously.
- In some patients, dilated cardiomyopathy develops as a result of myocarditis.
- Patient and family may be very anxious because of the diagnosis and the severity of the patient's condition.
- Patient condition may be changing fast; the patient and family will need guidance and support as they are trying to understand the disease, possible treatments, and long-term manifestations.

STRUCTURAL HEART DISORDERS

Cardiomyopathy

▶ Refers to a group of diseases that affect myocardial structure or function. It is classified as primary (idiopathic), involving the heart muscle only, or secondary, which is related to another condition. The cause may not be known. It can be a subacute or chronic disease. Although there are many types of cardiomyopathy, there are three major classifications: dilated, hypertrophic, and restrictive. Dilated cardiomyopathy will be discussed.

Dilated Cardiomyopathy

▶ Risk factors/etiology:
  - Most common type:
    - ▶ Causes:
      - Alcohol
      - Cocaine
      - Doxorubicin
      - Can develop after infectious myocarditis
      - Hypertension
      - Pregnancy
      - Valvular disease
      - CAD
      - Genetic, inherited
  - Inflammation and degeneration of myofibrils and interference with myocardial metabolism
  - Wall thickness normal
  - Cardiomegaly—enlarged chambers due to dilated atria and ventricles
  - Stasis of blood in ventricle—predisposes to clots
  - Impaired systolic function—predisposes to SCD

Assessment/Interventions/Education

▶ Medical history:
  - See above
  - May develop acutely or over long period of time
  - Fatigue; dyspnea on exertion (DOE)
  - Paroxysmal nocturnal dyspnea, orthopnea
  - Nausea, vomiting, anorexia
  - Chest discomfort, cough, palpitations

▶ Clinical manifestations:
  - Signs of heart failure: tachycardia, tachypnea, S3 and S4 heart sounds, murmurs
  - Peripheral edema, hepatomegaly, crackles
  - Stasis of blood in the heart can lead to clot formation and embolization
  - ECG—assessing for dysrhythmias, tachycardia, atrial fibrillation
  - Echocardiogram—dilated chambers, systolic dysfunction
  - BNP—elevated if patient has HF
  - Chest x-ray—may show cardiomegaly and pleural effusion
  - Cardiac catheterization—performed to determine whether there is coronary artery disease; may do endomyocardial biopsy to help determine cause
  - MUGA scan—performed to evaluate EF

> **Clinical Consideration**
>
> There may be a family history of SCA (sudden cardiac arrest) or SCD (sudden cardiac death) in patients with hypertrophic cardiomyopathy.

▶ Nursing diagnosis:
- Decreased cardiac output related to cardiac dysfunction
- Activity intolerance related to impaired cardiac function, increased preload and afterload and decreased contractility

▶ Treatment:
- Directed toward the cause if known (e.g., if related to alcohol, alcohol cessation; if related to CAD or HTN, optimize treatment for these conditions)
- See HF section on treatment
- Treat HF: increase CO, decrease preload and afterload:
  - Nitrates, diuretics, ACEIs, beta-blockers, aldosterone antagonists
  - May need infusion therapy
  - Dysrhythmias—antidysrhythmics—amiodarone (Cordarone)
  - Anticoagulation
- VAD—may be bridge to transplantation or may be destination therapy
- CRT and ICD for select patients
- Heart transplantation—many patients are not candidates or may die while waiting to get a donor heart because of lack of available hearts
- Palliative/hospice care may be the best option, depending on disease stage or classification

▶ Patient/family teaching:
- See HF section on patient teaching
- Related to patient specific treatment (e.g., devices; pre/post cardiac transplantation teaching)
- How to maximize and maintain functional status
- Hospice/end-of-life care perhaps

Question	Rationale
The nurse is teaching a patient who has been newly diagnosed with hypertrophic cardiomyopathy. Which of the following statements by the patient demonstrates understanding of the nurse's teaching? A. "I will take my nitroglycerin before I exercise." B. "I have to make sure that I have plenty of water and not let myself get dehydrated." C. "My heart enlarged after I had an infection." D. "I understand that this type of cardiomyopathy usually does not cause heart rhythm disturbances."	Answer: B There is impaired diastolic filling, so the patient has decreased preload. There is obstruction to outflow, so both of these can cause decreased cardiac output. Keeping hydrated and elevating the feet increase venous return to the heart. Nitroglycerin is contraindicated because it will decrease venous return to the heart and decrease output from the heart (which may worsen chest pain). The most common cause of SCD in healthy young adults is hypertrophic cardiomyopathy.

VALVULAR HEART DISEASE

The mitral and tricuspid valves are the AV valves. The aortic and pulmonic are the semilunar valves. These control blood flow through the heart; the closure of the valves is what creates the heart sounds we hear on the precordium with the stethoscope. Valve disease can be caused by stenosis, which is constriction or narrowing in the valve opening.

This causes a pressure difference on the two sides of the valve. The greater the difference between each side of the valve, the more severe the stenosis. Incomplete closure of valves is called "regurgitation" and the blood flows backward. This is also called "incompetence" or "insufficiency."

Types of Valvular Disorders

Mitral Stenosis (MS)

▌ Risk factors/etiology:
- Rheumatic fever (RF) most common cause; also congenital; may be found in those with rheumatoid arthritis, lupus
- Rheumatic endocarditis causes scarring and thickening and shortening of the valve leaflets and the chordae tendineae
- Valve can't open during diastole (filling phase), blood can't go from LA to LV, so the blood and volume increase in LA, and create back pressure in pulmonary vasculature, which can then cause increased pressure in lungs and RV (and pulmonary hypertension); pressure gradient (difference) exists between LA and LV.
- Atrial fibrillation may develop due to stretching of LA

▌ Medical history:
- DOE, hemoptysis, fatigue, palpitations, orthopnea
- History of rheumatic fever, strep infection, IE, MI, IV drug use

▌ Clinical manifestations:
- Low-pitched, diastolic murmur, heard best in the apex (mitral area)
- Loud S1 auscultated
- Assess for signs/symptoms of right-sided heart failure

▌ Diagnosis:
- TEE and Doppler imaging—structure, function of heart valves, chamber-sized, presence of vegetations/thrombi
- Chest x-ray
- ECG—perhaps atrial fibrillation
- Cardiac catheterization—determine pressure gradients across the valves, chamber sizes, size of valve openings

▌ Nursing diagnosis:
- Fatigue related to decreased CO
- Risk for decreased CO related to decreased forward flow of blood

▌ Treatment:
- Drug(s) used for rate control in atrial fibrillation—CCBs
- Drug or electrical therapy to convert atrial fibrillation
- Anticoagulation if patient has atrial fibrillation or thrombi
- Discuss antibiotic prophylaxis to prevent recurrent IE or rheumatic fever or if patient has prosthetic valve
- Percutaneous transluminal balloon valvuloplasty may be an option for some patients, depending on pathology
- Repair of valve not always an option
- Replacement of valve
  - Mechanical
    - Requires anticoagulation
    - More durable, lasts longer
  - Biologic
    - Usually no anticoagulation is needed unless patient is in atrial fibrillation or has other indication,
    - Bovine, porcine, or human with some man-made materials

▶ Patient teaching:
  - Regular appointments with HCP.
  - All patients should participate in exercise appropriate to their condition and with guidance from their HCP.
  - Report worsening dyspnea, fatigue, signs/symptoms of HF to HCP.
  - Pre/post procedure teaching.
  - Anticoagulation needed after mechanical-valve surgery.
  - Women with mitral stenosis should notify HCP immediately if they become pregnant, as pregnancy causes the heart to work harder.

Mitral-Valve Regurgitation (MVR)

▶ Risk factors/etiology
  - MI, rheumatic heart disease, mitral-valve prolapse, hypertrophic cardiomyopathy, ruptured chordae tendineae
  - Chronic: blood backs up from LV to LA; can cause LA enlargement/stretching and pressure transmits to pulmonary bed; LV hypertrophy and dilation, LV failure and decreased CO
  - Acute mitral regurgitation (MR) can happen quickly and cause pulmonary edema and shock

▶ Medical history:
  - Chronic—asymptomatic for many years
  - Fatigue, weakness, dyspnea, and palpitations, progressing to decreased exercise endurance, orthopnea, and paroxysmal nocturnal dyspnea

▶ Clinical manifestations:
  - Chronic—tachycardia, edema, JVD, hepatomegaly, edema
  - S3, loud holosystolic murmur at apex
  - Signs/symptoms of progressive heart failure and pulmonary hypertension
  - Acute MR—signs/symptoms of pulmonary edema and possibly shock

▶ Diagnosis:
  - Echocardiogram/TEE—abnormal valve-leaflet motion; LA enlargement
  - Exercise stress test
  - Cardiac CT scan to see whether the patient is a candidate for robotic surgery
  - Cardiac MRI
  - Chest x-ray to see the condition of the lungs
  - ECG—LA enlargement and LV hypertrophy; sinus tachycardia or atrial fibrillation

▶ Nursing diagnosis:
  - Activity intolerance related to imbalance between oxygen supply and demand
  - Fatigue related to decreased CO

▶ Treatment:
  - Depends of severity of MR:
    - May be watchful waiting
    - May replace or repair valve if patient has to have other heart surgery (e.g., coronary bypass)
    - Ideal to replace/repair valve before severe LV dysfunction develops and patient becomes too sick
  - Keep BP under control with medications, diuretics
  - Anticoagulant therapy if atrial fibrillation or if patient received mechanical heart valve
  - Treatment of atrial fibrillation
  - May be candidate for minimally invasive surgery, or may have open heart surgery procedure

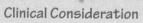

Clinical Consideration

Some of the blood is going backward into the atria instead of forward through the aortic valve.

- ▶ Patient teaching:
  - Risk-factor reduction
  - Notify HCP if having dental/invasive procedure; may need antibiotic prophylaxis
  - If patient has had replacement with mechanical valve, will need to be on lifelong warfarin (Coumadin), maintaining INR values between 2.5 and 3.5 therapeutic range (some HCPs may prefer slightly different ranges).
  - Notify HCP if any signs of infection, HF, or bleeding
  - Cardiac rehabilitation after procedure or surgery

Mitral-Valve Prolapse

- ▶ Risk factors/etiology:
  - Affects both genders equally
  - Genetic link; may affect those with Marfan syndrome or other conditions
  - Valve leaflets prolapse back into LA during systole
  - Generally a benign condition, but can lead to MR, IE, SCD, and HF
- ▶ Medical history:
  - Most patients are asymptomatic
  - Palpitations, light-headedness, syncope, dyspnea, fatigue
  - Stress can precipitate chest pain
- ▶ Clinical manifestations:
  - May have signs/symptoms of MR
  - Midsystolic click with or without a mid to late systolic murmur
- ▶ Diagnosis:
  - Echocardiogram reveals prolapse of valve leaflets into atrium during systole.
  - Exercise treadmill test might reveal chest pain and dysrhythmias.
  - Cardiac catheterization may be performed to see whether there are other abnormalities in the heart and to assess the amount of mitral regurgitation.
- ▶ Nursing diagnosis:
  - Fatigue related to abnormal regulation and decreased intravascular volume
  - Fear related to lack of knowledge about MVP
- ▶ Treatment:
  - May require beta-blockers to control palpitations and tachycardia.
  - If MR is severe, patient may require valve replacement or valve repair.
  - The AHA no longer recommends prophylactic antibiotics before certain dental or medical procedures for most people with mitral-valve prolapse or mitral regurgitation (Nishimura et al., 2017).
- ▶ Patient teaching:
  - Take medications per HCP recommendations.
  - Notify HCP if dyspnea, chest pain, palpitations, anxiety, fatigue have worsened.
  - Incorporate stress management into lifestyle modifications.
  - Maintain healthy eating, sleep, and exercise habits.

Aortic Stenosis

- ▶ Risk factors/etiology:
  - Congenital aortic bicuspid valve—usually found in childhood, adolescence.
  - Degeneration calcifications caused by mechanical stress, hypertension, diabetes, hypercholesterolemia, coronary artery disease.
  - Rheumatic fever can cause stenosis and calcification of both the aortic and mitral valves.
  - Obstruction of blood flow from LV during systole causes LV hypertrophy, decreased tissue perfusion, pulmonary hypertension, and HF.

▶ Medical history:

- Exertional dyspnea, angina, syncope are the most common symptoms; fatigue, paroxysmal nocturnal dyspnea, and palpitations have been reported.

▶ Clinical manifestations:

- Systolic murmur heard in aortic and pulmonic areas and radiate into carotids; S4 and diminished S2 heart sound; JVD, signs and symptoms of HF

▶ Diagnosis:

- Chest x-ray—valvular calcification, LV enlargement, pulmonary vascular congestion
- Cardiac CT/MRI
- Echocardiogram/TEE—thickened aortic valve and LV wall
- ECG—LV hypertrophy
- Cardiac catheterization—increased pressure gradient across aortic valve, increased LV pressures

▶ Nursing diagnosis:

- Decreased cardiac output related to cardiac dysfunction
- Ineffective breathing pattern related to pulmonary vascular disease

▶ Treatment:

- Depends on severity of patient condition.
- Care taken when administering SL NTG; can cause hypotension in patient with aortic stenosis (AS).
- Balloon valvuloplasty may be appropriate for some patients.
- Aortic-valve replacement—mechanical or biological tissue valve.
- Transcatheter aortic valve replacement (TAVR) for high-risk individuals; faster recovery.
- Post-TAVR care.
- Antibiotic prophylaxis if patient has had IE or has a prosthetic heart valve.

▶ Patient teaching:

- Keep mouth, teeth, and gums clean.
- Follow HCP recommendations for IE prophylaxis.
- Review care/medications after TAVR, valve replacement/repair surgeries.
- A patient with AS must balance rest with activity; avoid strenuous activities that cause fatigue and dyspnea.
- Cardiac rehabilitation after surgery or procedure.

Aortic Regurgitation (AR)

▶ Risk factors/etiology:

- Chronic: rheumatic fever, age, syphilis, hypertension, IE, congenital bicuspid valve, autoimmune diseases
- Acute: trauma, IE, dissecting aortic aneurysm
- Backward flow of blood from ascending aorta into LV during diastole; leads to volume overload, and pulmonary hypertension

▶ Medical history:

- Acute: sudden signs of dyspnea, chest pain,
- Chronic: asymptomatic for many years; fatigue, palpitations, exertional dyspnea, cough, angina, perhaps syncope

▶ Clinical manifestations:

- Acute: left ventricular failure, cardiogenic shock, CV collapse
- Chronic: soft S1, diastolic, blowing murmur at left sternal border; S3, S4
  - Apical impulse is palpable
  - Water hammer pulse with strong, quick upstroke that collapses quickly

- Exertional dyspnea, orthopnea, paroxysmal nocturnal dyspnea, edema, irregular pulse develop in chronic AS with disease progression
- Diagnosis:
  - Echocardiogram/esophageal echocardiogram—will display LV enlargement; alteration in MV movement
  - Exercise or pharmacologic stress test to see if there are signs/symptoms of aortic regurgitation during physical activity
  - Chest x-ray—assessing condition of lungs and to see if the heart or aorta are enlarged
  - ECG—sinus tachycardia; LV hypertrophy
  - Cardiac catheterization—will help determine if there are blockages in the coronary arteries; will show aortic regurgitation; increased LV end diastolic pressure
- Nursing diagnosis:
  - Decreased CO related to cardiac dysfunction
  - Activity intolerance related to fatigue, generalized weakness, and decreased CO
- Treatment:
  - Acute AR—surgical emergency; may need to replace part of aorta and the valve
  - Chronic AR—may have surgery without symptoms if, for example, patient has to have open heart surgery for coronary artery bypass; or watchful waiting monitoring for progression of symptoms
  - Repair—with catheter procedure or open chest procedure
  - Aortic valve replacement—with open chest procedure:
    - Biologic tissue valve:
      - No anticoagulation, unless patient is in atrial fibrillation
    - Mechanical valve:
      - Requires anticoagulation
- Patient teaching:
  - Postprocedure/postoperative care
  - Lifestyle modifications for heart healthy living
  - Teaching about all medications
  - Teaching about HF
  - Cardiac rehabilitation after surgery or procedure

Pulmonic Stenosis

- Risk factors/etiology:
  - RF, IE carcinoid syndrome, congenital
  - Orifice in valve is narrowed and decreased blood flow to pulmonary artery and lungs
- Medical history:
  - May be asymptomatic
  - Fatigue, dyspnea on exertion, chest pain, syncope
- Clinical manifestations:
  - Peripheral edema, JVD, hepatomegaly, dysrhythmias
  - Systolic murmur at left sternal border
- Diagnosis:
  - ECG—may show right ventricular hypertrophy (RVH) and right atrial hypertrophy; perhaps atrial fibrillation
  - Echocardiogram/TEE—evaluates degree of valvular stenosis and RV size
  - Cardiac catheterization—determines if mild, moderate, or severe stenosis and the pressures in the heart and pulmonary artery

◗ Nursing diagnosis:

- Excessive fluid volume related to cardiac dysfunction
- Risk for decreased cardiac output related to cardiac dysfunction

◗ Treatment:

- Antibiotics for recurrent IE; patient will need prophylactic antibiotics if history of IE or valve replacement
- Percutaneous transcatheter pulmonary valve replacement may be an option
- Open heart surgery; or minimally invasive repair/replacement of valve
- Diuretics

◗ Patient teaching:

- Postprocedure/postoperative care
- Lifestyle modifications for heart healthy living
- Cardiac rehabilitation after surgery or procedure

Tricuspid Regurgitation

◗ Risk factors/etiology:

- Cardiomyopathy, right-sided heart failure, IE, carcinoid syndrome, RF, congenital, radiation therapy to the chest, injury from pacemaker.
- Pulmonary hypertension is common cause.
- Tricuspid stenosis can be present also.
- Blood goes from the RV backward into the RA during systole (should be going forward).

◗ Medical history:

- Signs of pulmonary hypertension: fatigue, weakness, difficulty exercising, shortness of breath, palpitations; may report signs of right-sided HF: edema, ascites

◗ Clinical manifestations:

- May be asymptomatic
- Edema, JVD, ascites, hepatomegaly, possible S3, systolic murmur at lower left sternal border accentuated with inspiration
- Atrial fibrillation or other dysrhythmias

◗ Diagnosis:

- ECG—possibly atrial fibrillation or other dysrhythmias
- Echocardiogram/TEE
- Exercise/stress test
- Cardiac MRI
- Cardiac catheterization

◗ Nursing diagnosis:

- Fatigue related to impaired cardiac function
- Ineffective breathing pattern related to pulmonary vascular disease

◗ Treatment:

- Careful monitoring if not candidate for valve replacement or repair
- Antibiotics if secondary to IE
- Diuretics and HF treatment
- Repair or replacement of valve via open heart approach
- Patient may be candidate for catheter procedure to replace with biologic valve
- If patient has atrial fibrillation and is having valve repair or replacement, Maze procedure may be performed at same time to treat the dysrhythmias. The maze procedure uses cryotherapy or radiofrequency energy to induce scar tissue in and around the conduction system that will block rhythm pathways.

❱ Patient teaching:

- Postprocedure/postoperative care
- Lifestyle modifications for heart healthy living
- Teach about all medications
- Will need antibiotic prophylaxis for dental and other procedures if patient receives prosthetic heart valve
  - Patients with history of IE will need prophylactic antibiotics for certain dental and other procedures (Nishimura et al., 2017)

Question	Rationale
The nurse is caring for a patient newly diagnosed with mitral stenosis. The HCP suspects that it is related to rheumatic fever (RF), a preventable form of heart disease associated with: A. Direct infection of the endocardium by group B streptococcus. B. A viral infection of the heart. C. The body's immune response to group –A beta hemolytic streptococcus. D. IV drug use.	Answer: C RF is an acute inflammatory disease that can affect all layers of the heart. It can leave the patient with chronic scarring and destruction of the heart valves. It is related to the body's immune response to group A hemolytic streptococcus. Infection with this strain is the most common bacterial cause of pharyngitis. IV drug use is associated with infective endocarditis (IE), not RF.

Vascular Disorders

Peripheral Arterial Disease (PAD)

PAD is a disease that is caused by atherosclerosis and involves narrowing of the arteries in the upper and lower extremities. This disease often goes underrecognized and undertreated. The prevalence is higher in women, in African Americans, and in those from lower socioeconomic classes (Eraso et al., 2014).

❱ Risk factors/etiology:

- Age >65 years
- Age 50 to 64 years:
  - Diabetes
  - Smoking
  - Hyperlipidemia
  - Hypertension
  - Family history of PAD
- Age <50 years:
  - Diabetes
  - 1 or more cardiovascular risk factors.
  - Those with atherosclerotic disease elsewhere (e.g., coronary, carotid, subclavian, renal, mesenteric artery stenosis, or AAA). (Gerhard-Herman et al., 2016)
  - Femoral and popliteal arteries are most common sites of disease occurrence in nondiabetics.
  - In diabetics, PAD develops most often in arteries below the knee.

▶ Medical history:

- Symptoms depend on site, amount of blockage, and presence of collateral circulation.
- Intermittent claudication (IC)—fatigue, discomfort, cramping, or pain in the muscles of the lower extremities that is consistently induced by exercise and is relieved by rest within 10 minute; most likely due to femoral or popliteal occlusion
- Buttock or thigh pain—ischemia from iliac artery occlusion
- Paresthesia—burning, shooting pain, numbness, loss of feeling
- Can progress to pain at rest—especially at night when leg is elevated (may notice pallor); patient dangles leg over side of bed and pain goes away when dependent (may notice dependent rubor)
- Patient may report wounds that don't heal

▶ Clinical manifestations:

- See Table 9.8
- Critical limb ischemia—chronic (≥2 weeks) ischemic pain at rest, nonhealing wound/ulcers, or gangrene in one or both legs attributable to objectively proven arterial occlusive disease

▶ Diagnosis:

- Ankle brachial index (ABI)—objective screening tool for PAD; divide the ankle systolic BP by the higher of the left and right brachial systolic BPs:
  - Older adults and diabetics may have falsely elevated ABI because of calcification of arteries.
  - Normal ABI: 1.0 to 1.3
  - Mild PAD: 0.9 to 0.71
  - Moderate PAD: 0.7 to 0. 41
  - Severe PAD: <0.40
- Doppler ultrasound
- Segmental BPs using ultrasound—drop in BPs in leg >30 mm Hg indicates PAD
- Angiogram
- MRA/CTA
- CBC
- CMP, including BUN/creatinine to assess kidney function

▶ Nursing diagnosis:

- Chronic pain, intermittent claudication related to ischemia
- Ineffective peripheral tissue perfusion related to disease process
- Risk for impaired tissue integrity due to ineffective peripheral tissue perfusion

▶ Treatment:

- Risk-factor modification
- Aggressive lipid management—dietary and statin and fibric acid derivative (gemfibrozil [Lopid])
- ACEIs—to reduce risk of CV ischemic event
- Antiplatelet agent
- Cilostazol (Pletal)—inhibits platelet aggregation; vasodilator
- Supervised exercise program
- Revascularization bypass surgery for critical limb ischemia (CLI); endarterectomy; patch graft angioplasty
- Endovascular procedure—percutaneous transluminal angioplasty (PTA); stent; atherectomy
- Amputation if gangrene or chronic osteomyelitis, nonhealing ulcer

Clinical Consideration

Those with a nonhealing ulcer may be asked to decrease their activity to reduce oxygen demand and increase supply.

TABLE 9.8	COMPARING PERIPHERAL ARTERIAL DISEASE AND CHRONIC VENOUS INSUFFICIENCY	
Variable	Peripheral Arterial Disease	Chronic Venous Insufficiency
Pulses	Diminished or absent	Present
Capillary refill	>3 sec	<3 sec
Ankle brachial index (ABI) (normal, 1.0–1.30)	<0.90	>0.90
Skin color	Dependent rubor, elevation pallor	Brown, darkened, stained from hemosiderin; no change with positioning
Skin texture	Thin, shiny, may be fragile	Rough, thick, hard, dry
Skin temperature	Cool	Warm
Nails	Thick, yellow, brittle	May be thickened or normal for patient
Edema	Absent	Present
Hair	Absent	Present or absent
Ulcer location	Tips toes, heel, lateral ankle	Above medial ankle, but various locations on lower leg
Ulcer characteristics	Smooth margins; wound base may be pale or have black eschar: minimal drainage	Irregular margins; wound base dark red; moderate to large amount of drainage; can become infected
Pain	Possible manifestations depending on disease progression: paresthesias, intermittent claudication, pain at rest, critical limb ischemia	Ache, heaviness in legs; can be worse when in dependent position
(Lewis et. al., 2017)		

▶ Patient teaching:
- Goals: relief of pain, heal wounds, improve exercise tolerance, increase knowledge of disease
- CV risk factor modification
- Protection of extremity and prevention of further injury
- Avoid staying in one position too long
- Foot care and inspection of legs/feet daily
- Avoid cutting own nails—go to podiatrist

Raynaud's Phenomenon

▶ Episodes of vasospasms; vasoconstriction alternating with vasodilation of the small arteries in the fingers and toes
▶ Risk factors/etiology:
- Women (typically 15 to 40 years old)
- History of autoimmune disease (rheumatoid arthritis, lupus, scleroderma)
▶ Manifestations:
- Discoloration of fingers, toes:
  - Pallor from decreased perfusion
  - Blue from cyanosis
  - Rubor (red) when blood flow returns

- Sensation changes: numbness alternating with pain and tingling
- Triggers: smoking, caffeine, cold, emotions
- In severe cases, digital ulcerations and necrosis from ischemia
▸ Diagnosis
- No definitive diagnostic test
- Based on patient having persistent symptoms for >2 years
▸ Nursing diagnosis:
- Acute pain related to transient decease in blood flow
- Ineffective peripheral tissue perfusion related to decrease in blood flow
▸ Treatment:
- Avoidance of triggers and vasoconstrictive medications (cocaine, amphetamines, pseudoephedrine)
- Drug therapy:
  - CCBs: nifedipine (Procardia) may decrease attacks.
  - Nitroglycerin transdermal glyceral trinitrate (Nitro-Dur), if CCB not effective
- Only for significant advanced Raynaud's syndrome—sympathectomy (removal of a sympathetic nerve to prevent the stimulation of vasospasms)
▸ Patient teaching:
- Avoidance of triggers; caffeine; vasoconstrictive medications; smoking cessation
- Protection from the cold; wear loose, warm clothing and gloves
- Discuss stress management strategies and provide community resources

Buerger's Disease (Thromboangiitis Obliterans)

▸ A rare inflammatory disease of the arteries and veins, in the upper and lower extremities, causing a decrease in blood flow to the extremities
▸ Risk factors/etiology:
- Men <45 years old
- History of long-term use of tobacco and/or marijuana
- Long-term gum infections
▸ Manifestations:
- Tissue ischemia due to thrombosis and fibrosis
- Intermittent claudication; pain at rest is a sign of progressing disease
- Color, temperature, and sensation changes in extremities similar to Raynaud's syndrome
- Ulcerations on hands or feet
▸ Diagnosis—no definitive diagnostic test, based on symptoms
▸ Nursing diagnosis:
- Ineffective peripheral tissue perfusion related to disease process
- Acute/chronic pain: intermittent claudication related to ischemia
▸ Treatment:
- Cessation of tobacco and marijuana
- Decrease exposure to cold temperatures
- Drug therapy:
  - CCBs
  - Cilostazol (Pletal)—for vasodilation and decreasing coagulation effects
  - Sildenafil (Viagra)—for vasodilation effects
- Surgery:
  - Sympathectomy
  - Spinal cord stimulator

▶ Patient teaching:

- Continued tobacco or marijuana use may result in progression of the disease, requiring amputation of part of limb
- Avoidance of triggers
- Medication education

Acute Arterial Ischemia

▶ Risk factors/etiology:

- Embolism from heart:
  - IE, mitral-valve disease, atrial fibrillation, prosthetic heart valves
- Thrombosis in existing atherosclerosis
- Acute traumatic injury:
  - Related to procedure (e.g., angiography)

▶ Medical history/clinical manifestations:

- See Risk factors/etiology, above
- 6 Ps
  - Pain
  - Pulselessness
  - Paresthesia
  - Pallor
  - Paralysis
  - Poikilothermia (cool temperature in most situations)

▶ Diagnosis:

- Ultrasound
- Arteriogram
- CBC, CMP

▶ Nursing diagnosis:

- Ineffective tissue perfusion related to interruption of arterial flow
- Acute pain related to ineffective tissue perfusion

▶ Treatment:

- IV unfractionated heparin (UH) continuous drip, coumadin
- Catheter-guided or surgical thrombectomy
- Percutaneous catheter directed thrombolytic therapy with t-PA or urokinase if blockage is less than 14 days
- Surgical bypass or surgical repair

▶ Patient teaching:

- May require long-term anticoagulation to prevent reoccurrence
- Anticoagulation teaching
- Protection of extremity and prevention of further injury
- Avoid staying in one position too long
- Keep surgical site clean dry
- Observe surgical site for signs/symptoms of infection
- Notify HCP for signs/symptoms of infection, reocclusion, and bleeding

Aortic Aneurysm

▶ Risk factors/etiology:

- Age, male sex, hypertension, family history, tobacco, hypercholesterolemia, lower-extremity PAD, carotid artery disease, previous stroke, obesity, infection (e.g., HIV, chlamydia, syphilis), Marfan syndrome
- Permanent dilation of aortic arch, thoracic, or abdominal aorta

▶ Medical history:
- Thoracic aneurysm—less common; often asymptomatic
  - Chest pain, angina
  - Patient may report signs/symptoms of transient ischemic attack (TIA)
  - Coughing, shortness of breath, hoarseness
- Abdominal aortic aneurysm—most common site
  - Often asymptomatic
  - Back pain, nausea, vomiting, intermittant claudication, altered bowel elimination

▶ Clinical manifestations:
- Thoracic:
  - TIA—decreased blood flow to carotid arteries
  - Coughing, shortness of breath, hoarseness, dysphagia—pressure on laryngeal nerve
  - JVD
  - Possible loss of radial, femoral, carotid pulses
  - With rupture, tearing pain in back and chest, hemorrhage, shock, death
- Abdominal:
  - Pulsatile mass in umbilical area
  - Bruit over aneurysm
  - Change in peripheral pulses/perfusion
  - BUN/creatinine can increase if kidney perfusion is altered
  - Occasionally, embolization of plaque from aneurysm causing mottling appearance in feet
  - With rupture, severe abdominal or lower back pain; nausea and vomiting; Turner sign (bluish discoloration under skin secondary to internal hemorrhage); shock, and death

▶ Diagnosis:
- Incidental finding on workup for something else
- Chest x-ray—widening of mediastinum; calcification
- ECG to rule out MI—patient may present with chest pain
- Ultrasound—used for screening and surveillance of aneurysm
- CT scan—most accurate to determine size and presence of thrombus
- MRI/MRA—size and location can be determined accurately
- Angiography
- CBC—assessing for bleeding
- CMP—assessing BUN/creatinine

▶ Nursing diagnosis:
- Acute pain related to disease process
- Readiness for enhanced health maintenance

▶ Treatment:
- Early detection and immediate treatment:
  - Watchful waiting for AAA <4.0 cm; ultrasound every 2 to 3 years for AAA 4.0 to 5.4 cm without symptoms
    - Stop smoking, control hypertension; treat hyperlipidemia; increase physical activity
    - Beta-blocker, ACEI, statin
    - Ultrasound or CT every 6 to 12 months
  - AAA ≥5.5 cm, surgical repair; may be performed earlier in certain diseases and/or with rupture (Anderson et al., 2013)

- If concurrent CAD or carotid artery disease, patient may need treatment before AAA repair
- Open aortic repair with graft—more invasive open abdominal procedure with placement of synthetic graft; use of cross clamping of aorta during surgery; longer recovery period
- Minimally invasive endovascular aneurysm repair (EVAR):
  - Insertion of stent graft:
    - Shorter stay
    - Periodic imaging to monitor for endoleak and need for further surgical intervention
- Patient teaching:
  - Postprocedure instructions related to activity, medications, skin/incision care
  - Notify HCP about signs/symptoms of:
    - Decreased perfusion to extremities, decreased urine output, increased pain, sign/symptoms of infection

Chronic Venous Insufficiency

Older adults and those with chronic diseases such as diabetes, HF, varicose veins, post-thrombotic syndrome, and cardiovascular disease are susceptible to abnormalities of the venous system that predispose them to edema, skin changes, and/or venous leg ulcers.

- Risk factors/etiology:
  - Varicose veins and postthrombotic syndrome (PTS) can damage vein walls and valves; blood is not able to be pumped back to the right side of the heart; pressure increases in capillaries and venules, causing fluid and red cells to leak from them into surrounding tissues.
  - Edema, chronic inflammation persist
  - Enzymes break down red cells and release hemosiderin, causing brown discoloration in tissues
  - Fibrotic hard, dry tissue develops in legs
  - Susceptible to ulcer formation
- Medical history—see above
- Clinical manifestations:
  - See Table 9.8
  - Pain worse when in dependent position
  - Ulcers are not always infected
  - Ulcers may be chronic and lead to osteomyelitis
  - Some patients require amputation for chronically infected, nonhealing wounds
- Diagnosis:
  - Patient history and physical exam
  - Doppler ultrasound to rule out venous thromboembolism
- Nursing diagnosis:
  - Chronic pain related to impaired venous circulation
  - Impaired tissue integrity related to chronic venous congestion
- Treatment (see Chapter 18)
  - Compression therapy (as long as patient does not have severe PAD also)
  - Elevate legs
  - Must have adequate diet to maintain albumin levels
  - Antibiotics, only if infection is present
  - Consultation with wound specialist, if appropriate
  - Diuretics as ordered

▶ Patient teaching:

- Elevate legs; avoid standing or sitting too long in one place
- Use of compression therapy
- Cleanse dry, flaky skin on legs; apply topical moisturizer to dry, intact skin
- Foot and leg care to avoid trauma, injury, infection
- Nail care by professional to avoid injury
- Daily assessment for any new signs of breakdown, infection, injury
- Activity as guided by HCP

Venous Thromboembolism (VTE)

This inclusive term can describe deep vein thrombosis (DVT), which is usually formed in the iliac and/or femoral veins. VTE can also be used to describe pulmonary embolus (PE) which is associated with a thrombus in one or more pulmonary arteries.

▶ Risk factors/etiology:

- Virchow's triad contributes to formation of a DVT:
  - Venous stasis—advanced age, atrial fibrillation, prolonged bed rest, HF, fracture of leg or hip, orthopedic surgery (especially on lower extremity or hip), immobility, varicose veins, paralysis, obesity, pregnancy and postpartum period
  - Endothelial damage to vein—history of VTE, some IV drugs, intravascular catheterization, abdominal and pelvic surgery, burns, trauma, sepsis, diabetes, chemotherapy
  - Hypercoagulability—malignancies, hormone therapy, antiphospholipid antibody syndrome, antitrypsin III deficiency, dehydration, elevated clotting factors, high altitude, oral contraceptives, pregnancy and postpartum, sepsis, tobacco use
- Damage to the endothelium of the vein stimulates platelet aggregation and the coagulation cascade. A thrombus forms and can block the lumen of the vein. The thrombus can detach and form an embolus.

▶ Medical history:

- See previous discussion for possible precipitating factors
- Maybe no symptoms; silent

▶ Clinical manifestations:

- Maybe no symptoms
- Perhaps: unilateral leg edema, erythema, cramping pain, warm, tender to touch, paresthesias, fever
- Complications
  - Pulmonary embolus
  - Postthrombotic syndrome (PTS)
    - Chronic pain, heaviness, aching, tingling, paresthesia, pain with exercise, increased brownish pigmentation, ulcers
    - Chronic damage to vein wall and vein valves causes decrease in venous return and increase in pressure in veins; results from chronic inflammation and edema

▶ Diagnosis:

- Clinical assessment
- D-dimer—a fibrin degradation fragment produced by fibrin and clot lysis; screening test for VTE; if elevated, may suggest VTE
- Duplex ultrasound

▶ Nursing diagnosis:

- Acute pain related to vascular inflammation and edema

- Risk for impaired skin integrity related to altered peripheral perfusion
- Ineffective health management related to lack of knowledge about disorder and treatment

▶ Treatment:

- Goals of drug therapy:
  - Prevent new clot formation
  - Prevent the current clot from getting larger
  - Prevent embolization
  - Prevent bleeding (side effect of all these drugs)
- Be aware of agency-specific guidelines for administration of high-alert drugs
- Vitamin K antagonists:
  - Warfarin (Coumadin)—for long-term therapy; may need overlap (bridge) with parenteral anticoagulant (like UH [heparin sodium]) because therapeutic effect is not achieved for approximately 5 days
    - Daily INR is used to monitor therapeutic range of warfarin, generally considered to be between 2 and 3; may be less frequent once the INR is at the goal range of between 2 and 3.
    - Antidote is vitamin K.
- Thrombin inhibitors (indirect):
  - UH, heparin:
    - Can be given subcutaneously for VTE prophylaxis or via a continuous IV infusion for treatment for VTE
    - If given subcutaneously, do not aspirate or rub site after injection
    - Frequent monitoring of activated partial thromboplastin time (aPTT) needed for IV infusion
    - Heparin-induced thrombocytopenia (HIT) is an immune reaction to heparin:
      - Heparin antibodies can be measured in the blood, as can low platelet counts
      - Increase in thrombosis
      - Must stop heparin and place patient on nonheparin anticoagulant
    - Protamine sulfate is antidote for heparin
  - LMWH (Low molecuar weight heparin):
    - Enoxaparin (Lovenox)—more predictable response, longer half-life, fewer bleeding complications
    - Can be used to prevent or treat VTE
    - Less likely to cause HIT
    - No routine anticoagulation tests required
    - Adjust dose for renal disease
    - Do not eject bubble from prefilled syringe
- Thrombin inhibitors:
  - Bivalirudin (Angiomax; direct thrombin inhibitor)—given as IV infusion during PCI for those who may be at risk for HIT
    - aPTT and activated clotting time (ACT) monitor anticoagulant activity
    - No antidote
  - Argatroban (synthetic direct thrombin inhibitor)—same indication as bivalirudin
  - Dabigatran (Pradaxa)—synthetic direct thrombin inhibitor

> **Clinical Consideration**
> Heparin is a high-alert drug; refer to agency policy and procedures when administering.

- Used for VTE prevention after joint-replacement surgery, for stroke prevention in nonvalvular atrial fibrillation and as treatment option for VTE
- Idarucizumab (Praxbind) neutralizes effect of dabigatran
  - Anticoagulant effect can be monitored with aPTT and ACT.
- Factor Xa inhibitors:
  - Rivaroxaban (Xarelto); apixaban (Eliquis)—produce rapid anticoagulation
    - Used for VTE treatment and prophylaxis
    - Dose adjustment not needed; no need to monitor anticoagulant activity
    - Anticoagulant activity of drugs can be measured by anti-Xa assays
    - If uncontrolled bleeding, may use recombinant factor VIIa
  - Fondaparinux (Arixtra)—subcutaneous injection; do not expel air bubble in prefilled syringe
- Thrombolytic therapy:
  - Catheter-directed t-PA may be appropriate for some patients with low bleeding risk.
- Open venous thrombectomy with anticoagulation
- Percutaneous endovascular procedures in select patients:
  - Thrombectomy
  - Angioplasty with stent
  - Anticoagulation
- Vena cava interruption devices (e.g., Greenfield) placed in vena cava to trap clots and prevent PE.
  - Placed percutaneously for patients with contraindications for anticoagulation or for those in whom VTE developed with anticoagulation

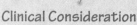

Clinical Consideration
VTE may be "silent" or subtle in many patients.

- Patient teaching:
  - Recognize and report signs and symptoms of VTE, PE, and side effects of drugs
  - If DVT, elevate legs
  - Teach VTE prevention to hospitalized patients:
    - Stay hydrated.
    - Stay active.
    - Wear sequential compression devices.
    - Mode of action, rationale, and potential side effects for anticoagulants.
  - Take all drugs as directed, same time each day
  - Fall prevention
  - Teach signs and symptoms of PE and chronic venous insufficiency and when to call EMS and/or HCP
  - If on anticoagulants:
    - Report any unusual bleeding, or blood in urine, stool, or vomit if on anticoagulants.
    - Be aware of activities that may cause bleeding.
    - Be aware of any blood test follow-up.
    - Inform all providers.
    - Do not take any new vitamins, herbal or other supplements, or over-the-counter medications without discussing with HCP.
    - Be aware of and avoid aspirin-containing drugs and ointments.
    - Be aware if and when blood tests are due to assess therapeutic effect of anticoagulant; be aware of goal therapeutic range.
    - If on Coumadin, be aware of need to avoid excessive amounts of vitamin K and maintain consistent eating patterns.
    - Medic Alert bracelet.

CASE STUDY

A 68-year-old female is admitted to your unit from the emergency department with acute decompensated heart failure. She has signs and symptoms of right- and left-sided heart failure. She reveals that she ran out of her medications and has not been taking all of them. She has been busy watching her grandchildren and has not "been taking care of herself."

Vital signs: temperature: 98.6°F; HR: 100 beats/min, irregular; respirations: 24 breaths/min; blood pressure: 138/90 mm Hg; SaO_2: 90% while breathing room air.

Medical history: Heart failure for 2 years, hypertension for 20 years, 30 pack-year smoker—quit 5 years ago

Her medications include:

Furosemide (Lasix) 20 mg by mouth daily

Carvedilol (Coreg) 12.5 mg by mouth twice daily

Enalapril (Vasotec) 10 mg by mouth twice daily

Aspirin 81 mg by mouth daily

1. **What diagnostic procedures do you expect the HCP to order? What is the rationale for these procedures and tests?**

    ▶ *Chest x-ray—to look at degree of heart failure, heart size, any signs of other issues in the lungs, such as pneumonia, widened mediastinum (patient with history of hypertension), COPD (patient with history of smoking).*

    ▶ *CBC—assess for signs and symptoms of anemia, which can decrease oxygen-carrying capacity to tissues; assess white-cell count to rule out infection.*

    ▶ *CMP—assess potassium—patient is taking ACEI that can cause hyperkalemia; patient is taking diuretic which can cause increased BUN/CR and also is potassium wasting diuretic assess BUN/creatinine, which are reflective of kidney function; in heart failure, there may be decreased perfusion to the kidneys, causing an elevation of BUN/creatinine and a decrease in estimated GFR.*

    ▶ *TSH—to make sure patient does not have hyperthyroidism or hypothyroidism that can contribute to her heart failure.*

    ▶ *BNP—elevated BNP greater than 100 pg/mL indicates that heart failure is present. The higher the BNP, the more severe the heart failure. This substance is released by the body in response to atrial and ventricular stretching. This is the body's attempt to compensate for the heart failure by blocking aldosterone and renin, thereby decreasing preload and afterload.*

    ▶ *Lipid profile—obtain after 10-hour fast; not always reliable when drawn from acutely ill patients. But if she does not have a baseline reading, this will be important to evaluate. She is not on a statin at this time.*

    ▶ *Cardiac troponins I and T—Make sure that she is not experiencing myocardial ischemia that could be causing the acute decompensated HF. In addition, when some patients go into HF, this increases the myocardial oxygen demand and can cause unstable angina, NSTEMI, or STEMI to develop.*

    ▶ *Urinalysis—to assess for protein or albumin in urine. This can be reflective of kidney disease.*

    ▶ *12-lead ECG—to assess the heart rhythm. Is she in atrial fibrillation, a common dysrhythmia in the elderly and in those with heart failure? Does she have ST/T-wave changes indicative of myocardial ischemia?*

    ▶ *Echocardiogram—to assess size/function of the heart chambers; valve function; function of the heart's pumping ability—estimated EF; any signs or symptoms of clots anywhere in the heart; assess thickness/size of heart muscle.*

    ▶ *Telemetry monitoring continuously*

2. **The patient asks you why she is taking the medications. She doesn't think they are helping.**

- *Carvedilol (Coreg)—beta-blocker to decrease BP, HR, and workload; will block SNS and renin; decreases mortality rate associated with HF; this drug also is a vasodilator, so the heart does not have to work harder than necessary to empty.*
- *Enalapril (Vasotec)—ACEI will block aldosterone; decreases afterload, so heart does not have to work harder than necessary; will prevent remodeling of heart and protect kidney function.*
- *Aspirin—will decrease platelet aggregation and is cardioprotective.*
- *Furosemide (Lasix)—potassium-wasting loop diuretic that will decrease preload and blood volume so the heart does not have to work harder than necessary.*

3. **What signs and symptoms of right- and left-sided heart failure will you review with your patient?**

- ***Right-sided heart failure:*** *right-upper-quadrant pain, anorexia, nausea, weight gain, hepatomegaly, peripheral edema, JVD, ascites*
- ***Left-sided heart failure****—dyspnea, orthopnea, paroxysmal nocturnal dyspnea, nocturia, frothy pink tinged secretions, S3, S4, PMI displaced to the left of the midclavicular line, restlessness, confusion*

4. **In addition to the medication teaching and signs and symptoms of right- and left-sided heart failure, what other teaching must be reviewed with this patient?**

- *The need to balance rest with activity*
- *This is a chronic disease and she needs to see her health care provider frequently.*
- *Low sodium, low fat diet; or DASH diet*
- *Read labels to be mindful of hidden sodium*
- *No added salt when cooking*
- *Regular exercise program, avoiding extremes in temperature; cardiac rehab*
- *Daily weights and notification if she gains 3 lb in 2 days or 3 to 5 lb in a week. Keep body-mass index (BMI) in desirable range so the heart does not have to work harder than necessary.*
- *Inform patient about keeping track of urine output. She may urinate more during night because more cardiac output is available to perfuse kidneys when the body is at rest.*
- *Recognize signs of atrial fibrillation: feeling faint, tired, palpitations, increased dyspnea, edema*
- *Monitor BP and pulse at home*
- *Annual flu vaccine and adult vaccinations*

Bibliography

Abraham, W.T., Adamson, P.B., Bourge, R.C., Aaron, M.F., Costanzo, M.R., Stevenson, . . . Yadav, J.S. (2011). Wireless pulmonary artery haemodynamic monitoring in chronic heart failure: a randomised controlled trial. *Lancet* 377, 658–666.

Ackley, B.J., Ladwig, G.B., and Flynn Makic, M.B. (2017). *Nursing Diagnosis Handbook: an Evidenced Based Guide to Planning Care,* 11th ed. (St. Louis: Elsevier).

American College of Cardiology (ACC)/American Heart Association (AHA). (2017). Heart risk calculator. Accessed June 7, 2018, from www.cvriskcalculator.com.

Anderson, J.L., Halperin, J.L., Albert, N.M., Bozkurt, B., Brindis, R.B., Curtis, L.H., …Win-Kuang, S. (2013). Management of patients with atrial fibrillation (compilation of 2006 ACCF/AHA/ESC and 2011 ACCF/AHA/HRS recommendations): a report of the American College of Cardiology/American Heart Association task force on practice guidelines. (2013). *Circulation* 127, 1916–1926.

Benjamin E.J., Blaha, M.J., Chiuve, S.E., Cushman, M, Das, S. R., Deo, R., ...Muntner, P. (2018). Heart disease and stroke statistics—2018 update: a report from the American Heart Association. *Circulation* 137, e67–e492.

Bibbins-Domingo, K. (2016). Aspirin use for the primary prevention of cardiovascular disease and colorectal cancer: U.S. preventive services task force recommendation statement. *Annals of Internal Medicine* 164, 836–845.

Burchum, J.R., and Rosenthal, L.D. (2016). *Lehne's Pharmacology for Nursing Care*, 9th ed. (St. Louis: Elsevier).

Burg, M.M., Edmondson, D., Shimbo, D., Shaffer, J., Kronish, I.M., Whang, W., ...Davidson, K.W. (2013). The 'perfect storm' and acute coronary syndrome onset: do psychosocial factors play a role? *Progress in Cardiovascular Diseases* 55, 601–610.

Cohen, B.E., Edmondson, D., and Kronish I. M. (2015). State of the art review: depression, stress, anxiety, and cardiovascular disease. *American Journal of Hypertension* 28, 1295–1302.

Elmoselhi, A. (2018). *Cardiology: An integrated approach* (New York: McGraw-Hill). Accessed April 1, 2018, from http://accessmedicine.mhmedical.com/content.aspx?bookid=2224&sectionid=171659224

Epocrates Plus for Apple iOS (Version 18.2.1). (2018). Cardiovascular Drugs. [Mobile application software]. Accessed March 27, 2018 from http://www.epocrates.com/mobile/iphone/essentials

Eraso, L.H., Fukaya, E., Mohler E.R. III, Xie, D., Sha, D., and Berger, J.S. (2014). Peripheral arterial disease, prevalence and cumulative risk factor profile analysis. *European Journal of Preventive Cardiology* 21, 704–711.

Fuster V, Harrington R.A., Narula, J, Eapen, Z.J., eds. (2017). *Hurst's the Heart*, 14th ed. (New York: McGraw-Hill). Accessed April 1, 2018, from http://accessmedicine.mhmedical.com/content.aspx?bookid=2046&sectionid=176545550

Gerhard-Herman, M.D., Gornik, H.L., Barrett, C., Barshes, N.R., Corriere, M.A., Drachman, D.E, ... Walsh, M.E. (2016). 2016 AHA/ACC guideline on the management of patients with lower extremity peripheral artery disease: executive summary: a report of the American College of Cardiology/American Heart Association task force on clinical practice guidelines. *The Journal of the American College of Cardiology*, 69(11), e71–e126, http://dx.doi.org/10.1016/J.jacc.2016.11.007.

Goff, D.C., Lloyd-Jones, D.M., Bennett, G., Coady, S., D'Agostino, R.B. Gibbons, R., ... Levy, D. (2014). 2013 ACC/AHA guideline on the assessment of cardiovascular risk: a report of the American College of Cardiology/American Heart Association task force on practice guidelines. *Circulation* 129, S49–S73.

Huether, S.E., McCance, K.L, Brashers, V.L., and Rote, N.S. (2017). *Understanding Pathophysiology*, 6th ed. (St. Louis: Elsevier).

January C.T., Wann, L.S., Alpert, J.S., Calkins, H., Cigarroa, J.E., Cleveland J.C., . . .Yancy, C.W. (2014). 2014 AHA/ACC/HRS guideline for the management of patients with atrial fibrillation: executive summary. *Journal of American College of Cardiology* 64, 2246–2280.

Kaspar, D., Fauci, A., Hauser, S., Longo, D., Jameson, J.L., and Loscalzo, J. (2015). *Harrison's Principles of Internal Medicine*, 19th ed. (New York: McGraw-Hill Education).

Levine, G.N., Steinke, E.E., Bakaeen F.G., Bozkurt, B., Cheitlin, M.D., Conti, J.B..., . Stewart, W.J. (2012). Sexual activity and cardiovascular disease: a scientific statement from the American Heart Association. Circulation, 125, 1058–1072.

Lewis, S.L., Bucher, L., Heitkemper, M., Harding, M.M., Kwong, J., and Roberts, D. (2017). *Medical-Surgical Nursing: Assessment and Management of Clinical Problems*, 10th ed. (St. Louis: Elsevier).

Mayo Clinic. Abdominal aortic aneurysm. Accessed March 20, 2018, from https://www.mayoclinic.org/diseases-conditions/abdominal-aortic-aneurysm/diagnosis-Treatment/drc-20350693

Merai, R., Siegel, C., Rakotz, M., Basch, P., Wright, J., Wong, B., and Thorpe P. (2016). CDC grand rounds: a public health approach to detect and control hypertension. *MMWR Morbidity Mortality Weekly Report* 65, 1261–1264.

Mescher, A.J. (2016). *Junqueira's Basic Histology*. (New York: McGraw Hill Education).

Mozzafarian, D., Benjamin, E.J., Go, A.S, Arnett, D. K., Blaha, M.J., Cushman, M., . . . Turner, M.B. (2015). Heart disease and stroke statistics—2015 update: a report from the American Heart Association. *Circulation* 131, e29–322.

National Heart Lung, and Blood institute. Cardiomyopathy. U.S. Department of Health and Human Services. Accessed March 29, 2018, from https://www.nhlbi.nih.gov/health-topics/cardiomyopathy

Nishimura, R.A., Otto, C.M., Bonow, R.O., Carabello, B.A., Erwin, J.P., Guyton, R.A.,...Thomas, J.D. (2014). 2014 AHA/ACC guideline for the management of patients with valvular heart disease: executive summary: a report of the American College of Cardiology/American Heart Association task force on practice guidelines. *Circulation* 129, 1–169.

O'Gara, P.T., Kushner, S.G., Ascheim, D.D., Casey, D.E., Chung, M.K., de Lemos, J.A., . . . Zhao, D.X. (2013). ACCF/AHA guideline for the management of ST-elevation myocardial infarction. *Circulation* 127, e362–425.

Pagana, K.D., Pagana, T.J., & Pagana, T.N. (2017). *Mosby's Diagnostic & Laboratory Test Reference*, 13th ed. (St. Louis: Elsevier).

Stone, N.J., Robinson, J., Lichtenstein, A.H., Bairey Merz, C.N., Blum, C.B., Eckel, R.H., . . . Wilson, P.W.F (2014). 2013 ACC/AHA guideline on the treatment of blood cholesterol to reduce atherosclerotic cardiovascular risk in adults: a report of the American College of Cardiology/American Heart Association task force on practice guidelines. *Circulation* 129, 1–85.

Weir, H. K., Anderson, R.N., Coleman King, S.M., Soman, A., Thompson, T. D., Hong Y., … Leadbetter, S. (2016). Heart disease and cancer deaths — trends and projections in the United States, 1969–2020. *Preventing Chronic Disease* 13, E157.

Whelton, P.K., Carey, R.M., Aronow, W.S., Casey, D.E., Collins, K.J., Dennison Himmelfarb, C. . . . Wright, J.T. (2018). 2017 AACC/AHA/AAPA/ABC/ACPM /AGS/APhA/ASH/ASPC/NMA/PCNA guideline for the prevention, detection, evaluation, and management of high blood pressure in adults: executive summary: a report of the American College of Cardiology/American Heart Association task force on clinical practice guidelines. *Journal of the American College of Cardiology,* 71(19), 2199–2269. DOI:10.1016/j.jacc.2017.11.005.

Yancy, C.W., Jessup, M., Bozkurt, B., Butler, J., Casey, D.E., Drazner, M.H., . . . Wilkoff, B.L. (2013). 2013 ACCF/AHA guideline for the management of heart failure: a report of the American College of Cardiology Foundation/American Heart Association task force on practice guidelines. *Circulation* 128, e240–e327.

Yancy, C.W., Jessup, M., Bozkurt, B., Butler, J., Casey, D.E. . . . Westlake, C. (2017). ACC/AHA/HFSA focused update of the 2013 ACCF/AHA guideline for the management of heart failure: a report of the American College of Cardiology/American Heart Association task force on clinical practice guidelines and the Heart Failure Society of America. *Circulation* 137, 1–129.

10

Diabetes

Donna Martin, DNP, RN, CMSRN, CDE, CNE

Diabetes is a chronic disorder that is caused by an absolute insulin deficiency or a relative deficiency of insulin production and insulin resistance. It is estimated that more than 30 million Americans have diabetes and 84 million have prediabetes (CDC, 2017).

OVERVIEW

▶ Type 1 diabetes is thought to be due to an autoimmune response in which there is destruction of the β cells in the pancreas, creating an absolute insulin deficiency. Approximately 5 to 10% of people with diabetes have type 1. These individuals tend to be younger at diagnosis and have a slim stature. Acute onset of symptoms includes polyuria, polydipsia, polyphagia, hyperglycemia, ketonuria, weight loss, weakness, and fatigue.

▶ Type 2 diabetes has several contributing factors. Insulin resistance and a progressive loss of β-cell function in the pancreas are the most significant causes. Onset typically occurs over several years, and the patient may not have any symptoms. These individuals account for 90 to 95% of persons with diabetes, are more likely to be diagnosed at an older age, and are typically overweight. Common manifestations at the time of diagnosis may include blurry vision, infections (skin, urinary, yeast), hyperglycemia, fatigue, and target organ damage.

▶ Prediabetes is defined as a blood glucose that is higher than what is considered normal, although not high enough to meet the criteria for diabetes. A person who has prediabetes is considered at high risk for the development of type 2 diabetes as well as other chronic diseases. Addressing prediabetes through education, medical nutritional therapy, exercise, and weight loss can reduce the risk of developing diabetes.

Question	Rationale
It is important for the nurse to understand that type 2 diabetes is primarily characterized by: A. Insulin resistance. B. Absolute insulin deficiency. C. Autoimmune destruction of β–cells. D. Insulin sensitivity.	Answer: A Insulin resistance is a significant characteristic of type 2 diabetes. Type 1 diabetes is noted for an absolute insulin deficiency due to the autoimmune destruction of β-cells.

DIAGNOSIS

▶ Diagnosis can be made if any of the following laboratory tests are abnormal: a fasting plasma blood glucose (FPG), a random plasma blood glucose, a 75-g oral glucose-tolerance test (OGTT), and a hemoglobin A_{1c} (glycosylated hemoglobin) (Table 10.1).

TABLE 10.1	DIAGNOSTIC CRITERIA			
	FPG (8 hour fast)	Random Plasma Blood Glucose (symptomatic)	2-Hour Plasma Glucose (75-g OGTT)	Hemoglobin A_{1c}
Prediabetes	100–125 mg/dL	NA	140–199 mg/dL	5.5–6.4%
Diabetes	≥126 mg/dL*	≥200 mg/dL*	≥200 mg/dL	≥6.5%

*In the absence of unequivocal hyperglycemia, results should be confirmed by repeat testing.
(American Diabetes Association, 2017b)
NA = not applicable.

TREATMENT

Lifestyle Management

▶ Goals:

- Maintain blood glucose levels in target range.
- Reduce the risk for acute and chronic complications associated with diabetes.
- Improve nutritional intake.
- Exercise
- Weight reduction:
  - Weight loss improves insulin sensitivity.
  - Metabolic/bariatric surgery is now considered a treatment for diabetes. Candidates include those with:
    - A BMI >40, regardless of glycemic control
    - A BMI >30 with uncontrolled blood glucose despite medications and lifestyle modifications.
- Smoking cessation

Medical Nutritional Therapy

▶ Goals:

- Improve glucose and lipid levels.
- Promote consistent day-to-day food intake.
- Consistent intake for each meal:
  - Carbohydrate, 40 to 60% of meal
  - Protein, 15 to 20% (reduced if client has renal disease)
  - Fat ≤30%:
    - ≤7% saturated fat
- Weight management
- Adequate nutrition across the lifespan.
- Vitamin and mineral requirements are the same as for the general population.

Exercise

▶ Exercising 150 minutes a week, over at least 3 days, is recommended. Blood glucose typically lowers during exercise and for several hours afterward.

▶ Benefits:
- Decreased blood glucose and improved insulin sensitivity in type 2 diabetes
- Improved lipid levels
  - Increases HDL
  - Decreases LDL
- Decreased blood pressure
- Increased oxygen consumption
- Improved blood flow
- Reduced cardiovascular risks
- Stress reduction
- Weight control

▶ Considerations:
- Complete a preexercise evaluation prior to beginning an exercise program.
- Wear proper footwear.
- Blood glucose must be checked prior to exercise, especially for individuals with type 1 diabetes:
  - If blood glucose >250 mg/dL and ketones are present, avoid exercise.
- If blood glucose <100 mg/dL, have a snack prior to exercise to prevent hypoglycemia.
- Have fast-acting glucose readily available.

> **Clinical Consideration**
> Exercise can cause a significant drop in blood glucose; monitor for hypoglycemia.

Question	Rationale
A patient with type 2 diabetes managed with oral medications, is scheduled for a follow-up visit. Which test would the nurse expect the provider to order to evaluate the effectiveness of the current treatment? A. Fasting blood glucose B. Oral glucose tolerance C. Glycosylated hemoglobin D. Urine dipstick for ketones	Answer: C The glycosylated hemoglobin reflects the previous 90 days of blood glucose control. The fasting blood glucose and oral glucose tolerance tests indicate a blood glucose at one point in time. Checking for urine ketones is done for patients with type 1 diabetes with blood glucose levels >250 mg/dL.

Blood Glucose Monitoring

▶ Point of care/blood glucose self-management
- Before meals—preprandial
- Bedtime
- 2 hours after meals—postprandial:
  - Primarily for individuals with gestational diabetes
  - Can be used for medication adjustments
- Hemoglobin A_{1c}
  - Indicates blood glucose control over the last 3 months
- Glycemic targets (ADA, 2017b)
  - 70–130 mg/dL preprandial
  - <180 mg/dL postprandial
  - Hemoglobin A_{1c} < 7.

> **Clinical Consideration**
> Frail and older adults have more liberal targets to prevent hypoglycemic events.

Medications

▶ Oral medications (Table 10.2):

- Used in type 2 diabetes:
- Classifications:
  - Increased insulin secretion
  - Increased insulin sensitivity
  - Decreased hepatic glucose production
  - Delayed absorption of carbohydrates
  - Increased urinary excretion of glucose

TABLE 10.2	ORAL DIABETES MEDICATIONS	
Oral Hypoglycemia Agent	Dosage Range (per day)	Patient Instructions/Monitoring
Sulfonylureas—help the pancreas release more insulin		
Glipizide (Glucotrol)	2.5–20 mg	Take 30 minutes before meal. The most common side effect is hypoglycemia.
Glipizide (Glucotrol XL)		
Glyburide (Micronase)		
Glimepiride (Amaryl)	1–8 mg	Take 30 minutes before first main meal of day.
Meglitinide D-Phenylalanine Derivative—helps pancreas release more insulin, especially after meals		
Repaglinide (Prandin)	0.5–4 mg (up to 16 mg each day)	Take 15–30 minutes before each meal, skip dose if no meal, with extra meal add a dose. Hypoglycemia is possible.
Nateglinide (Starlix)	60–120 mg (up to 360 mg each day)	
Biguanides—help liver hold glucose; makes insulin work more efficiently		
Metformin (Glucophage) Metformin (Riomet) [liquid form]	500–2550 mg 500 mg in 5 ml	Take with meals and take extended-release formulation with evening meal. May cause gas, diarrhea and bloating, and nausea and stomach pain. Not to be taken by people with heart and kidney failure. Withhold for 48 hours after surgery or diagnostic tests with contrast material.
metformin (Glucophage XR, Fortamet, Glumetza)	500–2000 mg 1000–2500 mg 500–2000 mg	
Thiazolidinediones—make insulin work more efficiently		
Rosiglitazone (Avandia)	2–8 mg	Take with or without meals. Liver tests before starting and at least every year thereafter. Assess for fluid volume overload. Takes up to 16 weeks to be most effective.
Pioglitazone (Actos)	15–45 mg	
Alpha-glucosidase inhibitors—slow down absorption in the gut, lowering after meal blood sugar		
Acarbose (Precose)	75–300 mg	Take with first bite of meal. Treat hypoglycemia with glucose tabs or 15g carbohydrate. Can cause gas and diarrhea so dose is increased gradually.
Miglitol (Glyset)	75–300 mg	
DPP4 Inhibitors—preserve pancreas's ability to make insulin and slow liver glucose production		
Sitagliptin (Januvia)	100 mg daily	Take with or without meals Dose reduced with kidney failure
Saxagliptin (Onglyza)	2.5–5 mg	Take with or without meals 2.5 mg dosing with kidney failure

(continued)

TABLE 10.2   (*Continued*)

Oral Hypoglycemia Agent	Dosage Range (per day)	Patient Instructions/Monitoring
Linagliptin (Tradjenta)	5 mg	Take with or without meals No dose adjustments required with kidney or liver failure
Alogliptin (Nesina)	6.2–25 mg daily	Take with or without meals Dose reduced with kidney failure
Combination Medications—combination of 2 of the above medications		
Glyburide/metformin (Glucovance)	Actos/metformin (Actoplusmet)	See previous information for each of the individual medications Reminder: All agents containing metformin should be taken with meals
nesina/metformin (Kasano)	Nesina/actos (Oseni)	
metformin/glucotrol (Metaglip)	Actos/glimepride (Duetact)	
Sodium-Glucose–Linked Transporter 2 (SGLT2) Inhibitors excrete excess sugar into the urine		
Canagliflozin (Invokana)	100 mg daily	Provider will watch kidney and cholesterol labs closely. Possible side effects include hypoglycemia yeast or urinary tract infections, decreased blood pressure, and increased low-density lipoprotein (LDL).
Dapagliflozin (Farxiga)	5 mg or 10 mg daily	
Empagliflozin (Jardiance)	10 mg or 25 mg daily	

Used and adapted with permission from Mercy Health Saint Mary's Diabetes Self-Management Education Program, Grand Rapids, MI.

Question	Rationale
A patient with type 2 diabetes just returned from having a computed tomographic (CT) scan of the head with contrast. Which order should the nurse question? A. Consistent carbohydrate diet B. Glargine (Lantus) 10 units subcutaneous at 9 pm C. Glyburide (Micronase) 2.5 mg daily D. Metformin (Glucophage) 1,000 mg twice a day	Answer: D Patients typically can resume eating after this type of procedure. Metformin is contraindicated for 48 hours after surgery, a diagnostic test with contrast material, or any other procedure that may impact kidney function. Lantus and Micronase would not be contraindicated in this situation.

◗ Noninsulin injectable medications (Table 10.3):
- Classifications:
  - Enhance production of glucose-dependent insulin
  - Assist insulin to work more efficiently
◗ Insulin (Table 10.4):
- Used in all individuals with type 1 and some individuals with type 2 diabetes
- High-alert medication—administer with caution, confirm dose with another nurse

TABLE 10.3	NONINSULIN INJECTABLES	
Exenatide (Byetta) (used with oral diabetes medications and/or basal insulin)	5- or 10-µg pen Taken twice a day within 60 minutes before meal	Enhances glucose-dependent insulin production, slows gastric emptying, decreases liver glucose release, promotes satiety. **Side effects:** Nausea and low blood sugar
Dulaglutide (Trulicity) (used with oral diabetes medications and/or basal insulin)	0.75 or 1.5 mg once every 7 days	
Albiglutide (Tanzeum) (used with oral diabetes medications and/or insulin)	30 mg once every 7 days	
Liraglutide (Victoza) (used with oral diabetes medications and/or basal insulin)	1.2–1.8 mg daily (using a pen) Administered once daily at any time, independent of meals	Actions similar to those of Byetta Patients with a personal or family history of medullary thyroid cancer or multiple endocrine neoplasia syndrome should not use Victoza. **Side effects:** Nausea and low blood sugar
Exenatide (Bydureon) (Used along with oral DM medications and/or basal insulin)	2 mg once every 7 days	Long acting form of Byetta Medication must be mixed prior to administration **Side effects:** Nausea and low blood sugar
Pramlintide acetate (Symlin) (used with insulin)	Vials or pens—dose titrated from 30 µg 3 times a day to 60 µg or 120 µg 3 times day Taken with each meal of 250 calories or 30 g of carbohydrates	Taken with mealtime insulin, but in a separate injection; helps insulin work more efficiently **Side effects:** Nausea and low blood sugar

Used and adapted with permission from Mercy Health Saint Mary's Diabetes Self-Management Education Program, Grand Rapids, MI.

> **Clinical Consideration**
>
> The term *sliding scale insulin* has been replaced with *correction insulin*, and the dose is based on blood glucose results.

> **Clinical Consideration**
>
> Do not administer scheduled meal bolus insulin if patient is NPO (non per os; nothing by mouth) or does not eat.

- Classifications:
  - Bolus insulin—used to cover meals and snacks and to correct an elevated blood glucose:
    - Rapid-acting
    - Short-acting
  - Basal insulin—used to provide background insulin:
    - Intermediate-acting
    - Long-acting
  - Combination
  - Inhaled:
    - Rapid-acting
    - Prepackaged cartridges (4-, 8-, 12-unit doses)
    - Contraindicated for people with chronic lung diseases (asthma, chronic obstructive pulmonary disease [COPD]), history of lung cancer, recent or current smoker, pregnant, and breastfeeding
- Insulin pens:
  - Prefilled pens with insulin
    - One pen per patient—**DO NOT use an insulin pen on more than one patient, or draw up insulin from the pen.**
    - Use a new pen needle each time and remove the pen needle immediately after use.

Insulin pump:

- Provides a continuous basal insulin dose for a patient who is able to administer a bolus of insulin for food or blood glucose correction.
- Patient must be able to cognitively and physically be able to do self-management in order to continue to use the insulin pump during hospitalization.
- There must be a physician order for the patient to use the insulin pump in the hospital. Basal rates, as well as all bolus doses, need to be documented.
- Patients need to provide their own insulin pump supplies during their hospital stay.
- Insulin pump site must be assessed daily; patient should change site every 3 days (per manufacturer's instructions).
- Nurses are responsible for documenting insulin pump doses in the medical record.

TABLE 10.4   INSULIN

Type	Color	Onset	Peak	Duration
Rapid-Acting				
Glulisine (Apidra)	Clear	5 minutes	1 hour	2–4 hours
Lispro (Humalog)	Clear	5 minutes	1 hour	2–4 hours
Aspart (Novolog)	Clear	5 minutes	1 hour	2–4 hours
Inhaled insulin (Afrezza)	4-, 8-, and 12-unit cartridges	12 minutes	35–45 minutes	1.5–4 hours (depending on dose)
Short-Acting				
Regular (Humulin R, Novolin R)	Clear	0.5–1 hour	2–5 hours	6–12 hours
Regular (U-500)	Similar action to regular insulin, 5 times more concentrated			
Degludec (Tresiba)	Clear	60 minutes	Peakless	42 hours
Intermediate-Acting				
NPH (Humulin N, Novolin N)	Milky-white	1–1.5 hour	4–12 hours	≥24 hours
Long-Acting				
Glargine (Toujeo)	Clear **Never Mix**	60 minutes	Peakless	27 hours
Glargine (Lantus)	Clear **Never Mix**	60 minutes	Peakless	24 hours
Detemir (Levemir)	Clear **Never Mix**	0.8–2 hours	Relatively flat	Up to 24 hours
Premixed				
Humalog 75/25	Milky-white	5 minutes	6–15 hours	≥22 hours
Humulin 70/30 Novolin 70/30	Milky-white	30 minutes	2–12 hours	24 hours
Novolog Mix 70/30	Milky-white	5 minutes	6–15 hours	≥22 hours

Used and adapted with permission from Mercy Health Saint Mary's Diabetes Self-Management Education Program, Grand Rapids, MI.

Question	Rationale
The patient received regular insulin 10 units subcutaneously at 8:30 a.m. for a blood glucose level of 244 mg/dL. The nurse plans to monitor this patient for signs of hypoglycemia during which time period? A. 8:40 a.m. to 9:00 a.m. B. 9:00 a.m. to 11:30 a.m. C. 10:30 a.m. to 1:30 p.m. D. 12:30 p.m. to 8:30 p.m.	Answer: C Regular insulin exerts peak action in 2 to 5 hours, making the patient most at risk for hypoglycemia between 10:30 a.m. and 1:30 p.m. Rapid-acting insulin's onset is between 10 and 30 minutes, with peak action and hypoglycemia most likely to occur between 9:00 a.m. and 11:30 a.m. With intermediate-acting insulin, hypoglycemia may occur from 12:30 p.m. to 8:30 p.m.

ACUTE COMPLICATIONS

Hypoglycemia

Hypoglycemia is defined as a blood glucose of <70 mg/dL and severe hypoglycemia is defined as a blood glucose <54 mg/dL (ADA, 2017b). It is important to collect the patient history, including:

▶ History of hypoglycemia and symptoms experienced
▶ Usual treatment for hypoglycemia
▶ Risk factors:
  • Oral diabetes medications
  • Insulin
  • Skipping meals
  • Exercise
  • Incorrect medication dose and timing
▶ Medication history and compliance review

Question	Rationale
A patient was given 10 units of lispro (Humalog) insulin 30 minutes ago. The patient reports feeling light-headed and sweaty. Which action should the nurse take first? A. Have the patient drink 4 ounces of orange juice. B. Obtain a glucose reading using a finger stick. C. Infuse dextrose 50% by slow IV push. D. Administer 1 mg glucagon subcutaneously.	Answer: B The first action would be to check the blood sugar. Based on the blood glucose, the nurse may then administer 4 ounces of juice, D50, or glucagon to treat the hypoglycemia.

Assessment/Analysis
▶ Blood glucose <70 mg/dL
▶ Autonomic symptoms of hypoglycemia:
  • Shaky
  • Sweaty
  • Tachycardia

- Palpitations
- Hungry
▶ Neuroglycopenic symptoms:
  - Confusion
  - Coma
  - Seizures

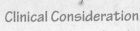

Intervention

▶ Check blood glucose
▶ If alert and able to swallow, treat with 15g of carbohydrate. Treat with one of the following:
  - Glucose tablets
  - Glucose gel
  - 4 oz juice
  - 8 oz milk
▶ If NPO or not alert enough to swallow, treat with one of the following:
  - D50 IV push
  - Glucagon subcutaneous or intramuscular
▶ Recheck blood glucose 15 minutes after treatment
▶ If blood glucose remains below 70 mg/dL, retreat with 15g of carbohydrate, recheck in 15 minutes. Continue this until blood glucose is >70 mg/dL (ADA, 2017b).

Evaluation

▶ Evaluate cause of hypoglycemic event
▶ Notify provider about the event for possible medication/insulin adjustments
▶ Patient teaching:
  - Reinforce appropriate administration and timing of diabetes medications.
  - Check blood glucose if symptomatic.
  - Treat with 15g of carbohydrate, recheck blood glucose 15 minutes after treatment, and repeat if necessary.
  - Notify provider about hypoglycemic events.

Diabetic Ketoacidosis (DKA)

DKA is hyperglycemia at a blood glucose level of >250 mg/dL with the presence of ketones and metabolic acidosis. It is important to collect the patient history, including:

▶ History of hyperglycemia and occurrences of DKA
▶ Presence of illness/infection
▶ Review of medication history and compliance
▶ Possible triggers:
  - Newly diagnosed type 1 diabetes
  - Omission of insulin doses
  - Insufficient amount of insulin administered
  - Illness/infection

Assessment/Analysis

▶ Blood glucose >250 mg/dL
▶ Presence of ketones in urine
▶ Metabolic acidosis: pH <7.35, HCO_3^- <22
▶ Kussmaul respirations (rapid, deep, and labored)
▶ Fruity odor to breath
▶ Dehydration

Clinical Consideration

Rapid administration of fluids—1 L of fluid can be administered over 30 minutes, for DKA in otherwise healthy individuals.

Intervention

- Isotonic IV fluids to restore volume
- IV insulin drip
- Frequent blood glucose monitoring (every hour initially)
- Monitor potassium levels
- Correct acidosis
- Possible transfer to critical care

Evaluation

- Fluid volume restored
- Blood glucose levels within normal range
- Potassium level in normal range
- Correction of metabolic acidosis (pH 7.35–7.45)
- Evaluate cause of event
- Patient teaching:
  - Reinforce appropriate insulin administration and doses.
  - Sick-day management
  - Notify provider about persistent hyperglycemia and ketonuria.

Question	Rationale
A patient admitted with type 1 diabetes has a glucose level of 320 mg/dL and a moderate level of ketones in the urine. While the nurse assesses for signs of ketoacidosis, what respiratory pattern would the nurse expect to find? A. Rapid, shallow respirations B. Hypoventilation C. Kussmaul respirations D. Cheyne–Stokes respirations	Answer: C In diabetic ketoacidosis, the lungs try to compensate for the acidosis by blowing off volatile acids and carbon dioxide. This leads to a pattern of Kussmaul respirations, which are deep and labored. Rapid, shallow respirations occurs with respiratory acidosis as the body tries to blow off additional CO_2. Hypoventilation and Cheyne–Stokes respirations do not occur with ketoacidosis.

Hyperosmolar Hyperglycemic Nonketotic Syndrome (HHNS)

HHNS is hyperglycemia at a blood glucose of >250 mg/dL without the presence of ketones and metabolic acidosis. It tends to occur in older individuals with type 2 diabetes. It is important to collect the patient history including:

- History of hyperglycemia
- History of illness/infection
- Chronic disease
- Medication history and compliance
- Possible triggers:
  - Uncontrolled type 2 diabetes
  - Illness/infection/sepsis

Assessment/Analysis

◗ Blood glucose >250 mg/dL

◗ Severe dehydration

Intervention

◗ Isotonic IV fluids to restore volume

◗ IV insulin drip

◗ Frequent blood glucose monitoring

◗ Monitor potassium levels

◗ Possible transfer to critical care

> **Clinical Consideration**
> Administer fluids with caution—may need to be administered slowly because of comorbidities to prevent fluid volume overload.

Evaluation

◗ Fluid volume restored

◗ Potassium level remains in normal range

◗ Evaluate cause of event

◗ Patient teaching:

- Reinforce appropriate insulin administration and doses.
- Sick-day management
- Notify provider about persistent hyperglycemia.

CHRONIC COMPLICATIONS

Microvascular Complications

Elevated blood glucose levels contribute to damage of the small blood vessels, resulting in long-term complications. Recommendations include maintaining target blood glucose levels and screening for these complications at various intervals.

◗ *Retinopathy*

- Very specific vascular complication associated with individuals with type 1 and type 2 diabetes; most frequent cause of new cases of blindness (ADA, 2017b)
- *Assessment/Intervention/Education*
  - When was last dilated eye exam?
  - Yearly dilated eye exam is necessary to assess for changes that are undetectable by the individual.
  - Panretinal laser photocoagulation therapy and intravitreous injections may be used to reduce vision loss.
  - Patient teaching:
    - Maintain glucose levels in target range.
    - Notify provider about changes in vision.
    - Have a yearly dilated eye exam.
    - Patients with known retinopathy should avoid activities that increase intraocular pressure.

> **Clinical Consideration**
> Treatment will not reverse damage; it will only slow progression.

◗ *Nephropathy*

- Disorder diagnosed by elevated urine albumin and declining glomerular filtration rate (GFR). Diabetes is the leading cause of new cases of end-stage renal disease (ADA, 2017b).
- *Assessment/Intervention/Education*
  - Optimizing blood glucose and blood pressure to decrease the risk and slow progression of kidney disease due to diabetes.
  - Monitor albuminuria and GFR regularly and refer to nephrologist if GFR <60 ml/min.

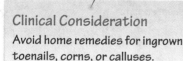

Clinical Consideration
ACE inhibitors have been shown to be kidney-protective for some patients.

- May be prescribed an angiotensin-converting enzyme (ACE) inhibitor or angiotensin-receptor blocker (ARB).
- Patient teaching:
  - Maintain blood glucose in target range.
  - Maintain blood pressure in target range.
  - Yearly testing for urine microalbumin.
  - Nutrition education—reduction of protein.
  - Avoid nephrotoxic substances.

▶ *Neuropathy*

- A group of disorders with diverse manifestations depending on the origin of the neuropathy. Glycemic control can slow the progression of neuropathies (ADA, 2017b).

- ***Assessment/Intervention/Education***
  - Peripheral neuropathy
    - Assess the location and characteristics of pain, paresthesias, foot drop, motor dysfunction, and loss of protective sensation.
    - Charcot deformity—a disorder that affects the bones, joints and tissues of foot and ankle (Rogers et al., 2011)
    - Use of medications to manage neuropathic pain:
      - Anticonvulsants:
        - Pregabalin (Lyrica)
        - Gabapentin (Neurontin)
        - Carbamazepine (Carbatrol, Tegretol)
      - Antidepressants:
        - Duloxetine (Cymbalta)
        - Venlafaxine (Effexor)
      - Narcotic analgesics:
        - Tapentadol (Nucynta)
        - Tramadol (Ultram)
      - Topical capsaicin
    - Foot inspection:
      - Daily foot inspection
      - Semmes–Weinstein monofilament examination (see Figure 18.6)
    - Foot care:
      - Notify provider immediately about any areas of concern on feet.
      - Always wear shoes or slippers; avoid going barefoot.
      - Keep nails trimmed.
    - Prevent amputations:
      - Daily foot inspection and excellent foot care are critical to preventing amputations.
  - Autonomic neuropathy:
    - Gastroparesis—delayed gastric emptying due to vagus nerve damage (ADA, 2017a):
      - Assess whether patient has bloating, nausea, or vomiting, especially after meals.
      - Small, low-fat, low-fiber meals may help.
      - May benefit from metoclopramide (Reglan).
      - Administer antiemetics.
    - Cardiac autonomic neuropathy (CAN)—may be asymptomatic with detection only with deep breathing and decreased heart rate variability or, in severe CAN, if resting tachycardia is present.

Clinical Consideration
Avoid home remedies for ingrown toenails, corns, or calluses.

- Orthostatic hypotension—CAN is a contributing factor:
  - Encourage adequate fluid volume intake.
  - Medications:
    - Midodrine (Proamatine)
    - Droxidopa (Northera)
- Erectile dysfunction and/or retrograde ejaculation:
  - Medications
    - Sildenafil (Revatio, Viagra)
    - Tadalafil (Adcirca, Cialis)
    - Avanafil (Stendra)
    - Vardenafil (Levitra, Staxyn)
  - Intracavernous or intraurethral prostaglandin injections
  - Vacuum devices
  - Penile prostheses
- Patient teaching:
  - Notify provider immediately about any problems.
  - Foot care:
    - Daily foot inspection.
    - Notify provider about any changes in feet.
    - Avoid going barefoot.
    - Cut nails straight across.
    - Keep skin moist, but do not put lotion between toes.
    - Wear cotton socks.
    - Wear well-fitting shoes.

Macrovascular Complications

Elevated blood glucose levels contribute to damage of the large blood vessels, resulting in long-term complications. Recommendations include maintaining target blood glucose levels and screening for these complications at various intervals. Macrovascular complications include:

▶ Cardiovascular disease

▶ Cerebrovascular disease

▶ Peripheral vascular disease

▶ Hypertension

▶ Hyperlipidemia

(see Chapter 9 for more in-depth review of these diseases)

- *Assessment/Intervention/Education*
  - Monitor blood pressure.
  - Monitor cholesterol levels.
  - Assess nutritional intake:
    - Fat intake
    - Sodium intake
    - Weight assessment
  - Patient teaching:
    - Maintain glucose levels in target range.
    - Importance of lifestyle modifications to reduce complications:
      - Exercise
      - Heart healthy dietary recommendations
        - Low fat; less than 30% of daily intake, less than 7% saturated fats
        - Sodium restriction

- Smoking cessation
- Stress reduction
- Maintaining blood pressure in target range

Question	Rationale
The nurse reviewed principles of foot care with a patient who has diabetes. Which statement indicates that the patient understands the principles of foot care? A. "I should only walk barefoot in nice dry weather." B. "I should look at the condition of my feet every day." C. "I can remove my ingrown toenails." D. "I can purchase shoes that are tight and will stretch as I wear them"	Answer: B Patients with diabetes need to inspect their feet daily for broken areas that are at risk for infection and delayed wound healing. Patients should not go barefoot because of the risk for injury. A podiatrist should be consulted for the care of ingrown toenails, corns, and calluses. Properly fitted (not tight) shoes should be worn at all times.

SPECIAL CIRCUMSTANCES

Geriatric Considerations

▶ Relaxed/individualized glycemic control targets based on cognition and comorbidities (Table 10.5)

▶ Consider comorbidities and medications.

▶ Prevent hypoglycemia.

▶ Poor glycemic control is associated with cognitive decline (ADA, 2017b).

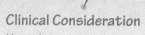

Clinical Consideration

Hypoglycemia may contribute to patient falls or injuries.

Surgery

▶ Reduce insulin doses the evening before and morning of surgery.

▶ Withhold metformin (Glucophage) 24 hours prior to surgery.

▶ Check blood glucose often during surgery and postoperative period.

▶ May need to consider IV insulin infusion to maintain control.

Hospitalization

▶ Blood glucose target 140 to 180 mg/dL

▶ Avoid using oral medications during hospitalization.

TABLE 10.5	GLYCEMIC TARGETS FOR OLDER ADULTS WITH DIABETES		
Health Status	Blood Glucose	Bedtime Blood Glucose	Hemoglobin A$_{1c}$
Fairly healthy, minimal comorbidities	90–130 mg/dL	90–150 mg/dL	<7.5%
Complex health, multiple comorbidities	90–150 mg/dL	100–180 mg/dL	<8.0%
Very complex, frail, poor health	100–180 mg/dL	100–180 mg/dL	<8.5%
American Diabetes Association (2017b)			

▶ Begin insulin for blood glucose >180 mg/dL

▶ May need an IV insulin infusion

▶ Basal/bolus insulin preferred

▶ Avoid using correction insulin as sole treatment

▶ Allow patient to use insulin pump if cognitively able to operate

> **Clinical Consideration**
> Basal/bolus insulin closely mimics normal insulin secretion.

Sick-Day Management

▶ Patient teaching:

- Blood glucose monitoring every 2 to 4 hours
- Carbohydrate intake every hour
- Insulin needs increase
- Urine ketone testing (type 1 diabetes)
- When to notify health care personnel:
  - Nausea and vomiting
  - Persistent hyperglycemia
  - Ketonuria
- Prevention of illness:
  - Influenza vaccine
  - Pneumococcal vaccine
  - Consider hepatitis B immunization
  - Home dental care
  - Dentist visit twice yearly

Glucocorticoid Therapy

▶ Causes an increase in blood glucose

▶ May require insulin to treat hyperglycemia

Parenteral / Enteral Feedings

- Continuous feedings:
  - Blood glucose testing every 6 hours with regular insulin coverage
                              or
  - Blood glucose testing every 4 hours with rapid-acting insulin
- Bolus enteral feedings
  - Test blood glucose and administer rapid-acting insulin with each bolus (ADA, 2017b).

CASE STUDY

A 62-year-old woman with a 15-year history of type 2 diabetes presents with symptoms of fatigue, difficulty losing weight, and "no motivation." She denies polyuria, polydipsia, polyphagia, blurred vision, and vaginal infections. Her medical history includes hypertension and hyperlipidemia, and she has begun to have symptoms of mild COPD. Current medications include:

▶ Metformin (Glucophage) 1000 mg twice a day

▶ Glargine (Lantus) insulin—12 units every morning

▶ Lispro (Humalog) insulin—5 units at breakfast and dinner

▶ Lisinopril (Prinivil) 10 mg daily

▶ Hydrochlorthiazide 25 mg daily

▶ Ipratropium (Atrovent) inhaler as needed

She states that she consistently takes her medications and checks her blood glucose before meals. The premeal blood glucose levels have been running higher lately. She retired 6 months ago and recently moved in with her niece. She admits that there has been a significant increase in her stress since the move and she has been eating whatever the family has for meals.

On physical exam, her height is 5'1" and her weight is 265 lb. Her blood pressure is 160/88 mm Hg, heart rate 68 beats/min, respirations slightly labored at a rate of 20 breaths/min, and diminished breath sounds were noted. Six months ago, her hemoglobin A$_{1c}$ was 7.2%; it is currently 8.1%. The provider instructs the patient to increase the lisinopril to 20 mg daily, increase the glargine insulin to 14 units, and increase the lispro insulin to 6 units with each meal (adding a lunchtime dose). In addition, the patient is referred to the diabetes educator. She is to return to the provider in 3 months.

The patient sees the diabetes educator a week later and receives education on meal planning, blood glucose testing, and signs and symptoms of hypoglycemia. Detailed medication instructions, including timing and administration, were reviewed. After several weeks of following the meal plan that she developed with the diabetes educator, the patient feels light-headed and shaky between 1 and 1.5 hours after breakfast and again after lunch. When she checks her blood glucose, the readings range between 58 and 67 mg/dL. She eats a candy bar and feels better shortly thereafter.

The patient returns for her follow-up visit 3 months after the initial visit and the nurse is reviewing her history and medications before the provider enters the room. Her weight is 254 lbs, blood pressure is 132/78, pulse 66, respirations are labored at 24, some audible wheezing noted, and her breath sounds are diminished with expiratory wheezing. Her A$_{1c}$ has decreased to 7.4%. She reports that sometimes she feels shaky after breakfast and lunch. The nurse suspects that she is having an exacerbation of her COPD and hypoglycemic episodes. There are no other significant physical assessment findings.

1. **What other information would be important to know?**
    - *Review her blood glucose records, look for trends of lowering blood glucoses, and specifically, check what her blood glucose levels have been prior to meals.*
    - *Inquire whether she is following the meal plan and check to see that she is eating three meals a day; review food records.*
    - *Review medication compliance, including doses and timing of insulin in relation to her meals.*
    - *Ask the patient about any exercise or physical activity, including time of day and duration of exercise/activity.*
    - *Does she check her blood glucose after she consumes candy, and if so what has her blood glucose been after treatment?*

2. **What information would you discuss with this patient?**
    - *Review importance of taking her mealtime insulin only if she is eating that meal.*
    - *Review more effective treatment options for hypoglycemia; 15g of carbohydrate (glucose tablets, glucose gel, 4 oz juice, or 8 oz milk) and then rechecking her blood glucose 15 minutes later.*
    - *Teach patient to avoid exercise or increased physical activity during the peak time of the lispro (Humalog) insulin. Insulin lispro peaks approximately 1 hour after administration.*
    - *Check blood glucose prior to exercise.*

The provider decides to adjust the mealtime lispro (Humalog) insulin doses to 4 units at each meal to prevent hypoglycemia, as well as start the patient on prednisone 10 mg daily for 5 days to treat her COPD exacerbation.

3. **What effect would you anticipate that the insulin dose changes and predni- sone would have on her blood glucose?**

 ◗ *Decreasing the lispro insulin doses before each meal should help to prevent hypoglycemic episodes after breakfast and lunch. The patient may have been receiving too much mealtime (bolus) insulin for her nutritional intake, especially since she saw the diabetes educator and has been adhering with the meal plan.*

 ◗ *Steroids typically will increase a person's blood glucose, with prednisone hav- ing an effect on the blood glucose for many hours after administration. It is not uncommon for someone taking steroids to need additional amounts of insulin to help reduce hyperglycemia.*

 ◗ *Blood glucose should be checked more frequently to evaluate the effectiveness of the insulin-dose changes and to assess the impact of the prednisone on blood glucose control.*

Discussion

It would be important to look at the patient's food intake as well as her activity levels, especially on the days that she has been feeling shaky and light-headed. Several lifestyle changes may have occurred since she received diabetes educa- tion, along with having her insulin doses increased and a lunchtime dose of insu- lin added. She most likely is experiencing hypoglycemia, so contributing factors need to be assessed. Is she receiving too much insulin, decreased or inadequate food intake, and/or increased activity? It may be a combination of all of these. It would also be important to have the patient check her blood glucose when she is experiencing these episodes, prior to treating, as well as after the treatment. The patient should be instructed to treat hypoglycemia with 15g of carbohydrate (fast-acting glucose is preferred) and then to recheck her blood glucose 15 minutes later. Decreasing the insulin doses to prevent further hypoglycemia makes sense, although the addition of steroids typically causes an increase in blood glucose levels. It will be important to monitor this patient's blood glucose levels closely, especially as prednisone doses are adjusted.

Bibliography

American Association of Diabetes Educators. (2016). Special considerations in the management and educa- tion of older persons with diabetes: AADE practice synopsis. Accessed June 9, 2018, from https://www. diabeteseducator.org/docs/default-source/legacy-docs/_resources/pdf/inpractice/aadepracticeadvisory_ older_adults.pdf?sfvrsn=2.

American Diabetes Association. (2017a). Living with diabetes complications: Gastroparesis. Accessed April 12, 2017, from http://www.diabetes.org/living-with-diabetes/complications/gastroparesis.html? loc=lwd-slabnav.

American Diabetes Association. (2017b). Standards of medical care in diabetes—2017. *Diabetes Care* 40(Suppl. 1), S6–S127.

Centers for Disease Control and Prevention. (2017). *National Diabetes Statistics Report, 2017.* Atlanta, GA: Centers for Disease Control and Prevention, US Department of Health and Human Services. Accessed June 9, 2018, from https://www.cdc.gov/diabetes/data/statistics/statistics-report.html

Garber, A.J., Abrahamson, M.J., Barzilay, J.I., Blonde, L., Bloomgarden, Z.T., Bush, M.A., … Umpierrez, G.E. (2017). Consensus statement by the American Association of Clinical Endocrinologists and American College of Endocrinology on the comprehensive type 2 diabetes management algorithm—2017 executive summary. *Endocrine Practice* 23, 207–238.

James, P.A., Oparil, S., Carter, B.L., Cushman, W.C., Dennison-Himmelfarb, C., Handler, J., … Ortiz, E. (2014). 2014 evidence-based guideline for the management of high blood pressure in adults: report from the panel members appointed to the Eighth Joint National Committee (JNC 8). *Journal of the American Medical Association* 311, 507–520.

Qaseem, A., Barry, M. J., Humphrey, L. L., and Forciea, M. A. (2012). Oral pharmacologic treatment of type 2 diabetes mellitus: a clinical practice guideline update from the American College of Physicians oral pharma- cologic treatment of type 2 diabetes mellitus. *Annals of Internal Medicine* 156, 218–231.

Rogers, L.C., Frykberg, R.G., Armstrong, D.G., Boulton, A.J., Edmonds, M., Ha Van, G., … Uccioli, L. (2011). The Charcot foot in diabetes. *Diabetes Care* 34, 2123–2129.

11

Endocrine System

Patricia Braida MSN, RN, AGPCNP-BC

OVERVIEW

▶ The endocrine system is responsible for maintaining homeostasis in the body. Its function is crucial in coordinating responses to dynamic changes in the internal and external environment. The endocrine system and the immune system are closely integrated and depend on each other to help control fluid balance, metabolism, growth, and development.

▶ The endocrine glands communicate with other organs through the nervous system, hormones, cytokines, and growth factors to regulate cellular and physiologic processes.

▶ Negative and positive feedback are features of the endocrine system. The hypothalamus, anterior pituitary gland (the "master gland"), and posterior pituitary gland regulate function of other endocrine glands and target tissues.

▶ Disease of the endocrine system is usually due to hormone excess, hormone deficiency, or hormone resistance.

▶ Only two of the endocrine glands are accessible to direct access (thyroid and gonads). To determine whether there is dysfunction, the provider must accurately assess signs and symptoms, family and social history, and exposure to medications and substances that affect the endocrine system.

▶ Laboratory testing plays a central role in evaluating hormone levels. Further diagnostic testing may be indicated if the hormone levels are abnormal.

▶ If a patient has an endocrine disorder, it must be determined whether there is pathology in the hypothalamus, pituitary gland, and/or target gland/tissue. A problem with any part of these axes can create disease.

ANATOMY AND PHYSIOLOGY

▶ The endocrine system is composed of the following (Table 11.1):
  • Hypothalamus:
    • Connected to the pituitary gland

TABLE 11.1 ENDOCRINE GLANDS AND HORMONES

Gland	Releasing Hormones	Tissue Affected	Hormones Released	Target	Action
Anterior Pituitary Hormones					
Hypothalamus	Growth hormone–releasing hormone (GHRH) or somatotropin-releasing hormone	Anterior pituitary gland	Growth hormone	All cells in the body	Growth hormone Promotes tissue growth, building/repair Promotes carbohydrate, lipid and protein metabolism and catabolism; Excess: acromegaly Deficient: decreased muscle mass and strength; weakness; fatigue; flat affect
Hypothalamus	Thyrotropin-releasing hormone	Anterior pituitary gland	Thyroid-stimulating hormone (TSH)	Thyroid gland	TSH stimulates the thyroid to produce and release: Thyroid hormones (free T_3 and T_4) T_3 and T_4 regulate metabolic rate, O_2 consumption, heat production; growth and development, carbohydrate and lipid metabolism, and brain and nervous system function. T_3 and T_4 are released to all cells of the body. Calcitonin helps regulate calcium and phosphorus levels; helps decrease serum calcium levels. Hypothyroidism: low T_3 and T_4, so pituitary releases more TSH (primary hypothyroidism) Hyperthyroidism: high T_3 and T_4, so pituitary releases less TSH (primary hyperthyroidism)
Hypothalamus	Corticotropin-releasing Hormone	Anterior Pituitary	Adrenocorticotropic hormone (ACTH)	Adrenal cortex	ACTH promotes growth of the adrenal cortex and secretion of these three hormones: Cortisol/corticosteroids—affect all body tissues; stress fighting hormone; promotes metabolism and has antiinflammatory effects Mineralocorticoids—regulate sodium, potassium–water balance Androgens/estradiol—promote growth spurt in adolescence, libido in both sexes and secondary sex characteristics Excessive cortical hormones can lead to Cushing syndrome. Deficient cortical hormones can lead to Addison's disease.
Hypothalamus	Gonadotropin-releasing hormone	Anterior pituitary	Follicle-stimulating hormone (FSH)	Ovaries Testes	FSH: Stimulates secretion of estrogen from the ovary; helps stimulate ovulation and development of ova Estrogen: Production stimulated by FSH Stimulates development of secondary sex characteristics; prepares uterus for fertilization and pregnancy Estrogen stimulates bone growth in women FSH stimulates sperm production in the testes
Hypothalamus	Gonadotropin-releasing hormone	Anterior pituitary	Luteinizing hormone (LH)	Ovaries Testes	LH: Stimulates secretion of estrogen and progesterone from ovaries Stimulates ovulation Progesterone: Maintains growth of uterine wall and maintains pregnancy; affects menstrual cycle; stimulates growth of mammary glands Stimulates testes to produce testosterone Testosterone: Produced by the testes and promotes development of secondary sex characteristics and production of sperm

Hypothalamus	Prolactin-releasing factor	Anterior pituitary	Prolactin	Ovary and mammary glands Testes	Prolactin: In lactating women, milk production is increased; Increases response to LH and FSH in follicles; Prolactin contributes to male reproductive health and testicular function

Posterior Pituitary Hormones

Hypothalamus	Oxytocin is produced in the hypothalamus and stored in the posterior pituitary	Posterior pituitary	Oxytocin	Mammary glands; uterus	Stimulates uterine contraction and secretion of breast milk
Hypothalamus	ADH (vasopressin) is produced in the hypothalamus and stored in the posterior pituitary gland	Posterior pituitary		Renal tubules, vascular smooth muscle	ADH: Released in response to decreased blood pressure, dehydration, and/or increased serum osmolality; Water is then reabsorbed by the kidneys; Syndrome of inappropriate antidiuretic hormone (SIADH)—too much ADH is produced, causing excessive fluid retention and hyponatremia; Diabetes insipidu (DI)—Not enough ADH, causing polyuria, polydipsia, dehydration, and hypernatremia

Parathyroid Gland Hormones

Parathyroid			Parathyroid hormone (PTH)	Bones, kidneys, small intestine	PTH: Release is regulated by negative feedback—when serum calcium level falls, PTH is secreted; When serum calcium level rises, PTH secretion decreases; Calcium level is increased by: Increasing bone resorption, Stimulating calcium reabsorption in kidneys, Stimulating kidneys to convert vitamin D to active form so intestinal calcium can be absorbed; PTH affects phosphorus level by: Reducing reabsorption of phosphorus in the kidney, Increasing bone release of phosphorus, Increasing absorption in the small intestine; Excessive PTH can cause bone pain/fracture, kidney stones, lethargy, weakness, and dysrhythmias secondary to hypercalcemia. Deficient PTH can cause tetany, laryngospasm, hypotension, muscle cramping, weakness, and fatigue secondary to hypocalcemia.

Adrenal Medulla Hormones

Adrenal medulla			Epinephrine and norepinephrine (catecholamines)	Alpha and beta cells throughout the body	Sympathetic nervous system (SNS) stimulates the medulla to release epinephrine and norepinephrine in response to stress and the "fight or flight" response. Pheochromocytoma is a caused by a tumor in the adrenal medulla. The patient exhibits signs and symptoms of excessive epinephrine and norepinephrine production: episodic hypertension, tachycardia, headaches, diaphoresis.

(Huether, McCance, Brashers, and Rote, 2017)

- Vasopressin (AVP) or antidiuretic hormone (ADH) and oxytocin synthesized here and transported to the posterior pituitary gland
- Sends inhibiting or stimulatory peptides to the anterior pituitary to allow for regulation of adrenocorticotropic hormone (ACTH), follicle-stimulating hormone (FSH), luteinizing hormone (LH), growth hormone (GH), prolactin, and thyroid-stimulating hormone (TSH)
- Anterior pituitary:
  - ACTH, FSH, LH, GH, TSH, and prolactin produced and released
- Posterior pituitary:
  - Stores and secretes ADH and oxytocin
- Adrenal glands:
  - Lie at superior pole of each kidney
  - Adrenal cortex:
    - Secretes the mineralocorticoid aldosterone as regulated by the renin–angiotensin–aldosterone system; also influenced by ACTH
    - Secretes the glucocorticoid cortisol in response to ACTH
    - Secretes adrenal androgens
  - Adrenal medulla:
    - Secretes catecholamines epinephrine and norepinephrine in response to stress
- Thyroid gland:
  - Two lateral lobes joined by an isthmus
    - Secretes thyroxine (T_4) and triiodothyronine (T_3) in response to TSH:
      - Dietary iodine necessary for synthesis of thyroid hormones.
      - Thyroid hormones control metabolism, heat production, and growth and development.
    - Secretes calcitonin in response to hypercalcemia.
- Parathyroid gland:
  - Four glands located behind the thyroid lobes, two on the right, two on the left:
    - Continuously monitor serum ionized calcium concentration independently; not directly affected by pituitary hormones:
      - If serum ionized calcium levels decrease, parathyroid hormone (PTH) is secreted.
      - If serum ionized calcium levels increase, PTH secretion is suppressed.
      - PTH inhibits renal calcium excretion.
      - PTH mobilizes calcium from bone.
      - PTH increases renal synthesis of the active form of vitamin D_2, which increases intestinal calcium absorption.
- Negative feedback is a defining feature of the endocrine system (Figure 11.1)

DIAGNOSTIC TESTS

- Radiology:
  - X-rays (skull, abdomen)
  - Ultrasound
  - Nuclear imaging

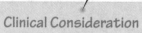

Clinical Consideration

Iodine deficiency is the most common cause of hypothyroidism worldwide. In the United States, iodized salt provides sufficient iodine to prevent deficiency. The most common cause of hypothyroidism in the United States is gland atrophy.

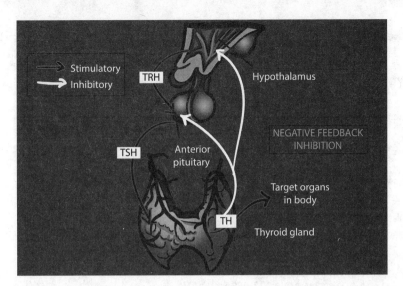

Figure 11.1 Thyroid gland: negative feedback loop. TH= thyroid hormone; TRH = thyrotropin-releasing hormone; TSH = thyroid-stimulating hormone.

- Computed tomography (CT)
- Magnetic resonance imaging (MRI)
▶ Screening:
  - It is recommended that adults over age 35 have a screening TSH exam every 5 years; if abnormal, further testing may be warranted.
  - If other routine diagnostic testing is abnormal (comprehensive metabolic panel [CMP], complete blood count [CBC], calcium, phosphorus, magnesium, for example), pathology of the endocrine system must be ruled out.
▶ Laboratory (Table 11.2):
  - GH:
    - Increased in acromegaly
    - If decreased in children, short stature/growth problems
    - If decreased in adults, can lead to osteoporosis
  - Plasma insulin-like growth factor 1 (IGF-1):
    - Increased in acromegaly
  - Oral glucose-tolerance test (OGTT):
    - May be used to evaluate patient with acromegaly or Cushing syndrome
  - Gonadotropins: FSH and LH:
    - Used to differentiate primary gonadal problems from pituitary insufficiency
    - FSH and LH levels would be high in primary gonadal problems
      - Negative feedback would cause the pituitary gland to continue to release high levels of FSH and LH if the ovaries and testes are unable to produce sufficient hormones.
      - Levels of FSH and LH would be low if the problem was due to the pituitary gland not being able to produce them.

TABLE 11.2	LABORATORY STUDIES FOR PITUITARY DISORDERS	
Test	Reference Range for Adults	Significance
Serum sodium	135–145 mEq/L	Increased in DI Decreased in SIADH
Growth hormone	Men: <5 ng/mL Women: <10 ng/mL	Increased in acromegaly Decreased in pituitary insufficiency Decreased with GH deficiency Decreased in dwarfism
Insulin-like growth factor 1	42–110 ng/mL	Increased in acromegaly Decreased in hypopituitarism
Follicle-stimulating hormone	Men: 1.42–15.4 mU/mL Women: Follicular phase: 1.37–9.9 mU/mL Ovulatory phase: 6.17–17.2mU/mL Luteal phase: 1.09–9.2 mU/mL Postmenopause: 19.3–100.6 mU/mL	Increased with gonadal failure Decreased with pituitary insufficiency
Luteinizing hormone	Men: 1.24–7.8 IU/L Women: Follicular phase: 1.68–15 IU/L Ovulatory peak: 21.9–56.6 IU/L Luteal phase: 0.61–16.3 IU/L Post menopause: 14.2–52.3 IU/L	Increased with gonadal failure Decreased with pituitary insufficiency
Antidiuretic hormone	1–5 ng/L	Increased in SIADH Increased in nephrogenic DI (secondary to primary renal disease) Decreased in neurogenic DI Decreased in surgical removal of pituitary gland
Serum osmolality	285–295 mOsm/kg	Increased in hypernatremia Increased in DI Decreased in SIADH Decreased in hyponatremia
Urine osmolality	Random: 50–1200 mOsm/kg After 12–14 hr. fluid restriction: >850mOsm/kg	Increased in SIADH Increased in Addison's disease Decreased in DI Decreased in aldosteronism
Oral glucose-tolerance test	2 hours <140 mg/dL	Increased in acromegaly Increased in Cushing's disease and syndrome Decreased in Addison's disease

(Pagana, Pagana, and Pagana, 2017)
DI = diabetes insipidus; SIADH = syndrome of inappropriate antidiuretic hormone.

- Free thyroxine (T_4), triiodothyronine (T_3):
  - Increased in Graves' disease (with suppressed TSH)
  - Decreased in primary hypothyroidism (with associated increased TSH)
- TSH:
  - Increased in primary hypothyroidism
    - Negative feedback of low thyroid hormone (free T_4) increases release of TSH from pituitary gland.
  - Decreased in secondary hypothyroidism:
    - Pathology of the pituitary gland causes decreased secretion of TSH, providing inadequate stimulation to the thyroid gland.

- Decreased in primary hyperthyroidism (Graves' disease)
  - Increased thyroid hormone secretion (T_3 and T_4) causes negative feedback to stop secretion of TSH from the pituitary.
- Thyroid autoantibodies:
  - Thyroid peroxidase (TPOAb)
    - May be present in hypothyroidism from autoimmune origin.
  - Thyroglobulin (TgAb)
  - TSH receptor antibody:
    - Increased in Graves' disease
- Thyroglobulin:
  - Used as tumor marker for those being treated for thyroid cancer
- Plasma cortisol levels:
  - Problems with the hypothalamus, pituitary gland, or adrenal glands can also cause too much or not enough cortisol to be produced.
  - Elevated in Cushing's disease
  - Decreased in Addison's disease
- Plasma ACTH levels:
  - Low levels from: primary pituitary dysfunction: secondary pituitary dysfunction (problem in the hypothalamus); or panhypopituitarism (deficiency of all anterior pituitary hormones)
  - Low level may lead to adrenal insufficiency.
  - Can have high levels from pituitary tumor or tissue overgrowth or from ACTH-producing tumors anywhere in the body.
  - High levels of ACTH can contribute to adrenal gland hyperfunction (Cushing's disease).
- Suppression tests:
  - Used in suspected hyperfunction
  - Dexamethasone-suppression test used to evaluate Cushing's syndrome
    - Dexamethasone (Decadron) given at 11 p.m. to suppress corticotropin-producing hormone.
    - High plasma cortisol levels drawn at 8 a.m. are considered abnormal findings consistent with Cushing syndrome.
- Stimulation tests:
  - Used to assess for endocrine's hypofunction
  - ACTH stimulation test with cosyntropin (Cortrosyn) assesses patient with adrenal insufficiency
    - Low plasma cortisol levels or failure to rise after receiving ACTH administration indicates primary adrenal insufficiency (Addison's disease).
- Serum calcium, free ionized calcium
- Vitamin D levels
- PTH levels
- Phosphorus levels
- Radiologic studies:
  - MRI of head, adrenal glands
  - CT scan of head, adrenal glands
  - Ultrasound of thyroid
  - Nuclear scan of thyroid, parathyroid
  - Radioactive uptake scan of thyroid and parathyroid

Clinical Consideration

Graves' disease is thought to be immune-mediated. Auto antibodies attach to the TSH receptors on the thyroid gland and simulate overproduction of the thyroid hormones.

- Thyroid biopsy:
  - Fine-needle aspiration (FNA)
  - Diagnosing cancer
- Electrocardiogram/echocardiogram:
  - An echocardiogram can reveal decreased ejection fraction due to heart failure or perhaps hypertrophy secondary to persistent hypertension.
- Urine studies:
  - 17-Ketosteroids—24-hour collection evaluates adrenocortical and gonadal function
  - Free cortisol—evaluates for hypercortisolism
  - Vanillylmandelic acid (VMA)—measures urinary secretion of catecholamine metabolites, which are increased in pheochromocytoma

Endocrine Disorders of the Anterior Pituitary Gland

▶ *Acromegaly*

- Rare disorder caused by hypersecretion of GH in adulthood that is almost always caused by a benign, GH-secreting pituitary tumor (adenoma).
- *Assessment/Intervention/Education*
  - Detailed medical history:
    - Insidious; family and patient often do not notice symptoms right away
    - Changes happen gradually over many years
  - Risk factors:
    - Average age at diagnosis in 40's
    - Occurs more often in females
    - Prognosis depends on age at diagnosis, when treatment was started, and size/extent of tumor
  - Clinical manifestations:
    - Protrusion of jaw and forehead
    - Overgrowth of tissue and bones in hands, feet, face, and skull
    - Joint pain, muscle weakness, atrophy
    - Enlarged tongue with speech and sleep difficulty
    - Deep voice, leathery skin
    - Pressure on optic nerve from tumor may cause vision changes, headache
    - Decreased level of consciousness, lethargy, fatigue
    - Sexual dysfunction
    - Body image disturbance, depression
    - Development of glucose intolerance due to excessive GH blocking action of insulin
    - Polydipsia, polyuria due to excessive GH and possibly increased glucose
  - Diagnosis (Table 11.2):
    - GH (increased)
    - IGF-1 (increased)
    - OGTT (increased blood glucose levels)
    - MRI (evaluate presence of pituitary adenoma)
  - Nursing diagnosis:
    - Fatigue related to muscle weakness and atrophy

- Disturbed body image related to physical changes
- Risk for sexual dysfunction
- Treatment:
  - Drug therapy—may be used in conjunction with radiation or surgery (Table 11.7):
    - Somatostatin analog—octreotide (Sandostatin):
      - Decreases GH:
        - Must monitor GH levels
    - Dopamine agonist—bromocriptine; alone or with somatostatin analog to decrease GH
    - GH antagonists-pegvisomant (Somavert)—blocks production of IGF-1, thereby decreasing GH
  - Radiation may be used with surgery and medications
    - Monitor for adverse effects of radiation
  - Surgery is treatment of choice:
    - Minimally invasive endoscopic transnasal approach or transsphenoidal hypophysectomy; craniotomy may be necessary depending on tumor size, location and other patient factors.
    - May result in loss of all pituitary hormones.
    - Lifelong replacement therapy of vasopressin (ADH), thyroid, sex hormones, and glucocorticoids may be necessary.
- Nursing management:
  - Monitor blood sugar levels.
  - Provide emotional support, as personality, physical, and fertility changes may occur.
  - Monitor response to medications.
  - If patient has had surgery:
    - Keep the head of the bed elevated at least 30 degrees.
    - Assess neurologic exam and vision.
    - Assess for signs and symptoms of increasing intracranial pressure (ICP)—headache, nausea, vomiting, change in level of consciousness.
    - Monitor intake and output (I&O) and electrolytes.
    - Monitor for signs of cerebrospinal fluid (CSF) leak—clear drainage from nose or reports of postnasal drip.
    - Monitor for signs and symptoms of meningitis.
- Patient teaching:
  - Lifelong hormone replacement therapy may be needed—vasopressin, gonadal hormones, cortisol and thyroid.
  - Encourage the patient to seek support from health care providers, family, friends, and support groups.
  - In postoperative phase, monitor for signs and symptoms of CSF leak.
  - Monitor for increased/decreased urine output.
  - For postoperative patients, teach to avoid blowing nose, brushing teeth, coughing, bending forward in first few weeks after surgery.
  - The patient and family should be taught signs and symptoms of hypo/hypernatremia.

Clinical Consideration

With surgery, bone growth can be stopped, tissue hypertrophy can be reversed, and the patient will notice changes in his or her appearance.

Clinical Consideration

This intervention helps decrease increased intracranial pressure and postoperative headache.

Clinical Consideration

These activities will prevent CSF leak and disruption of the surgical site in postoperative patients.

Question	Rationale
A patient underwent a transsphenoidal hypophysectomy for a pituitary adenoma 4 days ago. About which of the following would the nurse notify the provider immediately? A. A headache that is improving each day B. Clear drainage coming from both nares C. The patient is alert and oriented to person, place, and time D. The morning capillary blood glucose level is 190 mg/dl	Answer: B Rationale: A headache that is not getting any worse may be an expected finding for a patient who had this surgery. Although it would be important to notify the provider about the elevated blood glucose level, it is an expected finding since the patient is likely receiving corticosteroids. Clear drainage from the nose after cranial surgery is worrisome for possible CSF leak, and this would be the most important finding to notify the provider about. A thorough neurologic assessment must be performed and if this is CSF, this could place the patient at risk for the development of meningitis.

Disorders of the Posterior Pituitary Gland

▶ **Diabetes Insipidus (DI)**

- ADH causes the distal tubules and collecting ducts to reabsorb urine.
- Deficiency of ADH production or inability of the kidneys to respond to ADH leads to excretion of large volumes of dilute urine and dehydration.
- Central DI (neurogenic)—defect in ADH synthesis, transport, or release; caused by: hypothalamus or pituitary problem, brain tumor, head trauma, central nervous system (CNS) infection
- Nephrogenic DI—renal tubules don't respond to ADH; renal disease, drugs such as lithium carbonate (Eskalith) and demeclocycline (Declomycin)
- Primary DI—caused by: excessive water intake; psychologic disorder and lesion in thirst center are also possible causes
- *Assessment/Intervention/Education*
  - Detailed medical history/risk factors:
    - Surgery, head trauma, tumors, infectious processes, brain diseases
    - Medications
    - May be new/transient or lifetime condition
  - Clinical manifestations:
    - Polydipsia (as long as thirst mechanism is intact)
    - Polyuria—dilute; low specific gravity, low osmolality
    - Two to 20 L of urine may be produced in 24 hours
    - Hypotension, tachycardia—danger of hypovolemic shock if fluids are not replaced
    - Increased blood urea nitrogen (BUN), hemoglobin, hematocrit, sodium due to hemoconcentration
    - Dry skin, mucous membranes, poor skin turgor
    - Hyperthermia (fluids help maintain normal body temperature)
    - Possibly altered mental status—irritability progressing to lethargy/coma/seizures due to hyperosmolar state and hypernatremia
  - Diagnosis:
    - Based on clinical manifestations
    - Increased BUN, hemoglobin, hematocrit
    - Increased serum osmolality (>295 mOsm/kg)

Clinical Consideration
Hypernatremia causes brain cells to shrink. Cells in the brain are very sensitive to fluid and sodium changes and seizures may develop.

- Serum sodium may be elevated to >145 mEq/dl because of loss of free water; patient may be able to keep in the normal range by drinking enough water to keep up with the losses.
- Low urine specific gravity (<1.005)
- Low urine osmolality
- Water deprivation test; patient is deprived of water for 8–12 hours and then desmopressin acetate (DDAVP) is given subcutaneously or intranasally. If patient has central DI, the urine osmolality will increase and urine output will drop because the kidneys are responding normally. If the patient has nephrogenic DI, the kidneys will not be able to concentrate the urine and urine osmolality will stay the same or decrease.
- MRI (evaluate presence of pituitary adenoma, head trauma, other brain pathology)
- Lithium levels (if taking Lithium)
- Possible infection workup
- Nursing diagnosis:
  - Deficient fluid volume related to inability to conserve fluid
  - Ineffective health maintenance related to deficient knowledge regarding disease management and importance of medication adherence
- Treatment:
  - Treat underlying cause (brain tumor, injury, infection, drugs, etc.)
  - In acute central DI, hypotonic saline or 5% dextrose in water (D5W) is given to replace output
  - Increase oral intake to match output if able
  - Low-sodium (less than 3 g/day) diet for nephrogenic DI
  - Medications:
    - DDAVP (an analog of ADH) for central DI—given orally, intravenously (IV), subcutaneously, or as a nasal spray
    - Chlorpropamide (Diabinese) has antidiuretic activity, decreasing urine output and thirst
    - Carbamazepine (Tegretol) may be used for extreme thirst.
    - Thiazide diuretics for nephrogenic DI to reduce flow to distal tubules
- Nursing management:
  - Provide emotional support as personality and physical changes/discomfort may be occurring because of rapid changes in electrolyte and fluid status.
  - Frequent vital signs
  - I&O, daily weights
  - Monitor blood glucose, BUN, electrolytes, especially sodium
  - Monitor response to medications—urine specific gravity and urine osmolality
  - If patient has had surgery and/or head injury:
    - Assess neurologic exam and vision
    - Assess for signs and symptoms of increasing ICP—headache, nausea, vomiting, change in level of consciousness
    - Monitor for signs of CSF leak—clear drainage from nose or reports of postnasal drip
    - Monitor for signs and symptoms of meningitis
- Patient teaching:
  - Lifelong hormone-replacement therapy may be needed—DDAVP; may need instructions on how to administer if intranasal or by injection; importance of adherence, and signs and symptoms that may necessitate higher amounts of medication to be given (e.g., polyuria, polydipsia).
  - Patient must know what signs and symptoms to notify health care provider about (increasing polyuria, polydipsia, dehydration, hypernatremia).

Clinical Consideration
These are hypotonic solutions and they will hydrate the cells.

Clinical Consideration
After using the intranasal spray, the patient should not blow the nose for at least 1 hour to allow for absorption.

- Daily weight (same time, scale, and clothes) and keep track of I&O
- Drugs used to treat DI can cause fluid overload; if signs of water toxicity (weight gain, worsening headache, change in mental status), patient must be taught to seek medical care, or call 911
- Medical alert bracelet

Question	Rationale
The patient is receiving desmopressin (DDAVP) for treatment of diabetes insipidus. The nurse understands that the action of the drug is to: A. Increase insulin sensitivity B. Decrease tubular reabsorption of water C. Decrease the systemic blood pressure D. Increase the reabsorption of water in the tubules	Answer: D This drug does not affect insulin sensitivity. The drug is a synthetic type of ADH and it binds to kidney receptors and increases the reabsorption of water in the tubules, decreasing urine output. This is the desired outcome of the drug. However, the nurse must observe for, and teach the patient to observe for, signs of water intoxication and fluid overload that can occur if the patient is receiving too much DDAVP.

▶ **Syndrome of Inappropriate ADH (SIADH)**

This disorder occurs when ADH is released from the posterior pituitary gland despite normal or low plasma osmolality. Permeability of the distal tubules and collecting ducts is then increased and water is reabsorbed back into the circulation. Vascular fluid volume increases, plasma osmolality decreases, and sodium levels decrease.

- *Assessment/Intervention/Education*
  - Detailed medical history:
    - Patient may report weight gain, edema, decreased urine output
    - Initially may report thirst, dyspnea on exertion, fatigue, mild headache
    - Ask about mental status changes
    - Risk factors:
      - Cancers: small-cell lung, pancreatic, lymphoid, prostate, colorectal, thymus
      - CNS disorders: Head injury, stroke, brain tumors, meningitis, encephalitis, Guillain–Barré syndrome,
      - Drugs: carbamazepine (Tegretol), chlorpropamide (Diabinese); general anesthesia drugs; opioids; thiazide diuretics; selective serotonin-reuptake inhibitors (SSRIs); tricyclic antidepressants; some chemotherapy agents
      - Other: human immunodeficiency virus (HIV) infection, chronic obstructive pulmonary disease (COPD), hypothyroidism, lung infections
      - Self-limiting when secondary to head injuries or drugs, but may be chronic in patients with tumors or metabolic diseases
  - Clinical manifestations:
    - Low urine output with high specific gravity
    - Weight gain, dyspnea, fatigue
    - Mild hyponatremia—patient may experience nausea, anorexia, irritability, muscle cramping, headache
    - If serum sodium is <120 mEq/L, patient may experience muscle cramping/twitching, vomiting
    - May progress to cerebral edema, causing confusion, lethargy, seizures, and coma if hypoosmolality and hyponatremia are not treated

- Diagnosis:
  - Based on history, physical assessment findings
  - Serum sodium <134 mEq/L—dilutional hyponatremia
  - Serum osmolality <280 mOsm/kg
  - Urine specific gravity is greater than 1.025
- Nursing diagnosis:
  - Excess fluid related to altered regulatory mechanism
  - Risk for electrolyte imbalance related to increased intravascular fluid volume
  - Risk for injury related to decreased level of consciousness
  - Risk for acute confusion related to electrolyte imbalance
- Treatment:
  - Treat underlying cause
  - Discontinue medications that stimulate ADH release.
  - Fluid restriction if serum sodium >125 mEq/L.
  - If serum sodium is >125mEq/L, furosemide (Lasix) may be given to reduce fluid volume.
  - If serum sodium is <120 mEq/L, and in the presence of severe neurologic impairment, small amounts of 3% sodium chloride (hypertonic saline) may be given slowly IV.
  - Demeclocycline blocks effects of ADH on renal tubules.
  - Vasopressor receptor antagonist drugs block action of ADH:
    - Conivaptan (Vapriosol)—given IV
    - Tolvaptan (Samsca)—given orally
  - Daily weights, I&O, monitor serum electrolytes
  - Monitor for signs and symptoms of water excess: edema, fatigue, crackles in the lungs, dyspnea, hypertension, tachycardia.
  - Observe for signs and symptoms of hyponatremia.
  - Institute fall and/or seizure precautions if patient has altered neurologic status.
- Patient teaching:
  - If this is a chronic problem, teach the patient to check daily weight at same time in same clothes, and I&O; report weight gain, decreased urine output, and concentrated urine.
  - Teach signs and symptoms of low sodium that should be reported to the provider.
  - If the patient is on a fluid-restriction, teach to use ice chips sparingly, sugarless chewing gum, moisturizing mouth spray, and frequent oral care to help decrease thirst.

Question	Rationale
A patient has been treated for lung cancer. Which of the following would be included in the discharge teaching plan related to recognition of SIADH? A. Observe for signs and symptoms of low sodium, such as cracked lips and warm, flushed skin B. Notify the provider if weight loss is noticed C. Notify the provider if the urine output decreases and the urine looks concentrated D. Report to the provider immediately large amounts of dilute urine	Answer: C SIADH can occur in acutely ill patients, such as those with lung cancer. It is from excessive ADH secretion from the posterior pituitary gland. It results in low urine output, high urine osmolality, and hyponatremia. Cracked lips and warm, flushed skin are signs of hypernatremia. Typically the patient would gain weight. A patient with hyponatremia may exhibit muscle twitching, headaches, and possibly seizures.

DISORDERS OF THE ADRENAL GLANDS

▶ *Pheochromocytoma—Adrenal Medulla*

- Most of the catecholamine (norepinephrine and epinephrine)-secreting tumors occur in the adrenal medulla. They can also occur in any sympathetic ganglion in the body. Norepinephrine is the primary catecholamine; it causes hypertension. Only 10% of these tumors turn out to be malignant. The patient may experience episodic or persistent hypertension. The sympathetic manifestations of headache, tachycardia/palpitations, and sweating are common in these patients when the blood pressure is elevated. The clinical manifestations depend on the amount of epinephrine and norepinephrine secreted.

- *Assessment/Intervention/Education*
  - Detailed medical history:
    - Patient may report headache, palpitations, sweating, anxiety, nausea, fatigue, chest/abdominal pain, weight loss.
    - The symptoms can be episodic and can last for minutes to hours.
    - Risk factors that can precipitate symptoms:
      - Emotional stress
      - Smoking
      - Some medications: opioids, some antihypertensives, tricyclic antidepressants, contrast media dye
      - Exercise
      - Anesthesia
      - Intake of tyramine-containing foods
      - Anything that increases intraabdominal pressure—having bowel movement, sexual intercourse
  - Clinical manifestations:
    - Hypertension that comes and goes or may be persistent
    - Wide fluctuations in blood pressure
    - Hypertension does not respond to standard antihypertensive medications
    - Sweating
    - Tachycardia, chest and abdominal pain
    - Severe headache and vision disturbances when hypertensive
    - Tremor
    - Possible dysrhythmias
    - Hyperglycemia may occur with hypertension
  - Diagnosis:
    - CT scan or MRI
    - Plasma free metanephrine and normetanephrine levels elevated—most often used for diagnosis with clinical findings (Table 11.3)
    - 24-hour urinary fractionated metanephrines and catecholamines
  - Nursing diagnosis:
    - Decreased cardiac output related to hypertension
  - Treatment:
    - Avoid physical and emotional stress and stimuli in environment.
    - Monitor orthostatic blood pressure.
    - Assess for and treat hypertensive crisis.
    - Assess response to medications for blood pressure management, pain, and anxiety.
    - Avoid caffeine and foods containing tyramine.
    - Provide sufficient calories and monitor for hyperglycemia.

Clinical Consideration

This diagnosis is often missed.

TABLE 11.3   LABORATORY STUDIES FOR ADRENAL DISORDERS

Test	Reference Range for Adults	Significance
Cortisol, total (plasma)	8 a.m.: 5–23 µg/dL 4 p.m.: 3–13 µg/dL	Increased in Cushing's syndrome Increased from adrenal adenoma or carcinoma Increased from stress Increased from ACTH-producing tumors in body Increased in obesity Decreased in hypopituitarism Decreased in Addison's disease Decreased in congenital adrenal hyperplasia
Aldosterone	Male: 6–22 ng/dL Female: 5–30 ng/dL	Increased in primary aldosteronism Increased from adrenal adenoma, hyperplasia Increased in Cushing's syndrome Decreased in Addison's disease
Adrenocorticotropic hormone (ACTH, corticotropin)	Male: 7–69 pg/mL Female: 6–58 pg/mL	Increased in Addison's disease Increased in Cushing's disease (pituitary is overproducing) Increased from ACTH-producing tumor in the body Increased from stress Decreased with pituitary insufficiency Decreased with steroid administration Decreased with adrenal adenoma or cancer Decreased with Cushing's syndrome (feedback sent back to pituitary that there is enough cortisol)
ACTH stimulation with cosyntropin	Increase more than 7 µg/dL above baseline	Increased in hypopituitarism Increased with neuroendocrine tumor Increased with exogenous steroid ingestion Increased with adrenal hyperplasia Decreased in Addison's disease Decreased in adrenalectomy Decreased in adenoma or metastatic tumor of adrenal gland Decreased with chronic steroids
ACTH suppression with dexamethasone	Normal plasma cortisol after dexamethasone: <2 µg/dL	Increased in Cushing's syndrome and Cushing disease Increased in ACTH-producing ectopic tumors in the body Increased in bilateral adrenal hyperplasia
Metanephrine, Normetanephrine (plasma)	12–60 pg/mL 18–111 pg/mL	Increased in pheochromocytoma
24-hour urine 17-ketosteroids	Men: 6–20 mg/day Women: 6–17 mg/day	Increased in adrenal tumor Increased in Cushing's syndrome Increased in testicular cancer Increased in ovarian cancer Decreased in Addison's disease Decreased in hypopituitarism Decreased in myxedema
Urine, cortisol free	<100 µg/24 hr	Increased in Cushing's syndrome Increased in adrenal adenoma or carcinoma Increased with tumors elsewhere in body that secrete ACTH Decreased in Addison's disease Decreased in hypopituitarism Decreased in congenital adrenal hyperplasia
24-hour urine: Vanillylmandelic acid (VMA), homovanillic acid (HVA) and catecholamines (epinephrine, norepinephrine, dopamine, metanephrine, normetanephrine)	VMA: <6.8 mg/24 hr Free catecholamines: <100 µg/24 hr Epinephrine: <20 µg/24 hr Norepinephrine: <100 µg/24 hr Dopamine: 65–400 µg/24 hr Metanephrine: <1.3 mg/24 hr Normetanephrine: 15–80 µg/24 hr.	All are increased in pheochromocytoma, neuroblastoma Increased in severe stress

(Pagana, Pagana, and Pagana, 2017)

- Daily weights
- Medications:
  - Start α-blocker medications to control blood pressure before, during, and after surgery.
  - Once blood pressure is controlled, start β-blockers.
  - Patient may require sedatives or antianxiety medications.
- Laparoscopic adrenalectomy:
  - Routine postoperative care
  - Continue to monitor blood pressure carefully postoperatively, as hypertension can persist even when tumor is removed.
  - Monitor for signs and symptoms of possible adrenal crisis (see sections on "Cushing's Syndrome" and "Addison's Disease").
- Patient teaching:
  - Monitor blood pressure.
  - Avoid triggers for hypertensive episodes (see above).
  - Reduce stress in environment, promote rest.
  - Take prescribed medications consistently.
  - Discontinue smoking.
  - Post-operative care teaching (see section on "Cushing's Syndrome").

> **Clinical Consideration**
>
> If the adrenal gland is removed, the lack of glucocorticoids, mineralocorticoids, and androgens can precipitate adrenal crisis, shock, and perhaps death.

Question	Rationale
Which of the following may be reported by the patient who was admitted with a possible pheochromocytoma? A. Weight gain in the abdomen and dark, coarse hair on the face and arms B. Frequently urinating large amounts of urine that looks like water and feeling light-headed C. Constant feeling of fatigue and "brain fog," that does not go away after sleep or rest D. Headache, diaphoresis, and "racing heart"	Answer: D These symptoms are common findings in a patient with pheochromocytoma, especially when the blood pressure is elevated. The findings in answer A may be found in a patient who has Cushing's syndrome secondary to excessive amounts of cortisol. Polyuria may be secondary to diabetes insipidus. The resultant light-headedness may be secondary to dehydration. Fatigue and slowing down of all body processes may be noted in a patient with hypothyroidism.

Cushing's Syndrome (Adrenocortical Excess)

- The corticosteroid classes that are secreted by the adrenal cortex include glucocorticoids, mineralocorticoids, and androgen precursors. Cushing's syndrome manifests as a group of clinical signs and symptoms secondary to long-term exposure to excessive amounts of glucocorticoids. This can be secondary to a pituitary adenoma, secretion of ACTH by other tissues or tumors anywhere in the body, adrenal cortical carcinoma, adrenal cortical adenoma, nodular adrenal hyperplasia, or exogenous corticosteroid use. *Cushing's disease* refers to Cushing's syndrome caused by a pituitary adenoma.

- *Assessment/Intervention/Education*
  - Detailed medical history:
    - Patient may report the following signs and symptoms:
      - Coarse hair on face, chest, arms, back
      - Weight gain in abdomen, on top of back
      - Bruising
      - Proximal muscle weakness
      - Menstrual irregularities; sexual dysfunction
      - Increased blood sugar
      - Possible vision alterations
      - Alteration in mood
      - Impaired concentration and memory
      - Disturbed sleep patterns
      - Fractures
    - Medication history, including use of corticosteroids
  - Risk factors/possible causes:
    - Medical use of corticosteroids for immunosuppression or as antiinflammatory treatment
    - Adrenal tumors
    - Pituitary adenomas
    - Ectopic tumors in other parts of the body
  - Clinical manifestations:
    - Hypertension
    - Hypokalemia
    - Increased blood sugar
    - Edema
    - Midabdominal adiposity with purple striae
    - Fat accumulation on upper back and in face and neck area
    - Acne
    - Hirsutism
    - Fragile skin, bruising
    - Osteopenia, osteoporosis
    - Increased intraocular pressure
    - Susceptibility to gastrointestinal bleeding
    - Risk for infection
  - Diagnosis:
    - Skull x-ray, CT scan, MRI (if pituitary adenoma is suspected)
    - Serum electrolytes—hypokalemia, hyperglycemia
    - Increased 24-hour urinary free cortisol (Table 11.3)
    - Dexamethasone-suppression test—increased plasma cortisol levels
  - Nursing diagnosis:
    - Risk for infection related to excessive corticosteroids and immunosuppression
    - Disturbed body image related to changes in appearance
    - Disturbed sleep related to excessive corticosteroids
    - Risk for impaired skin integrity related to excessive corticosteroids

> **Clinical Consideration**
> Corticosteroids are the most common cause of Cushing's syndrome.

- Treatment:
  - Diet: high protein, low carbohydrate, low Na^+, high K^+, low calorie, and possible fluid restriction
  - I&O; daily weight
  - Fall risk
  - Strict handwashing and care to prevent infection
  - Medications may be used before or after surgery, or for those who are not surgical candidates:
    - Aminoglutethimide (Cytadren), metyrapone (Metopirone), mifepristone (Mifeprex), and ketoconazole can be used alone or in combination for adrenal blockade.
  - Surgery and/or radiation may be used for pituitary adenomas.
  - Surgery—for pituitary adenoma:
    - Endoscopic transsphenoidal hypophysectomy
    - See section on "Acromegaly" for care of postoperative patient.
  - Surgery—if caused by adrenal adenoma or adrenal cancer:
    - Adrenalectomy
    - Monitor vital signs carefully.
    - Monitor I&O.
    - Provide adequate fluid replacement.
    - Routine postoperative care of incision(s)
    - Be aware of slow wound healing and risk for gastrointestinal bleeding.
    - Monitor electrolytes (Na^+ and K^+) and blood glucose carefully.
    - Fall risk and concern for increased risk of fractures
    - Be aware of signs and symptoms of hormone deficiency due to removal of gland(s).
    - Provide for rest and decrease stress in environment.
    - Be aware of factors that can precipitate Addisonian crisis (stress, surgery, failure to provide adequate steroid replacement):
      - Signs and symptoms of Addisonian crisis:
        - Hypotension, tachycardia
        - Nausea, vomiting, diarrhea, abdominal pain
        - Fever
        - Hypoglycemia, hyperkalemia, hyponatremia
        - Weakness and dehydration and patient can go into shock, progressing to coma; fatal if inadequate treatment with hormone replacement
    - Surgery and/or radiation—for ectopic ACTH-secreting tumor somewhere else in body
    - If Cushing's syndrome is related to prolonged administration of exogenous corticosteroid therapy for an existing medical condition, perhaps decreasing the dose or a gradual taper and weaning off is possible.
- Patient teaching:
  - Importance of following prescribed diet regimen.
  - Routine postoperative care
  - Importance of knowing side effects from treatment and removal of glands.
  - Importance of lifelong monitoring blood pressure, blood sugar, electrolytes and levels of hormones.
  - Lifelong hormone-replacement therapy:
    - Glucocorticoid and mineralocorticoid replacement postadrenalectomy
    - Perhaps vasopressin, thyroid, glucocorticoid, mineralocorticoid replacement posthypophysectomy

Clinical Consideration

To meet the stress/extra demand, extra IV hydrocortisone must be given.

Clinical Consideration

Never abruptly stop exogenous corticosteroid therapy, especially if the patient has been on it for more than 2 weeks.

Question	Rationale
A female patient presents with gradual onset of weight gain, headaches, acne, and purple striae on her abdomen and upper arms. She is diagnosed with Cushing's syndrome. She is likely to have which of the following? A. Hyperkalemia, hyponatremia, hypoglycemia B. Hypokalemia, hyperglycemia, high serum cortisol levels C. Low serum cortisol, high T_4 level, hyperkalemia D. Hypotension, intact skin, heat intolerance	Answer: B These laboratory findings are typical in a patient with Cushing's syndrome. The findings in answer A represent Addison's disease. High cortisol levels are found in a patient with Cushing's syndrome. High T_4 levels and heat intolerance would be commonly found in a patient with hyperthyroidism, or Graves' disease. Patients with Cushing's syndrome have fragile skin that easily bruises. They have hypertension due to weight gain and fluid retention.

▶ Addison's Disease (Adrenal Insufficiency)

- Primary adrenal insufficiency can be due to destruction or dysfunction of the adrenal cortex. This is often caused by an autoimmune process. It can result in glucocorticoid (cortisol), mineralocorticoid (aldosterone), and androgen deficiency. The adrenal medulla is usually spared. Secondary adrenal insufficiency can be due to ACTH hyposecretion from the pituitary.
- **Assessment/Intervention/Education**
  - Detailed medical history:
    - See "Risk factors," below.
    - Weakness, fatigue
    - Anorexia, nausea, diarrhea, weight loss
    - Hyperpigmentation, bronze skin tone
    - Frequent infections or intolerance to stress
    - Cold intolerance
    - Loss of pubic/axillary hair in women
    - Menstrual irregularities; loss of libido
  - Risk factors:
    - Infections—human immunodeficiency virus/acquired immunodeficiency syndrome (HIV/AIDS), tuberculosis, cytomegalovirus
    - Autoimmune disorders
    - Congenital disorders
    - Drugs/medications that are known to suppress adrenal function
    - Surgical history—adrenalectomy, hypophysectomy
    - Hemorrhage, thrombosis, infarction of the adrenal gland
    - Cancer and infiltrative diseases
  - Clinical manifestations:
    - Proximal muscle weakness
    - Muscle/joint pain
    - Hypotension
    - Hypoglycemia
    - Hyponatremia

- Hyperkalemia
- Anemia
- Hypercalcemia
- Diagnosis:
  - CT scan of adrenal glands
  - Antiadrenal antibodies
  - Plasma cortisol levels decreased (Table 11.3)
  - ACTH stimulation test reveals low cortisol levels
- Treatment:
  - Avoid situations that can precipitate Addisonian (adrenal) crisis:
    - Physical and emotional stress
    - Extremes in temperature
    - Excessive exercise
    - Illness
    - Inadequate or sudden withdrawal of steroid-replacement therapy
  - Recognize signs and symptoms of adrenal crisis/shock (see section on "Cushing's Syndrome")—can develop rapidly and is life-threatening
  - *Treatment of Addisonian crisis*
    - Administer hydrocortisone (Solu-cortef) or dexamethasone.
    - Provide IV fluids.
    - Provide IV glucose if hypoglycemic.
    - If hyperkalemic, may need to administer insulin and 50% dextrose IV; and/or sodium–potassium exchange resin (such as polystyrene sulfonate Kayexalate)
    - Electrocardiography (ECG), vital signs, and frequent reassessment of potassium, glucose, sodium levels
  - Patient will be on lifelong hydrocortisone therapy (two-thirds administered in the morning and one-third in the afternoon) and synthetic mineralocorticoid fludrocortisone (Florinef) daily.
- Patient teaching:
  - Teach when to seek medical attention
  - Medical alert bracelet
  - Prevent infections
  - Must know medications and signs of too much or not enough medication
  - Carry emergency kit with intramuscular (IM) hydrocortisone and be aware of situations that warrant extra dosing (stress, illness, surgery, etc.).
  - Teach family how to administer IM hydrocortisone in case patient is unable to self-administer.
  - Monitor blood pressure.
  - Must take medications consistently and not abruptly stop medications (especially corticosteroids)

> ### Clinical Consideration
> IV insulin facilitates potassium movement into cells. This will decrease the blood sugar, so IV dextrose 50% is administered to prevent hypoglycemia.

> ### Clinical Consideration
> If the glucocorticoids are given too close to bedtime, the patient may not be able to sleep.

DISORDERS OF THE THYROID GLANDS

Hyperthyroidism (Graves' Disease)

- Elevated levels of thyroid hormones result in thyrotoxicosis. The clinical signs and symptoms result from the direct effects of increased thyroid hormones as well as an increased susceptibility to catecholamines. Graves' disease, toxic multinodular goiter, thyroid cancer, and increased secretion of TSH can cause hyperthyroidism. Severe thyrotoxicosis is called "thyroid storm," and it can be life-threatening. The normal feedback mechanisms that regulate thyroid hormone secretion are altered and the hyperfunction of the thyroid gland causes suppression of TSH (from the pituitary gland) and thyrotropin-releasing hormone (TRH) from the hypothalamus. The increased thyroid gland metabolism causes increase in the gland size and the thyrotoxic clinical signs and symptoms. It is thought that in Graves' disease, the body produces antithyroid antibodies that target the thyroid gland and cause it to overproduce thyroid hormones.

- *Assessment/Intervention/Education*
  - Detailed medical history:
    - Weakness and fatigue with some difficulty sleeping
    - Tachycardia, heart palpitations, maybe atrial fibrillation
    - Gastrointestinal (GI) problems:
      - Increased appetite
      - Unintentional weight loss
    - Decreased tolerance to heat
    - Thinning hair
    - Stare
    - Possible protrusion of the eyes (exophthalmos)
    - Diplopia, photophobia, eye irritation
    - Difficulty swallowing, change in voice, enlargement of the thyroid gland
  - Risk factors:
    - Women in the second through fifth decades of life
    - Familial history of autoimmune disease, or thyroid disease
    - Higher incidence in smokers
    - Recent viral infection
    - Recent stressful event(s)
  - Clinical manifestations:
    - Goiter (50% of patients will not have enlargement of the thyroid gland)
    - Tender neck
    - Periorbital edema
    - Exophthalmos
    - Flushing, warm skin
    - Hyperactive reflexes
    - Fine hand tremors
    - Exertional fatigue/exercise intolerance
    - Irritability
    - Nervousness
    - Inability to concentrate
    - Impotence and decreased libido
    - Menstrual irregularities
    - Depression and apathy
    - Urinary frequency and nocturia
  - Diagnosis (Table 11.4):
    - TSH (decreased in primary hyperthyroidism)
    - Free T_4, T_3 (increased)
    - Radioactive iodine (131-I) uptake (RAIU) scan (may or may not be done)
    - Thyroid ultrasound
    - Presence of thyroid stimulating antibodies (or immunoglobulins)
    - FNA thyroid biopsy
  - Nursing diagnosis:
    - Activity intolerance related to heat intolerance and fatigue
    - Fatigue related to increased metabolic rate

TABLE 11.4   LABORATORY STUDIES FOR THYROID DISORDERS

Test	Reference Range for Adults	Significance
Thyroid-stimulating hormone (TSH)	2–10 mU/mL	Increased in primary hypothyroidism Increased in thyroiditis Decreased in secondary hypothyroidism (pituitary dysfunction/pituitary hypofunction) Decreased in hyperthyroidism
Triiodothyronine (T$_3$), total	20–50 years old: 70–205 ng/dL Age >50 years: 40–180 ng/dL	Increased in Graves' disease Increased in acute thyroiditis Decreased in hypothyroidism Decreased in ablation or thyroidectomy Decreased in hypothalamic failure Decreased in pituitary insufficiency
Triiodothyronine (T$_3$), free	260–489 ng/mL	See T$_3$, total Measures active component of total T$_3$
T$_3$ uptake (T$_3$ resin uptake)	24–3 %	Increased in hyperthyroidism
Thyroxine (T$_4$), total	Adult male: 4.0–12.0 µg/dL Adult female: 5–12.0 µg/dL Age >60 years: 5–11 µg/dL	Increased in Graves' disease Increased in thyroid cancer Decreased in pituitary insufficiency Decreased in hypothalamic failure Decreased in Hashimoto's thyroiditis Decreased in ablation or thyroidectomy Decreased in myxedema
Thyroxine (T$_4$), free	0.8–2.8 ng/dL	See T$_4$, total Measures active component of total T$_4$ Better indicator of thyroid function than total T$_4$
Thyroid stimulating hormone receptor antibodies (TSHR)	<130% of basal activity	Increased in Graves' disease
Thyroid peroxidase (TPO) Ab (Antibodies)	< 35 IU/mL	Increased in Hashimoto's thyroiditis Increased in some patients with Graves' disease
Thyroglobulin	0.5–53.0 ng/mL	Increased in thyroid cancer Increased in residual thyroid tissue in neck after surgery

(Pagana, Pagana, and Pagana, 2017)

Clinical Consideration
Propranolol can precipitate bronchospasm in patients who have severe COPD or asthma.

- Hyperthermia related to increased metabolic rate
- Imbalanced nutrition: less than body requirements resulting from increased metabolic rate
- Treatment (Table 11.7):
  - β-blockers—propranolol (Inderal); or metoprolol (Lopressor):
    • Block the manifestations of overstimulation from the sympathetic nervous system (SNS)
  - Antithyroid medications (supersaturated potassium iodide [SSKI]), methimazole (Tapazole), propylthiouracil (PTU)
  - Perhaps irradiation and ablation (patient will need lifelong hormone-replacement therapy)—destroys thyroid tissue
    • RAI (radioactive iodine) may be the treatment of choice for most nonpregnant adults; this is a more reliable treatment for hyperthyroidism:

- Maximum effect not seen for 3 months, so patient may continue to be hyperthyroid until the effects of RAI are noted (low thyroid-hormone levels will be noted then).
- Outpatient procedure; pregnancy test is done prior
- May develop mouth sores, dry mouth and throat, and parotiditis
- Because the patient has ingested unsealed radioactive iodine, they must keep 6 feet away from people for 3 to 7 days, depending on how much radioactive material was administered.
- Avoid contact with children, pregnant women for 7 days and sleep in own bed
- Push fluids, frequent handwashing and showers
- Use disposable utensils, plates, cups
- For 3 to 7 days, the patient should not share utensils, food, bedding, or personal items or cook food for others
- Use own toilet and flush two to three times after each use
- Wash clothes frequently and separately from those of others in the household
- Be aware that any urine or stool has radioactivity in it and patient should take precautions to contain it and protect others from exposure

- Observe for and treat thyroid storm:
  - Extreme, life-threatening form of thyrotoxicosis
  - Death can occur from dysrhythmia, heart failure, and hyperthermia.
  - Can happen during/after thyroidectomy
  - Can occur in response to stress and lack of antithyroid medications
  - Care of the patient experiencing thyroid storm:
    - Maintain airway and ventilation.
    - Frequent vital signs, neurologic/physical assessment
    - Place on monitor and assess for dysrhythmias.
    - Provide IV hydration with normal saline.
    - Monitor temperature frequently and provide cooling blanket and anti-pyretics as needed.
    - Administer antithyroid drugs as prescribed: methimazole (Tapazole), or propylthiouracil (PTU)
    - Potassium iodide may be prescribed.
    - Administer propranolol (Inderal) and monitor heart rate and rhythm.
    - Hydrocortisone IV will be given until adrenal insufficiency can be ruled out.
- Surgery (total or subtotal thyroidectomy):
  - Potassium iodide and antithyroid medications are given preoperatively to shrink the vascular thyroid gland in order to avoid bleeding.
  - Head of bed elevated 30 degrees; support head and neck in midline, preventing strain on suture line and flexing neck
  - Tracheotomy set and suction at bedside
  - Care taken when swallowing; lozenges, humidifier
  - Check for Trousseau's and Chvostek's signs, which can be present if hypocalcemia develops after accidental removal of one or more parathyroid glands during surgery:
    - Trousseau's sign—flexion of the wrist noted when a blood pressure cuff inflated on upper arm
    - Chvostek's sign—noted when cheek is lightly tapped and facial muscles spasm
    - Patient may require IV calcium gluconate or calcium chloride replacement.
  - If entire gland removed, patient on lifelong levothyroxine therapy

- Patient teaching (Table 11.7):
  - Importance of taking medications at same time of day and following up with provider to monitor lab values
  - Patient who has undergone surgery or ablation will be on lifelong thyroid hormone-replacement therapy and free T_4 and TSH will need to be followed.
  - Take the same thyroid-replacement therapy consistently; do not switch back and forth between brand name and generic.
  - Take the levothyroxine on an empty stomach and do not eat/drink anything for 1 hour afterward.
  - If patient has not had surgery and is taking antithyroid drugs, they may be lifelong or may be discontinued by the provider; TSH, T_4 must be assessed lifelong.
  - Patient should be taught signs and symptoms of hyperthyroidism/hypothyroidism and when to notify provider.
  - If Graves' disease has not been treated, the patient should rest frequently, avoid stimulation, wear cool clothing, increase caloric and fluid intake, and avoid caffeine and other stimulants.
  - Adjust caloric intake as necessary for weight gain/weight loss.
  - Patient should undergo a baseline ophthalmology consultation:
    - If exophthalmos is present: encourage use of artificial tears and sunglasses to prevent dryness and irritation; elevate the head of the bed at all times; institute low-sodium diet to reduce swelling around the eyes; tape eyes shut at night if they do not close.
    - Patient may need other procedures, surgery, medications for exophthalmos.
  - Patient should be aware that hyperthyroidism can cause loss of bone density.
  - Nutritional therapy may include high-calorie, high-protein diet with frequent meals (may need to decrease calories when the patient becomes euthyroid).
- Geriatric considerations:
  - Signs and symptoms of thyrotoxicosis may be less tolerable than in younger patients because of preexisting heart and lung disease.
  - Teach older adult to report palpitations, chest pain, shortness of breath to provider immediately.
  - Check 12-lead ECG and possibly echocardiogram to assess for any changes in rhythm and left ventricular function. If patient is in atrial fibrillation, may need to undergo anticoagulation. The need for heart rate control must also be evaluated.
  - Heart failure can occur.
  - May present with anorexia, weight loss, confusion, depression

Hypothyroidism

- Hypothyroidism is a condition in which the body does not produce enough thyroid hormone. The most common cause of primary hypothyroidism is autoimmune Hashimoto's thyroiditis. Secondary hypothyroidism is less common but might be caused by a problem with the hypothalamus or pituitary gland or may be due to peripheral resistance to thyroid hormones. Acute bacterial and viral infections can cause acute thyroiditis and hypothyroidism, but are not common causes for hypothyroidism.
- Predisposing factors:
  - Occurs in women more than men
  - Women older than 40 years old are at highest risk
  - More likely if patient already has one autoimmune disease

- More likely if first-degree relative with thyroid disease and if family member with an autoimmune disease
- Can be secondary to radiation treatment or removal of gland to treat hyperthyroidism or cancer
- Iodine deficiency is cause in other countries
- Chromosomal disorders
- Drug-induced (amiodarone, interferon alfa, lithium)
- *Assessment/Intervention/Education*
  - Detailed medical history:
    - Weight gain
    - Fatigue/sluggishness/"brain fog"/difficulty concentrating
    - Short-term memory loss
    - Loss of hair
    - Irregular, heavy menses and infertility
    - Muscle aches and stiffness
    - Neck pain, tenderness in thyroid area, hoarseness, difficulty swallowing
    - Depression
  - Clinical manifestations:
    - Delayed reflexes
    - Coarse, dry, brittle hair that is falling out
    - Ataxia, exercise intolerance
    - Slow to respond
    - Cold intolerance
    - May be asymptomatic if subclinical
    - Goiter
    - Carpal tunnel syndrome
    - Periorbital edema
    - Myxedema coma if hypothyroidism untreated or undiagnosed:
      - Hypoventilation
      - Hypotension
      - Extreme weakness
      - Hypothermia
      - Stupor progressing to coma
      - Can be precipitated by infection, some medications and exposure to cold
      - Facial and periorbital edema and masklike appearance due to fatty material gathering in the dermis and tissues
      - Life-threatening
  - Diagnosis (Table 11.4):
    - Primary hypothyroidism - Elevated TSH, low free T_4
    - TSH and free T_4 both low, possibly secondary to pituitary or hypothalamus condition
    - Thyroid ultrasound
    - Thyroid scan
    - Biopsy if cancer is suspected
    - Thyroid antibodies (present in Hashimoto's thyroiditis)
    - Lipid panel (cholesterol elevated)
  - Nursing diagnosis:
    - Impaired memory related to decreased metabolic rate
    - Constipation related to decreased GI motility

- Activity intolerance related to fatigue
- Fatigue related to decreased metabolic rate
- Impaired swallowing related to obstruction from goiter

- Treatment:
  - If myxedema coma:
    - Support airway, give IV fluids, give IV levothyroxine, warming blanket
    - IV hydrocortisone administered until adrenal insufficiency ruled out
    - Frequent vital signs, neurologic assessment, and physical assessment
    - Aspiration precautions
    - Treat in intensive care unit (ICU)
  - Medications—lifelong (Table 11.7):
    - Levothyroxine (Synthroid), start low dose and titrate
    - Desiccated thyroid (Armour Thyroid)
    - Stool softener
    - Possibly anticholesterol medications
    - If acute thyroiditis, nonsteroidal antiinflammatory drugs (NSAIDs) and prednisone may be prescribed
  - Surgery if goiter is obstructing airway or if malignant thyroid nodule

- Patient teaching:
  - Treatment is lifelong
  - Take Synthroid same time each day, on empty stomach, and wait an hour before eating; do not frequently switch from brand name drug to generic, as they do not all have the same potency.
  - The patient won't feel the effects for several months, and any changes in dosage must be followed by checking serum TSH.
  - Review signs and symptoms of hypothyroidism or hyperthyroidism and what to report to provider.
  - Be careful with soaps that may dry the skin; use moisturizing lotions.
  - Treat and manage constipation.
  - Cholesterol-reducing drugs, calcium, aluminum, cholestyramine interfere with adsorption of thyroid hormone; take 6 hours apart from thyroid hormone
  - Fiber and caffeine interfere with the absorption of levothyroxine.
  - May need to incorporate strategies to promote weight loss: exercise, nutritional therapy.

- Geriatric considerations:
  - The thyroid gland can atrophy with age.
  - The basal metabolic rate decreases in older adults.
  - The older adult who presents with confusion, a fall, and depression should have the TSH level checked.
  - Some older adults who are hypothyroid (high TSH and low T_3/T_4) sometimes present with signs and symptoms of hyperthyroidism.
  - Any patient taking thyroid-replacement therapy, but especially the elderly, should report chest pain, shortness of breath, and palpitations immediately.
  - Start with the lowest dosage and titrate up carefully, checking TSH levels and assess for chest pain, shortness of breath, arrhythmias and myocardial infarction (could be caused by high thyroid hormone (T_3, free T_4) levels).
  - Watch for signs and symptoms of increasing lethargy, decreased level of consciousness, and decreased respirations which may be signs of myxedema coma

Clinical Consideration
Hypothyroidism can contribute to hypercholesterolemia.

Clinical Consideration
Goiter can cause hoarseness, sore throat, and dysphagia.

Clinical Consideration
The dose of the thyroid-replacement therapy may be too high, causing signs and symptoms of hyperthyroidism.

Question	Rationale
A patient is admitted with hypothyroidism. The nurse is aware that which of the following needs to be included in the plan of care: A. Observing for signs of decreased level of consciousness B. Assessing for tachycardia and palpitations C. Administering methimazole (Tapazole) as ordered D. Providing decreased stimuli in the room	Answer: A The patient with hypothyroidism has a decreased metabolic rate. If the condition worsens or goes without adequate treatment, the patient can progress to myxedema coma and can die from cardiac, respiratory, or neurologic complications. The patient with increased metabolic rate (as in hyperthyroidism) may experience nervousness, tachycardia, and palpitations. Methimazole (Tapazole) may be given to a patient with Graves' disease, or hyperthyroidism. It inhibits thyroid hormone synthesis.

DISORDERS OF THE PARATHYROID GLANDS

TABLE 11.5 COMPARISON OF HYPO AND HYPERPARATHYROIDISM

	Hypoparathyroidism	Hyperparathyroidism
Description	Lack of PTH or decreased effectiveness on target tissue Manifestations of low calcium are noted clinically Calcium is not absorbed from the intestines, released from the bone, or conserved by the kidneys Vitamin D absorption affected	Increased PTH causes reabsorption of calcium and excretion of phosphorus in the kidney Excessive PTH levels increase loss of calcium from the bones, decrease bone building and increase bone breakdown Calcium deposited in soft tissues Manifestations of high PTH and/or hypercalcemia noted clinically
Etiology/risk factors	Congenital Iatrogenic—accidental or intentional removal during surgery or damage during radiation therapy Autoimmune Secondary to hypomagnesemia, poor nutrition	Parathyroid adenoma (benign tumor) Parathyroid carcinoma Congenital hyperplasia PTH-secreting tumors in lung, kidney, or GI tract Vitamin D deficiency Chronic kidney disease with high PTH, hypocalcemia and hyperphosphatemia Long-term lithium therapy
Clinical signs and symptoms	Weakness, fatigue Dysrhythmias, low cardiac output; prolonged QT interval; hypotension Hyperreflexia Muscle spasms Tetany Laryngospasm Dysphagia Paresthesia lips, hands, feet Positive Chvostek's and Trousseau's signs Tremor Seizures Abdominal cramping; malabsorption Soft tissue calcifications Change in personality, irritability	Weakness, fatigue, lethargy Dysrhythmias, hypertension, angina, Decreased reflexes; personality changes; irritability Headache Memory impairment Poor coordination, gait abnormalities Muscle weakness Osteoporosis Fractures Bone pain Kidney stones Constipation Loss of appetite Abdominal pain, possible peptic ulcer disease due to increased secretion of gastrin

(continued)

TABLE 11.5	*(Continued)*	
	Hypoparathyroidism	Hyperparathyroidism
Lab and diagnostic procedure results	Decreased serum and ionized calcium Increased serum phosphorus Decreased serum magnesium Decreased serum PTH Decreased vitamin D (calciferol) Decreased cAMP in urine 24 hour urinary calcium low	Increased serum and ionized calcium Decreased serum phosphorus Increased serum magnesium Increased serum PTH May have increased cAMP in urine Increased alkaline phosphatase if bone disease DEXA scan may show T score of <2.5 24-hour urinary calcium high Nephrolithiasis (stones) on ultrasound, x-ray, or CT scan eGFR <60 mL/hr
Possible nursing diagnosis	Ineffective breathing pattern related to laryngospasm Risk for decreased cardiac output related to suppressed contractility secondary to hypocalcemia Imbalanced nutrition less than body requirements, related to effects of vitamin D deficiency and malabsorption Activity imbalance related to neuromuscular irritability Risk for injury related to decreased calcium and vitamin D levels	Acute pain related to effects of increased calcium on bones or possibly kidney stone development High risk for injury, falls related to weakness, pain, and bone demineralization Risk for imbalanced nutrition, less than body requirements related to nausea, anorexia, possible ileus
Treatment	Replace calcium, vitamin D, magnesium as necessary Emergency treatment of tetany after surgery requires IV calcium; must give calcium chloride slowly and observe for hypotension, dysrhythmias	Patients with symptoms: serum calcium greater than 1 mg/dL above upper end of normal; hypercalcuria; reduced bone mineral density on DEXA scan; decreased eGFR <60 mL/hr; neuromuscular changes; nephrolithiasis; and under the age of 50: recommended for partial or complete surgical removal of the parathyroid gland via endoscopic approach Patients who are asymptomatic or have mild symptoms: increase fluids; furosemide (Lasix) increases renal excretion of calcium; strain urine if calculi are suspected; take care when moving patient; fall precautions Bisphosphonates, such as pamidronate (Aredia), can lower serum calcium levels Phosphate can be given to patients with normal kidney function to lower calcium Cinacalcet (Sensipar) decreases PTH secretion in those with chronic kidney disease
Patient teaching	May need lifelong supplementation of calcium, vitamin D Foods high in calcium and low in phosphorus: dark green vegetables, kale, collard greens; yogurt, milk and some cheeses are high in phosphorus Should know signs and symptoms of low/high calcium Care taken to prevent fall or injury Medical alert bracelet	If parathyroid gland(s) removed surgically, patient may experience tetany or laryngospasm postoperatively; nurses must be aware of signs and symptoms and have IV calcium gluconate ready. The patient may have the surgery as an outpatient and be discharged home. Teach patient signs/symptoms of low calcium (tetany: tingling/paresthesias of lips/hands/feet). More severe muscle spasms or laryngeal spasms may occur, and patient must seek emergency care. Check Trousseau and Chvostek signs in postoperative patient to assess for signs/symptoms of hypocalcemia. If patient is still hypercalcemic, must adjust diet to low-calcium diet. Encourage patient to stay active to prevent bone loss. Review fall risk precautions. Encourage patient to increase fluids and fiber to prevent constipation.

cAMP = cyclic adenosine monophosphate; DEXA = dual energy x-ray absorptiometry eGFR = estimated glomerular filtration rate. Lewis et al., 2017; Kaspar, et al., 2015.

TABLE 11.6	LABORATORY STUDIES FOR PARATHYROID DISORDERS	
Test	Reference Range for Adults	Significance
Parathyroid hormone (PTH)	50–330 ng/L	Increased in hyperparathyroidism from adenoma or carcinoma of parathyroid gland Increased lung/kidney carcinoma Increased in chronic renal failure Increased in vitamin D deficiency Increased in hypocalcemia Decreased in hypoparathyroidism Decreased in hypercalcemia Decreased in hypomagnesemia
Calcium, total	8.6–10.2 mg/dL	Increased in hyperparathyroidism Increased because of PTH-producing tumors in body Increased in acromegaly Decreased in hypoparathyroidism Decreased in hypoalbuminemia Decreased in alkalosis Decreased in vitamin D deficiency
Calcium, ionized	4.5–5.6 mg/dL	See Calcium, total Free form of calcium unaffected by albumin levels
Phosphate	3.0–4.5 mg/dL	Increased in hypoparathyroidism Increased in renal failure Increased in acromegaly Increased with hypocalcemia Decreased in hyperparathyroidism Decreased with hypercalcemia Decreased in malnutrition, alcoholism Decreased in vitamin D deficiency

(Pagana, Pagana, and Pagana, 2017)

CASE STUDY

A 42-year-old woman presented to her health care provider (HCP) with the chief complaints of feeling "shaky, weak, with frequent palpitations, and difficulty sleeping."

Review of Systems

She reports that she has had unintentional 10-lb weight loss in past 2 months and frequent watery, brown bowel movements. She feels very hungry, "overheated," and "on edge" all the time. She reports that her menstrual periods have been irregular.

History

She has no allergies and no other medical problems. She has 2 children, ages 10 and 12, delivered by uncomplicated cesarean section. She does not smoke or drink alcohol. She drinks 2 cups of caffeinated coffee daily.

Vital Signs

The patient's vital signs are: temperature 99.8°F, pulse 104 beats/min and regular, respiratory rate 24 breaths/min, blood pressure 148/88 mm Hg, and SaO$_2$ 99% while breathing room air. The patient reports no pain.

Physical Assessment

- Eyes—no bulging, dryness, or redness
- Thin, soft hair
- Soft, moist, warm, flushed skin
- Thyroid slightly symmetrically enlarged to palpation; no bruit auscultated
- Peripheral pulses are bounding bilaterally; S1–S2 clear, distinct with 2/6 systolic flow murmur noted at the apex
- Deep tendon reflexes 4+ and equal bilaterally; fine tremors noted in hands at rest

A thyroid ultrasound shows an enlarged multinodular thyroid gland, consistent with Graves' disease.

The lab and diagnostic procedure results (see below) confirm the diagnosis of Graves' disease. The patient will be started on methimazole (Tapazole) 5 mg daily and propranolol (Inderal) 10 mg three times daily.

Lab/Diagnostic Procedure Results	Normal Range	Patient Result
Thyroid-stimulating hormone (TSH)	2–10 mU/L	0.1 mU/L
Triiodothyronine (T$_3$)	Age 20–50 years: 70–205 ng/dL >60 years: 40–180 ng/dL	350 ng/dL
Free thyroxine (T$_4$)	0.8–2.8 ng/dL	13 ng/dL
Radioactive iodine uptake nuclear scan (RAIU)	Measures amount of radiation that is taken up by the thyroid gland 5–35% is normal	99% uptake

Discussion:

1. **Correlate the signs and symptoms to the patient's underlying pathophysiology.**

   This autoimmune disease causes oversecretion of thyroid hormones. This can cause the thyroid gland to be symmetrically enlarged. Goiter develops in some patients. Metabolic rate is increased and the body is more sensitive to the effects of the sympathetic nervous system. The increased sympathetic nervous system stimulation has caused the patient to have elevated temperature, pulse, blood pressure, and respiratory rate. She has palpitations, insomnia, tremors, and increased DTRs (deep tendon reflexes). The increased sympathetic nervous system stimulation is also causing her to have increased cardiac output. She has bounding peripheral pulses and a "flow murmur," which can occur in high-output states. The weight loss is due to increased caloric expenditure and increased metabolic rate.

2. **The patient asks why her lab values are abnormal. How does the nurse explain the reason for the abnormalities?**

The body produces antibodies that attach to the TSH receptor on the thyroid gland and cause the thyroid gland to produce too much thyroid hormone. When the body has too much thyroid hormone (T_3, T_4), it sends a message back to the hypothalamus and the pituitary gland that blocks the release of thyrotropin-releasing hormone (TRH) and TSH. So, the TSH levels are very low or nondetectable. The T_3 and T_4 remain high because the thyroid gland keeps producing these hormones because of the antibodies' effects on the thyroid gland. The patient's nuclear radioactive iodine uptake scan showed high uptake of radioactive iodine in the metabolically hyperactive thyroid gland. The provider may also choose to test for the presence of thyrotropin receptor antibodies since Graves' disease is an autoimmune disease.

3. **What will the nurse teach the patient about the medications, propranolol (Inderal) and methimazole (Tapazole)?**

Propranolol (Inderal) is a nonselective β-blocker that will help block the effects of the sympathetic nervous system. This drug will decrease the heart rate, blood pressure, nervousness, tremors, and hyperactivity. She should start to see effects from this drug soon after starting it. She should be taught that this drug will decrease her pulse and blood pressure. She may want to check her heart rate and blood pressure and notify her provider if she feels any new/adverse signs or symptoms. The methimazole prevents thyroid hormone synthesis and should be taken with food. The drug begins to work in 1 to 2 weeks after starting it, but therapeutic results are not usually seen for 4 to 8 weeks. She will have her T_4 and/or TSH rechecked then to assess outcomes from the drug. The provider will decide whether to increase or decrease the dosage of the methimazole based on the results of her lab work and how she is feeling. The dose of the propranolol may be increased if she still has tachycardia or feels palpitations, nervousness, and tremors.

4. **What other teaching points will the nurse review with this patient?**

She must be taught to take her medications as directed. She will need to rest more, keep herself hydrated with plenty of water and make sure she gets sufficient calories to prevent more weight loss. She should avoid caffeine or other stimulants while the thyroid hormone levels are high. When her thyroid function returns to normal, she will need to adjust her caloric intake to prevent weight gain. She needs to keep herself from overheating because her metabolic rate is elevated, which elevates body temperature. Although she may feel "shaky" or nervous, it is important to walk, get some exercise (not overdoing it), and balance rest with activity. Her HCP may share with her that Graves' disease may be associated with remissions and exacerbations and can progress to destruction of the thyroid gland. Spontaneous remission occurs in 20 to 40% of patients. Some patients may need lifelong antithyroid medication therapy, or radiation therapy or surgery to treat the Graves' disease.

TABLE 11.7	DRUGS FOR ENDOCRINE CONDITIONS				
Drug Name	Drug Type and Use	Mode of Action	Dosage	Adverse Effects	Clinical Considerations/Patient Teaching
Drugs Related to Pituitary Function					
Octreotide (Sandostatin)	Somatostatin analog; growth hormone (GH) antagonist; used to treat acromegaly	Normalizes levels of GH and IGF-1	50–100 mg Subcutaneous (SC)/IV three times daily	Nausea, cramps, diarrhea, flatulence subside w/in 1–2 weeks	Dose adjusted and/or discontinued if patient has radiation and/or surgery. Monitor GH and IGF-1 levels May cause biliary tract abnormalities, cholelithiasis; Injection site pain
Pegvisomant (Somavert)	GH Receptor Antagonist; used to treat acromegaly	Inhibits GH receptor binding, decreasing IGF-1 and GH responsive proteins	10–30mg SC once daily;	Injection site irritation; flulike symptoms; nausea, diarrhea, chest pain; possible abnormal LFTs	Dosage may be adjusted and/or discontinued if patient has had surgery or radiation Dosage is titrated based on IGF-1 levels and patient signs and symptoms Monitor liver function. Opioids may reduce effectiveness
Bromocriptine (Parlodel)	Dopamine receptor agonist; used to treat pituitary adenoma and acromegaly	Activates dopamine receptors in the pituitary and reduces prolactin secretion; can also suppress tumor growth	20–30 mg orally once daily	Nausea, headache, dizziness, fatigue, lightheadedness, diarrhea	Take with food to minimize side effects
Desmopressin (DDAVP)	Synthetic arginine vasopressin (antidiuretic hormone) analogue; used for DI	Promotes renal conservation of water	1–2mg SC/IV twice daily; 0.1–1.1 – 1.2 mg Orally daily; Given via intranasal Spray also	Flushing, abdominal cramps, nausea, hyponatremia, diaphoresis, tremor, headache, rhinitis	• Smallest effective dose should be given due to cost and also excessive dosing can result in water intoxication • Teach patient to cut back on fluid intake since treatment with DDAVP prevents fluid loss and patient can develop water intoxication • Does not cause adverse cardiac effects because it is a weaker pressor agent
tolvaptan (Samsca)	Vasopressin Antagonist Used for SIADH	Blocks the effects of ADH in the kidneys and increase excretion of free water	15mg–60mg oral once daily	Thirst, xerostomia, polyuria, constipation, ALT elevated, weakness, hyperglycemia	• Since free water is excreted can cause sodium level to rise; if it rises too fast, can cause neuronal injury • Monitor sodium levels I & O, weight

Drugs Related to Adrenal Function

phenoxy-benza-mine (Dibenzyline)	Alpha adrenergic blocker; Used for blood pressure management before and after surgery for pheochromocytoma; (pheochromocytoma releases epinephrine and norepinephrine which raise heartrate and blood pressure)	Blocks alpha 1 and alpha 2 adrenergic receptors to decrease blood pressure;	20mg–40mg, orally, two to three times daily	Orthostatic hypotension, reflex tachycardia, nasal congestion, sexual dysfunction/inhibition of ejaculation	• Use before patient has surgery for pheochromocytoma to control blood pressure and also to prevent hypertensive crisis during surgery • Beta blockers are usually added to treatment plan for pheochromocytoma after the alpha blockers are started • Teach patient about orthostatic hypotension and need to change positions slowly
propranolol (Inderal)	Nonselective beta adrenergic blocker; used to decrease blood pressure and pulse in patient with pheochromocytoma (after alpha blockers are started); Also used to treat Graves' disease	Blocks beta 1 and beta 2 adrenergic receptors to decrease heart rate; blocks impulses through AV node; decreases ventricular contractility; so decreased cardiac output and oxygen demand ; Decreases renin secretion from kidney	20mg orally, three to four times daily; can titrate up to 60 mg/day in divided doses to control HR and blood pressure; available in extended release form	Fatigue, dizziness, bradycardia, hypotension, depression, bronchoconstriction; inhibition of glycogenolysis (by blocking beta 2 fibers in liver, diabetic patient can become hypoglycemic); also blocks beta 1 fibers so normal responses to hypoglycemia—tachycardia, shakiness, and diaphoresis—are blocked and patient may be unaware of hypoglycemia	• Check heart rate and may need to hold if heart rate and/or blood pressure become too low • Teach diabetic patients that normal signs/symptoms of hypoglycemia (from sympathetic nervous system) may be blocked • Monitor for bronchospasm in patients with COPD or asthma; they may need to be switched to beta 1 agent like metoprolol (Lopressor) • Monitor for AV block • Monitor for signs/symptoms of heart failure • Taper dose to discontinue
Metoprolol (Lopressor)	Beta 1 adrenergic blocker, Used with alpha blockers for pheochromocytoma; May be used in Graves' Disease	Selective Blockade of beta 1 receptors in heart to decrease heartrate, conduction through AV node and force of contraction, decreasing cardiac output and oxygen demand; reduces renin secretion from kidney	50–200mg orally, twice daily; Titrate to goal heartrate and blood pressure; Available in extended release form	See above for propranolol	• May be used instead of propranolol in patient with COPD or asthma • May produce bronchospasm in high doses • Give with food • Taper dose to discontinue • See above for propranolol

(continued)

TABLE 11.7   (Continued)

Drug Name	Drug Type and Use	Mode of Action	Dosage	Adverse Effects	Clinical Considerations/Patient Teaching
Ketoconazole (Nizoral)	Antifungal, used as adjunct treatment (in addition to surgery/radiation) for Cushing's disease caused by pituitary adenoma	Blocks production of glucocorticoids in adrenal cortex	200mg orally two to three times daily; may increase to 400mg three times daily	Liver toxicity, nausea, dizziness, diarrhea, abdominal pain, pruritus, rash, decreased libido/ erectile dysfunction, menstrual irregularities	• Check liver enzymes • Give with food • Monitor for signs/symptoms of acute adrenal insufficiency
Hydrocortisone (Cortef)	Glucocorticoid used for replacement therapy in adrenocortical insufficiency, Addison's Disease	Anti-inflammation; produces glucocorticoid and mineralo-corticoid effects	25 mg–30mg/day orally, divided twice daily; or may take all in a.m.	Impaired wound healing; susceptibility to infection; Cushingoid appearance; weight gain; emotional lability; sodium and fluid retention; hypertension; muscle atrophy; acne; thin, fragile skin; hyperglycemia, hypokalemia; insomnia; menstrual irregularities; susceptible to GI bleeding and osteoporosis	• Take with food • Lifelong therapy for those with chronic adrenocortical insufficiency • Do not stop suddenly • Patient may be instructed to increase dose to fight stressors of increased emotional stress, illness, procedure, surgery if they have chronic adrenal insufficiency • Learn how to give self IM injection of hydrocortisone if vomiting, or if need to give extra "stress dose" • Daily weights • Notify provider if other adverse effects
fludrocortisone (Florinef)	Mineralocorticoid that possesses glucocorticoid activity; used for primary adrenal insufficiency	Enhances sodium and water reabsorption in distal tubules and increases excretion of potassium	0.1–0.2mg orally daily	See above for hydrocortisone since med possesses glucocorticoid activity	• Give with food • Do not stop taking • May need to adjust dose; patient to consult with provider for specific instructions • Monitor weight, blood pressure, blood sugar, potassium, and sodium levels
Drugs Related to Thyroid Function					
methimazole (Tapazole)	Thionamide, Antithyroid; used to treat hyperthyroidism, Graves' Disease	Inhibits thyroid hormone synthesis by inhibiting binding of iodine to thyroid tissue	Initiate: 5mg–20mg orally three times daily; Maintenence: 5mg–15mg daily	Rash, urticaria, nausea, vomiting, dyspepsia, arthralgia, headache, vertigo, hyperpigmentation, agranulocytosis and possibly susceptible to infection; Signs and symptoms of hypothyroid if dose is too high	• Take evenly spaced throughout day every 8 hrs. daily maintenance dose taken in the a.m. • Monitor weight • Monitor for signs symptoms of hypo/hyper thyroid • Dose will be adjusted by HCP based on thyroid function tests and patient signs/symptoms • Assess CBC; patient should report sore throat or fever • Do not take if pregnant or breastfeeding; notify HCP immediately

Drug	Classification / Use	Action	Dosage	Side/Adverse Effects	Nursing Considerations
propylthiouracil (PTU)	Thionamide, Antithyroid; used to treat hyperthyroidism/ Graves' Disease, thyrotoxic crisis; can be given preoperatively; Short or long term use	Inhibits thyroid hormone synthesis by inhibiting binding of iodine to thyroid tissue; prevents Conversion of T4 to T3 in peripheral tissues	Initial: 300mg–500mg Orally divided every 8 hrs. Maintenance: 100mg–150mg /day oral in divided doses every 8 hrs	Reports of hepatotoxicity, Agranulocytosis, susceptible to infection; rash, pruritus, urticarial arthralgia, nausea, vomiting, signs and symptoms of hypothyroid if dose is too high	• Monitor LFTs, CBC • Increased risk for infection; report signs/symptoms of fever, sore throat • Take evenly spaced throughout day every 8 hrs. • Monitor weight • Monitor for signs symptoms of hypo/hyper thyroid • Dose will be adjusted by HCP based on thyroid function tests and patient signs/symptoms • Patient must notify HCP if any signs of liver problems (jaundice, bruising, bleeding, dark urine, pale stools etc.)
Saturated solution of potassium iodide (SSKI) Lugol's solution (nonradioactive)	NonRadioactive Iodine used in hyperthyroid patients, and before thyroidectomy to suppress thyroid function	Inhibits synthesis and release of thyroid hormone; reduces size and vascularity of thyroid	Prethyroidectomy 50mg–250mg orally, 3 times daily; Thyrotoxicosis: 50-500mg orally 3 times	Metallic taste, gingival/tooth soreness, sore throat, increased salivation, dyspepsia, fever, urticaria, skin eruptions, acne, headache, rhinitis	• Usually used short term in thyrotoxicosis or before thyroidectomy to prevent intra- and post-operative bleeding • Started 10–14 days before surgery • Mixed with juice • Take one hour after methimazole or propylthiouracil
levothyroxine (Synthroid)	Synthetic thyroid hormone preparation used for primary and secondary hypothyroidism, simple goiter, myxedema coma	Synthetic preparation of naturally occurring thyroxine	50–200 mcg orally daily in the morning	If dose too high, may develop signs and symptoms of hyperthyroid	• Take same time each morning on empty stomach, 30-60 minutes before breakfast • Lifelong therapy • Med alert bracelet • Don't switch brands; may have different affect • Patient must be aware of correct dosage and should not change dose or frequency unless directed by HCP • Start with lowest dose in elderly and in those with heart disease; adjust dosages slowly • HCP will titrate dosage according to TSH levels and patient signs and symptoms • HCP will re-check TSH every 4–8 weeks until levels are stable and monitor for signs/symptoms of hypo/hyperthyroid • Patient should know s/s of hypo/hyperthyroid • Patient should report chest pain/shortness of breath and seek immediate treatment • Don't take the following drugs within 4 hrs. of levothyroxine; can block absorption of levothyroxine: - PPIs, H2 blockers - Antacids - Calcium supplements - Magnesium - Iron supplements

(Burcham & Rosenthal, 2016; Epocrates, 2018)

Bibliography

Ackley, B.J., Ladwig, G.B., and Flynn Makic, M.B. (2017). *Nursing Diagnosis Handbook: An Evidenced Based Guide to Planning Care,* 11th ed. (St. Louis: Elsevier).

Bahn, R.S., Burch, H.B., Cooper, D.S., Garber, J.R., Greenlee, M.C., Klein. L., ... Stan, M.N. (2011). Hyperthyroidism and other causes of thyrotoxicosis: management guidelines of the American Thyroid Association and American Association of Clinical Endocrinologists. *Thyroid* 21, 593–646. Epub 2011 Apr 21.

Bilezikian, J.P., Brandi, M.L., Eastell, R., Silverberg, S.J., and Udelsman, R. (2014). Guidelines for the management of asymptomatic primary hyperparathyroidism: summary statement from the fourth international workshop. *Journal of Clinical Endocrinology and Metabolism* 99, 3561–3569.

Burchum, J.R. & Rosenthal, L.D. (2016). *Lehne's pharmacology for nursing care,* 9th ed. (St. Louis, MO: Elsevier).

Epocrates Plus for Apple iOS (Version 18.2.1). (2018). Endocrine/Metabolism. [Mobile application software]. Accessed June 8, 2018, from http://www.epocrates.com/mobile/iphone/essentials.

Garber, J.R., Cobin, R.H., Gharib, H., Hennessey, J.V., Klein, I., Mechanick, J.I, ... Woeber, K.A. (2012). Clinical practice guidelines for hypothyroidism in adults: co-sponsored by the American Association of Clinical Endocrinologists and the American Thyroid Association. *Endocrine Practice* 18, 988–1028.

Huether, S.E., McCance, K.L, Brashers, V.L., and Rote, N.S. (2017). *Understanding Pathophysiology,* 6th ed. (St. Louis: Elsevier).

Kaspar, D., Fauci, A., Hauser, S., Longo, D., Jameson, J.L. and Loscalzo, J. (2015). *Harrison's Principles of Internal Medicine,* 19th ed. (New York: McGraw-Hill Education).

Katznelson, L., Laws, E.R., Melmed, S., Molitch, M.E., Murad, M.H., Utz, A., and Wass J.A.H. (2014). Acromegaly: an Endocrine Society clinical practice guideline. *Journal of Clinical Endocrinology and Metabolism* 99, 3933–3951.

Lacroix, A., Feelder, R.A, Stratakis, C.A., and Nieman, L.K. (2015). Cushing's syndrome. *Lancet* 386, 913–927.

Lenders, W.M., Duh, Q.Y., Eisenhofer, G., Gimenez-Roqueplo, A.P., Grebe, S.K.G., Murad, M.H., ...Young, W.F. (2014). Pheochromocytoma and paraganglioma: An endocrine society clinical practice guideline. *Journal of Clinical Endocrinology & Metabolism,* 99(6), 1915-1942.

Lewis, S.L., Bucher, L., Heitkemper, M., and Harding, M.M., Kwong, J., and Roberts, D. (2017). *Medical-Surgical Nursing: Assessment and Management of Clinical Problems,* 10th ed. (St. Louis: Elsevier).

Mescher, A.J. (2016). *Junqueira's Basic Histology.* (New York: McGraw Hill Education).

Miller, B.A., Ioachimescu, A., and Oyesiku, N.M. (2014). Contemporary indications for transsphenoidal pituitary surgery. *World Neurosurgery* 82(6), S147–S151.

Neary N., and Nieman, L. (2010). Adrenal insufficiency: etiology, diagnosis and treatment. *Current Opinion in Endocrinology, Diabetes and Obesity 17,* 217–223.

NIH National Institute of Diabetes and Digestive and Kidney Diseases. (2014). Adrenal insufficiency and Addison's disease. Accessed June 10, 2018, from https://www.niddk.nih.gov/health-information/endocrine-diseases/adrenal-insufficiency-addison's-disease.

Pagana, K.D., Pagana, T.J., & Pagana, T.N. (2017). *Mosby's Diagnostic and Laboratory Test and Reference,* 13th ed. (St. Louis: Elsevier).

Zieger, M., Thompson, G.B., Duh, Q.Y., Hamrahian, A.H., Angelos, P., Angelos, P., ... Kharlip, J. (2009). The American Association of Clinical Endocrinologists and American Association of Endocrine Surgeons guidelines for the management of adrenal incidentalomas. *Endocrine Practice, 15* (suppl 1), 1–20.

12

Renal and Urologic System

Donna Martin, DNP, RN, CMSRN, CDE, CNE

OVERVIEW

⏺ The renal and urologic system plays an important role in several critical body functions. Filtration of blood, removal of waste products, production of hormones necessary for red-cell production, vitamin D utilization, and blood pressure (BP) control are all vital functions of the system.

ANATOMY AND PHYSIOLOGY

⏺ The renal and urologic system is composed of the kidneys, ureters, bladder, and urethra. Urine formed in the kidneys drains to the bladder through the ureters, and is excreted from the body by passage through the urethra (Figure 12.1).

- Kidneys:
  - Anatomy:
    - Renal artery:
      - Transports blood to the kidney for filtration
    - Nephrons (over one million in each kidney):
      - Glomerulus
      - Bowman's capsule
      - Tubular system (Figure 12.2):
        - Proximal convoluted tubule
        - Loop of Henle
        - Distal convoluting tubule
        - Collecting tubules
    - Renal vein:
      - Transports filtrate blood back into the vascular system
    - Adrenal gland on the top of each kidney

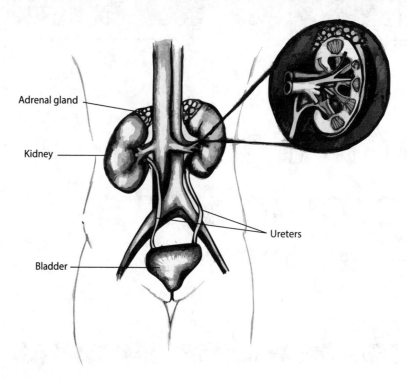

Figure 12.1 Renal System

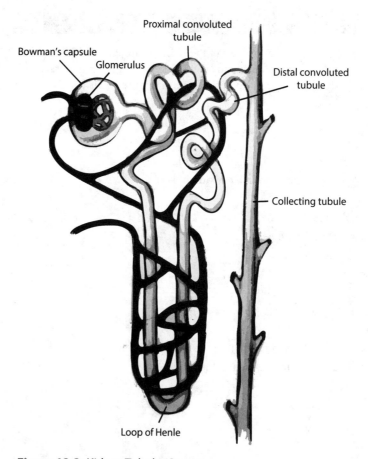

Figure 12.2 Kidney Tubular System

- Functions:
  - Regulates extracelluar fluid volume and electrolytes
    - Antidiuretic hormone (ADH) makes the distal tubules and collecting ducts more permeable to water.
    - Aldosterone causes reabsorption of sodium and water in the distal tubules.
    - Atrial natriuretic peptide (ANP) hormone is stimulated in response to stretching of the atria from an increase in plasma volume, causing an increase in sodium excretion resulting in an increased amount of urine.
    - The majority of electrolytes are reabsorbed in the proximal convoluted tubules.
    - Water reabsorption occurs in the distal convoluted tubules.
  - Excretes waste products from the body
  - Regulates BP control:
    - Prostaglandin synthesis in the kidney decreases systemic vascular resistance (SVR), lowering BP.
  - Maintains acid–base balance:
    - Impacts bicarbonate reabsorption and hydrogen (H^+) excretion.
    - Compensatory mechanism for respiratory acidosis and alkalosis.
  - Produces erythropoietin:
    - Stimulates red-cell production in the bone marrow.
  - Kidneys have vitamin D receptors and convert vitamin D into its active form, which helps balance calcium and phosphorus levels, and also helps regulate parathyroid hormone (PTH).
- Ureters:
  - Carries urine from the kidneys to the bladder
  - One-way valves prevent urine back-flow into the kidneys
  - Ureter lumens are narrowest at the junction where the ureter meets the bladder, most common site of obstructions
- Bladder:
  - Stretchable organ
  - Holds urine
  - Distention of the bladder stimulates desire to urinate
- Urethra:
  - Controls voiding
  - Passage to remove urine from the bladder
- Gerontologic considerations:
  - Age-related changes
    - Reduction in kidney size by up to 30%
    - Loss of glomeruli function by up to 50%
    - Alterations in hormones that impact renal function
    - Loss of bladder elasticity for women, increasing infections and incontinence
    - Increase in prostate size, causing urinary retention and infections
  - Other factors:
    - Atherosclerosis accelerates the reduction in kidney size and function

DIAGNOSTIC TESTS

- Radiology:
  - Kidneys, ureters, and bladder (KUB)—noninvasive x-ray that includes the named organs

- Computed tomographic (CT) scan—visualization of kidneys, ureters, and bladder to identify abnormalities and may be done with and without contrast
- Renal arteriogram—visualizes the renal blood vessels
- Renal ultrasound—noninvasive ultrasound that can detect masses and obstructions
- Intravenous pyelogram (IVP)—allows for visualization of the urinary tract after administration of IV contrast
- Retrograde pyelogram—x-ray of urinary tract after administration of IV contrast
- MRI—allows for visualization of the kidneys

▶ Endoscopy:

- Cystoscopy:

  - Allows for visualization of the bladder as well as for inserting urethral stent, removing renal calculi, obtaining bladder specimens, and stopping bleeding

▶ Laboratory:

- Blood:

  - Blood urea nitrogen (BUN)—measures the amount of urea nitrogen in the blood; renal diseases cause an accumulation of urea, and elevate the BUN above normal
  - Creatinine—excreted by the kidney and indicates kidney function; interpreted in conjunction with the BUN
  - BUN/creatinine ratio—measure of kidney and liver function
  - Glomerular filtration rate (GFR)—number of milliliters filtered by the nephrons per minute
  - Sodium (Na^+)—value indicates a balance between sodium and renal excretion
  - Potassium (K^+)—potassium excreted by the kidneys; values outside normal range may impact heart function
  - Calcium (Ca^{2+})—used to evaluate parathyroid function
  - Phosphorus (PO_4^{3-})—levels determined by parathyroid hormone and renal excretion
  - Bicarbonate (HCO_3^-)—measure of the metabolic (renal) component of the acid–base imbalance

- Urine:

  - Urinalysis—identifies the color, odor, and composition of the urine for protein, glucose, ketones, bilirubin, specific gravity, osmolality, pH, and red and white cells
  - Urine culture—identifies the organism causing infection; clean-catch or sterile technique used to decrease possibility of introducing contaminant bacteria into urine
  - Residual urine—assess for urine in bladder immediately after voiding, can be done by bladder scan

- Renal biopsy:

  - Renal tissue analyzed to determine the extent of kidney disease

Renal/Urologic Disorders

▶ *Urinary Incontinence (UI)*

- Urinary incontinence is defined as the involuntary leakage of urine. This is not a normal part of the aging process, although UI occurs more often in older adults.

- *Assessment/Intervention/Education*

  - Detailed medical history:
    - Mobility issues
    - Cognitive functions
    - Duration of urinary problems

- Risk factors:
  - Delirium
  - Depression
  - Infection
  - Restricted mobility
  - Polyuria
  - Polypharmacy
- Clinical manifestations:
  - Involuntary loss of urine
  - Types of incontinence:
    - Stress incontinence—increase in intraabdominal pressure causes leakage of urine
    - Urge incontinence—uncontrolled contraction of muscles with urinary urgency
    - Overflow incontinence—bladder becomes overfull due to an obstruction, causing urine to leak
    - Reflex incontinence—loss of urine with no stressor or warning
    - Functional incontinence—due to cognitive or environmental causes
- Diagnosis:
  - Based on symptoms
  - Urinalysis
  - Postvoid residual (PVR) volume
- Nursing diagnosis:
  - Functional urinary incontinence related to altered environment
  - Overflow urinary incontinence related to relaxation of pelvic muscles
  - Reflex urinary incontinence related to neurologic impairment
  - Stress urinary incontinence related to increased abdominal pressure
  - Situational low self-esteem related to inability to control urine leakage
- Treatment:
  - Maintain patient dignity
  - Scheduled voiding regimens
  - Pelvic floor exercises (Kegel)
  - Avoid bladder irritants
    - Caffeine
    - Alcohol
  - Medications (Table 12.1)
  - Biofeedback:
    - Feedback from monitoring can allow the person to increase control of urinary incontinence.
  - Antiincontinence devices:
    - Intravaginal support devices
  - Containment devices:
    - External collection devices
    - Absorbent products
  - Surgery:
    - Retropubic suspension/sling
- Patient teaching:
  - Kegel exercises
  - Void at regular intervals

TABLE 12.1 URINARY MEDICATIONS

Medication	Action
Anticholinergics Oxybutynin (Ditropan XL) Tolterodine (Detrol) Solifenacin (VESIcare) Darifenacin (Enablex)	Relaxes bladder to allow for greater storage of urine; decreases overactive bladder contractions
α-Adrenergic blockers Doxazosin (Cardura) Tamsulosin (Flomax) Alfuzosin (Uroxatral)	Reduces resistance to urinary outflow
5α-reductase inhibitors Finasteride (Proscar) Dutasteride (Avodart)	Causes epithelial atrophy and decreases prostate size
α-Adrenergic agonists Pseudoephedrine	Increase urethral resistance
$β_3$-Adrenergic agonists Mirabegron (Myrbetiq)	Improves bladder storage by relaxing bladder muscle
Tricyclic antidepressants Imipramine (Tofranil) Amitriptyline	Reduces overactive bladder contractions

(Lewis et al., 2017)

Question	Rationale
If a patient leaks urine while coughing, sneezing, or lifting, they are experiencing which type of incontinence? A. Overflow B. Urge C. Functional D. Stress	Answer: D Stress incontinence occurs when there is a sudden increase in intraabdominal pressure. Overflow incontinence occurs when the bladder is overfilled and urine leaks. Urge incontinence involves urine leakage due to an overactive bladder and is associated with a sense of urgency. Functional incontinence occurs when a patient is unable to recognize they need to urinate or they are unable to reach the toilet.

▶ *Urinary Retention*

- Urinary retention involves accumulation of urine in the bladder, inability to empty the bladder, or incomplete emptying of the bladder. Retention is due to obstruction or the inability of the bladder muscle to sufficiently force urine from the bladder.
- *Assessment/Intervention/Education*
  - Detailed medical history:
    - History of urinary problems
    - Benign prostatic hyperplasia (BPH)
  - Risk factors:
    - Recent surgery with general or spinal anesthesia
    - Spinal cord injuries
    - Stroke
    - Herpetic infection
    - Side effect of some medications

- Vaginal delivery
- Constipation
- Clinical manifestations:
  - Abdominal distention
  - Decreased urine output
  - Feeling of incomplete emptying of bladder
  - Increased frequency with small amounts of urine
- Diagnosis:
  - Based on symptoms
  - PVR volume
  - Digital rectal exam (DRE)
- Nursing diagnosis:
  - Urinary retention related to incomplete emptying of the bladder
- Treatment:
  - Timed voiding
  - Double voiding
  - Intermittent catheterization:
    - Relieves urinary retention
    - Sterile technique—one-time use
    - Clean technique—per patient at home
  - Indwelling catheter:
    - Sterile technique
    - Keep collection bag below the bladder
    - Provide perineal care regularly
    - Remove catheter as soon as possible
    - Anchor device to prevent injury to urethra
  - Medications:
    - α-Adrenergic blocker
  - Surgery:
    - Transurethral resection of the prostate (**TURP**)
    - Pelvic reconstruction
    - Bladder stimulator
    - Suprapubic catheter—urinary diversion tube that can be temporary or permanent
    - Ureteral catheter—catheter inserted surgically through the ureters to the kidney pelvis
    - Nephrostomy tube—temporary tube inserted surgically when a ureter is completely obstructed
- Patient teaching:
  - Discuss voiding problems with provider.
  - Teach patient to double void to increase bladder emptying.
  - If unable to void for 6 hours, seek medical attention.
  - Avoid over-the-counter cold remedies with a decongestant.
  - Avoid antihistamines, as they increase urinary retention.

▶ *Urinary-Tract Infection (UTI)*

- A urinary tract infection (UTI) is an infection involving any part of the urinary system, including the urethra, bladder, ureters, and kidneys. UTIs are the most commonly reported health-care–acquired infection (CDC, 2017).
- More common in women due to a shorter urethra; most common organism is *Escherichia coli* (*E. coli*).

TABLE 12.2	INDICATIONS/USES OF INDWELLING URETHRAL CATHETERS		
Appropriate	**Inappropriate**	**Alternatives**
Urinary obstruction Acute urinary retention Accurate urine output needed Surgery of the urinary system Patients with prolonged immobilization End of life comfort	For prolonged duration without appropriate indications For a patient with incontinence As a means for obtaining urine	Consider external catheters Consider intermittent catheterization

Adapted from CDC catheter-associated urinary tract infections (CAUTI) guidelines (CDC, 2017).

- Appropriate indications for indwelling catheter usage have been identified by the CDC (2017) for prevention of catheter-associated urinary-tract infections (CAUTI) (Table 12.2)
- *Assessment/Intervention/Education*
  - Detailed medical history:
    - Factors that cause urinary stasis
    - Use of urinary catheters
    - History of UTIs
  - Risk factors:
    - Urinary calculi
    - Hyperglycemia
    - Pregnancy
    - Poor personal hygiene
    - Menopause
  - Clinical manifestations:
    - Uncomplicated:
      - UTI in a normal urinary tract
      - Only bladder is involved
    - Complicated:
      - Recurrent UTIs
      - Urinary-tract abnormalities
      - Other urinary problems
      - Other comorbidities
        - Neurologic diseases
        - Diabetes
    - Lower UTI—urethra and bladder:
      - Frequency with urgency
      - Dysuria
      - Urine odor
      - Cystitis—inflammation of the bladder
      - Urethritis—inflammation of the urethra
      - No systemic manifestations
    - Upper UTI—kidney and ureter:
      - Fever
      - Chills
      - Flank pain
      - Pyelonephritis—inflammation of the renal parenchyma

- Older adults may be asymptomatic, leading to them not being treated:
  - Afebrile
  - Altered mental status
- Diagnosis:
  - Urinalysis:
    - Presence of nitrates
    - Increased white cells
    - Presence of leukocyte esterase
  - Urine culture and sensitivity:
    - Identify organism
    - Identify susceptible antibiotics
  - CT scan:
    - Determine obstructions
- Nursing diagnosis:
  - Ineffective health maintenance related to deficient knowledge of how to prevent urinary tract infections
  - Acute pain related to inflammation of bladder
- Treatment:
  - Adequate fluid intake
  - Medications:
    - Antibiotics—based on sensitivity:
      - Trimethoprim–sulfamethoxazole (Bactrim)
      - Nitrofurantoin (Macrodantin, Macrobid)
      - Ampicillin
      - Amoxicillin
      - Cephalosporins
    - Urinary analgesic:
      - Phenazopyridine (Pyridium)
- Patient teaching:
  - Adequate fluid intake
  - Finish antibiotics
  - Empty bladder regularly
  - Hygiene practices
  - Consider cranberry juice/tablets

> **Clinical Consideration**
> Some antibiotics cause an increased sensitivity to sunlight.

> **Clinical Consideration**
> Phenazopyridine may cause urine to turn orange or red and stain clothing.

Pyelonephritis

- Pyelonephritis involves inflammation of the renal parenchyma and renal pelvis that typically begins with an infection or colonization of bacteria in the lower urinary system. Patients in whom pyelonephritis develops also tend to have obstructive problems, in addition there may be a problem with retrograde reflux of urine from the lower to the upper urinary tract.
- Acute pyelonephritis is acute inflammation of the renal parenchyma and pelvis with recurrent acute episodes leading to chronic pyelonephritis. Chronic pyelonephritis causes the kidneys to become atrophic and fibrotic, with the end result a loss in kidney function.
- *Assessment/Intervention/Education*
  - Detailed medical history:
    - History of UTIs

- Urinary disorders:
  - Obstructions
  - Kidney stones
  - BPH
- Risk factors:
  - Indwelling urinary catheter
- Clinical manifestations:
  - Fever, chills
  - Nausea, vomiting
  - Malaise
  - Flank pain
  - Urinary frequency
  - Dysuria
- Diagnosis:
  - Laboratory:
    - Urine:
      - Urinalysis:
        - Pyuria
        - Bacteriuria
        - Hematuria
        - WBC casts indicate renal parenchyma involvement
      - Culture:
        - Presence of infection, typically bacterial
    - Serum:
      - Blood cultures
      - Complete blood count (CBC) with differential:
        - Leukocytosis with a shift to the left
  - Flank pain on percussion at costovertebral angle
  - Renal ultrasound identifies abnormalities
  - CT scan to determine size of kidney and detect fibrosis
  - Biopsy to indicate extent of disease
- Treatment:
  - Broad-spectrum antibiotics initially
  - Once culture result available, switch to appropriate antibiotics
  - Adequate hydration
  - Nonsteroidal antiinflammatory drugs (NSAIDs) or antipyretic medications
  - Monitor for symptoms of sepsis
- Patient teaching:
  - Disease process education
  - Complete antibiotics as ordered
  - Importance of follow-up to ensure infection has resolved
  - Prevention of reoccurrence
  - Encourage patient to drink at least eight glasses of fluid daily.

▶ *Glomerulonephritis*

- Inflammation of the renal glomeruli that is characterized as acute or chronic; glomerulonephritis that is not treated can lead to endstage renal disease (ESRD).
- Acute glomerulonephritis is most likely to occur after a streptococcal infection, occurs suddenly, and is usually reversible.
- Chronic glomerulonephritis is a slow progressive inflammation of the renal glomeruli that is irreversible and progresses to ESRD.

Clinical Consideration
Prompt diagnosis and treatment is important to prevent kidney damage and sepsis.

- *Assessment/Intervention/Education*
  - Detailed medical history:
    - Recent infections
    - Viral infections:
      - Human immunodeficiency virus (HIV)
      - Hepatitis B
      - Hepatitis C
    - Autoimmune disorders
    - Illegal-drug use
  - Risk factors:
    - Recent streptococcal infection (usually throat)
    - Infective endocarditis
    - Systemic lupus erythematosus
    - Scleroderma
    - Goodpasture syndrome—autoimmune disease that attacks the glomerular basement membrane
    - Diabetic nephropathy
    - Hypertension
  - Clinical manifestations:
    - May be asymptomatic
    - Periorbital edema
    - Smoky urine
    - Oliguria
    - Hematuria
    - Proteinuria
    - Flank or abdominal pain
  - Diagnosis:
    - Positive immune response to streptococci
    - Laboratory:
      - Urine:
        - Proteinuria
        - Urine sediment with erythrocyte casts
      - Serum:
        - Elevated BUN and creatinine
  - Treatment:
    - Acute:
      - Symptom relief
      - Rest
      - Sodium and fluid restriction if edema is present
      - Antibiotics if active infection is present
      - Antihypertensive medication if appropriate
      - Protein-restricted diet
    - Chronic:
      - Supportive
      - Symptomatic
      - Similar to the treatment for Chronic Kidney Disease (CKD)
  - Patient teaching:
    - Encourage early diagnosis of sore throats.
    - Take full course of antibiotics for streptococcal infections.

Question	Rationale
A college student is admitted with dark urine, fever, and flank pain and is diagnosed with acute glomerulonephritis. Which would most likely be in this student's health history? A. Renal calculi B. Renal trauma C. Recent sore throat D. Family history of glomerulonephritis	Answer: C Acute poststreptococcal glomerulonephritis is a common form of acute glomerulonephritis. This occurs a few weeks after a streptococcal infection. Renal calculi, trauma, and a family history of glomerulonephritis are not contributing factors in the development of glomerulonephritis.

▶ *Nephrotic Syndrome*
- A significant increase in glomerular membrane permeability, along with a constellation of symptoms that indicate kidney damage
- *Assessment/Intervention/Education*
  - Detailed medical history:
    - Systemic lupus erythematosus (SLE)
    - Diabetes
    - Recent infections
    - History of neoplasms
    - Drug use:
      - NSAIDs
      - Captopril (Capoten)
      - Heroin
  - Risk factors:
    - Infections:
      - Streptococcal
      - Syphilis
      - Hepatitis
      - HIV
      - Malaria
    - Hodgkin's lymphoma
    - Leukemia
    - Solid tumors
  - Clinical manifestations:
    - Peripheral edema
    - Ascites
    - Anasarca
    - Hypertension
    - Hyperlipidemia:
      - Elevated cholesterol >300 mg/dL
      - Elevated low-density lipoproteins
      - Elevated triglycerides
    - Foamy urine due to fatty casts
    - Significant proteinuria >3.5 g/day
    - Immune response altered, making patients more susceptible to infection

- Hypercoagulability with high incidence of thromboembolism
- Malnourished from loss of protein
- Diagnosis:
  - Laboratory results:
    - Cholesterol values
    - Protein
  - Clinical manifestations along with medical conditions
- Nursing diagnosis:
  - Disturbed body image related to edema
- Treatment:
  - Management of edema:
    - Salt restriction
    - Diuretics to manage edema
  - Excellent skin care to prevent breakdown from edema
  - Adequate nutrition to replace lost protein
  - Lipid-lowering medications
  - Anticoagulant therapy
- Patient teaching:
  - Avoid exposure to illnesses
  - Small frequent meals
  - Sodium intake restricted to 2 to 3 g/day
  - Daily weights
  - May need to monitor intake and output at home

Urinary Calculi (Kidney Stones)

- Formation of urinary calculi is the most common cause of upper urinary obstruction, with stones being formed from materials normally excreted in urine. Nephrolithiasis (kidney stones) is the third most common urinary disorder. There are four types of kidney stones:
  - Calcium (oxylate and phosphate):
    - 70 to 80% of kidney stones
    - Associated with increased concentration of calcium due to bone reabsorption from:
      - Immobility
      - Hyperparathyroidism
      - Bone disease
  - Magnesium ammonium phosphate (struvite):
    - Forms in alkaline urine when bacteria release the enzyme urease
    - Stones enlarge as the number of bacteria increases
    - Can enlarge to fill the entire renal pelvis
    - Often called "staghorn stones" because of their shape
    - Require surgical removal because of the large size of the stones
  - Uric acid (urate):
    - Develop in patients who have high concentrations of uric acid in the urine and those with gout
    - Form in an acidic environment
    - Not visible on x-ray films, as they are not radiopaque
  - Cystine:
    - Rare
    - Occur in people with a genetic defect in the transport of cystine, causing cystinuria

- **Assessment/Intervention/Education**
  - Detailed medical history:
    - Previous urinary calculi/stones
    - Family history of urinary calculi
    - Over-the-counter medications
  - Risk factors:
    - Immobilization
    - Urinary tract infections
    - Gout
    - Diffuse bone disease
  - Clinical manifestations:
    - Severe sudden pain due to stretching and dilation of the ureter:
      - Flank area
      - Lower abdominal pain
      - Back pain
    - Nausea and vomiting
    - Symptoms of UTI:
      - Fever
      - Chills
      - Dysuria
  - Diagnosis:
    - CT scan
    - Abdominal/renal ultrasound
    - Laboratory:
      - Urinalysis:
        - Hematuria
        - White cells—may have a UTI due to urinary stasis
        - Urinary pH
      - Blood:
        - Calcium
        - Phosphorus
        - BUN
        - Creatinine
  - Nursing diagnosis:
    - Acute pain related to passage of stones through urinary tract
  - Treatment:
    - Pain management—opioids
    - Small stones typically pass spontaneously—strain urine
    - Cystoscopy to remove small stones
    - Temporary stent placement to allow small/moderate stones or sediment to pass
    - Lithotripsy—ultrasonic waves to break up stones
    - Percutaneous nephrolithotomy—scope inserted through the back into the kidney pelvis; with tube(s) temporarily left in place
    - Open surgical procedure
  - Patient teaching:
    - Importance of hydration
    - Dietary restrictions
    - Instruct patient on type of stones present
    - Avoid the cause of stone formation (based on composition of stones)

Question	Rationale
The nurse is caring for a patient who was admitted with a diagnosis of renal calculi. The patient recently voided pink urine and is reporting increasing flank pain. Which intervention should be a priority? A. Strain all urine for stones B. Instruct patient to drink additional water C. Administer ordered pain medications D. Send stones to the lab for analysis	Answer: C While each of these nursing interventions is important when caring for the patient with renal calculi, when the patient is experiencing increasing pain, pain management should be the priority.

▶ *Strictures*
- Strictures can occur congenitally or from ureteral or urethral injury resulting in constricted opening along the ureters, urethra or at the meatus.
- *Assessment/Intervention/Education*
  - Detailed medical history:
    - Previous urinary disorders
    - Congenital defects
  - Risk factors:
    - Ureteral:
      - Scar tissue from previous injury:
        - Kidney stones
        - Surgery
        - Radiation
    - Urethral:
      - Fibrosis or inflammation:
        - Trauma
        - Gonococcal infection
        - Repeated catheterization
  - Clinical manifestations:
    - Ureteral:
      - Mild-to-moderate colic
    - Urethral:
      - Change in urine stream
      - Urinary retention
      - Inability to insert a urinary catheter
  - Diagnosis
    - symptoms
    - cystoscopy
    - retrogram urethrogram
  - Treatment:
    - Ureteral:
      - Temporary treatment:
        - Urinary stent placement
        - Nephrostomy tube insertion
      - Correction of stricture:
        - Dilation of ureter
        - Surgical incised endoscopically—endoureterotomy
        - Surgically excise stricture and reanastomosis of ureter—ureteroureterostomy

- Urethral:
  - Dilation of stricture:
    - Gradual dilation with progressively larger instruments
    - Patient may need to self-catheterize every few days to maintain patency.
  - Endoscopic procedures to open stricture
  - Surgical resection of stricture with reanastomosis
- Patient teaching:
  - When to notify provider
  - How to self-catheterize
  - Importance of sterile/clean technique to prevent infection

▶ *Acute Kidney Injury (AKI)*

- Sudden onset, over hours or days; slight to severe kidney function impairment that may be reversible
- *Assessment/Intervention/Education*
  - Detailed medical history:
    - Identification of precipitating cause
    - Sepsis
    - Conditions or diseases that cause decreased blood flow to the kidneys
    - Recently received nephrotoxins (medications or contrast dye)
    - Chronic obstructions in urine flow leading to hydronephrosis
  - Risk factors:
    - Result of other medical problems
    - Multiorgan failure
    - Prolonged hypovolemia
    - Hypotension
    - Nephrotoxic substances
  - Clinical manifestations:
    - Urinary changes:
      - Oliguria
      - Anuria
    - Azotemia—accumulation of urea nitrogen and creatinine in the blood
    - Hypovolemia
    - Metabolic acidosis
    - Decreased serum Na^+
    - Increased serum K^+
    - Increased white-cell count—infection
    - Increased BUN and creatinine
    - Mental status changes
  - Diagnosis:
    - Diagnostic changes may not be evident until >50% loss in kidney function
    - Renal ultrasound
    - Renal scan
    - CT scan
    - Urinalysis
    - Serum BUN and creatinine, GFR
  - Treatment:
    - Treat precipitating cause
    - Fluid restriction or fluid resuscitation, depending on cause

Clinical Consideration

Diagnostic tests using contrast dye can be fatal for the patient with AKI.

- Nutrition therapy:
  - Restrict potassium, sodium, and phosphate
  - Ensure adequate protein intake
- Dialysis if needed:
  - Urgent hemodialysis (see "Hemodialysis" in section on "Chronic Kidney Disease")
  - Continuous renal replacement therapy (CRRT)
    - Used in treatment of AKI
    - Slowly and continuously performs a process similar to hemodialysis
    - Depending on type of CRRT fluid, solutes or fluid or both may be removed from the body
    - CRRT may be done for up to 40 days
    - CRRT filter needs to be changed every 24 to 48 hours
- Monitor daily weights, intake and output
- Monitor daily labs for effectiveness

- Patient teaching:
  - Instruct patient on treatment plan.
  - Teach patient about factors that contributed to AKI and ways to prevent recurrence.
  - Nutritional teaching with dietary restrictions

Chronic Kidney Disease (CKD)

- Progressive, irreversible loss of kidney function that is not evident until there is significant loss of nephron function. The last stage of CKD is referred to as end-stage renal disease (ESRD) or CKD stage 5.

- **Assessment/Intervention/Education**
  - Detailed medical history:
    - Diabetes
    - Hypertension
    - History of urologic diseases
  - Risk factors:
    - Family history of CKD
    - Exposure to nephrotoxic drugs
    - Increasing age
    - Ethnicity
  - Clinical manifestations:
    - May be a symptomatic until GFR significantly declines; manifestations vary based on stage of kidney disease, age and comorbidities.
    - Clinical manifestations are related to retained water, electrolytes, urea, creatinine, hormones, and waste products.
    - As CKD progresses, all body functions are affected because of uremia:
      - Urinary system:
        - Oliguria
        - Anuria
      - Metabolic disturbances:
        - BUN and creatinine levels increased
        - Altered carbohydrate and lipid metabolism
      - Electrolyte and acid–base imbalances:
        - Various electrolyte alterations:
          - Hyperkalemia

- Sodium
- Magnesium
  - Metabolic acidosis due to inability to excrete acids
- Hematologic system:
  - Anemia due to decreased erythropoietin production by the kidneys
  - Bleeding susceptibility due to impaired platelet function
- Cardiovascular system:
  - Cardiovascular disease and CKD are closely linked.
  - Cardiovascular disease is the leading cause of death in patients with CKD.
    - Stroke
    - Myocardial infarction
    - Heart failure
    - Peripheral vascular disease
- Respiratory system:
  - Will be altered in an attempt to compensate for metabolic acid–base disturbances
- Gastrointestinal system:
  - Anorexia, nausea, and vomiting in ESRD
  - Constipation
- Neurologic system:
  - Central nervous system changes from waste products:
    - Lethargy
    - Inability to concentrate
    - Fatigue
    - Irritability
    - Seizures
  - Peripheral neuropathy
  - Restless legs syndrome
- Musculoskeletal system:
  - Bone disorders are common complications of CKD. This is called "mineral and bone disorder" (MBD) and is also related to inability to use vitamin D because the hormone that helps with this is absent.
    - Osteitis fibrosa:
      - Caused by increased parathyroid hormone in response to decreased serum calcium
      - Decalcification of the bone that is replaced by fibrous tissue
    - Osteomalacia:
      - Demineralization of bone with defective mineralization of new bone
    - Vascular and soft tissue calcifications:
      - Caused by increased calcium and phosphorus levels
      - "Uremic red eye" occurs because of calcium deposits in the eye.
- Integumentary system:
  - Pruritus
  - Bleeding or skin infections due to scratching of skin
  - Uremic frost is rare, occurs when BUN level is >200 mg/dL and urea crystalizes on the skin

TABLE 12.3	STAGES OF CHRONIC KIDNEY DISEASE (CKD)	
Stage	Criteria	Treatment
1	GFR >90 mL/min with persistent albuminuria	Screening for CKD risk factors CKD risk-factor reduction
2	GFR 60–89 mL/min with persistent albuminuria	CKD risk-factor reduction Slow progression of CKD
3	GFR 30–59 mL/min	Treat comorbid conditions Slow progression of CKD
4	GFR 15–29 mL/min	Treat complications Prepare for renal replacement therapy 　Dialysis 　　Kidney transplant list
5	GFR <15 mL/min	End-stage renal disease (ESRD) Renal replacement therapy

(KDIGO, 2013)

- Diagnosis:
  - CKD is defined by either a GFR <60 mL/min or the presence of kidney damage (KDIGO, 2013).
  - Laboratory:
    - Serum:
      - Decreased GFR
      - Increased BUN
      - Increased creatinine
      - Electrolytes
      - Lipids
      - Hemoglobin and hematocrit
    - Urine for protein
  - Renal ultrasound
  - Renal biopsy
- Nursing diagnosis:
  - Excess fluid volume related to impaired kidney function
  - Risk for electrolyte imbalance related to impaired kidney function
- Treatment:
  - Based on stage of CKD and clinical manifestations (Table 12.3)
  - Correct fluid balance
  - Nutritional therapy:
    - Restrict protein (depending on the stage of CKD)
    - Fluid restriction
    - Na^+ and K^+ restriction
    - Phosphate restriction
  - Dialysis:
    - Peritoneal dialysis (PD) uses the peritoneum as semipermeable membrane:
      - Process:
        - Instillation and drainage of prescribed dialysate to remove waste products—called "exchanges"

- Inflow—prescribed amount of dialysate is instilled into the peritoneum—typically 2 L
- Dwell—time in which the dialysate remains in the peritoneum allowing for diffusion and osmosis to occur—may last between 30 minutes and 8 hours
- Drain—dialysate is drained from the peritoneum and the process restarts with inflow of next exchange
  - PD systems:
    - Automated peritoneal dialysis (APD):
      - An automated device cycles several exchanges during the night while the patient sleeps
    - Continuous ambulatory peritoneal dialysis (CAPD):
      - Exchanges are typically performed several times a day
  - Access:
    - Catheter inserted through the abdominal wall and tunneled
  - Advantages:
    - Can be done at home
    - Portable system
    - Fewer dietary restrictions
    - Less stress on cardiovascular system
  - Disadvantages:
    - Infection, frequent peritonitis
    - Frequency of cycles
  - Contraindications:
    - Abdominal issues
    - Severe back pain
    - Abdominal scar tissue
  - Complications:
    - Infection
    - Peritonitis
    - Catheter can migrate
    - Problems with inflow/outflow
    - Can exacerbate or cause back pain or hernias
- Hemodialysis (HD):
  - Process:
    - Dialysis center:
      - Typically 3 days a week
      - 3 to 4 hours per session
    - Home HD:
      - Typically 5 days a week
      - 2 to 3 hours per session
      - Can be done at night
    - Blood is cycled through an artificial semipermeable membrane that allows for the filtration and osmosis of fluid and electrolytes and removal of waste products.
  - Access:
    - Access to large rapid blood flow is required

Clinical Consideration
Aseptic technique is critical to avoid infection!

- Temporary venous access:
    - Can be quickly inserted and used immediately
    - High rates of infection
    - Prone to dislodgment and malfunction
- Arteriovenous fistula (AVF):
    - Preferred access for HD
    - Surgical anastomosis of a vein into an artery
    - Need to wait at least 3 months for the fistula to mature
    - Assess bruit and thrill
- Arteriovenous graft (AVG):
    - Synthetic material that forms a bridge between an artery and vein
    - Typically need to wait several weeks before using
    - More prone to clotting, occlusion, and infection than AVF
    - More difficult to assess bruit and thrill
- Advantages:
    - Rapid fluid, electrolyte, and waste removal
    - Less protein loss
    - Lower serum triglycerides
- Complications:
    - Hypotension
    - Access problems
    - Muscle cramps
    - Blood loss
    - Hepatitis
    - Infection
- Kidney transplantation:
    - Highly successful
    - Donor kidney:
        - Compatibility studies a must
        - Live donor kidney:
            - Extensive workup of live donor
        - Cadaver kidney
    - Lifelong immunosuppressive therapy
- Patient teaching:
    - Dietary restrictions
    - Importance of completing dialysis treatments as ordered
    - Signs and symptoms of elevated electrolytes
    - Medication and side effects
    - When to notify health care provider
    - For transplant recipients:
        - Signs and symptoms of infection secondary to immunosuppressive therapy
        - Need to monitor drug levels and for adverse reactions from anti-rejection medications
        - Signs and symptoms of rejection
        - Antirejection medications lifelong

> **Clinical Consideration**
> Be sure to specify that NO blood pressures, blood draws or IVs are to be performed in the arm with the AVF or AVG.

Question	Rationale
The nurse is caring for a patient who is undergoing peritoneal dialysis. What should the nurse do if the return fluid is slowly draining? A. Check for kinks in the outflow tubing B. Ask the patient to cough C. Raise the drainage bag above the level of the abdomen D. Place the patient in reverse Trendelenburg position	Answer: A When there is a slow return of peritoneal fluid it is often related to the tubing. Other interventions that may help with fluid return include having the patient change positions or apply gentle pressure on the abdomen. Having the patient cough or placing the patient in the reverse Trendelenburg position will not help with fluid drainage. Raising the drainage bag above the abdomen may cause the fluid to flow back into the peritoneal cavity.

CASE STUDY

A 42-year-old African American with prediabetes (impaired fasting glucose), hypertension, and chronic kidney disease is admitted to the unit with peritonitis. He is currently on disability leave from a physically demanding job in a shipping warehouse for a printing company. He is married, with three children under 6 years old and lives in a two-bedroom apartment with his family. He was diagnosed with a congenital kidney disorder 15 years earlier and hypertension for the past 20 years. Currently, his blood pressure is 160/88 mm Hg. In the past few years his morning blood glucose levels have been running around 110 mg/dL and he was told he had prediabetes. He has been followed by his nephrologist closely over the past 15 years and has tried to follow a low-sodium diet and eat healthier but has found it challenging because of his job and having small children. Earlier this year, his GFR had rapidly declined to 18 mL/min and he was diagnosed with stage 5 CKD. He did not want to consider hemodialysis at that time, so a peritoneal dialysis (PD) catheter was inserted. He and his wife were trained on proper technique for PD and he began doing four exchanges a day. He felt better within a week of starting PD and he returned to work for a short time. Now he is admitted to your unit with a fever, a WBC of 27,000/mm³, and symptoms of abdominal pain. This is his second admission with peritonitis. His GFR has further declined to 9 mL/day, and it has been decided that he will need to undergo hemodialysis (HD) from this point on. Discussions were held regarding kidney transplantation, and it was decided that he would pursue evaluation to see whether he was a candidate.

1. **What are some factors that may be contributing to his recurrent peritonitis?**

   ▶ *Patient and wife using improper technique for connecting and disconnecting PD tubing and solution*

   ▶ *Hand hygiene and sterile/clean technique not being used*

   ▶ *Working in an environment that is not clean*

   ▶ *Less than optimal personal hygiene*

   ▶ *Assess to see whether blood glucose levels have been elevated*

2. **What education should be reviewed with this patient and his wife about HD?**

  ▶ *Temporary and permanent access:*

   i. *A temporary vascular device will be inserted and can be used immediately.*

   ii. *A permanent AVF or AVG will be surgically created but will not be able to be used until it heals and matures.*

   iii. *No blood pressures, IV lines, or venipuncture should be performed in the arm with the AVF or AVG.*

   iv. *Avoid injuries and tight clothing on the extremity that was or is to be used for the permanent access*

  ▶ *Procedure:*

   i. *Most patients go to an outpatient dialysis center for their scheduled treatments.*

   ii. *Two large-bore needles are inserted into the AVG or AVF for the procedure.*

   iii. *Treatments are typically 3 days a week and last 3 to 4 hours.*

   iv. *It is important not to miss treatments, as toxins will build up in the body and the patient will become ill.*

  ▶ *Complications:*

   i. *Hypotension during rapid removal of vascular volume*

   ii. *Muscle cramps during dialysis*

   iii. *Anemia due to small amount of blood loss with each treatment and to decreased production of erythropoietin from the CKD*

   iv. *Low possibility of contracting hepatitis B and hepatitis C*

  ▶ *Dietary:*

   i. *Protein intake needs to be sufficient to meet nutritional needs, avoid high-protein intake.*

   ii. *Fluid restriction to avoid no more than 1 to 3 kg weight gain between dialysis treatments (not all patients who go to dialysis are on fluid restriction)*

   iii. *Limit sodium intake to 2 to 4 g/day*

   iv. *Limit potassium intake to 2 to 3 g/day*

   v. *Limit phosphorus intake to 1 g/day*

3. **What medications would the nurse anticipate that this patient might be receiving now that he is receiving HD?**

  ▶ *Erythropoietin IV or subcutaneously to promote RBC production*

  ▶ *Iron supplements for RBC production*

  ▶ *Vitamin D supplements if serum levels are low*

  ▶ *Calcium if serum levels are low*

  ▶ *Phosphate binders to eliminate excess phosphorus from the body*

  ▶ *Statins or fibrates to lower cholesterol levels*

  ▶ *Folic acid and other water-soluble vitamins, such as B and C*

Discussion

This patient, as well as his family, will need education and support as he transitions to HD. Things to include in this patient's teaching are: adjust medications and withhold vasodilators or medications that will dialyzed out before going to dialysis (as per the dialysis physician and nurses' recommendations), monitor weight and blood pressure at home, and do not take over-the-counter medications unless he is aware of what is in them (e.g., vitamins/substances that could increase to dangerous levels in body). An interdisciplinary approach will be critical to a successful transition, as will being considered for kidney transplantation. This team must include case management/social worker, and a dietitian, in addition to nursing, medicine, and the transplant team.

Bibliography

Aschenbrenner, D.S., and Venable, S.J. (2012). *Drug Therapy in Nursing*, 4th ed. (Philadelphia: Wolters Kluwer).

Centers for Disease Control and Prevention. (2107). Catheter-associated urinary tract infections (CAUTI). Accessed November 11, 2017, from https://www.cdc.gov/hai/ca_uti/uti.html

Grossman, S., and Porth, C.M. (2013) *Pathophysiology: Concepts of Altered Health States*, 9th ed. (Philadelphia: Lippincott Williams & Wilkins).

Kidney Disease: Improving Global Outcomes (KDIGO) CKD Workgroup. (2013). KDIGO 2012 clinical practice guidelines for the evaluation and management of chronic kidney disease. *Kidney International Supplements* 3(1), 1–150.

Kidney Disease: Improving Global Outcomes (KDIGO) Glomerulonephritis Workgroup. (2012). KDIGO 2012 clinical practice guidelines for glomerulonephritis. *Kidney International Supplements* 2, 139–274.

Lewis, S.L., Bucher, L., Heitkemper, M., and Harding, M.M. (2017). *Medical-Surgical Nursing: Assessment and Management of Clinical Problems*, 10th ed. (St. Louis: Elsevier).

National Institute of Health. (n.d.). Bladder infection (urinary tract infection—UTI) in adults. U.S. Department of Health and Human Services. Accessed November 12, 2017, from https://www.niddk.nih.gov/health-information/urologic-diseases/bladder-infection-uti-in-adults/all-content

National Kidney Foundation. (2002). Clinical practice guidelines for chronic kidney disease: Evaluation, classification and stratification. *American Journal of Kidney Disease* 39(suppl 1), s1–s266.

Rowe, T.A., and Juthani-Mehta, M. (2014). Diagnosis and management of urinary tract infection in older adults. *Infectious Disease Clinics of North America* 28, 75–89.

13

Reproductive System

Stephanie Gedzyk-Nieman, DNP, MSN, RNC-MNN
Donna Martin, DNP, RN, CMSRN, CDE, CNE

OVERVIEW

▶ The primary purpose of both the male and female reproductive systems is the production of offspring, but they also play a role in the secretion of certain hormones.

▶ The male genitourinary system serves both urinary and reproductive functions.

ANATOMY AND PHYSIOLOGY

▶ The male and female reproductive systems consist of internal and external structures.

▶ Male reproductive system:
  - Penis:
    - Consists of the:
      - Glans (tip)
        - Contains many sensory nerves
        - Most sensitive portion of the penis
      - Prepuce (foreskin):
        - Loose skin that covers the glans
        - Removed during circumcision
      - Shaft composed of erectile tissues that become engorged with blood during erection:
        - Corpus cavernosum—two lateral sides of the penis
        - Corpus spongiosum—ventral side of the penis
  - Testes:
    - Pair of smooth firm organs
    - Male gonads that are responsible for:
      - Spermatogenesis—production of sperm in the seminiferous tubules
      - Testosterone and other male hormone secretions
    - Numerous sensory nerves fibers surround the testes

- Scrotum:
  - Houses the testes
  - Dartos muscle helps to maintain a constant temperature for sperm production
    - Contraction when cold
    - Relaxation when warm
- Accessory organs:
  - Transports and stores sperm:
    - Epididymides
    - Vas deferens
    - Ejaculatory ducts
- Accessory glands:
  - Produce and secrete semen to prepare sperm for ejaculation
    - Seminal vesicles
    - Prostate gland
    - Bulbourethral glands/Cowper glands
- Prostate:
  - Enclosed in a fibrous capsule
  - Located in the symphysis pubis with the posterior surface near the rectal wall
  - Surrounds the neck of the bladder and urethra
  - Portion of urethra passes through prostate—prostatic urethra
- Urethra:
  - Terminal portion of the male anatomy
  - Transports both urine and sperm
- Male hormones (androgens):
  - Testosterone:
    - Main testicular hormone
    - Responsible for the development of male sex characteristics
    - Promotes protein metabolism and musculoskeletal growth
    - Influences subcutaneous fat distribution
    - Promotes spermatogenesis and sperm maturation
    - Stimulation of erythropoiesis
  - Dihydrotestosterone (DHT)
    - 5α-reductase converts much of the testosterone to DHT
    - Similar actions as testosterone
  - Androstenedione:
    - Significant impact on body musculature
- Female reproductive system:
  - External structures
    - Mons pubis:
      - Layer of fat that lies over the symphysis pubis
      - May have coarse hair covering it
    - Labia majora:
      - Two, round folds of fatty tissue that extend downward from the mons pubis
      - May also have coarse hair covering them
      - Purpose—to protect the underlying structures
    - Labia minora:
      - Two, pink folds of hairless tissue that are visible by separating the labia majora
      - Purpose—lubrication and protection of underlying structures

- Clitoris:
  - Small, sensory-nerve–dense structure located anteriorly from the urethra and vaginal orifice
  - Becomes engorged during sexual arousal
- Skene glands:
  - Located on each side of the urethra
  - Purpose—mucus production to aid in vaginal lubrication
- Bartholin glands:
  - Located on posterior and lateral aspects of the vaginal opening
  - Purpose—mucus production to aid in vaginal lubrication
- Perineum:
  - Area between the posterior opening of the vaginal opening and the anus
- Internal structures:
  - Vagina:
    - 3 to 4 inches long; moist, tube-shaped structure
    - During reproductive years, consists of many folds (rugae) that allow for expansion during childbirth.
    - Estrogen deprivation during menopause, postchildbirth, and during lactation contribute to the rugae becoming smooth and to vaginal dryness.
    - Purpose—acidic secretions to keep bacterial counts low; passageway for menstrual flow, fetus, and for copulation
  - Uterus:
    - Muscular, pear-shaped organ located between the bladder and the rectum in the pelvic cavity
    - Size (in the woman who has never been pregnant): 2 to 3 inches long and 1.5 inches wide
    - Consists of the:
      - Fundus
        - Top of the uterus
      - Uterine wall:
        - Endometrium:
          - Highly vascular lining that is shed during menstruation
        - Myometrium:
          - Middle made of up of smooth muscle layers
        - Peritoneum:
          - Outer serosal layer
      - Cervix:
        - Lower portion of the uterus that connects the uterus to the vagina; consists of fibrous and elastic tissue
        - 0.8 to 1.6 inches long and tightly closed
        - Secretes different types of mucus based on estrogen and progesterone levels during the menstrual cycle to either enhance or prohibit sperm from entering the uterus
    - Purpose—houses and nourishes fertilized ovum (egg) during pregnancy; expulsion of fetus during childbirth; organ of menstruation during reproductive cycle
  - Fallopian tubes:
    - Bilateral tubes that extend from the uterine fundus to the ovaries
    - Purpose—allow a passageway for the ovum from the ovaries to the uterus and a place for fertilization of the ovum in reproduction

Clinical Consideration

These glands are usually not palpable upon exam, unless a cyst is present or if it is edematous from an infection.

Clinical Consideration

The cervix is made up of two types of endothelial cells. The area where these two meet, called the "squamocolumnar junction" (or "transformation zone") is where cells are sampled for a Pap test for cervical cancer screening.

- Ovaries:
  - Two, almond-shaped organs located bilaterally from the uterus and by the fallopian tubes
  - Purpose—release of an ovum (ovulation) for reproduction and the production of estrogen, progesterone, and androgen
- Breasts:
  - Paired mammary glands located from the second to the sixth rib and extending to the upper outer quadrant of the axilla
  - Each breast contains a nipple and dark pigmented area around the nipple (areola)
  - Fully matures during puberty into a dome shape with a smooth contour, but size may vary among women and based on cyclic hormone changes
  - Purpose—houses the mammary glands and ductal system for lactation
- Hormones and the menstrual cycle:
  - Monthly occurrence involving the ovaries, endometrium, pituitary gland, and hypothalamus
  - Purpose—to prepare the uterus for pregnancy
  - If there is no fertilized ovum, then menstruation occurs
  - Average cycle length: 28 days (but can vary from woman to woman)
  - First day of cycle is the first day of menstrual flow (documented as last menstrual period [LMP])
  - Duration of menstrual flow: 1 to 8 days; average blood loss of 50 mL
  - Cycles within menstrual cycle:
    - Hypothalamic–pituitary cycle
      - First half of cycle:
        - Hypothalamus secretes gonadotropin-releasing hormone (GnRH).
        - GnRH stimulates anterior pituitary gland to secrete follicle-stimulating hormone (FSH).
        - FSH stimulates follicle development in the ovary and increases production of estrogen in ovary.
      - Second half of cycle:
        - Luteinizing hormone (LH) peaks.
        - Ovum is released from ovary.
        - Progesterone production increases from the corpus luteum in the ovary.
        - If the ovum is not fertilized, estrogen and progesterone levels fall and cycle starts again.
    - Ovarian cycle:
      - Follicular phase (length varies from woman to woman):
        - FSH allows for the ovum (egg) to mature and estrogen production to increase
      - Luteal phase (14 days)
        - Begins immediately after ovulation and ends with menstruation.
        - LH surge causes ovulation and corpus luteum to increase progesterone production.
        - If implantation of fertilized ovum does not occur, corpus luteum degenerates, progesterone and estrogen levels fall, and menstruation occurs.
    - Endometrial cycle:
      - Menstrual phase (days 1 to 6):
        - Menstrual flow from endometrium is occurring
        - Estrogen and progesterone at their lowest

Clinical Consideration

There should be no discharge from the breasts except during pregnancy or lactation.

- Proliferative phase (days 7 to 14):
  - Due to increasing estrogen, endometrium is thickening
- Secretory phase (days 15 to 26):
  - Progesterone levels are rising.
  - Endometrial lining is reaching maximum thickness and vascularity.
- Ischemic phase (days 27 to 28):
  - If implantation does not occur, progesterone and estrogen levels decline.
  - Blood supply to the endometrium is blocked, causing necrosis, and shedding of the endometrium occurs again.

▶ Gerontologic considerations:
- General age-related changes:
  - Increased incidence of chronic diseases (hypertension, cardiovascular, diabetes)
  - Potential for multiple medications
  - Hormonal changes with aging
- Male:
  - Experiences gradual degenerative changes
  - Less dramatic changes than females
  - Testosterone levels decline
  - Prostate enlargement
  - Difficulty achieving/maintaining erection
  - Gynecomastia
- Female:
  - Decreased subcutaneous fat and increased fibrous tissue in the breasts
  - Decrease in ovarian function leads to decrease in estrogen and progesterone
  - Decreased myometrium thickness in the uterus can lead to uterine prolapse
  - Atrophy of vaginal tissue and dryness
  - Decrease in muscle tone and mucosal thinning of urethra possibly leading to urinary tract infections, urgency, frequency, dysuria, incontinence

DIAGNOSTIC TESTS

▶ Imaging:
- Male:
  - Transrectal ultrasound of prostate (TRUS):
    - With or without biopsy
  - Doppler ultrasound of the testes
  - Nuclear scan of the testes
- Female:
  - Mammogram
- Computed tomographic (CT) scan of pelvis
- Magnetic resonance imaging (MRI)

▶ Laboratory:
- Male:
  - Testosterone levels
  - Serum prostate-specific antigen (PSA)
- Female:
  - Pap smear
  - Human papillomavirus (HPV) screening
  - Estradiol levels:
    - Used to measure ovarian function and confirm perimenopausal status

- Progesterone levels:
  - Used to assess infertility and diagnose adrenal gland issues and some types of cancer
- FSH level:
  - Assesses gonadal function and confirms menopausal status (levels increase in menopause)
- LH level:
  - Used in assessment of infertility and menstrual irregularity
- Serum or urine human chorionic gonadotropin (HCG) level:
  - Used to detect pregnancy
- Serum prolactin level:
  - Used to assess problems with lactation, menstruation irregularities, and detect a prolactin producing pituitary tumor

SCREENINGS

▶ Male:
- Prostate:
  - Serum PSA
    - Men ages 55 to 69 consider screening (USPSTF, 2017)
      - If PSA <2.5 ng/mL, retest every 2 years.
      - If PSA >2.5 ng/mL, retest yearly.
  - Digital rectal exam (DRE)
▶ Female:
- Breast:
  - Self-exam:
    - No recommendation (AHRQ, 2014)
    - Not recommended for average-risk women (ACOG, 2017a)
  - Clinical exam:
    - No recommendation (AHRQ, 2014)
    - Every 1 to 3 years for average-risk women 25 to 39 years of age and annually for those ≥40 (ACOG, 2017a)
  - Mammogram:
    - Every 12 to 24 months for average-risk women ≥40 years or older (ACOG, 2017a; AHRQ, 2014) and continue until age 75 (ACOG, 2017a)
- Cervix/pelvic:
  - Annual examination of external genitalia for all women (ACOG, 2012)
  - Speculum and pelvic exams yearly, beginning at age 21, whether sexually active or not (ACOG, 2012):
    - May be deferred if asymptomatic and has undergone a total hysterectomy and bilateral salpingo-oophorectomy for benign indications and has no history of vulvar or cervical cancer, is not infected with human immunodeficiency virus (HIV), and is not immunocompromised (ACOG, 2012)
  - Pap smear (ACOG, 2017b; AHRQ, 2014):
    - Women 21 to 29 every 3 years
    - Women 30 to 65 every 3 to 5 years
  - Human papillomavirus (HPV) screening (ACOG, 2017b; AHRQ, 2014):
    - Women 21 to 29, screening not recommended
    - Women 30 to 65 every 5 years

Sexually Transmitted Infections (STIs)

▶ "Infectious diseases that are spread through sexual contact with the penis, vagina, anus, mouth, or sexual fluids of an infected person" (Lewis et al., 2017, p. 1227)

▶ Risk factors:
- Anyone who is sexually active
- High-risk populations:
  - Ages 15 to 24
  - Men who have sex with men (MSM)
  - Sexual assault victims
  - Residents of correctional facilities
- High-risk behaviors:
  - New or multiple sexual partners
  - Sexual partner who has multiple sexual partners
  - Incorrect or inconsistent use of barrier products, such as condoms
  - Intravenous (IV) drug use (self or sexual partner)
- Nursing diagnosis:
  - Impaired comfort related to infection
  - Ineffective health maintenance related to deficient knowledge regarding transmission, symptoms, and treatment of STIs
  - Social isolation related to fear of spreading disease
  - Fear related to illness, altered body function, stigma of having an STI

▶ Chlamydia:
- Bacterial infection (*Chlamydia trachomatis*)
- Most prevalent STI in the United States (CDC, 2017)
- Incubation period: 1 to 3 weeks
- ***Assessment/Intervention/Education***
  - Clinical manifestations:
    - May be asymptomatic (especially in females)
    - Males:
      - Dysuria
      - Urethral discharge
      - Epididymitis (rare)
    - Females:
      - Mucopurulent discharge
      - Vaginal bleeding
      - Dysuria
      - Painful intercourse
    - Rectal chlamydia:
      - Rectal pain
      - Discharge
      - Bleeding
  - Long-term complications:
    - Males:
      - Rare, but epididymitis can result in infertility
    - Females:
      - Risk for pelvic inflammatory disease (PID) increases with each infection

> **Clinical Consideration**
>
> All cases of syphilis and gonorrhea should be reported to the public health department and in some states so should chlamydial infections.

- Consequences of PID:
  - Infertility
  - Ectopic pregnancies
  - Chronic pelvic pain
- Diagnosis:
  - Swab of anatomic site of exposure
  - Most sensitive lab test is nucleic acid amplification test (NAAT)
- Treatment/management:
  - Should begin promptly to avoid long-term complications
  - Preferred drug therapy:
    - Azithromycin (Zithromax) or doxycycline
  - Alternative regimen:
    - Erythromycin, ofloxacin (Floxin), or levofloxacin (Levaquin)
- Patient teaching:
  - Abstain from sexual contact for 7 days after drug therapy is completed and asymptomatic.
  - Abstain from sexual contact until all sex partners within the past 60 days are also tested/treated.
  - Patient should also be tested for HIV, gonorrhea, and syphilis.
  - Recommend follow-up testing 3 months after treatment completion.
  - Encourage condom or barrier use at each sexual encounter.

▶ Gonorrhea:

- Bacterial infection (*Neisseria gonorrhoeae*)
- Second most prevalent STI in the United States (CDC, 2017)
- Incubation period: up to 1 week

Assessment/Intervention/Education

- Clinical manifestations:
  - May be asymptomatic (especially in women)
  - Males:
    - Dysuria
    - Purulent urethral discharge
    - Epididymitis
  - Females:
    - Dysuria
    - Urinary frequency
    - Vaginal discharge
    - Vaginal bleeding
  - Rectal gonorrhea:
    - Mucopurulent discharge
    - Bleeding
    - Painful bowel movements
    - Pruritus
  - Oral gonorrhea:
    - Sore throat
- Long-term complications:
  - Disseminated gonococcal infection (rare):
    - Skin lesions
    - Fever
    - Arthralgia

- Arthritis
- Endocarditis
- Males:
  - Rare, but epididymitis can result in infertility
- Females:
  - Symptoms of these long-term complications are usually the reason women seek care.
  - PID:
    - Infertility
    - Ectopic pregnancies
    - Chronic pelvic pain
  - Infection of Bartholin glands
- Diagnosis:
  - Swab of anatomic site of exposure
  - Most sensitive lab test is NAAT
  - Culture may also be used
- Treatment/management:
  - Can be difficult because of bacteria's ability to develop antibiotic resistance
  - Preferred drug therapy:
    - Ceftriaxone (Rocephin) intramuscularly (IM) with oral azithromycin (Zithromax)
  - Alternative drug therapy:
    - Cefixime (Suprax) with azithromycin (Zithromax)
- Patient teaching:
  - Abstain from sexual contact for 7 days after drug therapy is completed and asymptomatic.
  - Abstain from sexual contact until all sex partners within the past 60 days are also tested/treated.
  - Patient should also be tested for HIV, chlamydia, and syphilis.
  - Follow-up testing 14 days after treatment for oral infections that were treated with the alternative drug therapy option.
  - Encourage condom or barrier use at each sexual encounter.
- Genital herpes:
  - Chronic, lifelong viral infection
  - Two strains:
    - Herpes simplex virus type 1 (HSV-1)
    - HSV-2 (most common for genital herpes)
  - Incubation period: 2 days to 2 weeks
  - *Assessment/Intervention/Education*
    - Clinical manifestations:
      - Many are asymptomatic during the primary episode of the infection
      - Stages of symptoms (approximately 3 weeks in length)
        - Prodromal stage:
          - Burning, itching, tingling at infection site
        - Vesicular stage:
          - Painful vesical formation at infection site
        - Ulcerative stage:
          - Ruptured lesions form moist ulcerations
        - Final stage:
          - Crusting over and healing of the ulcerations

- May also experience flu-like symptoms
- Recurrent episodes tend to be less severe and shorter in length
- Long-term complications (rare):
  - Blindness
  - Aseptic meningitis
  - Encephalitis
- Diagnosis:
  - Lesion cultures
  - Blood test to detect antibodies for HSV-1 and HSV-2
- Treatment/management:
  - Topical therapy with antiviral drugs offers little benefit
  - First clinical episode:
    - 7 to 10 days of treatment, but can be extended if healing is not complete at end of the course:
      - Acyclovir (Zovirax)
      - Valacyclovir (Valtrex)
      - Famciclovir (Famvir)
  - Suppressive therapy:
    - Acyclovir
    - Valacyclovir
    - Famciclovir
  - Episodic therapy:
    - Initiated within 1 day of lesion onset or during the prodrome that precedes some outbreaks, so supply the patient with a supply of drug or prescription for the medication
      - Acyclovir
      - Valacyclovir
      - Famciclovir
  - Severe infection:
    - Acyclovir IV 2 to 7 days or until improvement, then oral therapy to receive a total of 10 days of therapy
- Patient teaching:
  - Greatest risk of transmission is during an episode, but still can transmit disease during asymptomatic periods
  - Abstain from sexual activity with uninfected partners when lesions or prodromal symptoms present
  - Importance of informing current and future sex partners about genital herpes
  - Correct and effective use of condoms
  - Proper care of lesions when they occur
  - Risk for neonatal HSV infection
  - Higher risk of acquiring HIV
  - Awareness of possible triggers for recurrence:
    - Stress
    - Fatigue
    - Sunburn
    - Immunosuppression
    - Menses
- Trichomonas:
  - Protozoan infection (*Trichomonas vaginalis*)
  - Incubation period: 1 week to 1 month, but can be much longer

Assessment/Intervention/Education

- Clinical manifestations:
  - Most infected persons are asymptomatic.
  - Untreated infections might last for months to years.
  - Urethra and cervix are the most commonly infected, the rectum rarely, and never the oropharynx.
  - Males:
    - Urethritis
    - Prostatitis
    - Epididymitis
  - Females:
    - Vulvar irritation
    - Yellow-green, malodorous vaginal discharge
- Long-term complications:
  - Higher likelihood of acquiring/transmitting HIV or another STI
  - Females:
    - PID—especially with HIV:
      - Infertility
      - Ectopic pregnancies
      - Chronic pelvic pain
- Diagnosis:
  - Swab of anatomic site of exposure
  - Most sensitive lab test is NAAT
  - Culture may also be used along with point-of-care testing and microscopic examination
- Treatment/management:
  - Preferred drug therapy:
    - Metronidazole (Flagyl)
    - Tinidazole (Tindamax)
- Patient teaching:
  - No alcohol consumption during treatment with nitroimidazoles:
    - Continue for 24 hours after completion of metronidazole or 72 hours after completion of tinidazole.
  - Abstain from sexual contact for 7 days after drug therapy is completed and patient is asymptomatic.
  - Abstain from sexual contact until all sex partners within the past 60 days are also tested/treated.
  - Patient should also be tested for other STIs, especially HIV.
  - Follow-up testing is not recommended for men.
  - Follow-up testing for all women 3 months after treatment because there is a high rate of reinfection.
  - Encourage condom or barrier use at each sexual encounter.
- Genital warts/HPV:
  - Over 40 types of the virus are sexually transmitted:
    - Some are oncogenic
    - Others cause genital warts and/or recurrent respiratory papillomatosis
  - Most sexually active people infected sometime in their lives, although most unaware
  - Incubation period: weeks, months. or years

- *Assessment/Intervention/Education*
  - Clinical manifestations:
    - Most individuals are asymptomatic and the virus resolves spontaneously within a few years
    - Single or clusters of papillary swellings
  - Long-term complications:
    - None a majority of the time, unless infected with the cancerous strains
  - Diagnosis:
    - Only definitive test is biopsy of the growth
    - Women may also may have abnormal Pap test results (if strain is cancerous)
  - Treatment/management:
    - Removal of the growths
    - Prevention via HPV vaccines:
      - Vaccines are not licensed or recommended for use in men or women >26 years of age in the United States
      - Can be administered regardless of history of warts, abnormal Pap/HPV tests, or anogenital precancer:
        - Human papillomavirus bivalent vaccine (Cervarix)
        - Human papillomavirus quadrivalent vaccine (Gardasil)
  - Patient teaching:
    - Reinforce that the types of HPV that cause genital warts are different from the types that can cause cancer.
    - Although condoms are helpful in reducing transmission, the most reliable form of prevention is abstinence, as HPV can infect areas not covered by a condom.
    - Removal of the warts does not guarantee that the virus cannot still be transmitted to others.
    - Even those with only one lifetime sex partner can contract HPV.
- Syphilis:
  - Bacterial infection (*Treponema pallidum*)
  - Incubation period: 10 to 90 days, with an average of 21 days
  - *Assessment/Intervention/Education*
    - Clinical manifestations:
      - Disease progresses through distinct stages, over a period of weeks to years, if left untreated.
        - Primary stage (3 to 6 weeks long):
          - Highly infectious
          - Chancres
          - Lymphadenopathy in infected region
        - Secondary stage (1 to 2 years long):
          - Highly infectious
          - Occurs after primary chancre has healed
          - Flu symptoms
          - Mucous patches in the mouth or on the cervix
          - Nonpruritic, symmetric rash on trunk, palms of the hands, and/or soles of the feet
          - Weight loss and/or hair loss
          - Moist, weeping papules in the anogenital area
        - Latent stage (lasts throughout life or until progresses to late stage):
          - Still infectious if <1 year since infected; noninfectious if ≥1 year since infected
          - Asymptomatic

Clinical Consideration

Cervarix can be given only to women, while Gardasil can be given to men and women.

- Late stage (chronic and potentially fatal):
  - Noninfectious
  - Gummas (chronic lesions that can form and impact any organ of the body)
  - Aneurysm
  - Heart-valve insufficiency
  - Heart failure
  - Aortitis
  - Neurosyphilis:
    - Dementia
    - Personality changes
    - Visual impairment
    - Nerve pain
    - Tabes dorsalis (progressive loss of muscle control/balance)
  - Long-term complications:
    - Mostly seen in late syphilis
    - Neurosyphilis can occur at any time
  - Diagnosis:
    - Microscopic exam of lesion tissue
    - Use of two blood tests:
      - Nontreponemal test:
        - Venereal Disease Research Laboratory (VDRL) or rapid plasma reagin (RPR)
      - Treponemal test:
        - Fluorescent treponemal antibody absorption test (FTA-ABS) or *T. pallidum* passive particle agglutination (TP-PA) assay
  - Treatment/management:
    - Preferred drug therapy (all stages):
      - Penicillin G
    - Alternative regimen (all stages):
      - Doxycycline or tetracycline
  - Patient teaching:
    - Treatment cannot reverse the damage present in the later stages of the disease.
    - All sexual partners within 90 days should be treated presumptively for syphilis, even if their serologic test results are negative.
    - Patient should also be tested for HIV.
    - Refrain from sexual activity until all treatment is completed, asymptomatic, and blood tests confirm disease is not present.
    - Reevaluation should occur at 6, 12, and 24 months after treatment.
    - Encourage condom or barrier use at each sexual encounter.

> **Clinical Consideration**
> Use of only one type of test is insufficient for diagnosis and can result in false negative results in persons tested during primary syphilis and false positive results in persons without syphilis.

> **Clinical Consideration**
> Jarisch–Herxheimer reaction, an acute febrile reaction frequently accompanied by headache, muscle pain, and fever, can occur within the first 24 hours of treatment. Patients should be informed about this possible adverse reaction and instructed to take analgesics and antipyretics if it occurs.

Question	Rationale
The VDRL and FTA-ABS lab tests for the patient are positive. The nurse will have to: A. Initiate the Gardasil vaccine series B. Administer acyclovir C. Administer ceftriaxone (Rocephin) with azithromycin (Zithromax) D. Notify the public health department	Answer: D A positive VDRL and FTA-ABS test indicate the patient has syphilis. Syphilis, as well as gonorrhea and sometimes chlamydia, must be reported to the public health department. The Gardasil vaccine series is used to *prevent* HPV and acyclovir is used to treat genital herpes. Ceftriaxone (Rocephin) with azithromycin (Zithromax) is used to treat gonorrhea.

▶ Bacterial vaginosis:

- Polymicrobial infection resulting from replacement of the normal hydrogen-peroxide–producing bacteria in the vagina with high concentrations of anaerobic bacteria.
  - *Assessment/Intervention/Education*
    - Clinical manifestations:
      - Characteristic strong, fish-like odor
      - Thin white, gray, or milky vaginal discharge
      - Pain, pruritus, or burning in or outside the vagina
    - Long-term complications:
      - Higher likelihood of acquiring/transmitting HIV or another STI
    - Diagnosis:
      - Gram stain
      - Clinical criteria require three of the following
        - Thin, smooth, white discharge coating the vagina
        - Clue cells on microscopic examination
        - pH of vaginal fluid >4.5
        - Whiff test (fishy odor released before or after addition of 10% potassium hydroxide (KOH) to vaginal secretions)
    - Treatment/management:
      - Preferred drug therapy:
        - Metronidazole (Flagyl) (orally or intravaginally)
        - Clindamycin (Cleocin) (orally or intravaginally)
      - Alternative regimen:
        - Tinidazole (Tindamax) (orally)
    - Patient teaching:
      - Avoid douching, as it increases the risk for this infection and may cause relapse.
      - Encourage condom or barrier use at each sexual encounter:
        - Clindamycin cream may weaken latex condoms and diaphragms for up to 5 days after treatment.
      - Sexual partners do not require treatment.
      - Follow-up is required only if symptoms persist or return.
      - Patient should also be tested for other STIs, as well as HIV.

Male Disorders

▶ Prostatitis:

- One of the most common urologic disorders that includes inflammatory and non-inflammatory disorders of the prostate gland. Prostatitis is classified into four categories with the most common type being nonbacterial:
  - Acute bacterial prostatitis
  - Chronic bacterial prostatitis
  - Chronic prostatitis or chronic pelvic pain syndrome
  - Asymptomatic inflammatory prostatitis
- *Assessment/Intervention/Education*
  - Detailed medical history
  - Risk factors
    - Male less than 50 years of age
    - Pelvic trauma
    - Prostate biopsy

Clinical Consideration

Alcohol consumption should be avoided during and for 24 hours after treatment with metronidazole. Also, avoid alcohol during and 72 hours after treatment with tinidazole.

- Clinical manifestations
  - Swelling and inflammation of the prostate gland
  - Painful urination
  - Pelvic/groin pain
- Diagnosis:
  - Expressed prostatic secretion evaluation and culture
    - Void just before and just after vigorous prostate massage
  - Laboratory:
    - Urinalysis
    - Urine culture
    - White-cell and blood cultures if fever present
  - Not diagnostic but used to rule out other causes of symptoms:
    - PSA (rule out prostate cancer)
    - Transrectal ultrasound (TRUS) (rule out abscess)
    - MRI (rule out abscess)
- Nursing diagnosis:
  - Acute pain/impaired comfort related to inflammation
  - Urge urinary incontinence related to irritation of the bladder, distention
- Treatment:
  - Acute and chronic bacterial prostatitis:
    - Antibiotics:
      - Up to 4 weeks for acute
      - 8 to 12 weeks for chronic
      - May be lifelong for immunocompromised patients
  - Pain management:
    - Nonsteroidal antiinflammatory drugs (NSAIDs)
    - α-Adrenergic blockers
    - Warm sitz bath
    - Prostatic massage
    - Ejaculation
  - Acute urinary retention
    - Prostatic massage
    - Ejaculation
- Patient teaching:
  - Drink adequate amount of liquids.
  - Signs and symptoms of infection
  - Signs and symptoms of prostatitis and when to seek medical attention

▶ Benign prostatic hyperplasia (BPH):
- Prostate gland is a muscular one surrounding the urethra at the base of the bladder. It grows throughout life, eventually causing hyperplasia. The primary hormone that stimulates prostate growth is dihydrotestosterone (DHT).
- The prostate enlarges beyond normal dimensions (4×5 cm) with a firmer consistency.
- BPH usually develops in the central area of the prostate and eventually encroaches on urethra.
- *Assessment/Intervention/Education*
  - Detailed medical history:
    - Urinary patterns
    - Elevated PSA level
    - Findings on digital rectal examination (DRE)

Clinical Consideration

Prostatic massage should not be done if a bacterial infection is suspected in order to avoid the risk of bacterial spread.

Clinical Consideration

An indwelling catheter is contraindicated in acute prostatitis.

- Risk factors:
  - Increased age
  - Obesity
  - Alcohol consumption
  - Erectile dysfunction
  - Smoking
  - Diabetes
- Clinical manifestations:
  - Increased frequency
  - Nocturia
  - Change in stream
  - Difficulty starting stream
  - Feeling of incomplete emptying
  - Intermittency
  - Urgency
  - Urinary leakage
- Complications:
  - Urinary retention
  - Frequent urinary-tract infections
  - Thickening of bladder wall
  - Hydroureter
  - Hydronephrosis
  - Kidney pelvis dilatation
  - Bladder calculi
- Diagnosis
  - Elevated PSA
  - Enlarged prostate noted on DRE
  - TRUS
  - Prostate biopsy—to rule out cancer
  - Ultrasound of kidneys and ureters
  - Cystoscopy
  - Residual urine—assess postvoid residual (PVR) by straight catheterization or bladder scan
  - Other labs that may be ordered
    - Urinalysis
    - Urine culture and sensitivity (C&S)
    - Blood urea nitrogen (BUN), creatinine, creatinine clearance
  - International Prostate Symptom Score (IPSS) survey
- Nursing diagnosis:
  - Urinary retention related to urethral obstruction
  - Impaired urinary elimination related to urethral blockage
- Treatment:
  - Watchful waiting:
    - Monitor for worsening symptoms
  - Medical treatment goals:
    - Slow prostate growth
    - Relax prostate muscle
    - Relieve retention

- Medications:
  - α-Adrenergic blockers:
    - Medications:
      - Tamsulosin (Flomax)
      - Doxazosin (Cardura)
      - Silodosin (Rapaflo)
    - Action:
      - Promotes smooth muscle relaxation in prostate
      - Facilitates urinary flow
      - Improvement in 2 to 3 weeks
    - Side effects:
      - Orthostatic hypotension and dizziness
      - Retrograde ejaculation
      - Nasal congestion
  - 5α-reductase inhibitors (androgen hormone inhibitor)
    - Medications:
      - Finasteride (Proscar)
      - Dutasteride (Avodart)
    - Action:
      - Decrease size of prostate gland
      - Improvement in 3 to 6 months
    - Side effects:
      - Decreased libido
      - Decreased volume of ejaculation
      - Erectile dysfunction (ED)
  - Erectogenic drugs:
    - Tadalafil (Cialis) 5 mg daily may be helpful when taken with other BPH medications.
- Minimally invasive procedures:
  - Intermittent catheterization to reduce symptoms and bypass obstruction
  - Laser prostatectomy
  - Transurethral microwave thermotherapy (TUMT)
  - Transurethral needle ablation (TUNA)
  - Balloon dilation
- Surgical procedures:
  - Transurethral resection of the prostate (TURP):
    - Most common procedure
    - Complications include bleeding and retrograde ejaculation.
    - Continuous bladder irrigation (CBI) is required postoperatively.
  - Transurethral incision of the prostate (TUIP)
  - Open prostatectomy:
    - Leads to greater risk of erectile dysfunction
- Preoperative care:
  - Use aseptic technique when using urinary catheter.
  - Administer antibiotics preoperatively.
- Postoperative care:
  - Provide patient opportunity to express concerns about alterations in sexual function.
  - Inform patient about possible complications of procedures.

- Postoperative bladder irrigation to remove blood clots and ensure drainage of urine
- Administer antispasmodics.
- Teach Kegel exercises.
- Observe patient for signs of infection.
- Discharge instructions for indwelling catheter.
- Managing incontinence
- 2 to 3 L fluids per day
- Signs and symptoms of urinary-tract infection (UTI), wound infection
- Stool softeners to prevent straining
- Patient teaching:
  - Urinate every 2 to 3 hours, or when urge begins.
  - Prevent constipation.
  - Avoiding heavy lifting.
  - Refrain from driving and intercourse after surgery as directed.
  - Sexual counseling if erectile dysfunction becomes a problem
  - Avoid bladder irritants; alcohol, caffeine.
  - Over-the-counter (OTC) medications may worsen symptoms of urinary retention:
    - Pseudoephedrine
    - Phenylephrine

Question	Rationale
A patient just returned from the recovery room after undergoing a TURP. He has a three-way Foley catheter with a 30-mL balloon. Continuous bladder irrigation with normal saline is infusing through the irrigation port. Soon he begins to report bladder spasms. The nurse should: A. Deflate the balloon to 10 mL to relieve pressure B. Explain that the feeling is normal and to avoid trying to urinate C. Slow down the irrigation fluid rate to reduce bladder spasms D. Encourage the patient to have a bowel movement to relieve pressure	Answer: B Explain to the patient that bladder spasms are typical after having a TURP. It would be important to administer antispasmodics as ordered to decrease the spasms. The nurse should NEVER deflate the balloon or remove the catheter after a TURP without a physician order. Slowing down the irrigation can predispose the patient to blood clots that may impair the flow of irrigation fluid and urine, creating a significant problem. Blood clot formation can cause the bladder to spasm. Having a bowel movement will not help relieve the spasms, and the patient should avoid straining in the immediate postoperative period.

- Erectile dysfunction (ED):
  - Inability to achieve or maintain an erection
  - *Assessment/Intervention/Education*
    - Detailed medical history:
      - Prostatectomy
      - Chronic diseases (see section on "Risk factors")
      - Blunt pelvic/perineal trauma

- History of smoking
- History of substance abuse
- Medications:
  - Antidepressants
  - Antipsychotics
  - Antiandrogens
  - Antihypertensive
- Risk factors:
  - Depression
  - Parkinson's disease
  - Stroke
  - Cerebral trauma
  - Decrease in androgen levels
  - Hypertension
  - Hyperlipidemia
  - Cigarette smoking
  - Diabetes
  - Pelvic radiation
  - Substance abuse (drugs, alcohol)
  - Vascular disease
- Clinical manifestations:
  - Inability to achieve an erection
  - Inability to maintain an erection
- Diagnosis:
  - Based on medical, sexual, and psychosocial history
  - International Index of Erectile Function (IIEF) screening tool
  - Laboratory tests
- Nursing diagnosis:
  - Sexual dysfunction related to altered body function
  - Situational low self-esteem related to changes in sexual function
- Treatment:
  - Psychosexual counseling
  - Androgen-replacement therapy
  - Medications
  - Vacuum constriction devices
  - Surgery:
    - Insertion of prosthetic device
    - Vascular surgery to restore adequate blood flow
- Patient teaching
  - Do not take the erectogenic drugs if taking vasodilator medication such as nitrates; can precipitate severe hypotension; talk to provider to ensure safety when taking these drugs with any prescribed medications.

▶ Priapism:

- Relatively uncommon disorder that involves persistent penile erection (>4 hours). Typically, only the corpora cavernosa are affected. This condition is considered a medical emergency because of the resulting ischemia of the corpora cavernosa and permanent damage.
- *Assessment/Intervention/Education*
  - Detailed history of onset and contributing factors
  - Clinical manifestations:
    - Prolonged erection (>4 hours)

- Diagnosis:
  - Usually self-diagnosed
  - Determine if ischemic or nonischemic priapism:
    - Provider examination
    - Duplex ultrasound
    - Cavernous blood gases
- Treatment:
  - Achieve detumescence—reversal of erection
  - Preserve erectile function
  - Use of a stepwise approach—least invasive to most invasive
    - Initial step—therapeutic aspiration (with or without irrigation)
    - Followed by intracavernous injection of sympathomimetic drugs:
      - Phenylephrine every 3 to 5 minutes for 1 hour
    - If aspiration and injections are unsuccessful, then cavernoglandular (corporoglandular) shunt may be required.
- Patient teaching:
  - Seek medical attention immediately for sustained erection (>4 hours).
  - Lack of treatment may result in permanent damage.
  - Patients with recurrent priapism may need to learn intracavernosal self-injection of phenylephrine.

▶ Epididymitis:
- Acute painful inflammatory process involving the epididymis
- ***Assessment/Intervention/Education***
  - Detailed medical history/risk factors:
    - Chlamydial or gonorrheal infections
    - BPH
    - Prostatitis
    - Scrotal trauma
    - Urinary reflux in vas deferens
  - Clinical manifestations:
    - Pain in scrotal/testicular region; possible redness and swelling
  - Diagnosis:
    - Urine culture
  - Nursing diagnosis:
    - Acute pain related to inflammatory process in scrotum
  - Treatment:
    - Antibiotics
    - Ice
    - Avoid standing
    - Analgesics
    - Support scrotum
  - Patient teaching:
    - Swelling and minor discomfort may last for several weeks
    - Complete course of antibiotics
    - Avoid sexual activity if due to infection
    - Ambulation increases pain

▶ Orchitis:
- Acute inflammation of the testes

- *Assessment/Intervention/Education*
  - Detailed medical history/risk factors:
    - Bacterial or viral infection
      - Mumps
      - Syphilis
      - Pneumonia
      - Tuberculosis
    - Epididymitis
    - Scrotal trauma
    - Infectious mononucleosis
    - Complicated urinary tract infection
    - Catheterization
  - Clinical manifestations:
    - Pain and tenderness in testes
    - Swollen testes
  - Diagnosis:
    - Urine culture
  - Nursing diagnosis, treatment, and patient teaching:
    - Same as for epididymitis

> **Clinical Consideration**
> Orchitis caused by mumps may result in infertility.

▶ Hypogonadism:
- Occurs because of a deficiency of the androgen hormones. Hypogonadism is classified as primary (gonadal problem), secondary (pituitary problem), or tertiary (hypothalamic problem) on the basis of the contributing cause.
- *Assessment/Intervention/Education*
  - Detailed medical history:
    - Obesity
    - Declining testosterone levels
  - Clinical manifestations:
    - Fatigue
    - Decreased libido
    - ED
    - Loss of secondary sex characteristics
    - Changes in body composition
    - Osteoporosis
    - Infertility
  - Diagnosis:
    - Two measurements of free testosterone
    - Sperm analysis
    - Pituitary hormones
    - Pituitary MRI
  - Treatment:
    - Testosterone-replacement therapy (TRT)
      - Intramuscular (IM):
        - Testosterone cypionate (Depo-Testosterone)
        - Testosterone enanthate (Delatestryl)
      - Transdermal
      - Buccal
      - Intranasally
  - Patient teaching:
    - Keep testosterone products out of reach of children.

- Women of childbearing age should avoid contact with testosterone products.
- Mood swings may be associated with IM injection route.
- Wash hands with soap and water after applying transdermal products.
- Transdermal products may cause skin irritation.
- Acquired problems:
  - Types:
    - Hydrocele
      - Fluid-filled mass (with lymphatic fluid) in the scrotum
      - Diagnosis by transillumination
      - No treatment unless the hydrocele becomes large and painful
      - Surgical repair may be required, but it is not recommended in younger men, as it may result in infertility.
    - Spermatocele:
      - Sperm-containing cyst of the epididymis
      - May be visible with transillumination
      - Cause is unknown
      - No treatment unless the spermatocele becomes large and painful
      - Surgical repair may be required, but it is not recommended in younger men, as it may result in infertility.
    - Varicocele:
      - Dilation of spermatic vein that drain the testes
      - Engorged veins may be palpable
      - Usually located on the left side of the scrotum
      - Treatment may include:
        - Injection of a sclerosing agent into the spermatic vein
        - Surgical ligation of the spermatic vein may be required, but it is not recommended in younger men, as it may result in infertility:
          - Open varicocelectomy
          - Laparoscopic varicocelectomy
          - Robotic surgery
          - Microsurgical varicocelectomy
    - Testicular torsion:
      - Spermatic cord becomes twisted; may occur spontaneously or result from trauma
      - Sudden onset of severe scrotal pain
      - Decreased blood flow shown on nuclear scan or Doppler of testes is diagnostic
      - Considered an emergency, as necrosis may occur if not resolved within 4 to 6 hours
      - May resolve spontaneously, otherwise surgery is indicated
    - Phimosis:
      - Can occur in uncircumcised males; the inability to retract the foreskin and may appear as a tight ring around the penis
      - Treatment may include:
        - Daily manual retraction
        - Circumcision
- Inguinal hernia
  - Intestinal protrusion into the inguinal canal due to a weakness in the abdominal wall

Female Disorders

- Candidiasis:
  - Fungal infection (*Candida albicans*)

- *Assessment/Intervention/Education*
  - Detailed medical history/risk factors:
    - Antibiotic therapy
    - Corticosteroid use
    - Immunosuppression
    - Pregnancy
    - Uncontrolled diabetes
    - Obesity
  - Clinical manifestations:
    - Vulvar and/or vaginal pruritus along with swelling and redness
    - Thick, white, lumpy vaginal discharge
    - Yeast-like or musty odor
  - Diagnosis:
    - Microscopic exam of vaginal discharge
    - Fungal culture of vaginal discharge
  - Nursing diagnosis:
    - Impaired comfort related to vulvar and/or vaginal pruritus
  - Treatment:
    - OTC medications
      - Clotrimazole cream, miconazole cream, or tioconazole ointment intravaginally
    - Prescription intravaginal agents:
      - Butoconazole or terconazole cream intravaginally
      - Fluconazole orally
  - Patient teaching:
    - Complete full course of treatment.
    - If menstruating, continue the medication but avoid tampon use.
    - Avoid sexual intercourse until treatment is completed.
- Mastitis:
  - Bacterial infection of the breast tissue; occurs most often in lactating women
  - Most common organism—*Staphylococcus aureus*
  - *Assessment/Intervention/Education*
    - Detailed medical history/risk factors:
      - Breastfeeding, especially with improper technique
      - Nipple trauma
    - Clinical manifestations:
      - Unilateral:
        - Breast pain
        - Redness
        - Axillary adenopathy
      - Fever
      - Chills
      - Fatigue
      - Malaise
    - Diagnosis:
      - Breast exam
    - Nursing diagnosis:
      - Acute pain related to breast-tissue inflammation
    - Treatment:
      - Antibiotics

- Patient teaching:
  - Despite having this infection, breastfeeding/emptying of the breasts should continue, as milk stasis exacerbates the problem.
  - Refer patient to a lactation consultant for breastfeeding assistance.
  - If not treated quickly, can lead to a breast abscess.

▶ Pelvic inflammatory disease (PID):

- "An infectious condition of the pelvic cavity that may involve the fallopian tubes, ovaries, and pelvic peritoneum" (Lewis et al., 2017, p. 1251)
- Most common organisms—*Chlamydia trachomatis* and *Neisseria gonorrhoeae*
- Not all cases of PID are due to an STI.
- *Assessment/Intervention/Education*
  - Detailed medical history/risk factors:
    - Use of intrauterine device (IUD)
    - Previous PID or other infections
    - Multiple sexual partners or new sexual partner
    - Infertility
    - Abortion or pelvic surgery
  - Clinical manifestations:
    - Lower abdominal/pelvic pain that increases with ambulation and sexual intercourse
    - Vaginal bleeding after sexual intercourse
    - Irregular bleeding
    - Purulent vaginal discharge
    - Fever
    - Chills
    - Painful and frequent urination
  - Complications:
    - Ectopic pregnancy
    - Infertility
    - Septic shock
    - Embolism
    - Peritonitis
    - Tubo-ovarian abscess
    - Perihepatitis (inflammation of the peritoneal coating of the liver)
  - Diagnosis:
    - Pelvic exam (possible transvaginal ultrasound):
      - Cervical motion tenderness
      - Uterine tenderness
      - Adnexal tenderness
    - Microscopic exam:
      - Abundant presence of white cells in vaginal fluid
    - Lab exam:
      - Pregnancy test (to rule out ectopic pregnancy)
      - Elevated erythrocyte sedimentation rate
      - Elevated C-reactive protein
      - Positive culture for *N. gonorrhoeae* or *C. trachomatis*
  - Nursing diagnosis:
    - Acute pain related to pelvic infectious process

- Treatment:
  - Broad-spectrum antibiotics:
    - Antibiotic treatment does not reverse any scarring that has already been caused by the infection.
- Patient teaching:
  - Notify health care provider if no improvement of symptoms within 72 hours after starting treatment
  - If cause of PID was gonorrhea or chlamydia, retest 3 months after treatment
  - Treat/test all sexual partners from 60 days prior to the onset of symptoms
  - Encourage condom/barrier device use

▶ Endometriosis:
- "Growth of endometrial tissue outside of the uterus" (Lowdermilk, Perry, & Cashion, 2014, p. 66)
- The tissue responds to cyclic hormonal stimulation and bleeding causing an inflammatory response, fibrosis, and adhesions to nearby organs.
- **Assessment/Intervention/Education**
  - Detailed medical history/risk factors:
    - Women in their 30s to 40s
    - Infertility
  - Clinical manifestations:
    - Secondary dysmenorrhea (menstrual cramps)
    - Pelvic pain
    - Painful sexual intercourse
    - Heavy menstrual bleeding
    - Bowel changes and/or pain
    - Dysuria
  - Complications:
    - Infertility
    - Chronic pain
  - Diagnosis:
    - Pelvic exam
    - Laparoscopy with biopsy
    - MRI
  - Nursing diagnosis:
    - Acute pain related to menstruation secondary to endometriosis
  - Treatment:
    - Based on severity of symptoms
    - Unless a hysterectomy is performed, 40 to 50% of women have disease recurrence
    - Mild pain, and pregnancy desired
      - NSAIDs
    - Severe pain and postponing pregnancy:
      - Oral contraceptives with a low estrogen-to-progestin ratio
      - GnRH agonist:
        - Leuprolide (Lupron)
        - Nafarelin (Synarel)
    - Surgical:
      - Laser therapy/laparotomy to remove endometrial tissue growths
      - Hysterectomy with bilateral salpingo-oophorectomy (BSO)

Clinical Consideration

Side effects from these drugs are the same as menopause (amenorrhea, hot flashes, vaginal dryness, bone loss).

- Patient teaching:
  - Discussion regarding treatment options, as well as disease recurrence
  - Counseling to address sexual difficulties and/or infertility
- Abnormal uterine bleeding (AUB):
  - "Any change in a woman's menstrual flow, including volume, duration, or cycle pattern" (Lewis et al., 2017, p. 1246)
  - Includes heavy menstrual bleeding (HMB) and intermenstrual bleeding (IMB)
  - May be chronic or acute
  - Potential causes in reproductive age women:
    - Leiomyomas (fibroids)
    - Polyps
    - Ovulatory dysfunction
    - Thyroid dysfunction
    - Endometrial problems
    - Cancer
    - Bleeding disorders
    - Medications
    - Eating disorders
    - Liver failure
    - Diabetes
  - Potential causes in postmenopausal women:
    - Endometrial cancer
  - *Assessment/Intervention/Education*
    - Detailed medical history:
      - Age at menarche
      - Pregnancy history
      - Birth control methods used
      - Current medications
      - Bleeding patterns (clots, perceived amount, duration)
      - History of STIs, sexually active
    - Clinical manifestations:
      - HMB:
        - More than 7 days in duration
        - Soaks through one or more tampons or pads every hour for several hours
        - Needing to wear more than one pad at a time to control menstrual flow
        - Needing to change pads or tampons during the night
        - Passing blood clots that are as quarter-sized or larger
      - IMB:
        - Bleeding in between menstrual cycles
    - Diagnosis:
      - Pelvic exam
      - Lab exam
        - Pregnancy test
        - Complete blood count (CBC)
        - Thyroid-stimulating hormone (TSH)
        - STI screening
        - Screening for bleeding disorders

- Imaging exam:
  - Transvaginal/pelvic ultrasound
  - MRI
  - Hysteroscopy
  - Endometrial biopsy
  - Saline infusion sonohysterography
- Nursing diagnosis:
  - Risk for disturbed body image related to menstrual disorder
  - Risk for infection related to prolonged use of superabsorbent tampons
- Treatment:
  - Depends on the causation of the AUB, whether children are desired in the future, patient's quality of life, and level of threat the AUB poses to the patient's health
  - Medications:
    - Oral contraceptives:
      - Estradiol valerate/dienogest (Natazia) is the only oral contraceptive approved for treatment of heavy menstrual bleeding.
    - Hormone therapy
    - GnRH agonists:
      - Used for only short periods (<6 months)
    - Tranexamic acid (Lysteda):
      - Cannot be taken with oral contraceptives
    - Levonorgestrel (Mirena) IUD
    - NSAIDs for pain
  - Surgical:
    - Endometrial ablation
    - Uterine artery embolization (UAE)
    - Myomectomy
    - Hysteroscopy
    - Hysterectomy
- Patient teaching:
  - If undergoing endometrial ablation, pregnancy can still occur but is very high risk. Must use some form of contraception until menopause occurs.
  - Teach signs and symptoms of toxic shock syndrome:
    - Fever
    - Diarrhea
    - Vomiting
    - Weakness
    - Myalgia
    - Sunburn-like rash

▶ Ectopic pregnancy:
- Implantation of the fertilized egg outside of the uterus, most commonly in the fallopian tube
- A life-threatening condition
- *Assessment/Intervention/Education*
  - Detailed medical history/risk factors:
    - Prior ectopic pregnancy
    - STIs

- IUD
- Prior pelvic or tubal surgery
- PID
- Infertility treatments
- Long-term complications:
  - Infertility
  - Recurrent ectopic pregnancy
- Clinical manifestations:
  - Before rupture:
    - Delayed menses
    - Abdominal pain
    - Abnormal vaginal bleeding (spotting)
  - After rupture:
    - Referred shoulder pain
    - Shock
    - Cullen's sign (ecchymotic blueness around the umbilicus)
- Diagnosis:
  - Pregnancy test
  - Transvaginal ultrasound
- Nursing diagnosis:
  - Acute pain related to ectopic pregnancy
- Treatment:
  - Medical:
    - Methotrexate (Rheumatrex, Trexall, Xatmep)
  - Surgical:
    - Salpingectomy
    - Salpingostomy
- Patient teaching:
  - Contraception method should be used for a minimum of three menstrual cycles
  - Contact Ob/Gyn as soon as patients suspects she might be pregnant; risk of recurrence
  - Provide support related to the pregnancy loss

▶ Uterine prolapse:
  - The displacement of the uterus into the vagina
  - *Assessment/Intervention/Education*
    - Detailed medical history/risk factors:
      - Vaginal birth
      - Pelvic trauma
      - Obesity
      - Straining for bowel movements
      - Chronic cough
      - Perimenopause
    - Clinical manifestations:
      - Pelvic pressure/fullness
      - Low backache
      - Vaginal protrusion
      - Fatigue
      - Urinary incontinence
      - Worsening symptoms after long periods of standing or after intercourse

- Diagnosis:
  - Physical/pelvic exam
- Nursing diagnosis:
  - Impaired comfort related to pelvic pressure secondary to uterine prolapse
  - Risk for stress urinary incontinence related to uterine prolapse
  - Risk for sexual dysfunction related to uterine prolapse
- Treatment:
  - Dependent on severity of prolapse and impact on patient's life
  - Kegel exercises
  - Medical:
    - Pessary (apparatus placed in the vagina by provider to provide uterine support)
  - Surgical:
    - Vaginal hysterectomy
- Patient teaching:
  - Improper use of pessary can lead to fistulas, erosion, and vaginal cancer.
- Cystocele and rectocele:
  - Weakening of the support between the vagina and nearby organ:
    - Cystocele—vagina and bladder
    - Rectocele—vagina and rectum
  - *Assessment/Intervention/Education*
    - Detailed medical history/risk factors:
      - Uterine prolapse
      - Vaginal birth
      - Obesity
      - Advanced age
    - Clinical manifestations:
      - Often asymptomatic
      - Cystocele:
        - Feeling of an object in the vagina
        - Urinary frequency
        - Urinary retention
        - Incontinence
        - Recurrent cystitis
      - Rectocele:
        - Feeling that pelvic organs are falling out, but sensation is gone when lying down
        - Difficulty having a bowel movement
    - Diagnosis:
      - Physical/pelvic exam
    - Nursing diagnosis:
      - Impaired comfort related to pelvic pressure secondary to cystocele/rectocele
      - Risk for stress urinary incontinence related to cystocele
      - Risk for constipation related to rectocele
      - Risk for sexual dysfunction related to cystocele/rectocele
    - Treatment
      - Depends on severity of prolapse and impact on patient's life
      - Kegel exercises
      - Medical:
        - Pessary (useful for cystocele)

- Surgical:
  - Colporrhaphy (tightening of the vaginal wall)
- Preoperative care:
  - Douche the morning of the surgery
  - Perineal shave
  - Enema (if for rectocele repair)
- Postoperative care:
  - Goal—to prevent infection and decrease pressure on the vaginal sutures
  - Perineal care twice daily minimum, as well as after each void/stool
  - Ice pack to perineum for comfort
  - Urinary catheter care (if for cystocele repair)
- Patient teaching:
  - Improper use of pessary can lead to fistulas, erosion, and vaginal cancer.
  - High-fiber diet and stool softeners/mild laxative (as needed)
  - Postoperative lifting and/or standing and intercourse restrictions
  - Postoperation—a temporary decrease in vaginal sensation sometimes occurs and can last for several months.
- Hysterectomy: (Table 13.1)
  - Nursing diagnosis:
    - Disturbed body image related to removal of reproductive organs
    - Acute pain related to surgical procedure
    - Grieving related to inability to bear children after removal of reproductive organs
  - Preoperative care:
    - Indwelling urinary catheter
    - Perineal or abdominal preparation
    - Possible vaginal douche and/or enema
  - Postoperative care:
    - Encourage ambulation to relieve abdominal distension

TABLE 13.1	COMMON TYPES OF HYSTERECTOMIES
Types of Hysterectomies	What It Entails
Total abdominal hysterectomy (TAH)	Low, transverse abdominal incision; uterus and cervix removed
Total Abdominal hysterectomy and bilateral salpingo-oophorectomy (TAH-BSO)	Same as above, except both ovaries and fallopian tubes are also removed
Radical hysterectomy	Removal of the uterus, ovaries, fallopian tubes, upper portion of the vagina, and cervix; partial removal of the pelvic lymph nodes; most invasive of all hysterectomies
Vaginal hysterectomy	Incision is made at the top of the vagina; uterus and cervix are removed
Laparoscopic-assisted vaginal hysterectomy (LAVH)	Same as above, except laparoscope is inserted through the abdomen to assist with surgery
Laparoscopic supracervical hysterectomy	Same as above, except the cervix remains

- Patient teaching:
    - Inform patient she will no longer menstruate and if the ovaries were removed, she will begin to experience menopause (if not already menopausal).
    - Abstain from sexual intercourse until healed (4 to 6 weeks).
    - Temporary loss of vaginal sensation is sometimes experienced with a vaginal hysterectomy but should return in a few months.
    - No heavy lifting for 2 months

Question	Rationale
A 35 year-old patient is being discharged after undergoing a total abdominal hysterectomy (TAH). Which of the following statements indicate that further teaching is necessary? A. "I will not have sex with my husband for at least 4 to 6 weeks." B. "I am ready for the symptoms of menopause to begin soon." C. "I am so glad I won't have my period anymore." D. "I am so glad my mom is visiting so she can lift my toddler out of the crib."	Answer: B The TAH procedure leaves the ovaries and fallopian tubes *intact*, so symptoms of menopause will not occur after the procedure. Her uterus and cervix were removed, so menstruation will cease. Heavy lifting is prohibited for 2 months and vaginal intercourse should not occur until fully healed (approximately 4 to 6 weeks after surgery).

▶ Polycystic Ovary Syndrome (PCOS):
- Ovarian disorder that causes a hormone imbalance and multiple, fluid-filled cysts in the ovaries
- Cause unknown
- ***Assessment/Intervention/Education***
    - Detailed medical history/risk factors:
        - Family history of PCOS
    - Long-term complications:
        - Type 2 diabetes
        - Cardiovascular disease
        - Infertility
    - Clinical manifestations:
        - Obesity
        - Irregular menstrual cycles or amenorrhea
        - Hirsutism
        - Hyperandrogenism
        - Acne
        - Male pattern baldness
    - Diagnosis:
        - Pelvic ultrasound
        - Labs to assess hormone levels
    - Nursing diagnosis:
        - Risk for disturbed body image related to hirsutism and obesity secondary to PCOS
        - Risk for disturbed personal identity related to infertility secondary to PCOS

- Treatment:
  - Oral contraceptives to regulate menstrual cycle
  - Spironolactone (Aldactone) to treat hirsutism
  - Flutamide (Eulexin) and leuprolide (Lupron) to treat hyperandrogenism
  - If seeking pregnancy, fertility drugs may also be used
- Patient teaching:
  - Weight management to reduce likelihood of developing diabetes and/or cardiovascular disease (insulin resistance is a potential complication)
  - Follow-up care importance to assess therapy effectiveness and monitor for complications

▶ Leiomyomas (uterine fibroids)
- Benign uterine tumors
- Most common in women 30 to 40 years old
- *Assessment/Intervention/Education*
  - Detailed medical history/risk factors:
    - Mother, sister, or identical twin with leiomyomas
    - Early menarche
    - African American race
    - Alcohol use
    - Diet high in red meat
    - Diet low in green vegetables
  - Clinical manifestations:
    - Most are asymptomatic
    - Abnormal uterine bleeding
    - Painful sexual intercourse/vaginal dryness
    - Frequent/painful urination
    - Constipation
    - Pelvic pain
  - Diagnosis:
    - Pelvic exam
    - Pelvic ultrasound
  - Nursing diagnosis:
    - Risk for altered tissue perfusion related to insufficient hemoglobin and hematocrit
    - Acute pain related to sexual intercourse secondary to fibroids
  - Treatment:
    - Depends on severity of symptoms
    - Medical:
      - Oral contraceptives
    - Surgical:
      - Myomectomy (surgical removal of fibroid)
      - Hysterectomy
      - Uterine artery embolization
  - Patient teaching:
    - The presence of fibroids does not increase the patient's risk of endometrial cancer.

▶ Menopause:
- Cessation of the menstrual cycle and ovulation due to a reduction in ovarian function:
  - Natural menopause is diagnosed after 12 months of no menses

- Average age: 52 years old
- Can be induced because of surgical removal of ovaries or use of certain drugs/therapies
- Perimenopause:
  - From the development of the first symptoms of menopause until menstruation ceases
- *Assessment/Intervention/Education*
  - Long-term health risks:
    - Osteoporosis
    - Stroke
    - Heart attack
  - Clinical manifestations:
    - Menstrual cycle changes/cessation
    - Hot flashes
    - Sleep issues
    - Night sweats
    - Vaginal dryness
    - Frequent vaginal infections
    - Frequent urinary tract infections
    - Change in mood
  - Diagnosis:
    - Consider other causes of symptoms first
    - FSH level:
      - Will be elevated in menopause
  - Nursing diagnosis:
    - Disturbed sleep pattern related to menopause symptoms
    - Sexual dysfunction related to painful sexual intercourse/vaginal dryness
    - Situational low self-esteem related to hormonal changes
  - Treatment:
    - Hormone therapy:
      - Estrogen:
        - Small increased risk of stroke, deep-vein thrombosis, and gallbladder disease
      - If uterus still present, estrogen and progestin reduce uterine and colon cancer risk
        - Small increased risk of heart attack, breast cancer, stroke, deep-vein thrombosis, and gallbladder disease
    - Bioidentical hormones:
      - Come from plant sources and made by a compounding pharmacist
      - "There is no scientific evidence that compounded hormones are safer or more effective than standard hormone therapy" (ACOG, 2015, p. 3)
    - Drug therapy:
      - Paroxetine (Paxil, Brisdelle), fluoxetine (Prozac, Sarafem), and venlafaxine (Effxor XR) to treat hot flashes
      - Clonidine (Catapres) and gabapentin (Neurontin) to treat hot flashes and/or sleep issues
      - Raloxifene (Evista) to treat hot flashes and vaginal dryness:
        - Also assists with preventing bone loss while reducing risk of uterine cancer
    - Herbal supplements:
      - Limited evidence on safety and efficacy

- Black cohosh:
  - Not recommended for use with liver disorders
- Soy:
  - May interact with warfarin (Coumadin)
  - Not recommended for use with history of breast, ovarian, or uterine cancer or endometriosis
- Patient teaching:
  - Include foods high in calcium and vitamin D to maintain bones.
  - Regular exercise, including weight-bearing, balance training, and strength training; also assists with bone maintenance, weight management, and overall health
  - Provide emotional support for this transitional moment in the patient's life.

▶ Hormonal contraceptives:
- Combined estrogen–progestin contraceptives
- Oral:
  - Monophasic:
    - Provide fixed doses of estrogen and progestin
  - Multiphasic:
    - Alter the doses of progestin, and sometimes estrogen
  - Side effects:
    - Common:
      - Nausea
      - Breast tenderness
      - Fluid retention
      - Chloasma (darkening of the skin around the eyes and bridge of the nose)
      - Increased appetite
      - Fatigue
      - Hirsutism
      - Nervousness
      - Oily skin/scalp
      - Bleeding irregularities
    - Serious:
      - Stroke
      - Myocardial infarction
      - Hypertension
      - Thromboembolism
      - Gallbladder disease
      - Liver tumors
  - Contraindications:
    - History or presence of:
      - Thromboembolic disorders
      - Cerebrovascular, coronary, or valvular heart disease
      - Breast cancer
      - Impaired liver function or tumor
      - Hypertension
      - Headaches with foci
      - Diabetes for past 20 years or longer with vascular disease

- Smoking
- Medications:
  - Anticonvulsants
  - Systemic antifungals
  - Antituberculosis drugs
  - Anti-HIV protease inhibitors
- Patient education:
  - Take the pill at the same time each day to enhance efficacy
  - Complications to report to provider:
    - Abdominal pain
    - Chest pain/shortness of breath
    - Headaches
    - Eye issues
    - Leg pain
- Transdermal:
  - Side effects
    - Same as oral
  - Contraindications:
    - Same as oral
  - Patient education:
    - Apply the patch on the same day of week for 3 weeks, then 1 week without the patch
    - Rotate sites
      - Upper, outer arm
      - Upper torso (excluding breasts)
      - Lower abdomen
      - Buttocks
    - May wear the patch for bathing, swimming, and exercise
    - Complications to report to provider:
      - Same as oral
- Progestin-only contraceptives:
  - Oral (minipill)
  - Injectable
    - Depot medroxyprogesterone acetate (DMPA, Depo-Provera)
      - Intramuscularly
      - Given during the first 5 days of the menstrual cycle
      - Repeat dose every 12 weeks
      - Side effects:
        - Decreased bone density:
          - Recommend use for maximum of 2 years because of this
        - Weight gain
        - Decreased libido
        - Lipid changes
        - Increased risk of thromboembolism
  - Implantable:
    - Effective for up to 3 years
    - Placed surgically with local anesthetic subdermally on the inner/upper part of nondominant arm

> **Clinical Consideration**
> Do not massage the site after injection, as this will affect absorption and shorten the period of effectiveness.

CASE STUDY

A 23-year-old male is seen in the clinic for an annual exam. Before the female health care provider comes in, he states to the nurse, "I have been having some weird stuff come out of my penis lately and it burns when I pee. I'm really embarrassed to ask the doctor about it, so I thought I'd mention it to you since you're a man. What do you think is wrong?"

1. **What questions should the nurse ask?**
    - *Onset of symptoms:*
      - *Color and/or odor of the discharge*
    - *Is he also experiencing:*
      - *Fever*
      - *Chills*
      - *Lesions and/or warts on his genitals and/or rash anywhere on his body*
      - *Genital itching*
      - *Urinary frequency/pain*
    - *Sexual history:*
      - *Number of partners/types of partners*
      - *New partner recently*
      - *His partner's sexual history*
      - *Use of condoms or barrier devices*
      - *Past diagnosis of STI, HIV*
    - *Other:*
      - *Alcohol, illicit drug, or polysubstance use*

He states, "I noticed it starting about 4 weeks ago or so. The stuff that comes out doesn't smell, but it is yellowish in color and looks pretty gross. Other than the burning when I pee, I'm not having any of those other problems. I only have sex with women. I would say about 6 of them in my lifetime. I'm not dating anyone right now, but did have a one-night stand a little over a month ago. I usually use condoms when I am with someone, but didn't have one with me this last time. This has never happened to me before and I'm kind of freaking out about it."

2. **What information that he shared puts him at risk for an STI?**
    - *Multiple sex partners*
    - *New sex partner*
    - *Unprotected sex*

The nurse shares that based on his symptoms and history, he may have contracted an STI such as chlamydia or gonorrhea. The nurse also explains that testing and treatment should begin promptly. The patient states, "Oh man, I am so embarrassed. What can I do to get rid of this and never have this happen again?"

3. **Once the diagnosis of an STI is made, what teaching should the nurse provide?**
    - *Take all of the medication as prescribed*
    - *Compete any recommended follow-up testing*
    - *Abstain from sexual contact for 7 days after drug therapy is completed and asymptomatic*
    - *Abstain from sexual contact until all of their sex partners from the past 60 days are tested/treated*
    - *Consider being tested for HIV and other STIs*
    - *Use a condom at each sexual encounter in the future*
    - *Ensure he knows the proper method of using a condom*

Bibliography

Ackley, B.J., Ladwig, G.B., and Makic, M.B. (2017). *Nursing Diagnosis Handbook: An Evidence-Based Guide to Planning Care*, 11th ed. (St. Louis: Elsevier).

Agency for Healthcare Research and Quality. (2014 June). *Guide to Clinical Preventive Services 2014*. Accessed June 15, 2018, from https://www.ahrq.gov/sites/default/files/publications/files/cpsguide.pdf

American College of Obstetricians and Gynecologists. (August 2012). Committee opinion no. 534: Well-woman visit. Accessed June 15, 2018, from https://www.acog.org/-/media/Committee-Opinions/Committee-on-Gynecologic-Practice/co534.pdf?dmc=1&ts=20180218T2230532384

American College of Obstetricians and Gynecologists. (2015 May). ACOG FAQ047: The menopause years. Accessed June 15, 2018, from https://www.acog.org/-/media/For-Patients/faq047.pdf?dmc=1&ts=20180309T0021000603

American College of Obstetricians and Gynecologists. (2016 June). ACOG FAQ193: *Heavy menstrual bleeding*. Accessed June 15, 2018, from https://www.acog.org/-/media/For-Patients/faq193.pdf?dmc=1&ts=20180225T2019060416

American College of Obstetricians and Gynecologists. (2017a July). *ACOG practice bulletin: Breast cancer risk assessment and screening in average-risk women*. Accessed June 15, 2018, from https://www.acog.org/-/media/Practice-Bulletins/Committee-on-Practice-Bulletins—Gynecology/Public/pb179.pdf?dmc=1&ts=20180218T2153314300

American College of Obstetricians and Gynecologists. (2017b September). *ACOG FAQ085: Cervical cancer screening*. Accessed June 15, 2018, from https://www.acog.org/-/media/For-Patients/faq085.pdf?dmc=1&ts=20180218T2253239218

American Urological Association. (2011). ED Clinical Practice Guidelines. Accessed January 29, 2018, from http://www.auanet.org/guidelines/erectile-dysfunction

American Urological Association. (2010). Management of priapism. Accessed March 11, 2018, from http://www.auanet.org/guidelines/priapism

Centers for Disease Control and Prevention. (2015). 2015 Sexually transmitted diseases treatment guidelines. Accessed February 13, 2018, from https://www.cdc.gov/std/tg2015/default.htm

Centers for Disease Control and Prevention. (2017). *Sexually transmitted disease surveillance 2016*. Accessed June 15, 2018, from https://www.cdc.gov/std/stats16/CDC_2016_STDS_Report-for508WebSep21_2017_1644.pdf

Grossman, S., and Porth, C.M. (2013). *Pathophysiology: Concepts of Altered Health States*, 9th ed. (Philadelphia: Lippincott Williams & Wilkins).

Lewis, S.L., Bucher, L., Heitkemper, M., and Harding, M.M. (2017). *Medical-Surgical Nursing: Assessment and Management of Clinical Problems*, 10th ed. (St. Louis: Elsevier).

Lowdermilk, D.L., Perry, S.E., and Cashion, K. (2014). *Maternity Nursing*, 8th ed. (Revised). Canada: Elsevier Mosby.

U.S. Preventive Services. (2017). Prostate cancer screening. Accessed June 15, 2018, from https://www.uspreventiveservicestaskforce.org/Page/Document/draft-recommendation-statement/prostate-cancer-screening1

14

Neurologic System

Elizabeth Pepe Greenlee, DHA, MSN, BSN, RN

OVERVIEW

▌ The primary function of the neurologic system or nervous system is to control activities of the essential physiologic functions of the body, such as breathing and digestion. It also controls the processes of the body that are based on the sensory information it gathers from internal and external sources.

ANATOMY

▌ The nervous system is composed of the:

- Central nervous system (CNS)—which is made of the following:
  - Brain:
    - Processes information from all stimuli and is responsible for voluntary and involuntary motor activity
    - The brain is made up of three parts:
      - Cerebrum:
        - Regulates language, problem solving, visual image interpretation, temperature, touch
          - Has a right and left hemisphere, each with four lobes: frontal, temporal, occipital, and parietal (Figure 14.1)

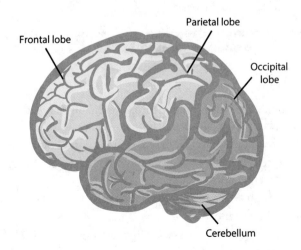

Figure 14.1 Brain lobes

- Brain stem:
  - Regulates bodily functions of the respiratory, auditory, and visual systems
- Cerebellum:
  - Regulates sensory and motor nerve pathways, maintains equilibrium, and coordinates muscle movement
- Spinal cord:
  - Connects the brain to the peripheral nervous system by way of nerve fibers that communicate through electrical impulses
  - Is approximately 18 inches long and is protected by the vertebrae in the spinal column
- Peripheral nervous system (PNS):
  - Is outside the brain and spinal cord and is comprised of the cranial nerves, peripheral nerves, and spinal nerves
  - Cranial nerves:
    - Olfactory nerve (I)—responsible for smell
    - Optic nerve (II)—responsible for sight
    - Oculomotor nerve (III)—responsible for movement of the eyeball, lens, and pupils
    - Trochlear nerve (IV)—responsible for movement of the superior oblique muscle of the eye
    - Trigeminal nerve (V)—controls the muscles used in chewing
    - Abducens nerve (VI)—controls the movement of the eye outward
    - Facial nerve (VII)—Controls muscles of the face used for smiling or frowning; accepts taste sensations from the anterior two-thirds of the tongue
    - Acoustic nerve (VIII)—also called the "vestibulocochlear nerve"; responsible for hearing and equilibrium
    - Glossopharyngeal nerve (VIX)—accepts taste sensation from the back of the tongue
    - Vagus nerve (X)—important nerve that controls the heart's sensory and motor functions, assists with digestion
    - Spinal accessory nerve (XI)—controls head and shoulder movement
    - Hypoglossal nerve (XII)—responsible for controlling the muscles of the tongue
- Autonomic nervous system (ANS):
  - Disseminated through the central and peripheral nervous systems
  - Made up of nerves that serve the involuntary structures of the body, including smooth muscles and the heart

PHYSIOLOGY OF THE NERVOUS SYSTEM

▶ Nervous system functions:
- Sensory input:
  - Information gathered through neurons (excitable nerve cells), neuroglia, and synapses (connectors between neurons).
  - Neurons conduct impulses from sensory receptors to the brain and spinal cord.
  - Neuroglia cells are not excitable and are found within tissues and help with myelination and ionic regulation.
  - Synapses are polarized to allow nerve impulses to travel between neurons.
- Integration of information:
  - Occurs when the brain processes all inputs from the CNS

Clinical Consideration
The ability of a synapse to function is decreased by a lack of oxygen, increased blood sugar levels, and anesthetics.

- Motor output:
  - After the integration of information in the brain, impulses are sent back out through the spinal cord to glands and muscles to tell them how to react.

Diagnostic Tests

▶ Imaging exams:
- Computed tomographic (CT) scanning:
  - Used to diagnose stroke and brain tumors and to identify degree of brain damage
- Computed tomographic angiography (CTA):
  - Used to provide images of cerebral blood vessels; identifies stenosis or occlusions with the assistance of IV contrast
- Computed tomographic perfusion:
  - Used to evaluate perfusion to the brain in the area of a stroke, and can help identify potential areas of the brain that can be salvaged
- Echocardiography:
  - Used to determine whether there are cardiac abnormalities
  - Two ways to perform this ultrasound test:
    - Transthoracic echocardiogram (TTE)—most common approach
    - Transesophageal echocardiogram (TEE)
    - Used to detect presence of clots
- Electroencephalography (EEG):
  - Monitors brain activity
  - Used to diagnose seizures and traumatic brain injury (TBI); confirm brain death
- Electromyography (EMG):
  - Used to diagnose spinal cord disease, nerve, and muscle dysfunction
  - Records electrical activity from the brain and/or spinal cord to peripheral nerve roots
- Magnetic resonance imaging (MRI)
  - Magnet and radio waves used to provide better images of soft tissue
  - Used to diagnose stroke, brain and spinal cord tumors, multiple sclerosis and to document brain injury from trauma.
  - Use a checklist to assess whether a patient may have any contraindications for the test.
- Magnetic resonance angiography (MRA)
  - Conducted using MRI scanner and MR contrast
  - Used to provide images of head and neck atherosclerotic lesions and carotid artery dissection
- Transcranial Doppler ultrasound:
  - Determines blood flow in the carotid arteries
  - Used to assess increased risk of stroke

▶ Laboratory:
- Blood glucose
- Blood lipid tests:
  - Cholesterol
  - Triglycerides
  - High-density lipoproteins (HDL)
  - Low-density lipoproteins (LDL)
- Cerebral spinal fluid (CSF)

> **Clinical Consideration**
> *Penumbra* is a term used to describe the tissue surrounding the area of ischemia in a stroke.

> **Clinical Consideration**
> Metal implants, pacemakers, and tattoos are contraindications for undergoing MRI.

> **Clinical Consideration**
> Check blood glucose level on all patients you suspect may have had a stroke, as hypo/hyperglycemia can mimic stroke symptoms.

- Complete blood count (CBC)
- Coagulation tests:
  - PT (prothrombin time)
  - PTT (partial thromboplastin time)
  - INR (international normalized ratio)
▶ Procedures:
- Lumbar puncture:
  - Also called a "spinal tap"; used to measure pressure in the brain and spinal canal and to collect CSF
  - The patient will be placed in a fetal position and may require assistance in maintaining this position. After a lumber puncture, patients may report a dull or pounding headache.
▶ Physical assessment:
- Glasgow Coma Score—an objective assessment of the conscious state of a patient
  - A lower score (3 to 8) indicates that the patient is unconscious and has no meaningful responses (Table 14.1).
- National Institutes of Health Stroke Scale (NIHSS)—an assessment tool used to determine neurologic deficits from stroke
  - A score of 0 indicates no stroke symptoms, while (Table 14.2) a score of 21 to 42 indicates a severe stroke
  - Specific training is required to complete this assessment

> **Clinical Consideration**
>
> To lessen the risk of developing a headache, have the patient lay quietly and keep the head of the bed flat for 2 hours after a lumbar puncture.

TABLE 14.1	GLASGOW COMA SCALE	
		Score
Eye-opening response	Spontaneous—open with blinking at baseline	4
	Opens to verbal stimuli, command, speech	3
	Opens to pain only (not applied to face)	2
	No response	1
Verbal response	Oriented	5
	Confused conversation, but able to answer questions	4
	Inappropriate words	3
	Incomprehensible speech	2
	No response	1
Motor response	Obeys commands for movement	6
	Purposeful movement to painful stimulus	5
	Withdraws in response to pain	4
	Flexion in response to pain (decorticate posturing)	3
	Extension response in response to pain (decerebrate posturing)	2
	No response	1
		http://www.glasgowcomascale.org/

TABLE 14.2 NIH STROKE SCALE

		Score
1a. **Level of Consciousness (LOC):** Arousal status	Alert (or awakens easily and stays awake)	0
	Drowsy (responds to minor stimulation but falls back asleep)	1
	Obtunded (responds only to deep pain or vigorous stimulation)	2
	Comatose (no response)	3
1b. LOC Questions: Month? Age?	Both questions answered correctly	0
	One question answered correctly	1
	Neither question answered correctly	2
1c. LOC Commands: Opens/closes eyes Opens/closes hands	Both commands performed correctly	0
	One command performed correctly	1
	Neither command performed correctly	2
2. **Eye Movements;** Horizontal eye movements	Normal	0
	Mild gaze paralysis (can bring eyes only over to midline)	1
	Complete gaze paralysis (deviated and unable to bring eyes over to midline)	2
3. **Visual fields:** Sees objects in four quadrants	Normal	0
	Partial hemianopia (upper OR lower quadrant)	1
	Complete hemianopia (upper AND lower quadrants)	2
	Bilateral hemianopia (total blindness)	3
4. **Facial:** Facial movements	Normal	0
	Minor paralysis (flattening of nasolabial folds)	1
	Partial paralysis (near or total paralysis of lower face)	2
	Complete paralysis (of upper and lower face)	3
5a. **Motor—Left Arm:** Hold arm straight out from chest	Normal (no drift at all)	0
	Drift (drifts downward but NOT to bed before 10 seconds)	1
	Drifts to bed within 10 seconds	2
	Movement, but not against gravity	3
	Complete paralysis (no movement at all)	4
	Amputation or joint fusion	NA
5b. **Motor—Right Arm:** Hold arm straight out from chest	Normal (no drift at all)	0
	Drift (drifts downward but NOT to bed before 10 seconds)	1
	Drifts to bed within 10 seconds	2
	Movement, but not against gravity	3
	Complete paralysis (no movement at all)	4
	Amputation or joint fusion	NA
6a. **Motor—Left Leg:** Keep leg off bed	Normal (no drift at all)	0
	Drift (drifts downward but NOT to bed before 5 seconds)	1
	Drifts to bed within 5 seconds	2
	Movement, but not against gravity	3
	Complete paralysis (no movement at all)	NA
	Amputation or joint fusion	
6b. **Motor—Right Leg:** Keep leg off bed	Normal (no drift at all)	0
	Drift (drifts downward but NOT to bed before 5 seconds)	1
	Drifts to bed within 5 seconds	2
	Movement, but not against gravity	3
	Complete paralysis (no movement at all)	NA
	Amputation or joint fusion	
7. **Limb Ataxia:** Finger–nose Heel–knee–shin	Absent (no ataxia, OR patient cannot move arm or leg)	0
	Present in one limb	1
	Present in two or more limbs (considered absent if patient cannot understand or is too weak to do)	2

(continued)

TABLE 14.2 *(Continued)*

		Score
8. **Sensory Hemisensory Loss:** Test on face, arm, and thigh	Normal, no sensory loss Mild to moderate loss Severe to total sensory loss (unaware of being touched)	0 1 2
9. **Language/Aphasia, Repetition, and Comprehension:** "Today is a bright sunny day."	Normal ability to use words and follow commands Mild to moderate (repeats/names with some difficulty) Severe aphasia (very few words correct or understood) Mute (no ability to speak or understand at all)	0 1 2 3
10. **Dysarthria:** Speech clarity (slurring)	Normal Mild to moderate slurred speech (some or most) Severe (unintelligible; not understandable) Intubated or other physical barrier	0 1 2 NA
11. **Neglect:** Ignores touch or vision to one side	No abnormality Mild (either visual or tactile; partial neglect) Profound (visual and tactile—complete neglect)	0 1 2
Total Score	0 = best, 42 = worst	

http://www.nihstrokescale.org/

Neurologic Disorders

▶ *Stroke*

- Ischemic:
  - Result of an occluded blood vessel in the brain or vessels leading to the brain
- Hemorrhagic:
  - Result of a ruptured blood vessel in the brain
- *Assessment/Intervention/Education*
  - Detailed medical history:
    - Identify the time the patient was last known to be well (without stroke-like symptoms)
    - Know the signs and symptoms. This acronym will help—BE FAST:
      - **B**alance—a sudden loss of coordination
      - **E**yes—double vision or loss of vision in one or both eyes
      - **F**ace—drooping of one side of the face
      - **A**rms—drift of one arm downward when held up
      - **S**peech—sudden difficulty speaking or slurred speech
      - **T**ime—it is an emergency—activate 911 in the community or call emergency response teams in the organization
  - Clinical manifestations:
    - Depends on the area of the brain where the stroke occurs and the presence of collateral circulation (Figure 14.2)
    - Ischemic stroke—may display some or all of the following: acute change in the level of consciousness; acute-onset weakness or paralysis on one side of the body; sensory changes on one side of the body; partial vision loss; difficulty with speech
    - Hemorrhagic stroke—same manifestations as ischemic strokes but could also see an acute onset of a headache and vomiting

Right-Sided Stroke (right brain injury)	Left-Sided Stroke (left brain injury)
• Left-sided hemiplegia (paralysis) • Left-sided neglect • Spatial–perceptual deficits • Denies/minimizes problems • Short attention span • Completes tasks rapidly • Impulsive • Impaired judgement • Impaired concept of time	• Right-sided hemiplegia (paralysis) • Impaired speech • Aphasia (receptive, expressive, or global) • Unable to discriminate between right and left • Overly cautious • Completes tasks slowly • May be depressed or anxious • Aware of deficits • Impaired language and math skills

Figure 14.2 Clinical Manifestations of Stroke

- Diagnosis:
  - Rapid assessment—time is critical, as is the need to identify the time last known to be well.
  - NIHSS provides a quantifiable metric of stroke-induced impairments.
  - CT scan to determine whether stroke is ischemic or hemorrhagic
  - Blood glucose to confirm this is not related to hypoglycemic event
  - Baseline electrocardiographic (ECG) assessment and troponins in patient with acute ischemic stroke
- Nursing diagnosis:
  - Impaired physical mobility related to loss of balance and coordination
  - Self-care deficits related loss of function, decreased strength and endurance
  - Impaired swallowing related to weakness or paralysis of affected muscles
  - Impaired verbal communication related to aphasia
  - Deficient knowledge related to prognosis, care and treatment plans, signs and symptoms of stroke, and prevention of future events
- Treatment:
  - Varies depending on the type and severity of stroke
    - Ischemic stroke:
      - May be candidate for fibrinolytic therapy with alteplase if diagnosis can be made within 3 hours (4.5 hours at some centers) of the last time they were last known to be well and after obtaining a thorough history and neurologic examination
        - Many contraindications for alteplase therapy
        - If receiving alteplase, observe for side effects of bleeding and angioedema
      - Patient may be candidate for mechanical retrieval of clot
      - The primary cause for the ischemic stroke will need to be determined and treated. For example, the patient may have atrial fibrillation that requires management.
      - Cardiac monitor for at least 24 hours in acute stroke
      - Additional treatment will be required based on the symptoms and deficits:
        - Airway support and ventilator assistance may be needed if decreased level of consciousness or compromised airway
        - Supplemental oxygen therapy to keep oxygen saturation (SaO_2) above 94%

> **Clinical Consideration**
> The NIHSS is completed by a nurse or physician who has completed a certified training program.

> **Clinical Consideration**
> Verify the organization's policy on consent for and administration of thrombolytic therapy.

- Correct hypovolemia and hypotension to maintain perfusion of vital organs
- If blood pressure is elevated, lower it slowly
- If receiving alteplase, blood pressure must be <185 mm Hg systolic or <110 mm Hg diastolic
- To save as much penumbra as possible, keep blood glucose levels and temperature within normal limits.
- A patient with swallowing difficulty may need a temporary feeding tube or a percutaneous endoscopic gastrostomy (PEG) tube for nutritional intake.
- Intermittent pneumatic compression devices on legs, unless contraindicated
- Assess for depression
- Skin assessments are necessary; special mattresses, wheelchair cushions, special seating devices may be required.
- Ongoing assessment for signs and symptoms of brain edema, seizures, and increased intracranial pressure (ICP)

- Hemorrhagic stroke:
  - May be more difficult to treat; requires a neurosurgeon to evaluate treatment options
  - As with the ischemic stroke, will need to identify the cause of the stroke and treat any deficits that may exist.

- Patient teaching:
  - Educate patient and caregivers about stroke deficits and how to manage them.
    - After a stroke, a patient may experience behavioral or emotional changes/outbursts, such as incontrollable crying.
    - Medications such as antidepressants can lessen the frequency of outbursts.
  - Explain the risk factors for stroke that are considered modifiable and the need to follow physician recommendations for managing these risks:
    - High blood pressure
    - Smoking tobacco products
    - Diabetes
    - Hyperlipidemia
    - Obesity
    - Atrial fibrillation
    - Effects of sedentary lifestyle, alcohol/substance abuse
  - Explain the signs and symptoms of a stroke and the need to call 911 for emergency treatment.
  - Review all medications and their purpose, side effects, and any special instructions related to taking them.
  - For patients with a noncardioembolic ischemic stroke, an antiplatelet agent is recommended for secondary stroke prevention.
  - For those with embolic stroke, possible anticoagulation will be discussed. (Powers et al., 2018).
    - More than two-thirds of stroke survivors require rehabilitation after hospitalization, and many have residual functional deficits. (Weinstein et al., 2016).
    - The residual effects of the stroke may impact the ability for a patient to independently perform some or all activities of daily living (ADLs):
      - Depression, apathy, fatigue
      - Motor issues

> **Clinical Consideration**
>
> Deficits may be difficult to diagnosis, so educating the patient and caregivers about the need to tell the physician of these symptoms is important.

- Cognitive/memory problems
- Swallowing disorder
- Communication disorders
- Sexual dysfunction
- Can patient return to work?
  - Patients are at a greater risk of falling.
  - Variety of rehabilitation care settings are available, but choice of setting is based on functional abilities, rehabilitation potential, and other factors
  - Multidisciplinary team approach
  - Goal is to achieve highest level of function possible
- Gerontologic considerations:
  - Residual deficits after a stroke can profoundly alter the life of an older adult.
  - Hospitalization and recovery can be challenged by preexisting medical problems, comorbidities, and the changes that occur with aging.
  - Sensory, motor, cognitive, perceptual, and emotional changes can contribute to significant disability after stroke.
  - The patient, caregiver, and family will need help with coping and possibly placement after a stroke.
  - The patient may need care in the hospital; may be transferred home, to intermediate- or long-term care, or to a rehabilitation facility. Multiple transfers may produce physiologic and emotional stress for the older adult.
  - Sensory and cognitive problems may make it challenging for the older adult and the spouse to manage the complex care needs after a stroke.
  - Significant concern as to whether the patient can regain and maintain independence
  - Adaptive equipment may need to be installed in the home. Mobility aides, transfer devices, and other supplies may need to be ordered.
  - The patient's spouse may be chronically ill and may not be able to assume the caregiver role. Perhaps the patient's spouse has passed away and the adult children do not live nearby.
  - The older adult may need to pay caregivers to provide care in the home. Perhaps they need to be transferred to assisted- or long-term care. For many older adults, these options may represent a financial burden.

▶ *Transient Ischemic Attacks (TIAs)*

- A TIA is similar to a stroke in that it occurs from an occluded blood vessel in the brain or vessels leading to the brain. However, the signs and symptoms are shorter in duration as the blood flow returns and the symptoms resolve.
- A TIA may be a predictor of subsequent stroke.
- *Assessment/Intervention/Education*
  - Detailed medical history:
    - Determine whether there have been other incidents during which symptoms come and go.
  - Clinical manifestations:
    - Same as stroke but for shorter duration
    - Acute change in the level of consciousness, acute-onset weakness or paralysis on one side of the body, partial vision loss, and/or difficulty with speech
  - Diagnosis:
    - Rapid assessment—time is critical, as is the need to identify the time of last time known to be well.
    - NIHSS provides quantifiable metric of stroke-induced impairments
    - CT scan to determine whether stroke is ischemic or hemorrhagic
    - Blood glucose to confirm that this is not related to hypoglycemic event

- Nursing diagnosis:
  - See Nursing diagnosis in section on "Stroke."
  - Risk for ineffective cerebral tissue perfusion related to clot, emboli, or hemorrhage
- Treatment:
  - As most of the time symptoms have resolved by the time the patient arrives at the hospital, treatment becomes an assessment of the cause.
  - Testing should include:
    - Echocardiogram
    - Carotid artery studies
    - CTA
    - MRI/MRA
- Patient teaching:
  - Explain the risk factors of stroke that are considered modifiable and the need to follow physician recommendations for managing these risks.
  - Signs and symptoms of a stroke/TIA and need to call 911 for emergency treatment
  - Review all medications, their purpose, side effects, and any special instructions related to taking them.

Epilepsy/Seizures

- Epilepsy is a disorder of the CNS that causes seizures. Seizures occur when the neurons in the brain send erroneous messages.
- Types of seizures:
  - Focal:
    - Simple—the patient may experience small twitches, become dizzy, or smell or taste something odd.
    - Complex—the patient may experience a loss of consciousness but will appear awake.
  - General:
    - Grand mal (tonic–clonic)—body becomes stiff, jerks, often incontinence of bladder and/or bowel
    - Petit mal—last only a few seconds and the patient will have a vacant stare and likely not remember the event
    - Clonic—last for a few minutes and most often are muscle spasms in the face
    - Tonic—last only a few seconds; muscles in the arms and legs become rigid
    - Atonic—last only a few seconds; muscles in the arms and legs become flaccid
    - Myoclonic—muscles shudder suddenly

Assessment/Intervention/Education

- Detailed medical history:
  - A description of the seizure is helpful in determining what type the patient may be experiencing.
  - How long the seizure lasts
  - Important to assess responses after seizure
  - Other causes of a loss of consciousness (such as syncope) need to be ruled out.
- Clinical manifestations:
  - Confusion
  - Loss of consciousness
  - Uncontrollable movement of the arms and/or legs
- Diagnosis:
  - Epilepsy may take time to diagnose and may require multiple tests to determine the type of seizure

- EEG is conducted to look for abnormalities in the brain's electrical impulses.
- CT scan or MRI may be performed.
- A lumbar puncture may be performed to rule out meningitis and encephalitis.
- Nursing diagnosis:
  - Risk for injury related to environment during seizure activity
  - Acute confusion related to postseizure state
  - Readiness for enhanced knowledge related to seizure treatment
- Treatment:
  - Anticonvulsant medications are usually not given if the patient experiences only one seizure.
  - Medications administered vary depending on the type of seizures and are narrow or broad spectrum (Table 14.3).

TABLE 14.3	COMMON MEDICATIONS FOR THE TREATMENT OF SEIZURES			
Drug Name	Drug Type and Use	How It Works	Manufacturer's Recommended Dosage	Common Side Effects
Narrow-Spectrum Drugs—used to prevent seizures that have been identified to a specific location of the brain				
Carbamazepine (Carbatrol, Tegretol)	Anticonvulsant Treat grand mal seizures originating in the temporal lobe of the brain; trigeminal neuralgia and bipolar disorder	Blocks sodium uptake to reduce abnormal electrical activity	Adults, begin with 200-mg tablet twice daily May increase up to a maximum daily dose of 1600 mg	Nausea, vomiting, drowsiness, dizziness; serious side effects include increase in suicidal thoughts.
Diazepam (Valium)	Benzodiazepine Treat seizures and anxiety; typically used to stop seizures and patient is placed on other long-acting medication to prevent recurrence.	Increases GABA, which inhibits neurotransmissions	Adults, 2- to 10-mg tablet, 2 to 4 times a day	Drowsiness, headache, dry mouth, constipation; serious side effects include increase in seizure activity, depression, or confusion.
Divalproex (Depakote)	Used to treat simple and complex absence seizures; complex partial seizures; bipolar disorder; migraines	Increases GABA, which inhibits neurotransmissions	Adults: Extended release tablets—10 to 15 mg/kg daily Delayed release tables—10 to 15 mg/kg three times daily	Nausea, headache, drowsiness; serious side effects include bleeding abnormalities, high ammonia levels, hypothermia
Gabapentin (Neurontin)	Can be used to treat partial seizures, restless legs syndrome; PHN and chronic pain	Influences transport of GABA and affects Ca²⁺ channels	300–600 mg three times daily; may increase to 1200 mg three times daily	Increased appetite, ataxia, irritability, dizziness, fatigue, weight gain
Lacosamide (Vimpat)	For partial and generalized seizures	Blocks sodium channels and decreases brain excitability	50 mg twice daily; increase to maintenance of 100–200 mg twice daily	Dizziness, memory/mood changes, diplopia, fatigue, headache
Oxcarbazepine (Trileptal)	For partial seizures as monotherapy, or as adjuvant therapy; not effective against absence or myoclonic seizures	Blocks sodium channels, stabilizes neural membranes, inhibits repetitive firing, and decreases synaptic impulse propagation	Start slowly and increase to 600 mg twice daily	Risk of hyponatremia, SIADH; sedation; diplopia; nausea, vomiting; headache; dizziness; sedation; rash; Stevens–Johnson syndrome; toxic epidermal necrosis
Phenobarbital	Barbiturate Used to treat clonic, tonic, and tonic–clonic seizures	Controls abnormal electric activity in the brain	Adults, 60- to 200-mg tablet daily	Drowsiness, dizziness, headache; serious side effects include increase in suicidal thoughts.
Phenytoin (Dilantin)	Antiepileptic Used to treat tonic–clonic seizures	Blocks spread of seizure activity in the neurons	Adult, 100-mg extended-release capsule 3 times daily	Slurred speech, dizziness, nausea, vomiting, constipation, gingival hyperplasia, rash; serious side effects include increase in suicidal thoughts.

(continued)

TABLE 14.3 (*Continued*)

Drug Name	Drug Type and Use	How It Works	Manufacturer's Recommended Dosage	Common Side Effects
Pregabalin (Lyrica)	Antiseizure medication used as adjunct therapy for partial seizures; PHN; neuropathy; fibromyalgia	Binds α_2-delta subunit of calcium channels, reducing neurotransmitter release; produces antinociceptive and antiseizure effects	For seizures may start at 150 mg/day and titrate up to 600 mg/day	Dizziness, somnolence, weight gain; xerostomia; peripheral edema; impaired coordination; blurred vision
Broad-Spectrum Drugs—used to prevent seizures in multiple locations				
Clonzaepam (Klonopin)	Long-acting benzodiazepine Used to treat myoclonic seizures	Increases GABA, which inhibits neurotransmissions	Adults, 0.5-mg tablet 3 times a day May increase up to a maximum daily dose of 20 mg in divided dose	Dizziness, drowsiness, depression; serious side effects include increase in suicidal thoughts
Lamotrigine (Lamictal)	Anticonvulsant Treats partial seizures; generalized tonic–clonic seizures; bipolar disorder	Inhibits sodium channels, decreasing presynaptic glutamate and aspartate release	May titrate up to 400 mg/day in divided doses; take with food or just after a meal.	Dizziness, drowsiness, ataxia, diplopia, headaches, nausea, vomiting
Levetiracetam (Keppra)	Anticonvulsant Used to treat myoclonic, partial, or grand mal seizures	Blocks spread of seizure activity in the neurons	Adults, 500-mg tablet twice daily May increase up to a maximum daily dose of 3000 mg	Dizziness, drowsiness, irritability; serious side effects include hallucinations, confusion, rash
Valproic acid (Depakene)	Anticonvulsant Partial and absence seizures	Increases GABA, which inhibits neurotransmissions	Adults, 10-mg/kg tablet daily as beginning dose; increase to maximum of 60 mg/kg daily	Diarrhea, dizziness; serious side effects include increase in suicidal thoughts, chest pain.

https://www.ninds.nih.gov/Disorders/All-Disorders/Epilepsy

GABA = gamma aminobutyric acid; PHN = postherpetic neuralgia; SIADH = syndrome of inappropriate antidiuretic hormone.

- Surgery (lobectomy) may be an option after treatment with medications is not successful or there is an identified lesion or location where the seizure begins.
- Nerve stimulator—used for patients who are not surgical candidates and who do not respond to medications:
  - Vagus nerve stimulator—attached to vagus nerve with device implanted in chest
  - Responsive stimulation device—attached to brain where seizure originates, with device implanted in skull
- Patient teaching:
  - Avoid activities that may trigger a seizure.
  - Depression is common in patients with seizures, they may be referred to counselors for learning ways to adapt to changes in lifestyle.
  - Many states restrict driving privileges of patients with seizures and may require a provider note indicating the patient is safe to drive.
  - Prevention:
    - No way to prevent a seizure, but dietary changes may reduce frequency.
      - High-fat and low-carbohydrate or ketogenic diet has been shown to improve seizure activity by 50% (NIH National Institute of Neurological Disorders and Stroke, 2017)
- Gerontologic considerations for seizures:
  - Older adults respond well to antiseizure drugs when they have more than one stroke, recurrent seizures, or a disease process that is likely to produce recurrent seizures.
  - They are more sensitive to the action of the drugs and will experience side effects at lower doses of the drug.

- Age-related changes in liver function can alter the way the liver metabolizes phenytoin (Dilantin), for example.

- Great care should be taken when older adults receive drugs such as phenobarbital, carbamazepine (Tegretol), and primidone (Mysoline), as they can cause drowsiness and cognitive impairment. Oxcarbazepine (Trileptal), phenytoin (Dilantin), phenobarbital, carbamazepine (Tegretol), primidone (Mysoline), and topiramate (Topamax), and levetiracetam (Keppra) may affect bone health in older adults.

- The following drugs may be safer for older adults, and have fewer side effects and interactions with other drugs:

  • Gabapentin (Neurontin)
  • Lamotrigine (Lamictal)
  • Oxcarbazepine (Trileptal)
  • Levetiracetam (Keppra)

Question	Rationale
The nurse enters a patient's room and witnesses a tonic–clonic seizure just starting. What is the priority action by the nurse? A. Stabilize the patient's head to prevent injury. B. Clear away anything that may cause the patient harm. C. Assess the first thing that happens at the beginning of the seizure. D. Ask the patient to describe the pain.	Answer: C Identifying the first thing that happens at the time of a seizure may assist with diagnosing the location of the seizure activity in the brain.

▶ *Alzheimer's Disease*

• Alzheimer's disease is a type of dementia caused by blood vessel changes that result in damage to brain neurons. The disease affects not only a person's bodily functions such as walking, but also memory and moods. According to the Centers for Disease Control and Prevention (CDC, 2017), it is the sixth leading cause of death and affects more than 5 million Americans.

Mild (early stage)	Moderate (middle stage)	Severe (late stage)
• Still independent • Forgetfulness beyond what is seen in a normal person • Trouble remembering names • Problems coming up with the right words • Problems remembering what they just read • Losing or misplacing a valuable object • Difficulties with planning or organizing • May be unable to do simple math problems	• Longest stage • May have difficulty remembering address and phone number • Confusion becomes more obvious • May begin having episodes of incontinence • Changes in sleep patterns • Lose track of where they are • May begin to wander or get lost • Behavior and personality changes may become apparent	• Significant cognitive decline • Very poor memory, unable to recognize family and friends • Difficulties talking and understanding others • Unable to process new information • Changes in physical abilities • Requires help from others for self-care activities • May require 24-hour caregiver

Figure 14.3 Stages of Alzheimer's Disease

Clinical Consideration
The onset of Alzheimer's disease is marked by memory loss and is often mistaken for conventional signs of aging.

- *Assessment/Intervention/Education*
  - Detailed medical history:
    - Ask family members about changes in behavior or the ability to perform ADLs
  - Clinical manifestations:
    - Usually diagnosed around the age of 65
    - Loss of memory that interferes with ADLs
    - Confused as to place and time
    - Changes in judgment and the ability to solve problems
    - Mood changes, including increased agitation and aggressive behaviors
  - Diagnosis:
    - No definitive test to diagnose Alzheimer's disease (Table 14.3)
    - Tests completed to rule out other causes of symptoms:
      - CT scan of the brain
      - MRI of the brain
      - Blood and urine testing
      - Neuropsychologic evaluation/test for problem-solving ability
  - Nursing diagnosis:
    - Impaired memory related to disease process
    - Self-care deficits related to loss of cognitive function
    - Caregiver role strain related to interrupted family processes
    - Powerlessness related to deteriorating condition
  - Treatment:
    - Focus is to delay progression of symptoms and manage behavioral manifestations
    - Symptom management:
      - Medications can be used to delay the worsening of symptoms (Table 14.4).
    - Preventing complications:
      - Certain medications should be used with caution:
        - Sleep aids such as zolpidem (Ambien) or eszopiclone (Lunesta)
        - Antipsychotics such as quetiapine (Seroquel) or risperidone (Risperdal)
        - Antianxiety medications such as lorazepam (Ativan)
        - Anticonvulsants such as sodium valproate (Depakote)
  - Patient teaching:
    - Family and caregivers need to understand that worsening symptoms will require increased assistance.
    - Ensuring a safe environment:
      - Prevent falls
      - Unintentional medication dosing errors
      - Accidents in the kitchen
    - Encourage a daily routine and physical activity, such as walking.

▶ *Parkinson's Disease*

- Parkinson's disease is a movement disorder in which there is progressive disability; there is no cure. It is the most common neurologic disorder, and it occurs when neurons die in the substantia nigra of the midbrain. As the neurons die, there is a decrease in the production of dopamine, leading to movement issues.
- *Assessment/Intervention/Education*
  - Detailed medical history:
    - Ask patient and family members about changes in: arm or leg movement or gait; dizziness; lack of facial expressions; soft voice; sleeplessness; small handwriting (micrographia); constipation; change in sense of smell

TABLE 14.4	COMMON MEDICATIONS FOR THE TREATMENT OF ALZHEIMER'S DISEASE			
Drug Name	Drug Type and Use	How It Works	Manufacturer's Recommended Dosage	Common Side Effects
Donepezil (Aricept)	Cholinesterase inhibitor prescribed to treat symptoms of mild, moderate, and severe Alzheimer's disease	Prevents the breakdown of acetylcholine in the brain	Initial dose, 5-mg tablet once a day May increase dose to 10 mg/day after 4–6 weeks if well tolerated, then to 23 mg/day after at least 3 months	Nausea, vomiting, diarrhea, muscle cramps, fatigue, weight loss
Rivastigmine (Exelon)	Cholinesterase inhibitor prescribed to treat symptoms of mild to moderate Alzheimer's (patch is also for severe Alzheimer's disease)	Prevents the breakdown of acetylcholine and butyrylcholine (chemical similar to acetylcholine) in the brain	Initial dose, 3-mg capsule per day (1.5 mg twice a day) May increase dose to 6 mg/day (3 mg twice a day), 9 mg (4.5 mg twice a day), and 12 mg/day (6 mg twice a day) at minimum 2-week intervals if well tolerated	Nausea, vomiting, diarrhea, weight loss, indigestion, muscle weakness
Memantine (Nameda)	NMDA antagonist prescribed to treat symptoms of moderate to severe Alzheimer's disease	Blocks the toxic effects associated with excess glutamate and regulates glutamate activation	Initial dose, 5-mg tablet or oral solution once a day May increase to 10 mg/day (5 mg twice a day), 15 mg/day (5 mg and 10 mg as separate doses), and 20 mg/day (10 mg twice a day) at minimum 1-week intervals if well tolerated	Dizziness, headache, diarrhea, constipation, confusion
Memantine extended-release and donepezil (Namzaric)	NMDA antagonist and cholinesterase inhibitor prescribed to treat symptoms of moderate to severe Alzheimer's disease (for patients stabilized on both memantine and donepezil taken separately)	Blocks the toxic effects associated with excess glutamate and prevents the breakdown of acetylcholine in the brain	28 mg memantine extended-release capsule + 10 mg donepezil once a day	Headache, nausea, vomiting, diarrhea, dizziness
Galantamine (Razadyne)	Cholinesterase inhibitor prescribed to treat symptoms of mild to moderate Alzheimer's disease	Prevents the breakdown of acetylcholine and stimulates nicotinic receptors to release more acetylcholine in the brain	Initial dose, 8-mg tablet per day (4 mg twice a day) May increase dose to 16 mg/day (8 mg twice a day) and 24 mg/day (12 mg twice a day) at minimum 4-week intervals if well tolerated	Nausea, vomiting, diarrhea, decreased appetite, dizziness, headache

https://www.nia.nih.gov/health/how-alzheimers-disease-treated

NMDA = N-methyl-D-aspartate.

- Clinical manifestations:
  - Symptoms:
    - Tremors
    - Changes in gait:
      - Slow movement (bradykinesia)
      - Stiff limbs and trunk with minimal arm swing
      - Trouble with balance (postural instability)
      - Festination—shuffling, short, rapid steps when walking
      - Freezing—stops in place, giving the appearance of being stuck
    - Cognitive changes—As the disease progresses, patients may demonstrate:
      - Memory loss
      - Inability to maintain attention
      - Hallucinations
      - Dementia
- Diagnosis:
  - Medical history and physical examination
  - No laboratory test to diagnose Parkinson's disease

Clinical Consideration

Subtle symptoms in the beginning stages of the disease and may be confused with normal signs of aging; family members may be the first to recognize these changes.

- Unsuccessful treatment with medications for related diseases helps in determining that the patient has Parkinson's disease.
- Demonstrated at least two of the four following signs over a period of time:
  - Shaking or tremors
  - Bradykinesia
  - Stiffness or rigidity
  - Postural instability
- Nursing diagnosis:
  - Imbalanced nutrition: less than body requirements related to tremors that cause difficulty eating
  - Risk for injury related to tremor, unsteady gait, slowed reactions
- Treatment:
  - No cure; administration of levodopa increases dopamine levels in the brain
  - Medications (Table 14.5)
  - Surgical treatments:
    - Deep-brain stimulators
    - Ablation surgery
    - J-tube insertion for administration of a gel form of carbidopa/levodopa (Duopa) that is administered continuously during the day by a small handheld pump
  - Exercise:
    - Regular exercise
    - Physical therapy to help with gait disorders
    - Occupational and speech therapy may help symptoms

> **Clinical Consideration**
>
> If a patient who is taking levodopa suddenly stops the medication, they may experience an inability to move or respiratory difficulties.

TABLE 14.5	COMMON MEDICATIONS FOR THE TREATMENT OF PARKINSON'S DISEASE		
Class	Drug	How It Works	Common Side Effects
Levodopa preparations	*Immediate release:* carbidopa/levodopa (Sinemet) *Immediate/extended release:* carbidopa/levodopa (Rytary) *Intestinal infusion:* carbidopa/levodopa (DUOPA)	Synthesized to dopamine in the brain	Nausea, vomiting, loss of appetite, light-headedness, hypotension, confusion
Dopamine agonists	*Oral:* pramipexole (Mirapex), ropinirole (Requip) *Transdermal:* rotigotine transdermal system (Neupro) *Injectable:* apomorphine (Apokyn)	Mimics the effects of dopamine	Excessive sleepiness, confusion, compulsive behaviors, and lower-extremity edema
Antivirals	*Immediate release:* amantadine (Symmetrel) *Extended release:* amantadine (Gocovri)	Reduces tremors and reduces dyskinesias that are associated with the use of levodopa	Nausea, light-headedness, insomnia, confusion, hallucinations
COMT inhibitors	Entacapone (Comtan) Tolcapone (Tasmar)	Prolongs the effect of levodopa	Exaggerate dyskinesias; confusion, hallucinations, hematuria
MAO inhibitors	Selegiline/deprenyl (Eldepryl, Zelapar) Rasagiline (Azilect)	Blocks an enzyme in the brain that breaks down levodopa, increasing the amount of available dopamine	Nausea, dry mouth, light-headedness, confusion, hallucinations
Anticholinergics	Trihexyphenidyl (Artane) Benztropine mesylate (Cogentin)	Reduces dystonia, may reduce tremors and alleviate rigidity and bradykinesia	Blurred vision, confusion, hallucinations, dry mouth, urinary retention, constipation
	http://parkinson.org/Understanding-Parkinsons/Treatment/Prescription-Medications		

COMT = catechol-omicron methyltransferase; MAO = monoamine oxidase.

- Patient and family teaching:
  - Ensure a safe environment to prevent falls that could result from balance and gait disorders.
  - Encourage the use of assistive devices such as a cane.
  - Family education and support on the importance of medication administration, providing safe environments, and the progression of the disease process.
  - Education about the importance of adequate nutrition to avoid malnutrition and constipation, possible impaired swallowing, and appropriate interventions.
  - Patients may be challenged by motor symptoms, but also with nonmotor symptoms such as apathy, depression, constipation, sleep disturbances, loss of sense of smell, and cognitive impairment
  - Each patient is evaluated to determine which drug or combination of drugs works best
  - Teach about motor fluctuations and "off time" related to the medications and to take medications at consistent times

Question	Rationale
What common cognitive impairment is associated with Parkinson's disease? A. Depression B. Loss of memory C. Learning disabilities D. Slurred speech	Answer: B Parkinson's disease is a progressive neurologic disease in which there is deterioration of neurons. This can lead to motor symptoms (tremors). In later stages of the disease, cognitive symptoms such as a loss of memory and the ability to retrieve information often occur.

▶ *Myasthenia Gravis (MG)*

- MG is a chronic autoimmune neuromuscular disease in which patients experience muscle weakness.
- MG results from destruction or blockage of receptors of acetylcholine (ACh), a neurotransmitter that activates muscles and produces contraction. The individual's own immune system creates the antibodies that block or destroy the receptors.
- In adults with MG, the thymus gland is atypically large. As part of the body's immune system, it is this gland that produces the antibodies that block or destroy acetylcholine receptors.
- *Assessment/Intervention/Education*
  - Detailed medical history:
    - Assess the patient's history related to difficulty swallowing, use of arms or hands, blurred vision, or drooping eyelids
    - Determine whether there are factors that influence increases in muscle weakness, such as emotional upsets or weather changes
  - Clinical manifestations:
    - Symptoms may be seen first as ptosis (drooping eye lid) due to muscle weakness.
    - Blurred vision may also be seen in the initial stages
    - This is often followed by progressive weakness of other muscles, such as hands, arms, and legs

- Some patients may experience swallowing difficulties or changes in speech.
- Fatigue may increase the symptoms of MG.
- Myasthenic crisis results when respiratory muscles weaken, and a patient may require mechanical ventilation.

- Diagnosis:
  - Physical examination to determine muscle strength, eye movements, and coordination
  - Blood tests to determine ACh receptor antibody levels; results will be abnormally high for patients with MG
  - EMG to determine whether the patient has impaired nerve/muscle transmissions

- Nursing diagnosis:
  - Deficient knowledge related to disease process and treatment options
  - Ineffective airway clearance related to diminished ability to cough and swallow
  - Impaired swallowing related to muscle weakness, neuromuscular impairment
  - Self-care deficits related to visual impairment or generalized weakness

- Treatment:
  - MG has no known cure and is usually controlled with medications.
    - Acetylcholinesterase (AChE) medications:
      - Pyridostigmine bromide (Mestinon) is the most common drug used; it prevents the ACh from breaking down.
    - Immunosuppressant medications—reduce the production of antibodies
      - Prednisone—very effective for treatment; however, has significant side effects
      - Azathioprine (Imuran) or cyclophosphamide (Cytoxan) are medications originally developed for use in organ transplantation but have been shown to provide a decrease in symptoms for immune-related diseases such as MG
      - Monoclonal antibodies—rituximab (Rituxan): intravenous injection used when MG not responsive to other medications
  - Intravenous immunoglobulin (IVIg)
    - Used for treatment of worsening MG, but offers only short-term effects
    - IV treatment of normal antibodies from donated blood
  - Plasmapheresis:
    - Used for treatment of severe MG, but offers only short-term effects
    - Plasma exchange that removes all antibodies from the blood
  - Thymectomy (removal of the thymus gland) may reduce the symptoms.
  - Diet and exercise:
    - Being overweight can add stress to the body and cause worsening of symptoms.

- Patient teaching:
  - Ensure that the patient understands the importance of taking medications as directed and on time
  - Instruct patients to notify their dentist of their MG, as many local anesthetics may worsen the symptoms of MG.
  - Instruct patients on methods to reduce fatigue while maintaining physical activity.

Clinical Consideration

Patients with myasthenia gravis need to understand the importance of correctly administering AChE inhibitor drugs.

Clinical Consideration

This includes taking the medication on time and at least 60 minutes prior to a meal.

Question	Rationale
A patient has just been diagnosed with myasthenia gravis and is being started on pyridostigmine bromide (Mestinon) therapy. The nurse should instruct the patient on which priority intervention? A. Eat large meals that are considered ketogenic. B. Take medication on time to maintain therapeutic blood levels. C. Exercise at the same time each day to maintain muscle strength. D. Develop a psychologic treatment plan to deal with fatigue.	Answer: B Mestinon is an AChE drug that increases the body's ACh level by blocking the enzyme that usually breaks it down. By maintaining a therapeutic level, the ACh can become concentrated in the muscle receptor, which leads to improved transmission of messages from nerves to muscles.

▶ *Migraine Headaches*

- Migraine headaches are throbbing headaches due to rapid constriction of blood vessels in the brain; they are frequently accompanied by sensory disturbances, such as sound or light sensitivity.
- Decreases in serotonin levels may cause changes to the trigeminal nerve that result in pain associated with migraines.
- *Assessment/Intervention/Education*
  - Detailed medical history:
    - Determine what symptoms the patient experiences with headaches and what may trigger an event.
  - Clinical manifestations:
    - Symptoms may begin gradually.
    - Lasts at least 4 hours
    - Progresses through four stages, although some patients may not experience all stages:
      - Prodrome—patient may experience difficulty concentrating and/or nausea for a few days to hours before the migraine begins
      - Aura—visual disturbances such as flashes of light that may appear within an hour before the migraine begins
      - Headache—lasts 4 to 72 hours, throbbing pain, patient may experience light or sound sensitivities
      - Postdrome—lasts 24 to 48 hours after the migraine ends; patient may be tired and lack ability to concentrate
  - Diagnosis:
    - The Headache Classification Committee of the International Headache Society (2013) recommends the following guidelines to diagnose migraines:
      - Presence of an aura
      - Headaches lasting 4 to 72 hours
      - Variable frequency
      - Unilateral and pulsating moderate to severe pain
      - Headache worsened by movement
      - Nausea and/or vomiting and photophobia
      - No runny nose or watery, red eyes

- Nursing diagnosis:
  - Ineffective health maintenance related to deficient knowledge about treatment and prevention of headaches
  - Acute pain: headache related to vasodilation of cerebral vessels
- Treatment:
  - Treatment plans fall into two categories: prevention and relief of symptoms during a migraine:
    - Prevention:
      - Identify events that may trigger a migraine, such as hormonal changes during menstruation, stress, insomnia, dehydration, changes in weather, foods, food additives, or even loud noises.
      - Medications that may prevent migraines:
        - Antiseizure medications, such as gabapentin
        - Medications to treat hypertension, such as β-blockers or calcium-channel blockers, metoprolol, or verapamil
    - Relief of symptoms during a migraine, medications that will increase serotonin levels:
      - First-line treatment:
        - Combination analgesics containing aspirin, caffeine, and acetaminophen
        - Ibuprofen at standard doses
      - Ergotamine tartrate (Cafergot)
      - Triptans (serotonin receptor agonist)
        - Sumatriptan (Imitrex)
- Patient teaching:
  - Keep a headache diary.
  - Seek immediate medical attention for the following symptoms:
    - Abrupt, unexpected headache
    - Headaches that are accompanied by a fever, a stiff neck, or difficulty speaking
    - The above symptoms may be associated with a stroke or meningitis.
  - Instruct patients on the side effects of medications. For example, Cafergot may cause sudden weakness on one side of the body, confusion, or bradycardia. Imitrex may cause chest pain or irregular heartbeats.

Question	Rationale
A patient is being started on Imitrex (sumatriptan) for migraine headaches. Of the following, which is the most important for the patient to report to the health care provider prior to starting this medication? A. A history of projectile vomiting B. Bilateral headache pain C. A recent myocardial infarction D. A history of hemorrhoids	Answer: C Imitrex is contraindicated for patients with a history of a recent myocardial infarction, coronary artery disease, or arterial vasospasm. Medications in the triptan class of drugs, such as Imitrex, constrict blood vessels to stop migraine headaches. In patients with heart disease, this vasoconstriction may lead to a decrease in blood flow to areas of the heart and may cause additional cardiac damage.

▶ *Guillain–Barré Syndrome (GBS)*

- GBS is an uncommon, acute autoimmune disease in which the body's immune system attacks the peripheral nervous system.
- The destruction of the myelin sheath disrupts the transmission of nerve impulses, and the patient begins to experience numbness and weakness in the lower extremities.
- There is no treatment, and most patients recover completely over 4 to 6 months (maybe up to 2 years); however, some have permanent neurologic deficits.
- *Assessment/Intervention/Education*
    - Detailed medical history:
        - Determine whether the patient had a recent history of infection such as pneumonia or intestinal virus. The infection or virus may trigger changes in the immune system that lead to the destruction of the myelin sheath.
        - Review the patient's medical history for several weeks prior to their. Has the patient received any immunizations recently? Symptoms may be present for 2 to 4 weeks prior to seeking medical attention.
    - Clinical manifestations:
        - Progressive muscle weakness that can progress to paralysis
        - Weakness begins in lower extremities and progresses to upper body.
        - Patient may lose bladder and bowel control.
        - As the disease progresses, the patient may have difficulty breathing and may require mechanical ventilation.
        - Symptoms usually level off at 4 weeks, and full recovery may take as long as 12 months.
    - Diagnosis:
        - Usually determined by the patient's symptoms
        - Lumbar puncture may reveal CSF with an increased level of protein.
        - Nerve conduction studies may be completed to determine the presence of injury to the myelin sheath.
    - Nursing diagnosis:
        - Impaired physical mobility related to paralysis
        - Ineffective breathing pattern related to weakened respiratory muscles
    - Treatment:
        - Plasmapheresis:
            - Plasma exchange that removes all antibodies from the blood
        - IVIg:
            - An IV treatment of normal antibodies from donated blood
        - Mechanical ventilation if the patient experiences respiratory failure
        - Physical therapy to maintain muscle strength during the illness and to regain strength during recovery
        - Nutritional therapy
    - Patient teaching:
        - Remain as regular with activities and exercise programs as possible to improve muscle strength
        - Educate the patient on the importance of notifying the nurse about increased efforts to breath, inability to urinate, and worsening weakness.
        - Use incentive spirometer or deep breathing exercises to maintain respiratory function.
        - Encourage patient and family regarding recovery from GBS.

Question	Rationale
A patient with GBS was admitted to the medical-surgical unit and has had worsening symptoms for the past 2 days. Which of the following is the priority nursing assessment? A. Monitor vital signs, including O2 saturation. B. Monitor frequency of voids and bowel movements. C. Monitor skin integrity. D. Monitor dietary intake.	Answer: A While all these assessments are important for the GBS patient, most important is to assess the vital signs and O2 saturation. A fluctuating blood pressure (usually hypertension), tachycardia, and decreasing O2 saturation are all clinical signs of significant deterioration that may require transfer to higher level of care and mechanical ventilation support.

▌ *Multiple Sclerosis (MS)*

- MS is an immune-mediated process targeting the CNS and characterized by disseminated demyelination of nerve fibers of the brain and spinal cord. The immune system attacks the myelin sheath surrounding peripheral nerves and the nerve fibers themselves. The damaged myelin forms scar tissue, or sclerosis. Nerve impulses traveling to and from the brain and spinal cord are changed or interrupted.

- *Assessment/Intervention/Education*
  - Detailed medical history:
    - Determine whether the patient had a recent history of swallowing difficulty, inability to complete simple tasks, or stumbling while walking.
  - Clinical manifestations vary and may include:
    - Muscle cramps and twitching
    - Stiff muscles
    - Muscle weakness
    - Slurred speech
    - Swallowing difficulties
    - Vision problems
    - Fatigue
    - Numbness, tingling
    - Bowel, bladder problems
  - Diagnosis:
    - Usually determined by the patient's symptoms
    - EMG
    - Nerve conduction studies may be completed to determine the presence of injury to the myelin sheath.
    - MRI to rule out other illnesses, such as spinal cord tumor, that may cause symptoms
    - MRI to confirm that damage in at least two separate areas of the CNS (brain, spinal cord, optic nerves) has occured at two different points in time.
  - Nursing diagnosis:
    - Impaired physical mobility related to neuromuscular changes
    - Urinary retention related to inhibition of the reflex arc

- Treatment:
  - Medications (Table 14.6)
    - Modify disease course—medications may reduce the number or relapses, delay the progression of the disease, and slow new disease activity.
    - Managing relapses—for severe relapses, corticosteroids may resolve the relapse more quickly.
    - Managing symptoms—a variety of medications may be used to treat the symptoms of MS listed here:
      - Bladder dysfunction, bladder infection
      - Bowel dysfunction
      - Depression
      - Emotional changes
      - Fatigue
      - Gait difficulties
      - Itching
      - Pain
      - Spasticity
      - Tremors
      - Vertigo
  - Physical and occupational therapy to maintain muscle strength
  - Speech therapy—may need text-to-speech devices
  - Nutritional therapy—to ensure adequate diet with swallowing difficulties:
    - Mechanical ventilation if the patient experiences respiratory failure
- Patient teaching:
  - Adhere to treatment plan to maximize effectiveness.
  - Remain as regular as possible with activities and exercise programs to improve muscle strength.
  - Important to notify nurse about increased efforts to breath or muscle weakness
  - Consult with social workers and palliative care teams, as appropriate.

TABLE 14.6	COMMON MEDICATIONS FOR THE TREATMENT OF MULTIPLE SCLEROSIS
Class	**Medication**

Modify disease course	Injectable:
	    Interferon beta-1a (Avonex, Rebif)
	    Interferon beta-1b (Betaseron, Extavia)
	    Glatiramer acetate (Copaxone, Glatopa)
	    Peginterferon beta-1a (Plegridy)
	Oral:
	    Teriflunomide (Aubagio)
	    Fingolimod (Gilenya)
	    Dimethyl fumarate (Tecfidera)
	Infused:
	    Alemtuzumab (Lemtrada)
	    Mitoxantrone (Novantrone)
	    Ocrelizumab (Ocrevus)
	    Natalizumab (Tysabri)

Managing relapses	Intravenous:
	    Methylprednisolone (Solu-Medrol)
	Oral:
	    Prednisone (Deltasone)
	Injectable:
	    Adrenocorticotropic hormone (H.P. Acthar Gel)

	https://www.nationalmssociety.org/Treating-MS/Medications

▶ *Amyotrophic Lateral Sclerosis (ALS)*

- ALS is a disease in which there is a progressive loss of neurons that control voluntary muscles.
- Also known as Lou Gehrig disease
- No cure or effective treatment
- *Assessment/Intervention/Education*
  - Detailed medical history:
    - Determine whether the patient had a recent history of progressive muscle weakness, swallowing difficulty, weakness in one limb, or muscle twitching.
  - Clinical manifestations:
    - Muscle cramps and twitching
    - Trips and falls
    - Muscle weakness
    - Slurred speech
    - Swallowing difficulties
    - Breathing difficulties
    - Difficulty maintaining good posture or holding up head
    - May have pseudobulbar affect
  - Diagnosis:
    - Usually determined by the patient's symptoms; every patient presents differently
    - May take a very long time to establish a diagnosis
    - EMG to determine active and chronic damage to nerves that control muscles
    - MRI to rule out other illnesses, such as spinal cord tumor, that may cause symptoms
  - Nursing diagnosis:
    - Anxiety related to impending progressive loss of function
    - Decisional conflict: ventilator therapy related to personal values or beliefs, deficient knowledge
    - Impaired swallowing related to muscle weakness
  - Treatment:
    - Medications:
      - Riluzole (Rilutek):
        - Taken daily
        - Slows progression of disease
      - Edaravone (Radicava):
        - IV infusion for 10 to 14 days a month
        - Decreases decline in ADLs
    - Physical and occupational therapy to maintain muscle strength and provide adaptive home equipment
    - Speech therapy—may need assistance with communication; text-to-speech devices; assistance with swallowing difficulties
    - Nutritional therapy—ensure adequate diet with swallowing difficulties; may require feeding tube
    - Respiratory therapy treatments/devices to help keep lungs clear, assisting with cough, expectorating secretions
    - Continuous positive airway pressure (CPAP)/bilateral positive airway pressure (BiPAP)
    - Mechanical ventilation if the patient experiences respiratory failure

- Patient teaching:
  - Remain as regular with activities and exercise programs as possible.
  - Important to notify nurse about increased efforts to breath or muscle weakness.
  - Multidisciplinary approach is needed; consult with social workers, pulmonary specialists, speech and language therapists, physical/occupational therapy, and palliative care teams.
  - Discuss patient and family wishes related to home care, nutrition, need for mechanical ventilation, and end-of-life care.

CASE STUDY

A 70-year-old male is admitted to the surgical unit to prepare for colon surgery in the afternoon. He has a large tumor that requires removal; however, his wife was not able to assist with the required treatment to prepare him for surgery at home. The patient has a medical history of colon polyps, hypertension, hyperlipidemia, chronic lower back pain, and diabetes. Current medications include:

Atorvastatin (Lipitor) 40 mg orally daily

Lisinopril (Zestril) 5 mg orally daily

Docusate sodium (Colace) 100 mg orally daily

Hydrocodone/Acetaminophen 5 mg/300 mg, one tablet, three times a day as needed for severe pain

Gabapentin (Neurontin) 300 mg orally every night at bedtime

Metformin (Glucophage) 500 mg orally twice a day

Multivitamin, one tablet daily

Upon admission to the medical-surgical unit, assessment reveals that he is afebrile, blood pressure 170/86 mm Hg, heart rate 99 beats/min, respiratory rate 20 breaths/min, and O_2 saturation 95% while breathing room air. He is awake, alert, oriented x4 (person, place, time, and situation) and states his low back pain level is 3 of 10 and tolerable for him to complete his bowel preparations. He states he feels a "little off" but thinks it may be nerves.

An hour later, the nurse returns to the room to begin his bowel prep. The patient now has a left-sided facial droop and he is not able to answer questions. The nurse calls for assistance from the charge nurse and begins to take vital signs. The blood pressure is 186/96 mm Hg, heart rate 120 beats/min, respiratory rate 16 breaths/min, and O_2 saturation 90% while breathing room air. The charge nurse brings the blood glucose monitor, and the patient's blood sugar is 102.

1. **Based on assessment findings what diagnosis might the nurse expect?**

   ▶ *The patient is demonstrating symptoms of a stroke. The inability to speak and the facial droop are symptoms of a stroke. At this time it cannot be determined whether it is ischemic or hemorrhagic.*

2. **What other information would be important to know?**

   ▶ *The nurse will need to recall the last time she saw the patient well. What was his baseline assessment when admitted to the unit?*

   ▶ *Many organizations have established programs that will require nurses to call for a rapid response team or stroke team to assist with further care of the patient.*

3. **What diagnostic tests would the nurse anticipate the provider to order?**
   ▶ *Stat CT Scan of the head*
   ▶ *CBC*
   ▶ *Chemistry*
   ▶ *Coagulation studies*
   ▶ *12-lead ECG*
   ▶ *Place the patient on telemetry monitoring*

4. **What education would be provided to this patient?**
   ▶ *It is important to educate the patient on the plan of care, including the rapid assessment with the CT scan, and that he may be transferred to another unit.*
   ▶ *Later in the hospital stay, education will focus on the risk factors for stroke. The level of care after the hospital stay will depend on the severity of the stroke, functional abilities, and the potential need for physical therapy, speech therapy and other specialized treatments.*

The rapid response team arrives, conducts a NIHSS assessment, and takes the patient to imaging, where a CT scan of the brain is completed. The results indicate no hemorrhage; therefore, it is determined that he had an ischemic stroke and is a candidate for thrombolytic therapy. The patient is transferred to critical care, where he receives alteplase and is monitored for the next 36 hours. After this, he returns to the medical surgical unit. The patient has slurred speech and is not able to eat, as he has failed a swallowing evaluation. There are currently no other neurologic deficits.

1. **Based on assessment findings, what nursing diagnoses might be included in the plan of care for this patient?**
   a. *Impaired swallowing related to stroke injury*
   b. *Imbalanced nutrition due to swallowing difficulties*
   c. *Self-care deficit related to loss of function*
   d. *Impaired verbal communication related to slurred speech*
   e. *Deficient knowledge related to prognosis, care and treatment plans, signs and symptoms of stroke, and prevention of future events*

2. **What education will this patient and his family need?**
   a. *These required topics:*
      i. *Activation of emergency medical system*
      ii. *Follow-up after discharge*
      iii. *Medications prescribed at discharge*
      iv. *Risk factors for stroke*
      v. *Warning signs and symptoms of stroke*
      vi. *Swallow precautions*
      vii. *Fall precautions*
   b. *Additional topics may include:*
      i. *Emotional changes, that may include depression*
      ii. *Community resources available for the patient and caregivers*
      iii. *Fatigue, apathy*
      iv. *Changes in role in the family*
      v. *Losses associated with stroke*

Bibliography

Black, J.M., and Hawks, J. (2009). *Medical-Surgical Nursing: Clinical Management for Positive Outcomes*, 8th ed. (St. Louis: Saunders).

Centers for Disease Control and Prevention. (2017). Alzheimer's disease. Accessed October 29, 2017, from https://www.cdc.gov/dotw/alzheimers/index.html

Glasgow Coma Scale. Accessed June 17, 2018, from http://www.glasgowcomascale.org/

Headache Classification Committee of the International Headache Society. (2013). The international classification of headache disorders, 3rd ed. (beta version). *Cephalalgia* 33, 629–808.

Jarvis, C. (2015). *Physical Examination & Health Assessment*, 7th ed. (St. Louis: Elsevier).

Lewis, S.L., Bucher, L., Heitkemper, M., and Harding, M.M. (2017). *Medical-Surgical Nursing: Assessment and Management of Clinical Problems*, 10th ed. (St. Louis: Elsevier).

National Multiple Sclerosis Society. (n.d.). Medications. Accessed March 11, 2018, from https://www.nationalmssociety.org/Treating-MS/Medications

NIH National Heart, Lung, and Blood Institute. (2017). Stroke. U.S. Department of Health and Human Services. Accessed November 20, 2017, from https://www.nhlbi.nih.gov/health/health-topics/topics/stroke

NIH National Institute on Aging. (2017). Epilepsy information page. Accessed November 20, 2017, from https://www.ninds.nih.gov/Disorders/All-Disorders/Epilepsy

NIH National Institute on Aging. (2017). Guillain–Barré syndrome. Accessed November 23, 2017, from https://www.ninds.nih.gov/Disorders/Patient-Caregiver-Education/Fact-Sheets/Guillain-Barr%C3%A9-Syndrome-Fact-Sheet

NIH National Institute on Aging. (2017). Myasthenia gravis. Accessed November 23, 2017, from https://www.ninds.nih.gov/Disorders/Patient-Caregiver-Education/Fact-Sheets/Myasthenia-Gravis-Fact-Sheet

NIH National Institute of Neurological Disorders and Stroke. (2018). Amyotrophic lateral sclerosis (ALS) fact sheet. Accessed January 13, 2018, https://www.ninds.nih.gov/Disorders/Patient-Caregiver-Education/Fact-Sheets/Amyotrophic-Lateral-Sclerosis-ALS-Fact-Sheet

NIH National Institute of Neurological Disorders and Stroke. (2017). Patient and caregiver education Accessed November 20, 2017 from https://www.ninds.nih.gov/Disorders/Patient-Caregiver-Education/Hope-Through-Research/Epilepsies-and-Seizures-Hope-Through#3109_32

NIH National Institute on Aging. (2017). Treatment of Alzheimer's disease. Accessed November 20, 2017, from https://www.nia.nih.gov/health/how-alzheimers-disease-treated

NIH National Institute on Aging. (2017). Treatment of Parkinson's disease. Accessed November 23, 2017, from https://www.nia.nih.gov/health/parkinsons-disease

NIH Stroke Scale International. (2017). Accessed November 20, 2017 from http://www.nihstrokescale.org/

Pagana, K.D., Pagana, T.J., and Pagana, T.N. (2017). *Mosby's Diagnostic and Laboratory Test Reference*, 13th ed. (St. Louis: Elsevier).

Parkinson's Foundation. (2018). Accessed March 2, 2018 from http://parkinson.org.

Powers, W.J., Rabinstein, A.A., Ackerman, T., Adeoye, O.M., Bamibakidis, N.C., Becker, K. … Tirschwell, D.L. (2018). 2018 guidelines for the early management of patients with acute ischemic stroke: A guidelines for healthcare professionals from the American heart association/American Stroke association. Stroke, 49 (3), e46–e99. doi:10.1161/STR.000000000000

Teasdale, G., and Jennett, B. (1974). Assessment of coma and impaired consciousness: a practical scale. *Lancet* 2, 81–84.

Weinstein, C.J., Stein, J., Arena, R., Bates, B., Cherney, L.R., Cramer, S.C. … Fisher, B. (2016). Guidelines for adult stroke rehabilitation and recovery: A guidelines for healthcare professionals from the American heart association/American stoke association. Stroke, 47, e98–e169. doi:10.1161/STR.0000000000000098

15

Musculoskeletal System

Ida Anderson MSN, RN, ONC

OVERVIEW

▶ The primary function of the musculoskeletal system is to provide humans the ability to move. The musculoskeletal system supports movement by providing stability, support, and structure. The musculoskeletal system protects vital organs and allows motion. In addition, bones are the primary storage site for calcium and phosphorus.

▶ The musculoskeletal system is comprised of bones and muscles that are attached to provide a stable structure for the body.

▶ Diseases and disorders of the musculoskeletal system can be difficult to diagnose and create complex medical conditions that impact multiple body systems.

ANATOMY

▶ The musculoskeletal system is composed of the:
- Bones:
  - Shapes: Long bones, short bones, flat bones, irregular bones
  - Function:
    - Provide rigid framework and support for the body
    - Protect vital organs
    - Store minerals, calcium and phosphate ions, lipids, and marrow elements
    - Form new red cells and other blood elements
- Skeletal muscles:
  - Characteristics: Irritability, contractility, extensibility, elasticity
  - Function:
    - Produce movement
    - Maintain posture
    - Guard entrances to and exits from digestive and urinary system
  - Action:
    - Controlled by central nervous system
    - Complex, variable, and often involuntary
    - Contractions: isometric and isotonic
  - Nerve supply:
    - Derived from spinal nerves

- Joints:
  - Gross structure—cartilage, synovial membrane, synovial fluid
  - Classifications—gliding, ball and socket, hinge, saddle, pivot, and condyloid
  - Motions—flexion, extension, hyperextension, abduction, adduction, circumduction, rotation, eversion, inversion, pivot, pronation, supination
- Skull—comprised of cranial and facial bones
- Thoracic cage:
  - Ribs—12 pairs
  - Sternum
- Spine–vertebral column:
  - Cervical—7 vertebrae between skull and thorax
  - Thoracic—12 vertebrae between cervical and lumbar regions
  - Lumbar—5 vertebrae, fused
  - Sacrum—5 vertebrae, fused
  - Coccyx—4 vertebrae, usually fused
  - Sagittal curvatures of vertebral column: cervical, thoracic, lumbar and sacrum
  - Abnormal curvatures: kyphosis, lordosis, scoliosis
- Extremities:
  - Upper: humerus, radius, ulna, wrist, hand, fingers
  - Lower: hip, femur, knee, tibia, fibula, feet, toes

▌ Gerontologic considerations:
- Age-related changes:
  - Bone density decreases
  - Muscles become smaller and less elastic
  - Decreased tolerance for exercise and repetitive movements
  - Decreased ability to recover from injuries
  - Ligaments may lose tensile strength (the force it can withstand without breaking)
  - Joint cartilage can become less elastic and damaged, and osteoarthritis can develop.
  - Decreased range of motion
  - Musculoskeletal changes can cause decreased coordination, loss of strength, and risk for falls.
  - Pain is not a normal process of aging.

NURSING ASSESSMENT AND CONSIDERATIONS

▌ Comprehensive health history:
- Chief symptom—explore all symptoms, have patient explain what caused him or her to seek treatment
- Usual state—physical, social, psychological, spiritual
- History of present illness—chronology of symptom progression
- Medical history—previous episodes related to current symptoms, previous remedies, treatments, surgeries, and/or hospitalizations
- Current health status—smoking, alcohol, medications, allergies, nutrition, exercise
- Family history
- Review of systems
- Special considerations—trauma, chronic, congenital:
  - Examine specifics of current problem—sequence of the development of symptoms
  - What, where, and how injury occurred
  - Onset of pain

- Direction of force, if applicable
- Symptoms continuous or intermittent:
  - Exacerbated by movement?
  - What helps?
  - Response to heat/cold?
  - What position causes pain?
- Impact on activities of daily living?
▸ General physical exam techniques—inspection, palpation, range of motion
  - Neurovascular assessment:
    - Sensation:
      - Normal, increased, decreased
      - Pain—constant, intermittent, sharp, dull, burning, aching, with activity, at rest
    - Movement:
      - Appropriate for limb
      - Reflexes—present, absent
    - Circulation:
      - Color
      - Temperature
      - Capillary refill
      - Edema
      - Pulses
  - Gait patterns:
    - Observe walking 10 to 20 feet.
    - Look for scraping of shoe at the toe, stomping, shuffling, or unequal step rhythm.
    - Abnormalities often related to pain, muscle weakness, instability or structural deformity
  - Presence of crepitus; clicking or popping during movement
  - Inspect for asymmetry or asymmetrical movements, swelling, deformity and abnormal limb size (Table 15.1)
  - Palpate for muscle spasms, painful areas, joint effusion, instability, and warmth
  - Test muscle strength

Question	Rationale
When assessing a patient for neurovascular deficits, which finding listed below is the most significant? A. Numbness B. Lack of pulse C. Cool to touch D. Paralysis	Answer: B While all of the options are important and require additional intervention, absence of a pulse is a catastrophic condition that can lead directly to loss of limb.

DIAGNOSTIC TESTS

▸ Imaging studies:
- Angiography
- Computed tomography (CT) scan
- Magnetic resonance imaging (MRI)

TABLE 15.1	POSITIONS AND MOVEMENTS OF MUSCULOSKELETAL SYSTEM
Anatomic position	Standing with back, legs and arms straight, palms facing forward
Anterior	Ventral, front, or abdominal side of the body
Posterior	Dorsal or back side of the body
Ventral	Anterior or front side of the body
Dorsal	Back or posterior side of the body
Superior	Above and closer to the top of the body
Inferior	Beneath or below another structure; farther from the top of the body
Medial	Nearer the middle of the body, toward the center
Lateral	Distal from the center of the body, to the side
Proximal	Closer to the center of the body
Distal	Further from the center of the body
Supinate	Turn the hand and forearm for the palm to face upward
Pronate	Turn the hand and forearm for the palm to face downward
Dorsiflexion	Movement of the foot toward the top or dorsum of the foot
Plantar flexion	Movement of the foot toward the bottom or plantar of the foot
Extension	Movement that brings the extremity to a straight position; increasing the angle of a joint
Flexion	Movement that bends an extremity, decreasing the angle of a joint
Supine	Lying on the back with face and anterior body facing upward
Prone	Lying horizontally with anterior body and face downward
Ligament	Strong fibrous tissue connecting bone to bone at joint areas
Tendon	Strong fibrous tissue connecting muscles to bone at joint areas
Meniscus	Fibrous crescent-shaped cartilage within the joint
Medulla	Bone marrow
Synovial membrane	Lining the capsule of a joint
Synovial fluid	Lubricating fluid within a joint
Articular cartilage	Cartilage formed at the articulating ends of bones

- Arthrography
- Bone scan – detects metastatic cancer to the bone
- Dual-energy absorptiometry (DEXA)—measures bone mineral density
- Myelography
- X-ray
▸ Specialty diagnostic testing:
- Arthroscopy
- Bone marrow aspiration
- Nerve conduction studies
- Joint aspirations
- Lumbar epidural venography—used to diagnose disk herniations

- Bone biopsies
- Muscle biopsies

▌ Blood:

- Antinuclear antibody (ANA)—used to detect presence of anti-nucleoprotein factors associated with certain autoimmune disorders
- Creatine kinase (CK)—reliable measure of skeletal muscle disease such as muscular dystrophy
- C-reactive protein (CRP)—evaluates inflammatory response
- Hematocrit—measures percentage of red-cell mass to blood volume
- Hemoglobin—index of oxygen-carrying capacity of the blood; often used to determine the need for blood transfusion
- Serum calcium
- Vitamin D_3
- Serum phosphorus
- Alkaline phosphatase
- Lactate dehydrogenase (LDH), aspartate aminotransferase (AST)
- Erythrocyte sedimentation rate (ESR)

▌ Urine:

- Bence-Jones protein
  - Found in 40% of multiple myeloma cases, tumor metastasis to the bone, chronic lymphocytic leukemia, amyloidosis, and macroglobulinemia
- Urine calcium:
  - Evaluates calcium metabolism
  - Monitors excretion levels
  - Identifies deficiency

OSTEOARTHRITIS

▌ Slowly progressive, noninflammatory disorder of movable joints characterized by gradual loss of cartilage, occurrence of bony outgrowths, and mild, chronic, non-specific synovial inflammation; sometimes called "degenerative joint disease" (DJD). Associated with overuse injuries (Table 15.2).

▌ Etiology:

- No apparent initiating factor
- Obesity major factor
- Can be secondary to trauma, long-term repetitive movements, joint instability
- Susceptibility increases with age, female sex, genetic predisposition, smoking

▌ Pathophysiology:

- Multistage progression
- Early pain, stiffness related to changes in synovium and joint capsule
- Classification based on joint involvement—not generally considered bilateral or symmetric:
  - Localized—1 to 2 joints
  - Generalized—3 or more joints
  - Affects weight-bearing joints, hands, and spine

▌ Lifespan considerations:

- Impact on mobility is the major contributor to disruption of lifestyle
- Impact on gait increases fall risk
- Emotional and social problems commonly related to chronic pain and physical limitations

TABLE 15.2	COMPARISON OF RHEUMATOID ARTHRITIS AND OSTEOARTHRITIS	
Characteristic	Rheumatoid Arthritis	Osteoarthritis
Age at onset	20s–50s	40s–50s
Gender	Females 3:1 Normalizes after age 60 to 1:1	Females 2:1 after age 55
Disease course	Exacerbations, remissions	Progressive, variable
Symptoms	Systemic	Local
Commonly affected joints	Small joints first (hands and feet), then wrists, knees, cervical spine	Weight-bearing joints (hips and knees) then small joints, cervical and lumbar spine
Morning stiffness	First hour to all day	10–30 minutes with first activity
Joint involvement	Symmetric	Asymmetric
Effusions	Common in superficial joints; rare in deep joints	Uncommon
Synovial fluid	Decreased viscosity; white cells present	Normal viscosity, minimal white cells
Synovium	Thickened, often severely inflamed	Possible localized inflammation with point tenderness
Nodules	Rheumatic nodules over bony prominences	Heberden nodes; Bouchard nodes
X-rays with disease progression	Global narrowing of joint space, erosions, dislocations, osteoporosis related to corticosteroid use	Asymmetric narrowing of joint space; joint cysts and sclerosis

▶ Assessment:
- History and physical exam:
  - Localized symptoms (nonsystemic)
  - Reduced range of motion
  - Deformities/instability:
    - Heberden and Bouchard nodes (Figure 15.1)
  - Joint warmth
▶ Diagnostic tests:
- Laboratory tests:
  - Testing done to rule out autoimmune disorders
  - ESR may be minimally elevated
- Radiographs
  - Confirm disease progression
  - X-rays, MRI, CT
- Synovial fluid analysis—clear, high viscosity, low white-cell count
▶ Nursing diagnosis:
- Activity intolerance related to chronic pain
- Impaired physical mobility related to joint impairment
▶ Common treatment methods:
- Goals:
  - Manage pain
  - Maintain functional mobility

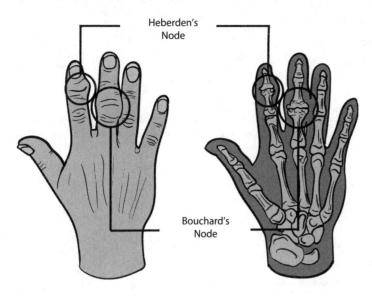

Heberden's
Node

Bouchard's
Node

Figure 15.1 Osteoarthritic Nodes

- Cope with and accept chronic illness
- Develop an individualized therapeutic regimen
- Nonpharmacologic management:
  - Rest, immobilization
  - Heat and cold therapy
  - Stimulation with electrical device (transcutaneous electric nerve stimulator [TENS])
  - Orthotic devices
  - Weight reduction
  - Exercise
  - Mobility aids
  - Acupuncture
  - Dietary supplements—glucosamine/chondroitin
  - Collaborate with physical and occupational therapists
- Pharmacologic management:
  - Nonopioid analgesics:
    - Nonsteroidal antiinflammatory drugs (NSAIDs), cyclooxygenase 2 (COX-2) inhibitors:
      - Doses of acetaminophen may need to be reduced in cases of liver disease, history of alcohol abuse, and the elderly
      - Teach patient correct dosing of acetaminophen (no more than 4 g daily)
  - Opioid analgesics:
    - Opioids are not a front-line medication, but are frequently a part of the overall plan.
  - Neuroleptics:
    - Gabapentin (Neurontin)
    - Pregabalin (Lyrica)
  - Local therapies:
    - Capsaicin creams and other topicals
    - Corticosteroid injection into joint
    - Hyaluronic acid injection into joint

> **Clinical Consideration**
> Maximum daily dose of acetaminophen is 4000 mg daily.

- Surgical management:
  - Joint surgery:
    - Arthroplasty—resurfacing of the joint
    - Replacement—partial or total joint replacement
- Patient teaching:
  - Primary nursing intervention—patient teaching is the single most important nursing intervention. Increased self-care knowledge is tied directly to positive patient outcomes:
    - Disease progression
    - Body mechanics
    - Impact of weight reduction
  - Medication reconciliation
  - Medication side effects
  - Facilitate family support
  - Fall risk/injury prevention
  - Self-care deficit needs

RHEUMATOID ARTHRITIS

- Chronic, progressive, systemic inflammatory disease that manifests primarily in joint spaces with unexplained alternating periods of exacerbation and remission (Table 15.2)
  - Arthritis Foundation defines as "an autoimmune disease in which the body's immune system attacks joint tissue, causing inflammation of the joint lining" (www.arthritis.com)
- Etiology—Multifactorial, abnormal immune response in genetically predisposed population; more common in women and in smokers
- Pathophysiology—Autoantibodies are formed that attack the synovial joints and cause inflammation; multistage progression of disease, systemic involvement
  - Characteristic deformities (Figure 15.2):
    - Rheumatoid nodules—bony prominences over joints
    - Boutonniere deformity—middle finger joint bends toward the palm, while outer finger joint may bend in the opposite direction

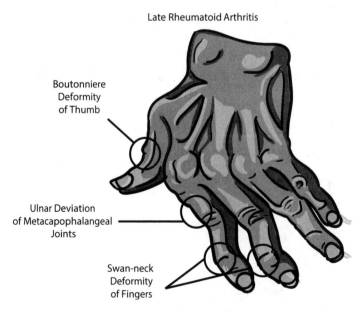

Late Rheumatoid Arthritis

Boutonniere Deformity of Thumb

Ulnar Deviation of Metacapophalangeal Joints

Swan-neck Deformity of Fingers

Figure 15.2 Rheumatoid Deformities

- Swan-neck deformity—base of the finger and distal joint bend, while middle finger joint straightens
- Hitchhiker's thumb—thumb flexes at the metacarpophalangeal joint and hyper-extends at the interphalangeal joint below the thumbnail (also called "Z-shaped deformity of the thumb")
- Claw toe deformity—toes are either bent upward from the ball of the foot, downward at the middle joints, or downward at the top toe joints and curl under the foot
- Painful, swollen, warm joints
- Symmetrical patterns of inflammation (bilateral)

▶ Lifespan considerations:

- Slower progression with early onset
- Acute and widespread manifestation when age at onset is >60

▶ Complications:

- Increased risk of death, double that of general population when disease not well controlled
- Bony erosion above and below joints
- Increased risk of masked infection related to side effects of steroid treatments
- Increased risk of osteoporosis
- Increased risk of heart disease
- Increase risk of lung disease

▶ Diagnostic tests:

- Diagnosed primarily by medical history and physical findings:
    - Anticitrullinated protein antibody (ACPA), rheumatoid factor (RF), ANA, ESR, serum complement
    - Joint inflammation must be present.
    - Radiographs often not needed.
    - Bone scans reveal early joint changes and confirm diagnosis.
    - Synovial fluid positive for white cells.

▶ Nursing diagnosis:

- Chronic pain related to joint deterioration
- Disturbed body related to joint abnormalities

▶ Common treatment methods:

- Goals:
    - Pain relief
    - Slow progression of joint damage
    - Prevent disability
    - No known cure
- Medication:
    - Disease-modifying antirheumatic drugs (DMARDs):
        - Help to preserve joints by blocking inflammation
        - Most important part of care plan
        - Common medications—hydroxychloroquine (Plaquenil), sulfasalazine (Azulfidine), methotrexate, NSAIDs, corticosteroids
        - Potential to mask infection because of blocked inflammatory response
    - Biologic response modifiers:
        - Stimulate the body's own immune system to fight arthritis
        - Genetically engineered to act like natural proteins within the immune system
        - Common medications—adalimumab (Humira), etanercept (Enbrel)

- Therapeutic exercise—range of motion, strengthening, and endurance exercises:
  - Low resistance
  - Heat and cold therapies can provide comfort.
  - Splints may reduce inflammation during exacerbation.
- Medicinal oils:
  - Omega-3 fatty acids may reduce inflammation
- Diet:
  - No specific dietary recommendations
  - Alcohol is contraindicated with most rheumatic arthritis (RA) medications
- Complementary or alternative therapies

▶ Nursing considerations:
- Patient teaching:
  - When to report adverse symptoms to health care provider
  - How to address a missed medication dose
  - Abrupt cessation of steroids is contraindicated.
- Self-care needs at home:
  - Assistive devices
  - Adaptive clothing
  - Mobility aids
  - Environmental modifications
- Pain management plan:
  - Reinforce consistent compliance with comprehensive plan
  - Analgesic use
  - Positioning, protecting joints
  - Heat and cold therapies
  - Relaxation techniques—imagery, breathing, music, distraction
- Social support:
  - Educate family members
  - Encourage maximized independence
  - Collaborate with patient
  - Identify community resources
- Maximize sleep and rest
- Promote coping strategies:
  - Active participation in decisions about treatment
  - Discussion related to impact of disease on sexuality, strategies to mitigate disruption of sexual function
  - Workplace adaptations
  - Encourage active participation in support groups such as the Arthritis Foundation

BACK PAIN

▶ Divided into four regions:
- Cervical
- Thoracic
- Lumbar
- Sacral

▶ Etiology—can originate from muscles, nerves, bones, joints, or spine structures. May occur from referred pain originating from internal organs such as gallbladder, pancreas, aorta, or kidneys.

Clinical Consideration
Back pain occurs in 9 out of 10 adults at some point during their life.

▶ Risk factors:

- Obesity
- Sedentary lifestyle
- Absence of routine exercise

▶ Diagnostic tests:

- Generally, treatment begins based on reported symptoms because back pain frequently resolves after a few weeks
- Lab tests:
  - Elevated ESR could indicate infection, malignancy, chronic disease, inflammation, or trauma
  - Elevated CRP associated with infection
- Imaging:
  - MRI
  - CT

▶ Nursing diagnosis:

- Acute/chronic pain related to back injury
- Impaired physical mobility related to back injury

▶ Common treatment methods:

- Management goals center on reducing pain rapidly to return to normal function
- Emergency surgical intervention is considered in specific conditions
  - Cauda equina syndrome:
    - Damage to the bundle of nerves at the base of the spinal cord
    - Symptoms include numbness around the anus with absence of anal reflex, loss of bowel and bladder control, pain radiating down the legs, sexual dysfunction, saddle paresthesia (numbness or tingling of the groin and inner thigh)
  - Cause—usually disk herniation

▶ Nonpharmacologic management:

- Initial treatment of choice for conservative management
  - Heat therapy helpful with muscular spasms
  - Massage
  - Gentle stretching and exercise
  - Core strengthening
  - Spinal manipulation—widely used, however, no definitive evidence of long-term benefit
  - Acupuncture

▶ Pharmacologic management:

- NSAIDs
- Muscle relaxers
- Single-dose steroid injections
- Epidural corticosteroid injection

▶ Patient teaching:

- Teach patient to use proper body mechanics to prevent subsequent injuries
- Refrain from doing activities that increase pain
- Encourage smoking cessation

> **Clinical Consideration**
> Tobacco use can contribute to back pain; circulation to the intervertebral disks is impaired with tobacco use.

THE SPINE

▶ Common conditions:

- Scoliosis—lateral curvature of the spine with vertebral rotation
- Kyphosis—increased convexity of the thoracic spine >45°

- Herniated disk—protrusion of the center of the intervertebral disk
- Spinal stenosis—narrowing of the spinal canal or intervertebral foramen
▸ Assessment:
  - History and physical examination—gait, range of motion, strength, reflexes, sensation
  - Symmetry
▸ Diagnostic tests:
  - Radiographic testing—primary source for definitive diagnosing
▸ Nursing diagnosis:
  - Impaired physical mobility related to restricted movement, curvature of the spine
  - Ineffective health maintenance related to deficient knowledge regarding treatment, restrictions, follow-up
▸ Common treatment methods:
  - Conservative—decreasing pain and maximizing function are primary goals of treatment; strength and conditioning, physical therapy, and aquatic therapy
  - Surgical intervention—release pressure on spinal column, repair herniations, cement microfractures, stabilize with plates or rods

TRAUMA

Sprains/Strains

▸ Traumatic injury to a muscle, ligament, or tendon caused by overstretching, indirect force, or overuse
▸ Pathophysiology:
  - Acute—includes a range of injury from mild to severe overstretching with possible tearing of muscles/tendons
  - Chronic—most often results from improper care of an acute strain or repeated use of a muscle beyond its normal capacity
▸ Incidence:
  - Can occur in any age group. Most common injuries sustained from sports activities.
▸ Lifespan considerations:
  - Shoulder tendons in the elderly are more prone to injury than in younger people
  - Upper arm strain more common in middle-aged and elderly males
  - Ankle and knee injuries common in any age group
▸ Complications:
  - At risk for recurrence once a sprain/strain has occurred
  - At risk for increased severity of sprain/strain with recurrence
▸ Assessment:
  - Mechanism of injury—sudden versus gradual onset; report of feeling a sudden tearing, snapping, or burning sensation
  - Edema or ecchymosis
  - Loss of range of motion
  - Point tenderness
▸ Diagnostic tests:
  - X-rays to rule out fracture
▸ Nursing diagnosis:
  - Acute pain related to physical injury
  - Impaired walking related to injury

▶ Common treatment methods:
- Rest, ice, compression, elevation (RICE):
  - Rest—reduced activity is key treatment. May include use of a sling, immobilizer, splint, or crutch. Immobilization decreases pain, reduces inflammation, and allows any tears to approximate.
  - Ice—cryotherapy decreases bleeding from injured blood vessels. The more blood that accumulates at injury site, the longer it takes the injury to heal.
    - Ice applied in 20-minute increments
    - Always assess skin for integrity under cryotherapy
    - Provides analgesic effect
  - Compression—applying some form of compression limits swelling at the injury site. Uncontrolled swelling can cause additional tissue injury and delay healing:
    - Elastic (Ace) bandages are most common
    - Should be applied after icing
    - Should be wrapped tightly; however, must not impair neurovascular function or arterial blood flow
  - Elevation—raise injured area above the level of the heart
    - Allows gravity to drain off excess fluid
    - Reduces pressure from injury site
    - Decreased edema facilitates analgesia and allows the area to move more freely
    - Elevation is contraindicated when arterial damage or deficiency is present.
▶ Patient teaching:
- Patient education regarding self-care, skin assessment under compression dressings, activity restrictions, assistive devices, and signs/symptoms of infection under the skin
- Emphasize to patient the need for rest and immobilization to prevent further injury

Dislocations

▶ Displacement of a bone from its normal joint position
▶ Etiology—force applied to a joint either directly or indirectly
▶ Complications:
- Nerve and blood vessel injuries
- Ligament laxity
- Avascular necrosis of the head of the femur due to loss of circulation when dislocated
- Possible fractures
- Elbow dislocations constitute emergency related to potential loss of limb
▶ Assessment:
- Neurovascular status
- Pain and tenderness on movement
- Obvious deformity
▶ Diagnostic tests
- X-rays—always bilateral for comparative analysis
- MRI—if soft-tissue damage is suspected
- Arteriography for suspected vascular injury
▶ Nursing diagnosis:
- Acute pain related to physical injury

Type of Bone Fractures

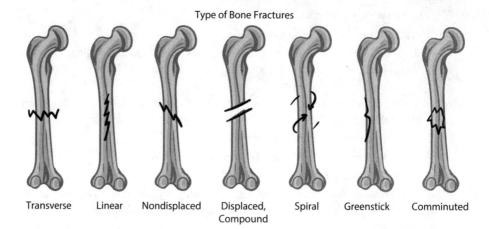

Figure 15.3 Fractures

▶ Common treatment methods:
- Closed reduction
- Traction
- Immobilization depends on affected joint
- Complex dislocations may require surgical intervention

▶ Nursing considerations:
- Impaired mobility
- Neurovascular status

▶ Patient education:
- Potential for recurrence
- Types of movements/activity to be avoided
- Maintaining functionality of unaffected side

Fractures

▶ Break or disruption in the continuity of the bone (Figure 15.3)

▶ Etiology—occurs when bone is subjected to more stress than can be absorbed

▶ Classification of fractures—incomplete, complete, open, closed (Table 15.3)

▶ Lifespan considerations—can occur at any age:
- Children have immature musculoskeletal systems:
  - Most treated with closed reduction and casting
  - Injuries affecting the growth plate can lead to significant complications such as:
    - Limb length discrepancy
    - Joint incongruity
    - Angular deformities
- Elderly:
  - Have increased risk of occurrence because of falls
  - Osteoporotic bone heals more slowly

▶ Diagnostic tests:
- Radiographs essential to differential diagnosis
- Laboratory tests indicated for severe injures (local vs. systemic)
  - Urine for occult blood
  - Complete blood count (CBC)

TABLE 15.3	FRACTURE CLASSIFICATIONS
Fracture	Definition
Complete	Break across the entire section of the bone, dividing it into separate fragments; frequently displaced.
Incomplete	Break occurs partially through the bone (e.g., greenstick fracture)
Open	Bone is broken through the skin. Graded by severity
Closed	Skin remains intact
Nondisplaced	Bone fragments aligned at fracture site
Avulsion	Separation of small fragment of bone at insertion site of ligament of tendon
Compression	Unusual force applied to bone causing it to buckle and eventually crack
Stress fracture	Occurs with repetitive minor stress
Pathologic fracture	Fracture occurs in absence of trauma or minimal trauma after pathologic process has weakened the bone
Comminuted	More than one fracture line with multiple fragments (e.g., crushed or shattered)
Spiral	Fracture line twists around bone shaft

- CK
- Pathologic fractures require additional testing

▎ Nursing diagnosis:

- Impaired physical mobility related to limb immobilization
- Acute pain related to muscle spasms, trauma
- Risk for peripheral neurovascular dysfunction—mechanical compression, treatment of fracture

▎ Stages of bone healing—6 to 8 weeks total healing time

- Reactive phase—7 to 9 days; inflammation stimulates granulation and tissue formation
- Reparative phase—10 days to 4 weeks; cartilage callus forms, which transforms into lamellar bone. Lamellar bone begins forming as tissue is mineralized and transforms into trabecular bone.
- Remodeling phase—4 to 8 weeks; trabecular bone transforms into compact bone.

▎ Common treatment methods:

- Closed reduction—align bone fragments manually without surgical intervention, generally under anesthesia; fix externally with cast or splint.
- Open reduction—align bone fragments with surgical intervention; fix internally with pins, wires, screws, rods, nails, or other type of hardware.
- Antibiotics and debridement for open fractures
- Traction
- Casts

▎ Complications:

- Impaired mobility
- Loss of limb
- Neurovascular compromise
- Malunion or nonunion
- Post-traumatic arthritis
- Infection—osteomyelitis

- Skin breakdown under splints or casts
- Compartment syndrome (Figure 15.4)
- Rhabdomyolysis
- Fat embolism syndrome
- Venous thromboembolism

▶ Patient teaching:

- Maintain mobility following prescribed activity program, assistive device use, pin site care if applicable
- Unusual symptoms—fever, swelling, severe pain, changes in sensation, burning, or drainage from area
- Cast care:
  - Do not get cast wet
  - Elevate extremity for first 48 hours
  - Notify provider of any problems; increased pain, burning or swelling under the cast, discoloration of exposed skin, foul odor from cast
- Traction care:
  - Monitor pin sites for redness or drainage
  - Ensure weights are free hanging

WOLFF'S LAW

- Bone in a healthy person will adapt to the loads under which it's placed.
- Weight bearing stimulates bone remodeling.
- The inverse is also true—reduction in bone density and weakness occurs with prolonged immobility and the absence of weight-bearing activity.

TUMORS

▶ Tumors of the musculoskeletal system are either benign or malignant.

- Sarcoma—malignant neoplastic bone tumor
  - Primary sarcomas are malignant tumors originating in bone or soft tissue.
  - Benign tumors and tumor-like conditions can also originate in bone or soft tissue.
  - Nonneoplastic bone and soft-tissue tumors are called "tumor-like."

▶ Pathophysiology:

- Sarcomas differ from carcinoma by cell origin; sarcomas arise from muscle, bone, fat, fascia, or cartilage.
- Sarcomas may be fast- or slow-growing

▶ Diagnostic tests:

- Radiographic testing
- Ultrasound to rule out cystic tumor
- Arteriogram to identify vessel involvement
- CBC with differential to rule out infection
- Sedimentation rate, liver-function tests (LFTs), serum electrolytes, calcium, phosphorus, and alkaline phosphate
- Bone scan to assess for metastatic disease

▶ Nursing diagnosis:

- Acute pain/chronic pain/Impaired comfort related to disease process, metastatic cancer
- Ineffective coping/grieving/powerlessness related to treatment, disease progression
- Spiritual distress related to test of spiritual beliefs

▶ Common treatment methods:

- Biopsy
- Excision
- Limb-salvage or limb-sparing procedures
- Amputation
- Radiation (see Chapter 19)
- Chemotherapy (see Chapter 19)

OSTEOMYELITIS

▶ Infection of the bone and surrounding tissue that can be difficult to treat and can result in chronic recurrence, loss of function and mobility, possibly amputation, and even death

▶ Etiology:

- Acute—generally spread through vascular system into the bone and synovial tissue
- Chronic—can be caused by any microorganism

▶ Lifespan considerations:

- Children—if growth plates involved, may develop limb-length discrepancies and deformities
- Recurrences are possible even years after initial treatment

▶ Diagnostic tests:

- Radiographic tests
- Sedimentation rates are generally elevated
- CBC—leukocytosis
- Blood cultures:
  - Positive 50 to 60% of the time in acute osteomyelitis
  - Generally negative for chronic osteomyelitis
- Aspiration or bone biopsy for culture and sensitivity

▶ Nursing diagnosis:

- Deficient knowledge related to treatment, long-term antibiotics, prevention of recurrence
- Ineffective thermoregulation related to infectious process

▶ Common treatment methods:

- Antibiotics—4 to 6 weeks of parenteral treatment
- Surgical drainage of soft-tissue and bone abscesses as needed
- Hyperbaric oxygen therapy—adjunctive therapy for patients with immune compromise
- Antibiotic depots—antibiotic beads may be placed directly on the site

▶ Nursing considerations:

- Hospital:
  - Teach importance of taking antibiotics as prescribed
  - Mobilization with appropriate limitations of weight bearing
  - Wound care, dressing, hand washing
- Office:
  - Physical therapy as appropriate
  - Reinforce hospital instructions
  - Potential referral to specialty wound center
- Home care:
  - Activity instructions, mobilization
  - Wound care
  - Clean techniques and hand washing

AMPUTATIONS

▶ Removal of part of limb above, below, or through a joint
  - Used for treatment of sarcomas when limb-sparing surgery not possible
  - Necessary when limb is not viable because of advanced infection, crush injury, or sudden severing without possibility of reattachment

▶ Types:
  - Closed amputation—skin flap covers the surgical site to create a stump
  - Open amputation (guillotine)—surgical site is left open because of an infection; second surgery required to close surgical site

▶ Amputation levels:
  - Symes—Proximal to the ankle
  - Below-the-knee (BKA)
  - Above-the-knee (AKA)
  - Knee disarticulation (KD)
  - Hip disarticulation (HD)
  - Below-elbow (BEA)
  - Above-elbow (AEA)
  - Forequarter amputation

▶ Potential complications:
  - Flexion contractures—consider sandbag during initial healing to maintain flexibility of joint proximal to amputation
  - Pressure injuries to distal stumps from prosthetic devices
  - Neuroma at the site of the amputated nerve
  - Wound dehiscence
  - Infection
  - Excessive swelling—due to improper wrapping or not wearing stump sock
  - Phantom sensation/pain
  - Bone overgrowth, especially in children

▶ Nursing diagnosis:
  - Disturbed body image related to amputation
  - Grieving related to loss of body part
  - Acute pain related to postoperative pain, phantom (residual) pain

▶ Patient teaching:
  - Monitor residual limb site for redness, swelling and drainage.
  - Do not elevate residual limb.
  - Keep residual limb clean and dry, do not apply lotions to stump.
  - Keep compression bandage on initially to reduce swelling and prepare residual limb for prosthesis.

▶ Recovering amputated parts:
  - Place part in slightly dampened normal saline or dry sterile gauze (if available).
  - Place part in watertight, sealed bag or container.
  - Do not place amputated tissue in water/saline or any solution.
  - Place watertight, sealed bag/container on ice
  - Note time elastic bandage applied and when cooling of tissue begins

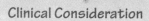

Clinical Consideration

Phantom (residual) limb pain occurs in many amputees; usually subsides as patient recovers and begins to ambulate.

Clinical Consideration

Elevating the residual limb is a major cause of flexion contractures.

OSTEOPOROSIS

▶ Common metabolic disease of the bone in which the rate of bone resorption is faster than the rate of bone formation:

- Severe reduction in the skeletal bone mass
- Increase susceptibility to fractures

▶ Etiology—exact cause unknown, contributing risk factors include:

- Immobilization
- Endocrine disorders
- Advanced age
- Nutritional abnormalities
- Smoking
- Low body weight, thin build
- Low calcium, low vitamin D
- Parental history
- Estrogen or androgen deficiency
- Certain drugs:
  - Corticosteroids
  - Heparin
  - Anticonvulsants
  - Immunosuppressants
  - Alcohol

▶ Pathophysiology—disturbance of normal osteoblastic and osteoclastic balance, loss of trabecular bone, medullary widening and decreased bone density

▶ Lifespan considerations:

- Calcium supplementation recommended for both premenopausal and postmenopausal women and men because calcium intake in all age groups is generally found to be deficient.
- Regular weight-bearing exercise regimen is recommended.
- Incidence of fractures increases in elderly.

▶ Assessment:

- History:
  - Family history of osteoporosis
  - Excessive height loss or fractures from minor trauma
  - Dietary calcium intake, vitamin D
  - Medication history
  - Physical examination

▶ Diagnostic tests:

- Urinary calcium may be elevated
- Serum osteocalcin is elevated
- Radiographic findings:
  - Osteoporotic changes are not apparent until >30% of bone mass lost
  - Diffuse radiolucency of bones
  - Old and/or recent compression fractures commonly found
- Bone mineral density:
  - DEXA
  - Quantitative ultrasound

▶ Nursing diagnosis:

- Imbalanced nutrition—less than body requirements, related to inadequate intake of calcium and vitamin D
- Risk for injury; fracture, reduced bone mass

▶ Common treatment methods:

- Prevention and early detection should be initiated before bone loss occurs to promote best outcome.
- Active treatment required if prevention fails.

▶ Pharmacologic management:

- Estrogen-replacement therapy (controversial)
- Antiresorptive therapy
  - Alendronate (Fosamax)
  - Risedronate (Actonel)
  - Calcitonin
  - Monthly bisphosphonate ibandronate (Boniva)
  - Teriparatide (Forteo)
  - Denosumab (Prolia)
- Calcium supplementation and adequate vitamin D

▶ Patient teaching:

- Exercise—weight-bearing regimen
- Fall-prevention strategies
- Medications:
  - Potential side effects—serious allergic reactions, low blood calcium, increased risk of fracture, heartburn, bloating, mild nausea, or vomiting
  - Administration instructions
  - By mouth, nasal spray, injections
- Drug interactions—review current regimen for interactions
  - Common interactions with alcohol consumption

RHABDOMYOLYSIS

▶ Syndrome stemming from direct or indirect muscle injury. Death of muscle tissue releases myoglobin, a damaging protein, into the blood stream

▶ Pathophysiology:

- Large-protein molecules damage renal cells and can lead to renal failure.

▶ Lifespan considerations:

- More common in males

▶ Assessment:

- Signs and symptoms can be hard to identify.
- Classic triad:
  - Muscle pain
  - Red or brown urine with decreased urine output
  - Muscle weakness

▶ Diagnostic tests:

- Creatine kinase elevated
- Urinalysis—presence of myoglobin
- Serum potassium—often significantly elevated
- Increased blood urea nitrogen
- Increased creatinine
- Decreased estimated glomerular filtration rate (eGFR)

- Nursing diagnosis:
  - Impaired physical mobility related to myalgia and muscle weakness
  - Risk for deficient fluid volume—reduced blood flow to kidneys
- Common treatment methods:
  - Vigorous fluid resuscitation
  - Supportive care for renal failure and coagulopathies
- Nursing considerations:
  - Maintain strict intake and output measurements
  - Daily weights
  - Pain management

FIBROMYALGIA

- Syndrome of diffuse musculoskeletal (nonjoint) pain and tenderness, often accompanied by subjective symptoms such as fatigue, memory difficulties, and irritable bowel symptoms.
- Etiology—overall unknown, attributed to human stress response and abnormalities in sensory processing.
- Pathophysiology—believed to be either an inflammatory or psychiatric condition, but no evidence supports either theory. Environmental factors may include psychological stress, trauma, or presence of infection. Appears to result from processes in the central nervous system. Medically unexplained.
- Lifespan considerations:
  - Highest incidence between ages 60 and 79
  - Onset in adolescence occurs predominantly in girls
  - May overlap with chronic fatigue syndrome, making differential diagnosis difficult
- Assessment:
  - History and physical exam:
    - Diffuse and burning pain that waxes and wanes; difficult to describe if in muscles, joints, or soft tissues
    - Extreme fatigue, weakness
    - Frequent absence from work
    - Positive point of tenderness in virtually all parts of the body
  - Localized erythema may manifest during palpation
  - Weary look, with flat or anxious affect
  - Fibromyalgia classification criteria established by the American College of Rheumatology (ACR) in 1990 includes history of widespread pain in all four quadrants of the body for a minimum of 3 consecutive months and pain in at least 11 of 18 designated tender points when pressure is applied. (Wolff et al., 1990)
  - New diagnostic criteria developed by the ACR in 2010 does not use pressure points, but focuses on pain being widespread accompanied by additional symptoms such as sleep disturbances, fatigue, and cognitive disruption. (Wolff et al., 2010)
  - Physicians must rule out other causes of widespread pain before diagnosing fibromyalgia.
- Diagnostic tests:
  - Primarily for purposes of ruling out other conditions
  - No specific diagnostic tests for definitive diagnosis
  - Routine laboratory analyses reveal little to no differential information.
  - Serologic assays should be avoided unless there is strong evidence of autoimmune involvement related to a low predictive value with fibromyalgia syndrome.

▶ Common treatment methods:
- Coordinated and collaborative approach vital, as long-term follow-up generally reveals little to no consistent symptom improvement.

▶ Nonpharmacologic management:
- Massage or reflexology may alleviate symptoms.
- Acupuncture or chiropractic manipulation has been shown to produce positive results in some studies.
- Local heat therapy often provides relief.
- Meditation to decrease sensory overload.

▶ Pharmacologic management:
- Variety of medications approved for treatment to address pain and improve sleep:
  - Pregabalin (Lyrica)
  - Duloxetine HCl (Cymbalta)
  - Milnacipran HCl (Savella)
- Not generally responsive to corticosteroids; minimally responsive to NSAIDs.
- Tramadol (Ultram) has been associated with effective analgesia.
- Adjunctive medications may be used in low doses to decrease pain and improve sleep:
  - Low-dose tricyclic antidepressants
  - Low-dose selective serotonin-reuptake inhibitors (SSRIs)
  - Benzodiazepines
  - Muscle relaxants
- Localized pain can be treated with topical ointments (e.g., capsaicin cream) or by injections at tender points
- Anecdotal reports that herbal therapies provide relief:
  - St. John's wort
  - Chromium picolinate
  - Melatonin or Calms Forté
  - Peppermint oil to help with irritable bowel
- Higher-dose SSRIs, other antidepressants for depression if needed

▶ Patient teaching:
- Reinforce basics of sleep hygiene
- Reinforce value of consistent exercise plan for relief of symptoms
- Educate regarding potential triggers:
  - Caffeine
  - Cereals made from wheat or corn
  - Dairy products
  - Yeast
  - Citrus
- Promote utilization of both nonpharmacologic and pharmacologic pain-management strategies.

GOUT

▶ Disorder in purine metabolism characterized by monosodium urate crystal deposits in joints and surrounding tissues that lead to acute attacks of arthritis.

▶ Etiology:
- Excess production of uric acid and/or decreased renal excretion of uric acid
- 10% of patients experience secondary gout resulting from drug therapies or other medical conditions:
  - Hemolytic anemia, psoriasis, chronic kidney disease

- Hypertension
- Metabolic syndrome
- Type 2 diabetes mellitus
- Thiazide and loop diuretics
- Obesity or starvation
- Lead toxicity
- Organ transplant recipients who take cyclosporine

▶ Pathophysiology—Uric acid is a normal end product of purine metabolism. When an excess exists, crystal deposits occur:

- Lower temperature of distal extremities thought to contribute to crystal deposition in metatarsals
- May also be related to repetitive minor trauma in sites where crystal deposition occurs

▶ Lifespan considerations:

- Duration and extent and age at onset of hyperuricemia directly correlate with likelihood of gouty arthritis developing.
- Initial onset can be followed by long periods (decade) of asymptomatic hyperuricemia.
- Older adults with decreased renal function who use diuretics are particularly susceptible.

▶ Complications:

- Soft-tissue damage and deformity
- Joint destruction with crippling deformity
- Nerve-compression syndromes
- Uric acid nephrolithiasis, chronic urate nephropathy, acute uric acid nephropathy
- Hypertension, hyperlipidemia

▶ Assessment:

- Swelling, pain, decreased range of motion of affected joints. Typically found in metatarsal joint in great toe; also, fingers, knees, ankles, wrists, elbows
- Tophi may be found in bone, joint, bursa, soft tissue
- Other possible findings—fever, headache, hypertension

▶ Diagnostic tests:

- Radiologic findings:
  - Normal findings in early gout
  - Asymmetric swelling seen in affected joint
  - Baseline films can help identify disease progression
- Synovial fluid aspiration
  - Demonstrates characteristic monosodium urate crystals
  - May be therapeutic as well as diagnostic
- Serum urate levels
- Evaluation of renal, cardiac, and vascular systems

▶ Nursing diagnosis:

- Impaired physical mobility related to musculoskeletal impairment
- Chronic pain related to inflammation of affected joint

▶ Nonpharmacologic management:

- Weight reduction
- Decreased alcohol consumption
- Decreased consumption of foods high in purine:
  - Alcoholic beverages (all types)
  - Fish/seafood such as anchovies, sardines, herring, mussels, codfish, scallops, trout, and haddock
  - Some meats, such as bacon, turkey, veal, and venison, and organ meats such as liver

- Control of hypertension, hyperlipidemia
- High fluid intake (>2 L/day)
▶ Pharmacologic management:
  - NSAIDs drug of choice
  - Colchicine effective alternative to NSAIDs
  - Intraarticular injections of corticosteroids
  - Systemic steroids
  - Prevention:
    • Antihyperuricemic therapy:
      - Allopurinol (Zyloprim)
▶ Patient teaching:
  - Patient must have high level of understanding regarding dietary guidelines:
    • Decreased intake of red and organ meats
    • Decreased alcohol intake
    • Avoid sudden, severe dietary modifications
  - Patient must have high level of understanding regarding gout medications and their potential interactions with other medications.
  - Encourage ice and elevation for relief.

COMPARTMENT SYNDROME

▶ Condition in which progressive pressure within a confined space (muscle compartment) compromises circulation within the space. Can lead to tissue death.
  - Classified as acute or crush syndrome/rhabdomyolysis
  - Acute—medical emergency, generally occurs after trauma
  - Crush syndrome/rhabdomyolysis—can be exacerbated by hypovolemia due to frank hemorrhage or trapped fluids. Aggressive treatment is necessary to prevent prolonged multiorgan failure and death. Acute renal failure a major complication.
▶ Etiology—Increased capillary pressure within the compartment
  - Increased volume in compartment:
    • Vascular injury after fracture or a coagulation defect with bleeding into compartment
    • Postischemic swelling following trauma
    • Reperfusion injury after restoration of tissue perfusion
    • Arterial clot
  - External pressure—tight cast, or crushing injury
  - Decreased compartment size—excessive traction
  - Contributing factors—acute trauma, fracture, infection, tibial nailing, insensate extremity, significant venous obstruction, significant IV infiltration, frostbite, venomous bite
▶ Pathophysiology:
  - Compartments are surrounded by tough facial tissue. Swelling increases the pressure within the compartment, which decreases capillary blood perfusion. Tissue hypoxia and cell death result (Figure 15.4).
  - Muscle damage is irreversible after 4 to 8 hours of ischemia.
  - Nerve damage is irreversible after 8 hours of ischemia if pressure is unrelieved.
  - Tissue pressure may be measured with Stryker device; however, must be certain that device is within affected compartment.

Clinical Consideration

A medical emergency; can be limb-threatening.

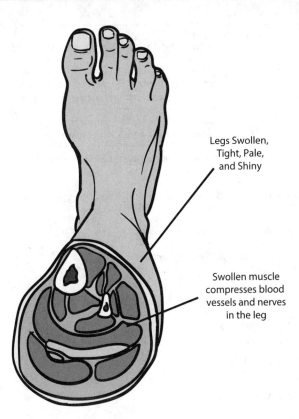

Legs Swollen,
Tight, Pale,
and Shiny

Swollen muscle
compresses blood
vessels and nerves
in the leg

Figure 15.4 Compartment Syndrome

▌ Lifespan considerations:
- Children have decreased cell viability at a lower pressure than adults. Intervention is mandatory when compartment pressure exceeds 30 mm Hg of mean arterial pressure. 18-gauge needle (typical in Stryker device assessment) is too large for use in children.

▌ Complications:
- Volkmann's contracture—rapidly forming flexion deformity of the wrist and fingers
- Sensory and motor deficits
- Muscle necrosis
- Infection
- Rhabdomyolysis
- Amputation
- Limb deformity/contractures
- Acute kidney injury (AKI)
- Hyperkalemia secondary to crush syndrome rhabdomyolysis

▌ Preventive strategies:
- Avoid external pressure to affected areas
- Monitor for early symptoms of tight cast, splint, or dressing:
  - Increased pain
  - Increased swelling
  - Numbness
  - Paresthesia
- Provide adequate hydration to maintain mean arterial pressure

TABLE 15.4	COMPARTMENT SYNDROME
6 Ps	Assessment
Pain	Primary early indicator; unrelieved with appropriate narcotics; progressive, out of proportion to what is expected for injury
Pressure	Palpable tightness of compartment; sometimes shiny appearance; difficult to assess with deep compartments
Pallor	Unhealthy, pale appearance; cool temperature when compared to opposite limb
Paresthesia (late indicator)	Decreased topical sensation; burning and tingling in affected area; indicative of decreased perfusion
Paralysis (late indicator)	Progressive decrease in motor strength and motion
Pulselessness (late indicator)	Tissue death imminent

▶ Assessment (Table 15.4)
▶ Diagnostic tests:
  • Primary test related to differential diagnosis is measurement of intracompartmental pressure.
  • Not mandatory for definitive diagnosis
▶ Nursing diagnosis:
  • Ineffective tissue perfusion related to increased pressure within extremity compartment
  • Acute pain related to compromised extremity
▶ Common treatment methods:
  • Relieve pressure:
    • Bivalve cast, remove splint, remove or loosen constrictive bandage, release or decrease traction
  • Maintain extremity at heart level. Elevating above heart level reduces arteriovenous pressure, which may lead to further compromise of perfusion.
  • Surgical intervention—relieve compartmental pressure via fasciotomy:
    • Wound remains open to prevent "rebound" compartment syndrome.
    • Skin graft frequently needed to achieve closure.
  • Amputation if severe neuromuscular damage has occurred
▶ Nursing considerations:
  • Assess neurovascular function frequently to identify subtle changes for early interventions.
  • Administer analgesics in timely manner and assess response to pain interventions.
  • If fasciotomy occurs—teach wound care with signs and symptoms of infection.
  • Reinforce activity restrictions.

FAT EMBOLISM SYNDROME (FES)

▶ FES is the presence of fat globules in the pulmonary circulation system, which become trapped in the lung capillaries causing a blockage of blood circulation.
▶ Etiology—fatty marrow is released into circulation following long-bone fracture; high incidence with multifracture or crush injuries:
  • Long bones include femur, tibia, and fibula.
▶ Pathophysiology—multiple theories exist; exact pathophysiology unknown

- Mechanical theory:
  - Fat embolized by direct entry into circulation
  - Fracture disrupts intramedullary compartment releasing fat cells into circulation
  - Cerebral signs and petechiae caused by direct obstruction of capillaries in brain and skin
  - Hypoxia and progressive distress caused by obstruction of the vessels in the lungs
- Biochemical theory:
  - Increased fatty acid circulation
  - Lysis of triglycerides may occur at time of injury, mobilizing free fatty acids
  - Release of catecholamines after major injuries may increase amount of circulating free fatty acids
  - Interaction with CRP with triglycerides may lead to increased formation of fat globules within the bloodstream.
- Effects:
  - Acute mechanical obstruction of pulmonary arteries causes right heart failure
  - Inflammatory cascade causes interstitial pulmonary edema leading to adult respiratory distress syndrome (ARDS)
  - Hypoxia causes cerebral decompensation, death
- Lifespan considerations:
  - Uncommon in children
  - Most common in males
- Prevention strategies:
  - Stabilization of long-bone fractures to avoid excessive movement before fixation
  - Aggressive fluid resuscitation to prevent hypovolemia
  - Minimal delay to surgical fixation—within 24 to 48 hours
- Assessment:
  - Classic triad of symptoms:
    - Hypoxemia—sense of impending doom, severe apprehension, restlessness
    - Neurologic abnormalities—agitation, anxiety, mental status changes
    - Petechial rash—skin and mucosa, frequently anterior side of chest and neck extending down to navel
- Diagnostic tests:
  - Characteristic serum laboratory results:
    - Sudden decrease in hemoglobin/hematocrit with onset of symptoms
    - Decreased platelets
    - Free fatty acids elevated
    - Increased ESR
  - Chest x-ray shows a diffuse snowstorm pattern (small granular opacities).
- Common treatment methods:
  - Primarily supportive interventions:
    - Oxygen therapy; intubation and ventilatory support as indicated
    - Fluid resuscitation
    - Airway management
    - Intensive-care-unit monitoring
- Nursing considerations:
  - Immediate intervention with onset of symptoms
  - Adequate air exchange with airway management
  - Caregiver support

Question	Rationale
What finding would be consistent in the assessment of a geriatric patient? A. Increased fine motor dexterity B. Decreased joint stiffness C. Quicker reflex response D. Slowed reaction time	Answer: D It is not unusual for the geriatric patient to have a decrease in fine motor dexterity, increased joint stiffness, and a slowed reaction time.

PAIN MANAGEMENT

▶ In orthopedics, pain is the most frequent symptom that brings a patient in for treatment.

▶ "An unpleasant sensory and emotional experience associated with actual or potential tissue damage" (International Association for the Study of Pain, 2018):

- Acute pain
- Chronic pain

▶ Effect of unrelieved pain:

- Negative physiologic and psychologic consequences
- Increased health care costs/lengthened hospital stays, increased use of health care
- Decreased patient satisfaction
- Significant impact on quality of life
- Depressed immune response
- Increased risk of falls in the elderly
- Can lead to death
- Can lead to chronic pain syndromes
- Complex regional pain syndrome

▶ Cross-cultural considerations:

- Culture has significant impact on personal reactions and adaptations to pain

▶ Ethical principles:

- Autonomy—patient's right to self-determination; nurse has obligation to inform the patient of options, including risk, benefit, and cost.
- Beneficence—nurses' responsibility to benefit the patient with safest and most reasonable method to control pain.
- Nonmalfeasance—nurse must avoid causing harm; must protect patient from harm; pain management can impact mortality.
- Veracity—nurse must be truthful in providing patient care. The use of a placebo to test for legitimacy of pain abuses the relationship between patient and caregiver indefensibly unethical.
- Justice—Limited resources in a high-cost environment obligates all members of team to use the least costly method of relieving pain.

▶ Principles of assessment:

- Person experiencing pain is the true source for assessment.
- Believe the patient's report of pain.
- Reassess after every intervention.
- Individualize pain-management plan.
- Assess and plan for constipation for all patients receiving opioids.

- Never use placebos.
- Recognize and treat side effects.
- Be aware of development of physical dependence and prevent withdrawal.
- Communicate pain management plan to others; provide continuity from one health care setting to another.
- Administer around the clock when pain is continuous:
  - Long-acting medications can increase risk of accidental overdose
- Give adequate doses and titrate to effect
- Immediate-release opioids for use in breakthrough pain
- Assess for constipation

▶ Potential complications of pain medication:

- Withdrawal—when physical or psychological dependence is present, the body develops withdrawal symptoms when medication is discontinued abruptly.
  - Emotional symptoms:
    - Anxiety, restlessness, irritability, insomnia, depression, isolation
  - Physical symptoms:
    - Sweating, nausea, vomiting, diarrhea, racing heart, palpitations, tremors
  - Dangerous withdrawal symptoms:
    - Grand mal seizures
    - Hallucinations
    - Delirium tremens
    - Myocardial infarction
    - Stroke
- Dependency:
  - Physiologic—body makes changes to adapt to medication; cause withdrawal symptoms when medication abruptly discontinued
  - Psychologic—emotional need for a drug that has no underlying physical need
- Tolerance—as the body adapts to the medication, increased dosing becomes necessary to produce the same effect.
- Ceiling effect—the phenomenon when a drug reaches a maximum effect so that increasing the dosage does not increase the effectiveness.

▶ Regional analgesia:

- Epidural steroid injections
- Nerve blocks—injection of local anesthesia directly into tissue to block sensation
- Bier block—intravenous regional anesthesia
- Implantable long-term analgesia pumps

▶ Common nonpharmacologic treatment methods:

- Therapeutic touch
- Massage
- Immobilization/support of involved part
- Elevation
- Thermal interventions—heat and cold application
- TENS
- Alternative methods:
  - Distraction
  - Deep breathing
  - Hypnosis

- Relaxation
- Spiritual interventions
- Acupuncture
- Imagery
- Humor
- Biofeedback
- Herbal

▶ Nursing considerations:
- Teach patient and family about analgesic pain relievers
- Titration of doses and dosage intervals
- Assessment and reassessment after interventions
- Clear communication between patient and nurse
- Persistence in attempting to provide optimal pain relief

▶ Gerontologic considerations—unrelieved pain increases fall risk and risk of delirium

▶ Myths and barriers to adequate pain relief:
- Inadequate assessment and reassessment of pain
- Inadequate knowledge of pain management
- Patient's resistance to report pain because of fear of addiction
- Physician's reluctance to prescribe pain medication
- Nurse's reluctance to administer opioids
- Patient's fear of side effects
- Knowledge deficit in patients and providers understanding that pain management is a right
- Institutional, procedural, and legal barriers

PERIOPERATIVE ASSESSMENT AND TEACHING

▶ Definition:
- Preoperative—begins with patient's decision to have surgery and ends when patient enters the operating room
- Intraoperative—begins with patient's transfer into the operating room and ends when the patient is admitted to the postanesthesia care unit
- Postoperative—begins with discharge from the operating room and ends with termination of treatment

▶ Preoperative assessment:
- Complete history, including previous surgical and anesthesia experiences with any complications
- Complete medication history—including over-the-counter medications and herbal supplements
- Allergy history—medications, anesthesia drugs; those with banana, avocado, kiwi, chestnut allergies are probably also allergic to latex
- Physical exam—absence of skin breakdown, neurovascular baseline, vitals
- Family history—specific attention to malignant hyperthermia or pseudocholinesterase deficiency
- Social history:
  - Presence of help after discharge and potential for financial burden
- Site marking

- Time-out
- Informed consent
- Laboratory studies:
  - Blood type and screen if blood loss anticipated
  - Electrolytes, urinalysis, chest x-ray and electrocardiogram as determined based on age and medical history
- May need other diagnostic procedures or laboratory tests depending on risks, medical history, and comorbidities

▸ Intraoperative considerations:
- Potential complications of general anesthesia:
  - Pulmonary aspiration
  - Hypovolemia
  - Cardiac arrhythmias
  - Hypothermia
  - Hypotension
- Positioning:
  - Optimal exposure of surgical site
  - Prevent pressure injury
  - Assess for neurovascular impairment
  - Prevent nerve injuries
  - Tourniquet safety—calibrate gauges, select appropriate cuff size, monitor time, document air pressures and release times
- Skin preparation:
  - Begin at the cleanest part and move outward
  - Avoid pooling of solutions under the patient
  - Hair removal—clip only if interferes with surgical area
- Infection prevention:
  - Aseptic technique—maintaining sterile field
  - Limiting traffic patterns in operating room
  - Airflow and filtration
  - Surgical counts—critical for safety, prevention of retention of foreign objects

▸ Postoperative considerations:
- Phase 1 recovery—maintain airway patency, air exchange, and circulation
- Phase 2 recovery—assessment upon admission to the inpatient unit:
  - Level of consciousness, vitals, nausea/vomiting, neurovascular assessment of extremities, status of incision, status of tubes, dressing and drains, comfort level, positioning, intake and output
- First void—prevent retention
- Patient teaching—preparing for self-care after discharge
- Discharge instructions:
  - Activity
  - Diet
  - Medication
  - Bathing restrictions
  - Wound care
  - Follow-up care/complications—when to call physician
  - Home care considerations, equipment needs, adaptive devices

CASE STUDY

A 76-year-old male was admitted through the emergency department because of a fall at home, where he lives with his wife. Patient reports severe pain in his left lower extremity, which is shortened and externally rotated. Medical history includes atrial fibrillation, hypertension, and arthritis.

Current medications include:

Hydrochlorothiazide 25 mg daily

Warfarin 2.5 mg daily

Ibuprofen 400 mg three times a day as needed for pain

1. **Based on assessment findings what diagnosis might be expected?**
   - *The patient presents with obvious signs of a fractured hip, shortened and externally rotated leg.*
   - *Radiographs are necessary for definitive diagnosis.*

2. **What other information would be important to know?**
   - *Circumstances surrounding the fall: physiologic symptoms or mechanical barrier?*
   - *Time since last food intake?*
   - *When was the last dose of warfarin?*
   - *Did the patient strike his head?*
   - *Were any other injuries noted?*

3. **What diagnostic tests would the provider probably order?**
   - *Bilateral hip anteroposterior and lateral radiographic studies*
   - *Current coagulopathy studies: risk for bleeding before and after surgical intervention*
   - *Blood type and cross match*
   - *Urinalysis*

4. **What education would be provided to this patient?**
   - *Preoperative teaching:*
     - *Importance of early mobilization after surgery*
     - *Pain-management strategies*
     - *Coughing and deep breathing, incentive spirometer (IS)*
   - *Preventing postoperative complications:*
     - *Infection: antibiotics, hand hygiene*
     - *Atelectasis: coughing, deep breathing, IS 10 times every hour while awake*
     - *Deep-vein thrombosis: early mobility, compression device usage, Lovenox or Heparin*
     - *Constipation: stool softener, laxative*
   - *Fall prevention strategies in the hospital and after discharge:*
     - *Environment free of clutter, remove throw rugs*
     - *Adequate lighting*
     - *Appropriate assistive devices as indicated*

The patient is diagnosed with a fractured hip and is scheduled for surgical repair with open reduction internal fixation.

1. **Following the immediate postoperative recovery period, the most important nursing intervention is:**
   a. *Providing hydration*
   b. *Ensuring proper nutrition*

   c. *Promoting safe mobilization*

   d. *Assessing bowel and bladder elimination*

Answer: c. Mobilization. Mobility prevents blood clots, decreases risk of pulmonary complications, decreases fall risk, and stimulates bone growth.

2. **Before mobilizing the patient, the nurse must assess and verify:**

   a. *Mentation*

   b. *Weight-bearing status*

   c. *Availability of assistive devices*

   d. *Level of function prior to surgery*

Answer: b. Weight-bearing status. Depending on the outcome of the repair in surgery, the physician determines any weight restriction for the limb. Generally, "weight bearing as tolerated" is the preferred status, as a patient will naturally protect the limb if there is pain. However, when severe osteoporosis is present or there are multiple fractures, it may be necessary to limit pressure on the healing bone for a period of time.

3. **On postoperative day 3, the patient declares that "nothing keeps him down for long and he'll be back on the golf course in 2 to 3 weeks". The appropriate response from the nurse is:**

   a. *Good for you! A great attitude goes a long way to improving your health.*

   b. *Bones are slow to heal. Be sure to pay careful attention to your physician's recommendations on the timing of returning to normal activity.*

   c. *Everyone heals differently, I hope you meet your goal.*

   d. *Golf is a great physical activity to get you back in shape.*

Answer: b. Bones are slow to heal. Patients are often surprised at the length of recovery after a fracture. Setting clear expectations around minimum healing times can assist patients in coping with injury.

Discussion

Nursing care plans for patients with musculoskeletal conditions include: pain control and mobility interventions. After treatment, mobilization becomes the primary nursing intervention to prevent complications and promote return to function. Pain control can be a barrier to mobilization, and careful planning for pain management can facilitate maximum mobility for a patient postoperatively. Safe patient handling is a necessary skill for nurses assisting patients with mobility issues following a musculoskeletal injury. Appropriate assistive devices provide the necessary support for patients to achieve maximum function.

Bibliography

International Association for the Study of Pain. (2018). Terminology. Accessed July 22, 2018 from http://www.iasp-pain.org/terminology?navItemNumber=576#Pain

Murphy, A.C., Muldoon, S.F., Baker, D., Lastowka, A., Bennett, B., Yang, M., and Bassett, D.S. (2018). Structure, function, and control of the human musculoskeletal network. *PLoS Biology 16*, e2002811.

NAON. (2016). *Core Curriculum for Orthopaedic Nursing*, 7th ed. (New York: Pearson Custom).

Potter, P.A., Perry, A.G., Stockert, P.A., and Hall, A.M. (2017). *Fundamentals of Nursing*, 9th ed. (St. Louis: Elsevier/Mosby).

Shekelle, P.G., Newberry, S.J., FitzGerald, J.D., Motala, A., O'Hanlon, C.E., Tariq, A., ... Shanman, R. (2017). Management of gout: a systematic review in support of an American College of Physicians Clinical Practice Guideline. *Annals of Internal Medicine 166*, 37–51.

The Joint Commission. (2012). *Universal Protocol for Safe Surgical Procedures*. Accessed February 15, 2018, from https://www.jointcommission.org/assets/1/18/UP_Poster1.PDF

Wolfe, F., Clauw, D. J., Fitzcharles, M., Goldenberg, D. L., Katz, R. S., Mease, P., ... Yunus, M. B. (2010), The American College of Rheumatology Preliminary Diagnostic Criteria for Fibromyalgia and Measurement of Symptom Severity. *Arthritis Care Res, 62*: 600–610. doi:10.1002/acr.20140

Wolfe, F., Smythe, H. A., Yunus, M. B., Bennett, R. M., Bombardier, C. , Goldenberg, D. L., ... Sheon, R. P. (1990), The american college of rheumatology 1990 criteria for the classification of fibromyalgia. *Arthritis & Rheumatism, 33*: 160–172. doi:10.1002/art.1780330203

Woodard, D., and Van Demark, R.J. (2017). The opioid epidemic in 2017: are we making progress? *South Dakota Medicine: The Journal of The South Dakota State Medical Association* 70, 467–471.

16

Hematologic System

Donna Martin, DNP, RN, CMSRN, CDE, CNE

OVERVIEW

▌ The hematologic system consists of organs that are responsible for the production of blood cells. The organs that make up this system include the lymph nodes, spleen, thymus, and bone marrow.

ANATOMY AND PHYSIOLOGY

▌ Structure and functions:
- Lymph nodes:
  - Located throughout the body
  - Connected through the lymph vessels
  - Macrophage action removes foreign particles at the lymph tissue
- Spleen:
  - Macrophage and immune response to bloodborne antigens
  - Recycles iron from destroyed red cells for future use in the body
  - Conditions immature erythrocytes
- Thymus:
  - Secretes hormones that play a role in the maturation of peripheral T cells
- Bone marrow:
  - Yellow marrow (adipose):
    - No role in blood-cell production
    - Stores adipocytes; triglycerides can serve as source of energy
  - Red marrow (hematopoietic):
    - Actively produces blood cells
    - Located in long bones, pelvic bones, vertebra, sacrum, sternum, ribs
- Blood performs three major functions:
  - Transport:
    - Oxygen from the lungs to the cells

- Nutrients to the cells
- Waste products from the cells for excretion by the lungs, liver, and/or kidneys
- Regulate:
    - Oncotic pressure
    - Fluid–electrolyte balance
    - Acid–base balance
- Protect:
    - Maintain homeostasis (clotting factors)
    - Prevent infection (white cells)
- Blood components:
- Plasma:
    - 55% of blood volume
    - Contains:
        - Water
        - Proteins:
            - Albumin
            - Globulin
            - Fibrinogen
        - Gamma-globulin with antibody immunoglobulins; essential for defending against microorganisms:
            - Immunoglobulin (Ig) M
            - IgG
            - IgA
            - IgD
            - IgE
- Blood cells:
    - 45% of blood volume
    - Erythrocytes (red cells): (Figure 16.1)
        - Lifespan, 120 days
        - Transport oxygen to cells and carbon dioxide to lungs
        - Assist with acid–base balance
    - Leukocytes (white cells):
        - Granulocytes—primary function is phagocytosis
        - Neutrophils—increased in acute inflammatory process
        - Eosinophils—increased in allergic response and parasitic infections
        - Basophils—increased in allergic and inflammatory reactions
        - Monocytes
        - Lymphocytes
    - Thrombocytes (platelets):
        - Lifespan, 8 to 10 days
        - Initiatesclotting response
- Normal clotting mechanisms:
- Critical process in minimizing blood loss
- Process activated by a vascular injury and subendothelial exposure:
    - Local vasoconstriction
    - Adhesion of platelets to glycoproteins

- Activation of fibrinogen receptors on platelets, causing aggregation
- Thrombin converts fibrinogen into fibrin
- Platelet plug formed as a result of strengthened clot
- Clot retraction and dissolution as the area of injury heals

▶ Gerontologic considerations:
- Age-related changes
  - Decline in red-cell mass
- Other factors:
  - Decreased nutritional intake
  - Comorbidities
  - Cancer

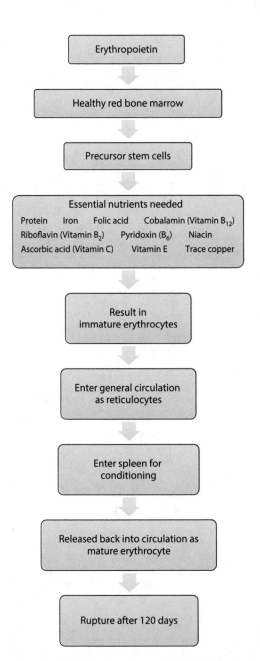

Figure 16.1 The Process of Red-Cell Production—Erythropoiesis

DIAGNOSTIC TESTS

▶ Laboratory:
- Complete blood count (CBC) with differential: (Table 16.1)
  - Red cells—total number circulating
  - Hemoglobin (Hgb)—oxygen-carrying pigment of red cells
  - Hematocrit (Hct)—percent volume of red cells in whole blood
  - Red-cell indexes (used in determining cause/type of anemia):
    - Mean corpuscular volume (MCV)—determines relative size of red cells
    - Mean corpuscular hemoglobin (MCH)—red-cell saturation/weight
    - Mean corpuscular hemoglobin concentration (MCHC)—red-cell saturation
  - White cells—total number
  - White-cell differential:
    - Neutrophils—acute inflammatory reaction
    - Eosinophils—parasite infections, allergic reactions
    - Basophils—allergic and inflammatory reactions

TABLE 16.1	DIAGNOSTIC TESTS
Test	Normal Value*
Red-cell count	Male: 4.7–6.1 Female: 4.2–5.4
Hemoglobin (Hgb)	Male: 13.2–17.3 g/dL Female: 11.7–15.5 g/dL
Hematocrit (Hct)	Male: 39–50% Female: 35–47%
Reticulocytes	0.5–2%
Platelet count	150,000–400,000/mm³
Red-cell indices	
Mean corpuscular volume (MCV)	80–95 fL
Mean corpuscular hemoglobin (MCH)	27–31 pg
Mean corpuscular hemoglobin concentration (MCHC)	32–36%
White-cell count	5000–10,000/mm³
White-cell indices	
Neutrophils	55–70% 2500–8000/mm³
Lymphocytes	20–40% 1000–4000/mm³
Monocytes	2–8% 100–700/mm³
Eosinophils	1–4% 50–500/mm³
Basophils	0.5–1% 25–100/mm³
*Values may differ by laboratory.	
	Pagana, Pagana, and Pagana (2017)

  - Lymphocytes—viral and chronic bacterial infections
  - Monocytes—chronic inflammatory disorders
- Peripheral blood smear, morphology—determines size and shape of red cells
- Reticulocyte count—number of immature red cells
- Platelet count—number of available platelets
- Serum folic acid levels
- Iron levels:
  - Serum iron
  - Total iron-binding capacity (TIBC)—measures proteins available to bind with iron. This value is increased in most patients with an iron deficiency.
  - Ferritin—the major iron storage protein that indicates available iron stores in the body.
- Serum vitamin B_{12}
- Coagulation studies:
  - Prothrombin time (PT)
  - Partial prothrombin time (PTT)
  - Bleeding time
- Bone marrow analysis:
  - Obtained by:
    - Aspiration
    - Bone marrow biopsy (see Table 16.2 for nursing responsibilities)
    - Surgical removal
  - Microscopic examination of the bone marrow tissue:
    - Number of cells
    - Size of cells
    - Shape of cells
    - Developmental stages of red and white cells and platelets

TABLE 16.2	NURSING RESPONSIBILITIES WHILE CARING FOR A PATIENT UNDERGOING A BONE MARROW BIOPSY
Preprocedure	Explain procedure to patient • Posterior iliac crest is the most common site • Will need to lay on side • May experience brief sharp or stinging pain for aspiration • May experience aching, tugging, or pulling sensation with biopsy • Instruct patient to remain very still during the procedure Obtain consent Administer preprocedure analgesic, as ordered
During procedure	Pain management Assist provider with procedure and possible IV sedation Monitor patient status
Postprocedure	Apply pressure to the puncture site Monitor vital signs Assess for excess drainage or bleeding Administer analgesics as needed Patient teaching • Lay on side of biopsy for 30–60 minutes to apply pressure • Small amount of bleeding is normal • Avoid getting the dressing wet for 24 hours • Avoid rigorous activity or exercise for 24 hours • May experience tenderness at site for several days

HEMATOLOGIC DISORDERS

▶ *Anemia*
- Contributing factors:
  - Dietary deficiency
  - Blood loss:
    - Acute hemorrhage:
      - Trauma
      - Surgery
    - Slow chronic blood loss:
      - Menstruation
      - Gastrointestinal (GI) bleed
      - Cancer
  - Problems with red-cell production:
    - Poor nutritional status:
      - Decreased iron
      - Decreased cobalamin
      - Decreased folic acid
    - Renal disease:
      - Decreased erythropoietin
    - Liver disease:
      - Decreased iron availability due to depleted iron stores and/or inability to synthesize transferrin
    - Medications that may suppress bone marrow production:
      - Corticosteroids
      - Cytotoxic agents
      - Antiinflammatory drugs
      - Radiation
  - Increased red-cell destruction:
    - Hemolytic anemia
    - Prosthetic heart valve
    - Incompatible blood
  - Poor quality of hemoglobin:
    - Abnormal shape:
      - Sickle cell
- Interpretation of laboratory results:
  - Step 1: Look at Hgb quantity—if decreased, anemia is present.
  - Step 2: Look at red-cell quality—this helps to determine the cause of anemia. (Table 16.3)
- Pathophysiology varies with each type of anemia but all result in:
  - Decreased oxygen-carrying capacity:
    - Leading to hypoxia
- ***Assessment/Intervention/Education***
  - Detailed medical history:
    - Nutritional intake and dietary habits
    - Alcohol use
    - Bleeding disorders/previous hematologic disorders
    - Autoimmune disease
    - Pregnancy

TABLE 16.3	QUALITY OF RED CELLS HELPS DETERMINE CAUSE OF ANEMIA

MCV—indicates red-cell size

Small size	-	Microcytic
Normal size	-	Normocytic
Large size	-	Macrocytic

MCH/MCHC—indicates red-cell concentration

Pale color	-	Hypochromic
Normal color	-	Normochromic
Dark color	-	Hyperchromic

- Menstruation history
- Family history of hematologic disorders
- Liver disease
- Recent surgery or trauma
- Recent/current anticoagulant or thrombolytic use:
  - Prescription
  - Over-the-counter medications
  - Herbal supplements
- Recent/current use of medications that may cause anemia:
  - Glyburide
  - Methyldopa
  - Antibiotics
  - Immunosuppressive drugs
- Risk factors:
  - Occupational exposure:
    - Radiation
    - Chemicals
- Clinical manifestations:
  - Dependent on severity and speed of onset
  - Generalized signs/symptoms:
    - Weak
    - Fatigued
    - Dizziness
    - Fainting
  - Cardiac system:
    - Low blood pressure
    - Tachycardia
    - Palpitations
    - Chest pain
    - Systolic murmur
  - Respiratory system:
    - Shortness of breath
    - Tachypnea
    - Decreased oxygen saturation

- Neurologic system (vitamin B deficiencies):
    - Paresthesias, numbness
    - Glossy tongue
    - Confusion, agitation
- Integumentary:
    - Cool skin
    - Pale color
    - Jaundice (due to rapid destruction of red cells)
    - Spoon nails (long-term iron deficiency)
- Nursing diagnosis:
    - Various nursing diagnoses are appropriate for patient experiencing hematologic disorders. Some examples include:
        - Altered tissue perfusion r/t decreased blood volume
        - Fatigue r/t inadequate oxygenation
        - Activity intolerance r/t inadequate oxygenation and decreased blood volume
        - Risk for injury r/t fatigue, weakness
        - Imbalanced nutritional intake: less than body requirements r/t inadequate nutritional intake
        - Deficient knowledge related to medical condition, diagnosis, and treatment
        - Risk for bleeding related to medical condition

Question	Rationale
A 65-year-old female patient underwent a total hip replacement and experienced an intraoperative hemorrhage yesterday. Which test result would you expect to find? A. Hgb 12.2 g/dL B. Hct 38% C. Decreased white-cell count D. Elevated reticulocyte count	Answer: D The hemoglobin and hematocrit are in normal range for a female and the white-cell count should not be impacted by the hemorrhage. Because of the acute blood loss, there would be an increase in the number of reticulocytes as the body tries to replace the lost red cells.

- *Types of anemia*:
    - **Acute blood loss:**
        - Etiology:
            - Sudden hemorrhage/loss of blood resulting in a reduction in vascular volume
        - Clinical manifestations:
            - Hypotension
            - Tachycardia
            - Decreased cardiac output
            - Shortness of breath
            - Hypovolemic shock (Table 16.4)
            - Lactic acidosis

TABLE 16.4	ADVANCED TRAUMA LIFE SUPPORT (ATLS) SHOCK CLASSIFICATION LEVELS	
Classification	Blood Loss	Findings
Class I	<15% blood loss	Mild tachycardia, blood pressure (BP) normal
Class II	15–30% blood loss	Tachycardia, tachypnea, decreased pulse pressure
Class III	30–40% blood loss	Decreased BP, significant tachycardia, narrow pulse pressure
Class IV	≥40% blood loss	Marked tachycardia, BP
		Kahsai (2015)

- Diagnosis:
  - Hgb/Hct may be normal initially, then low once plasma volume is replaced
  - Normocytic (normal size)
  - Normochromic (normal color)
- Treatment:
  - Identify source of bleeding and stop it
  - Replace vascular volume:
    - Blood transfusion
    - IV fluids:
      - Lactated Ringer's
      - Dextran
      - Albumin
  - Erythropoietin, subcutaneous:
    - To be effective, patient must have healthy red bone marrow capable of producing red cells and sufficient nutrients
- Patient teaching:
  - Teach patient about diagnostic tests and treatment
  - Injury/fall prevention
- **Iron deficiency anemia:**
  - Most prevalent hematologic disorder
  - Iron is needed to form healthy red blood cells
  - Etiology:
    - Dietary:
      - Decreased iron intake
      - Malabsorption
    - Chronic blood loss (every 2-mL blood loss = 1 mg iron)
      - As little as 2 to 4 mL/day
      - Peptic ulcers
      - Gastroesophageal reflux disease (GERD)
      - Hemorrhoids
      - Cancer
      - Gastritis
    - Excessive demands for red-cell production

- Diagnosis:
  - Low Hgb/Hct
  - Microcytic
  - Hypochromic
  - Increased TIBC
  - Decreased serum iron
- Treatment:
  - Treat underlying cause:
    - Blood loss
    - Malnutrition
  - Iron replacement:
    - Oral:
      - Depending on severity, three to four doses a day
      - May need to take long-term supplement
    - Intramuscular (IM):
      - Use different needle for drawing up and administration to prevent staining of skin
      - Use Z-track injection method
    - Intravenous piggyback (IVPB)
      - Monitor for allergic/anaphylactic reaction
  - Transfusion of packed red cells if anemia is severe and/or patient is symptomatic
- Patient teaching:
  - Dietary education on foods that are high in iron
  - Alcohol abstinence
  - Take oral iron 1 hour before eating.
  - Vitamin C and ascorbic acid help with absorption.
  - Avoid taking with milk or other dairy products, as these decrease absorption of iron.
  - Side effects of iron may include nausea, vomiting, constipation, black/tarry stools.
  - Concern for accidental overdose—keep away from children, and ensure child-proof cap
- **Pernicious anemia:**
  - Most prevalent form of vitamin B_{12} deficiency
  - Etiology:
    - Autoimmune disorder that leads to malabsorption of vitamin B_{12} because of an absence of intrinsic factor (IF) in gastric secretions
    - Decreased absorption of vitamin B_{12} in terminal ileum
    - Decreased gastric acid production
  - Manifestations may include:
    - Gastrointestinal:
      - Weight loss
      - Loss of appetite
      - Abdominal distention
      - Diarrhea
      - Constipation
      - Steatorrhea

- Neurologic:
  - Numbness/paresthesia of hands and feet
  - Poor gait
  - Memory loss
- Diagnosis:
  - Low Hgb/Hct
  - Macrocytic
  - Normochromic
  - Low reticulocyte count
  - Low vitamin B_{12} level
  - Elevated homocysteine and methylmalonic acid (MMA) levels
  - Presence of intrinsic factor (IF) and parietal-cell antibodies
  - Bone marrow biopsy
- Treatment:
  - IM vitamin B_{12} injections:
    - Daily for the first 1 to 2 weeks
    - Then monthly for life
  - May be able to take vitamin B_{12} orally if some IF present
- Patient teaching:
  - There is no cure
  - Treatment is lifelong
  - May be a problem in some people who have had gastric bypass surgery because of difficulty with absorption
  - Long-term proton-pump inhibitor (PPI) use may impair vitamin B_{12} absorption
- **Folic acid deficiency anemia:**
  - Folic acid is a critical element in the production of healthy red cells
  - Etiology:
    - Dietary deficiency:
      - Lacking green leafy vegetables
      - Eating disorders
      - Malabsorption causes:
        - Celiac disease
        - Crohn's disease
        - Small-bowel resection
      - Chronic alcoholism
      - Sometimes occurs with vitamin B_{12} deficiency
    - Dialysis:
      - Folic acid loss
    - Medications that interfere with folic acid absorption/use:
      - Anticonvulsants
      - Methotrexate
      - Some oral contraceptives
  - Diagnosis:
    - Low Hgb/Hct
    - Macrocytic
    - Normochromic
    - Folic acid level

> **Clinical Consideration**
> Many of the causes are the same as those for pernicious anemia; therefore, the provider should rule out pernicious anemia in addition to folic acid anemia.

- Treatment:
  - Folic acid supplement daily
  - Increase intake of green leafy vegetables and fruits
- Patient teaching:
  - Dietary education on foods that are high in folic acid
- **Aplastic anemia:**
  - Etiology:
    - Decreased red cells, white cells, and platelets (pancytopenia)
    - May be idiopathic or autoimmune response
    - Manifestations may be mild to severe
    - Abrupt, or possibly slow, onset of symptoms
  - Risk factors:
    - Exposure to chemical agents
    - Radiation
    - Viral and bacterial infections
    - Certain medications:
      - Alkylating agents
      - Antimetabolites
      - Antiseizure medications
      - Antimicrobials
      - Nonsteroidal antiinflammatory drugs (NSAIDs)
  - Clinical manifestations:
    - General manifestations of anemia
    - May have neutropenia
    - May have thrombocytopenia
  - Diagnosis:
    - Low Hgb/Hct
    - Normocytic
    - Normochromic
    - Decreased reticulocyte count
    - Decreased white cells
    - Decreased platelets
    - Bone marrow biopsy:
      - Hypocellular marrow
      - Increased yellow marrow
  - Treatment:
    - Identifying and removing cause
    - Neutropenic precautions
    - Thrombocytopenic precautions
    - Immunosuppressive therapy:
      - Antithymocyte globulin (ATG)
      - Cyclosporine
      - High dose cyclophosphamide
    - Hematopoietic stem-cell transplantation (HSCT)
  - Patient teaching:
    - Infection prevention
    - Bleeding prevention

- **Anemia of chronic disease:**
  - Etiology:
    - Causes:
      - Chronic inflammation
      - Chronic disease:
        - Chronic kidney disease
        - Heart failure
      - Autoimmune and infectious disorders:
        - Human immunodeficiency virus (HIV)
        - Malaria
        - Hepatitis
      - Malignant diseases
      - Bleeding episodes
    - Pathophysiology:
      - Underproduction of red cells
      - Shorter red-cell lifespan
  - Clinical manifestations:
    - Anemia occurs within a few months after development of the underlying disorder.
  - Diagnosis:
    - Elevated serum ferritin
    - Increased iron stores
    - Normal folate level
    - Normal cobalamin level
  - Treatment:
    - Correct the underlying disorder
    - May require a blood transfusion
  - Patient teaching:
    - Importance of following treatment plan for underlying disorder
- **Hemolytic anemia:**
  - Etiology:
    - Excessive destruction/hemolysis of red cells faster than the body can manufacture new ones
  - Risk factors:
    - Intrinsic:
      - Hereditary defects in red cells:
        - Sickle cell disease
    - Extrinsic:
      - Healthy red cells damaged by external factors:
        - Prosthetic heart valves
        - Disseminated intravascular coagulopathy (DIC)
        - Thrombotic thrombocytopenic purpura (TTP)
        - Antibodies against red cells
        - Infectious agents
  - Clinical manifestations:
    - General manifestations of anemia
    - Jaundice
    - Enlarged liver and spleen

- Diagnosis:
  - Low Hgb/Hct
  - Normocytic
  - Normochromic
  - Increased reticulocytes
  - Increased bilirubin
- Treatment:
  - Maintain renal function
  - Eliminate cause
  - Hemolytic crisis:
    - Hydration
    - Electrolyte replacement
    - Corticosteroids
    - Blood transfusion
    - Splenectomy
  - Chronic hemolytic anemia:
    - Folic acid
    - Decrease red cell destruction:
      - Immunosuppressive drugs
- Patient teaching:
  - Importance of following treatment for underlying disorder
  - Recognize symptoms
  - Notify provider immediately if experiencing any symptoms
- **Thalassemia:**
  - Autosomal recessive genetic disease
    - Thalassemia minor—heterozygous type
      - Individual has one thalassemic gene and one normal gene
      - Mild condition of the disease
      - Thalassemia minor does not require treatment
    - Thalassemia major—homozygous type:
      - Individual has two thalassemic genes:
        - Develops in childhood
        - Impacts physical and mental growth in children
      - Severe condition
      - Life-threatening disease:
        - Splenomegaly
        - Hepatomegaly
        - Cardiomyopathy from iron overload
        - Pulmonary disease
        - Hypertension
        - Thrombosis
  - Etiology:
    - Decreased erythrocyte production due to inadequate production of normal hemoglobin
    - Red-cell production stimulated in bone marrow

- Hemolysis of excess immature erythrocytes
- Causes enlargement of the bone marrow space and chronic bone marrow hyperplasia
- Spleen becomes enlarged due to excessive clearing of damaged red cells
  - Diagnosis:
    - Low Hgb/Hct
    - Microcytic
    - Hypochromic
    - Increased serum iron
    - Decreased TIBC
    - Increased bilirubin
  - Treatment for thalassemia major:
    - Transfusion management:
      - Blood transfusions or exchange transfusion to maintain a Hgb level of 10 g/dL
      - Iron-binding agents to prevent hemochromatosis
      - Folic acid for hemolysis
    - Splenectomy
    - HSCT
  - Patient/family teaching:
    - Lifelong treatment needed for thalassemia major
    - Importance of monitoring organ function (heart, liver, lung) for complications
- **Sickle cell anemia:**
  - Etiology:
    - Autosomal recessive disorder
    - Abnormal erythrocytes:
      - Stiff and elongated
    - Sickle-shaped cells have difficulty passing through the small vessels and capillaries, leading to tissue injury, vasospasms, and hypoxia.
  - Clinical manifestations:
    - Vary based on severity of disease
    - Asymptomatic except during episodes
    - Pain from tissue ischemia
    - Skin changes may include:
      - Pallor
      - Gray cast
      - Jaundice
    - Involvement of body organs with recurrent episodes:
      - Spleen:
        - Decreased size from repeated scarring (autosplenectomy)
      - Hepatobiliary:
        - Hepatomegaly
        - Gallstones
      - Lung disorders:
        - Pulmonary hypertension

- - Acute chest syndrome
    - Pneumonia
  - Heart failure
  - Renal failure
  - Thrombosis:
    - Stroke
    - Stasis ulcers of extremities
- Ophthalmologic:
  - Retinal detachment
  - Hemorrhage
  - Retinopathy
  - Blindness
- Diagnosis:
  - Low Hgb/Hct
  - Presence of hemoglobin S (Hgb S)
  - Decreased reticulocytes
  - Peripheral-blood smear:
    - Sickle shape
  - Elevated bilirubin
- Treatment:
  - Prevention of episodes of sickle cell crisis
  - Managing clinical manifestations:
    - Effective pain management
    - Oxygen administration
    - Rest
  - Aggressively treat infections:
  - Venous thromboembolism (VTE) prophylaxis
  - Medications:
    - Hydroxyurea (Hydrea):
      - May reduce number of pain crises
      - Improved quality of life
      - Lower incidence of acute chest syndrome
      - May decrease need for blood transfusions
    - Antihistamines to manage itching
    - Opioids/nonopioids for pain management
  - Minimize organ damage
  - Total red cell exchange transfusion
- Patient teaching:
  - Avoid high altitudes, as they may trigger an episode
  - Smoking cessation
  - Alcohol avoidance
  - Maintain adequate fluid intake
  - *Streptococcus pneumoniae* vaccine
  - Complications screening:
    - Annual screening for renal disease

- Notify provider:
  - Changes in respiratory status
  - Infections
  - Temperature >101.3°F

Question	Rationale
The nurse understands that the patient with pernicious anemia will have which distinguishing laboratory finding? A. An negative Schilling test B. Absent intrinsic factor (IF) C. Elevated reticulocyte count D. Decreased granulocytes	Answer: B Pernicious anemia is due to a lack of IF. This prevents the person from being able to absorb vitamin B_{12}, which is needed for the production of healthy red cells. The Schilling test is no longer the standard for diagnosing pernicious anemia. There would not be an increased reticulocyte count, and the granulocytes would not be impacted.

▶ *Blood Transfusions*
- Types of blood products:
  - Whole blood:
    - Composed of red cells, plasma, and plasma proteins
    - Rarely indicated
  - Packed red cells:
    - Replacement of red cells
    - Compatibility considerations
  - Platelets:
    - Crossmatch testing not required
    - 6 to 10 units may be pooled for administration
    - Interacts with clotting proteins to stop/prevent bleeding
  - Fresh frozen plasma (FFP):
    - Rich in clotting factors
  - Cryoprecipitate:
    - Rich in clotting factors
  - Granulocytes:
    - Used for infections unresponsive to antibiotic therapy
  - Albumin:
    - Protein used to move water from the extravascular to the intravascular space
  - Factors VIII and IX:
    - Rich in clotting factors
- Types of transfusions:
  - Homologous/donor
  - Autologous
  - Blood salvage
  - Most common type of transfusion is packed red cells

TABLE 16.5	ABO BLOOD AND Rh COMPATIBILITY	
ABO Blood Type	Who can they receive blood from?	Who can they donate blood to?
O	O	O, A, B, AB "universal donor"
A	O, A	A, AB
B	O, B	B, AB
AB	O, A, B, AB "universal recipient"	AB
Rh Type		
Rh-negative	Rh-negative only	Rh-negative or positive
Rh-positive	Rh-negative or positive	Rh-positive only

- Evidence-based recommendations for transfusing blood:
  - Considerations:
    - Hemoglobin level:
      - Not indicated until the hemoglobin level is 7 g/dL for hospitalized adult patients who are hemodynamically stable.
      - These recommendations do not apply to patients with acute coronary syndrome, severe thrombocytopenia (patients treated for hematologic or oncologic reasons who are at risk for bleeding), and chronic transfusion-dependent anemia (Carson et al., 2016).
    - Clinical condition:
      - Is the patient:
        - Hemodynamically stable?
        - Preoperative?
        - Postoperative?
    - Patient preferences:
      - Jehovah's Witnesses may decline transfusions
    - Alternative options:
      - Volume expanders
      - Growth factors:
        - Erythropoietin (Epogen)
      - Nutritional intake/supplements:
        - Iron
        - Folic acid
        - Vitamin B$_{12}$
- Process for blood transfusion (packed red cells):
  - Type and screen
  - Type and crossmatch
  - Blood consent
  - Obtain venous access
  - Use "Y" blood tubing with filter and 0.9 normal saline
  - Baseline vitals
  - Premedication (if ordered)
  - Double-check blood identification
  - Start the transfusion within 30 minutes of leaving blood bank

Clinical Consideration

The most crucial step is confirming compatibility and patient identification.

- Start infusion slowly
- Closely monitor patient for first 15 minutes of transfusion
- Check vital signs 15 minutes after the blood is started and every hour thereafter
- Complete transfusion within 4 hours
- Transfusion complications:
  - Immediate transfusion reaction:
    - Usually within first 15 minutes or 50 mL
    - Chills, fever
    - Rash, itching, flushing
    - Headache, anxiety
    - Back pain, muscle pain
    - Hypotension
  - When a reaction is suspected:
    - Stop transfusion immediately
    - Keep IV line open—use all new tubing
    - Notify provider and blood bank
    - Monitor vital signs
    - Send blood bag, tubing, and entire setup to blood bank for testing
  - Delayed reaction:
    - Fever
    - Jaundice
    - Rash
    - Hepatitis B virus (HBV), hepatitis C virus (HCV), and HIV
  - Fluid overload
  - Hypocalcemia

> **Clinical Consideration**
> A unit of blood can be split if the transfusion needs to be infused over more than 4 hours because of comorbidities, such as heart failure.

> **Clinical Consideration**
> It is extremely rare for HBV, HCV, or HIV to develop with today's improved screening methods.

Question	Rationale
A new patient is admitted to the medical surgical unit with symptoms of increasing fatigue, shortness of breath, and tachycardia. A laboratory workup reveals microcytic–hypochromic anemia. What type of anemia would the nurse suspect this patient has? A. Pernicious B. Sickle cell C. Aplastic D. Iron deficiency	Answer: D In iron deficiency anemia the red cells are small and pale (microcytic–hypochromic). Red cells are macrocytic–normochromic in pernicious anemia, misshapen in sickle cell anemia, and normocytic–normochromic in aplastic anemia.

▶ **Hemochromatosis**

- Hemochromatosis is caused by an excess of iron in the blood.
- **Assessment/Intervention/Education**
  - Detailed medical history:
    - History of anemia
    - Liver disease
    - Chronic blood transfusion
    - Genetic defect, autosomal recessive disorder

- Clinical manifestations:
  - Symptoms usually appear after age 40
  - Early symptoms:
    - Nonspecific
    - Weight loss
    - Abdominal pain
    - Arthralgia (joint pain)
    - Impotence
  - Late symptoms:
    - Multiple organ failure due to iron deposits:
      - Liver and spleen enlargement
      - Cirrhosis
      - Diabetes
      - Skin pigment darkening
      - Cardiac changes
      - Arthritis
- Diagnosis:
  - Elevated serum iron, ferritin, and TIBC
  - Genetic testing
  - Liver biopsy
- Treatment:
  - Lower serum iron level:
    - Regular phlebotomy for iron removal
    - Medications
      - IV or subcutaneous
        - Deferasirox
      - Oral:
        - Deferasirox
        - Deferiprone
  - Manage organ failure
- Patient teaching:
  - Teach patient about disease and treatment
  - Dietary instruction to decrease iron intake

▶ *Polycythemia*

- Rare disorder in which the person has two to three times the normal blood volume because of excessive bone marrow production of erythrocytes, leukocytes, and platelets. The increased blood viscosity and increased total blood volume contribute to severe congestion of the organs and tissues.
- *Assessment/Intervention/Education*
  - Etiology:
    - Primary polycythemia (polycythemia vera):
      - Chronic myeloproliferative disorder
      - Genetic mutations over time
      - Erythropoietin production is low to normal
      - Increased blood viscosity and volume
      - Predisposed to clotting
    - Secondary polycythemia:
      - Erythropoietin production is increased
      - Hypoxia-driven—causing increase in red-cell production
        - High altitude
        - Cardiovascular disease

- Pulmonary disease
- Tissue hypoxia
- Ineffective oxygen transport
  - Hypoxia-independent:
    - Erythropoietin production stimulated by tumors
- Clinical manifestations:
  - Ruddy complexion
  - Hypervolemia
  - Vascular:
    - Thrombus formation
    - Intermittent claudication
  - Cardiovascular:
    - Hypertension
    - Heart failure
    - Acute myocardial infarction (MI)
  - Neurovascular:
    - Paresthesias
    - Stroke
    - Headache
    - Visual disturbances
    - Pruritus
- Diagnosis:
  - Elevated Hgb and red cells
  - Elevated white cells
  - Elevated platelets
  - Elevated leukocyte alkaline phosphatase
  - Elevated uric acid level
  - Elevated cobalamin level
  - Elevated histamine level
  - Bone marrow biopsy
- Treatment:
  - Phlebotomy to reduce volume
  - Hydration to reduce viscosity
  - Myelosuppressive drugs
  - Radiation therapy:
    - May cause acute leukemia
  - VTE prevention:
    - Activity as tolerated
    - Anticoagulants/antiplatelets
- Patient teaching:
  - Long-term treatment required
  - Side effects of drugs
  - Increased activity/ambulation helps to prevent VTE formation.

Thrombocytopenia

- Condition characterized by an abnormally low platelet disorder that is inherited or acquired
- Types of thrombocytopenia:
  - Immune thrombocytopenic purpura (ITP)
    - Autoimmune disease
    - Infections may contribute to this disease
    - Lifespan of platelets is shortened due to macrophage destruction

- Thrombotic thrombocytopenic purpura (TTP)
  - Uncommon syndrome
  - Plasma enzyme deficiency that destroys the von Willebrand clotting factor (vWF)
- Heparin-induced thrombocytopenia (HIT)
  - Typical onset 5 to 10 days after heparin therapy initiated
- *Assessment/Intervention/Education*
  - Detailed medical history:
    - Recent hemorrhage, excessive bleeding
    - Cancer
    - Chemotherapy
    - Cirrhosis
    - DIC
    - Recent infections:
      - Viral (HCV, HIV)
      - Bacterial
    - Medications:
      - Cytotoxic drugs
      - Valproic acid (Depakote)
      - Furosemide (Lasix)
      - Penicillin
      - NSAIDs
  - Clinical manifestations:
    - May be asymptomatic
    - Bleeding:
      - Epistaxis
      - Gingival bleeding
    - Skin:
      - Petechiae
      - Purpura
      - Superficial ecchymosis
    - Hemorrhage:
      - Internal
      - External
  - Diagnosis:
    - Platelet count <150,000/mm^3
    - D-dimer
    - ITP-antigen–specific assay
    - Platelet-activation/function assay
    - Bone marrow biopsy
  - Treatment:
    - ITP:
      - Corticosteroids
      - High doses of IV immunoglobulin
      - Splenectomy
      - Rituximab (Rituxan)
      - Immunosuppressive therapy
      - May consider platelet transfusion for <10,000/mm^3

- TTP:
  - Identify and treat cause
  - Plasmapheresis
  - Corticosteroids
  - Splenectomy
  - Rituximab (Rituxan)
  - Immunosuppressive therapy
  - Chemotherapy
- HIT:
  - Discontinue heparin administration
  - Maintain anticoagulation:
    - Direct thrombin inhibitor
    - Indirect thrombin inhibitor
  - Warfarin (Coumadin) if platelets >150,000/mm^3
  - Plasmapheresis
- Platelet transfusion for platelets <10,000/mm^3
- Thrombocytopenic precautions:
  - Avoid injections
  - No enemas, suppositories, or rectal temperatures
  - Fall precautions
  - Stool softeners
- Patient teaching:
  - Avoid trauma or injury
  - Notify provider of any bleeding
  - Prevent bleeding:
    - Do not forcibly blow nose.
    - Avoid constipation; do not strain to have a bowel movement.
    - Use a soft-bristle toothbrush.
    - Use an electric razor for shaving.
    - Discourage over-the-counter medications (e.g., aspirin).

> **Clinical Consideration**
> Discontinue heparin immediately upon diagnosis of HIT.

Question	Rationale
A postoperative patient is receiving a transfusion of packed red blood cells. Thirty minutes after the infusion is started, the patient becomes anxious and develops chills, fever, and headache. After stopping the transfusion, what action should the nurse take? A. Administer the PRN Benadryl (diphenhydramine) B. Draw blood for a new type and crossmatch C. Administer PRN Tylenol (acetaminophen) D. Place patient upright with feet in a dependent position	Answer: C A nonhemolytic febrile reaction is the most common transfusion reaction; management consists of antipyretics, specifically acetaminophen. Diphenhydramine would be used for a mild allergic reaction such as flushing, itching, pruritus, and urticaria (hives). A patient experiencing circulatory overload would be positioned upright with the lower extremities in a dependent position.

▶ *Hemophilia*
- Condition characterized by a recessive genetic disorder, resulting in insufficient thrombin, which causes profound spontaneous bleeding
- Types of hemophilia:
  - Hemophilia A (HA):
    - Most common form of hemophilia (80%)
    - Factor VIII deficiency
    - Coagulation time prolonged, bleeding time normal
    - Typically occurs in males
  - Hemophilia B (HB):
    - Also known as "Christmas disease"
    - Factor IX deficiency
    - Coagulation time prolonged, bleeding time normal
    - Typically occurs in males
  - von Willebrand disease:
    - Most common congenital bleeding disorder
    - Defect of the von Willebrand factor (vWF)
    - Coagulation and bleeding time prolonged
    - Low levels of factor VIII
    - Affects both males and females
- *Assessment/Intervention/Education*
  - Detailed medical history
  - Risk factors:
    - Parents are carrier of genetic disorder
  - Clinical manifestations:
    - Excessive bleeding at an early age
    - Hemarthrosis (bleeding in joints):
      - Leads to deterioration of joints
      - Joints become deformed
    - Slow persistent bleeding from minor trauma, cuts, scratches
    - Recurrent hematoma formation
    - Severe epistaxis
  - Diagnosis:
    - Laboratory:
      - Quantitative assays for factor deficiency:
        - VIII
        - IX
        - XI
        - XII
        - vWF
      - Coagulation studies:
        - PT
        - PTT
      - Bleeding time
      - Platelet count
    - Genetic testing
  - Treatment:
    - Stop bleeding quickly
    - Early factor replacement based on type of factor deficiency
    - Antihemophilic factor (AHF) therapy

- Analgesics
- Corticosteroids to reduce joint pain and swelling
- Patient teaching:
  - Review manifestations of bleeding and need to seek treatment immediately
  - May need to learn IV infusion administration for home
  - When to contact provider
  - Avoid contact sports, invasive procedures, and activities that may result in a fall.
  - Avoid trauma or injury
  - Notify provider of any bleeding.
  - Prevent bleeding:
    - Do not forcibly blow nose.
    - Avoid constipation; do not strain to have a bowel movement.
    - Use a soft-bristle toothbrush.
    - Use an electric razor for shaving.

▌ *Neutropenia*
- Significant decrease in the number of circulating neutrophils, creating an increased susceptibility to infection
- *Assessment/Intervention/Education*
  - Detailed medical history:
    - Neoplasms involving the bone marrow:
      - Leukemia
      - Lymphoma
    - Chemotherapy/cytotoxic drugs
    - History of anemia
    - Autoimmune diseases
    - Medications that depress bone marrow production
    - Radiation exposure
  - Clinical manifestations:
    - Asymptomatic
    - Infection:
      - Malaise
      - Chills
      - Fever
      - Extreme weakness
    - Sepsis
  - Diagnosis:
    - Decreased white cells
    - Decreased absolute neutrophil count (ANC)
      - ANC <1000/mm^3
      - ANC <500/mm^3 (severe neutropenia)
  - Treatment:
    - Identify and eliminate cause (if possible)
    - Culture potential sources of infection
    - Antibiotics
    - Allogenic bone marrow transplant (BMT) for irreversible severe neutropenia
    - Institute neutropenic precautions:
      - Handwashing
      - Private room
      - Excellent oral care

Clinical Consideration
Do not administer aspirin or aspirin-containing medications.

Clinical Consideration
A temperature of >100.4°F (38°C) and a neutrophil count of <500/µL is considered a medical emergency.

- Avoid raw foods (cook all fresh foods)
- Avoid fresh flowers/plants
- Patient teaching:
  - Neutropenic precautions
  - Avoid crowds
  - Stay away from people who are sick or recently received live/attenuated immunizations (smallpox, chickenpox, measles/mumps/rubella [MMR], shingles).
  - Notify provider of:
    - Low-grade fever
    - Cough, sore throat
    - Chills/sweating
    - Frequent/painful urination
  - A temperature of 100.4°F is considered an emergency.

▶ *Disseminated Intravascular Coagulation (DIC)*

- DIC involves both bleeding and clotting defects that are stimulated by another disease or condition that creates a complex medical emergency.
- *Assessment/Intervention/Education*
  - Detailed medical history:
    - Malignant disorders
    - Autoimmune diseases
    - Blood transfusions
    - Organ transplantation with rejection
  - Risk factors:
    - Shock
    - Sepsis
    - Hemolytic disorders
    - Obstetric conditions
    - Tissue damage
    - Hepatitis
    - Glomerulonephritis
    - Pulmonary emboli
    - Fat emboli
  - Clinical manifestations:
    - Bleeding manifestations:
      - Petechiae, purpura, ecchymosis
      - Prolonged bleeding
      - Excessive bleeding from mucous membranes
      - Hematuria
      - GI bleeding
      - Uncontrolled bleeding
      - Mental status changes, headache
    - Thrombotic manifestations:
      - Acute renal failure
      - Thrombosis:
        - Pulmonary emboli
      - Tissue ischemia/necrosis
      - Cyanosis

- Acute respiratory distress syndrome (ARDS)
- Paralytic ileus
- Diagnosis:
  - Decreased platelets
  - Prolonged PT, PTT, activated PTT (aPTT)
  - Decreased fibrinogen
  - Elevated D-dimer
  - Peripheral-blood smear
- Treatment:
  - Treat underlying problem
  - Depends on severity:
    - Heparin
    - Transfusions—use with caution:
      - FFP
      - Cyroprecipitate
      - Platelets
      - Red cells
    - Hemodialysis
  - Follow thrombocytopenic precautions:
    - Avoid injections
    - No enemas, suppositories, or rectal temperatures
    - Fall precautions
    - Stool softeners
- Patient teaching:
  - Explain all tests, procedures, and treatment options.
  - Avoid trauma or injury.
  - Notify provider of any bleeding.
  - Prevent bleeding:
    - Do not forcibly blow nose.
    - Avoid constipation; do not strain to have a bowel movement.
    - Use a soft-bristle toothbrush.
    - Use an electric razor for shaving.
    - Discourage over-the-counter medications (e.g., aspirin).

Question	Rationale
The nurse is caring for a patient who is thrombocytopenic. Which action should be included in the plan of care? A. Avoid IM injections B. Limit visitors to adults C. Nutrition consult D. Emergency phlebotomy education	Answer: A The patient with thrombocytopenia is at increased risk for bleeding, so the plan of care should avoid any procedures that may cause bleeding, including IM injections. Neutropenia requires limiting exposure to others who are ill. A nutrition consult may be needed for some types of anemia, and an emergency phlebotomy may be required for a patient with polycythemia.

CASE STUDY

The nurse is caring for a 92-year-old male who was admitted with symptoms of fatigue, shortness of breath, and chronic back pain. He has resided in an assisted living facility since his wife passed away. He has recently stopped participating in community activities, has been missing meals, and is sleeping more than usual. His medical history includes hypertension, chronic obstructive pulmonary disease (COPD), osteoporosis, and a compression fracture in the lumbosacral spine. His vital signs are: pulse 86 beats/min, temperature 98.2°F, respirations 20 breaths/min, BP 112/64 mm Hg, and oxygen saturation 92% while breathing room air.

Upon admission, labs were ordered with the following results:

- WBC's: 5400/mm^3
- Red cells: 2.95
- Hgb: 8.7 g/dL
- Hct: 26%
- MCV: 89 fL
- MCH: 29.4 pg
- MCHC: 3.3%
- Platelets: 289,000/mm^3
- Glucose: 86 mg/dL
- Blood urea nitrogen (BUN): 20 mg/dL
- Sodium: 139 mEq/L
- Potassium: 4.3 mEq/L
- Chloride: 104 mmol/L
- Carbon dioxide: 27 mmol/L
- Creatinine: 0.9 mg/dL
- Calcium: 8.7 mg/dL
- Glomerular filtration rate (GFR): >60 mL/minute/1.73 m^2

1. **What problem would be suspected based on these labs?**

   - *The low red-cell count, Hgb, and Hct indicate that the patient has normocytic, normochromic anemia. Acute blood loss would be suspected since the red cells are normal size and color.*

2. **What other tests would most likely be ordered?**

   - *Although the initial labs came back with normal red-cell indexes (MCV, MCH, MCHC), it will be important to evaluate and rule out other causes of anemia. This could be done by ordering iron studies (serum iron, ferritin, and TBIC), serum folate level, and a vitamin B$_{12}$ level. A reticulocyte count will help to determine bone marrow function and erythropoietic activity. Since the patient may be experiencing a chronic blood loss, checking stool for occult blood would be appropriate.*

The following labs were ordered: iron studies (serum iron, ferritin, and TIBC), serum folate level, a vitamin B$_{12}$ level, reticulocyte count, and stool for occult blood. The stool was positive for occult blood, serum iron and ferritin levels were low, and TIBC was elevated. All other labs were unremarkable. The provider orders a colonoscopy, and several polyps were removed and biopsied.

3. **What type of anemia might this patient have? Why?**

 ▶ *Often older adults may have several contributing factors for anemia. This patient appears to have anemia related to an iron deficiency and chronic blood loss.*

 ▶ *The patient's medical history indicates that he has not been eating well and the labs indicate that the patient does not have adequate serum iron or ferritin stores in his liver.*

 ▶ *The colonoscopy revealed several polyps, which may have contributed to a chronic blood loss, as indicated by positive occult blood test.*

4. **Would it be appropriate for a blood transfusion to be ordered for this patient?**

 ▶ *Evidence-based practice states that transfusions are not indicated until the hemoglobin level is 7 g/dL for hospitalized adult patients who are hemodynamically stable. This patient appears to be hemodynamically stable at this time.*

Discussion

This patient is elderly, with multiple medical problems. It is important to evaluate all possible causes for anemia in older adults because of their comorbidities and the aging process itself. The older adult may present with vague symptoms, making it difficult to determine the cause without diagnostic testing. Based on evidence-based practice guidelines, this patient should not receive a transfusion at this time. Careful monitoring of the patient's symptoms, clinical assessment, and laboratory values will help to determine whether the patient may need a transfusion. Oral iron supplements may be appropriate for this patient, along with a nutrition consult to determine the best food choices. Adding a stool softener proactively and having the patient take iron with vitamin C (orange juice) will help to decrease some of the complications associated with iron supplementation.

Bibliography

Aschenbrenner, D.S., and Venable, S.J. (2012). *Drug Therapy in Nursing*, 4th ed. (Philadelphia: Wolters Kluwer).

Black, J.M., and Hawks, J.H. (2009). *Medical-Surgical Nursing: Clinical Management for Positive Outcomes*, 8th ed. (St. Louis: Elsevier).

Bonanno, F. G. (2012). Hemorrhagic shock: the "physiology approach." *Journal of Emergencies, Trauma, and Shock* 5(4), 285–295.

Carson, J.L., et al. (2016). Clinical practice guidelines from the AABB red blood cell transfusion thresholds and storage. *Journal of American Medical Association* 316, 2025–2035.

Grossman, S., and Porth, C.M. (2013) *Pathophysiology: Concepts of Altered Health States*, 9th ed. (Philadelphia: Lippincott Williams & Wilkins).

Kahsai, D. (2015). Acute anemia. *Medscape*, July 15, 2015. Accessed January 14, 2018, from https://emedicine.medscape.com/article/780334-overview#showall

Lewis, S.L., Bucher, L., Heitkemper, M., and Harding, M.M. (2017). *Medical-Surgical Nursing: Assessment and Management of Clinical Problems*, 10th ed. (St. Louis: Elsevier).

Moreno Chulilla, J.A., Romero Colás, M. S., and Gutiérrez Martín, M. (2009). Classification of anemia for gastroenterologists. *World Journal of Gastroenterology* 15, 4627–4637.

Pagana, K.D., Pagana, T.J., and Pagana, T.N. (2017). *Mosby's Diagnostic and Laboratory Test Reference*, 13th ed. (St. Louis: Elsevier).

National Heart, Lung, and Blood Institute. Pernicious anemia. U.S. Department of Health and Human Services. Accessed December 30, 2017 from https://www.nhlbi.nih.gov/health-topics/pernicious-anemia

U.S. Department of Health and Human Services National Institute of Health, and National Heart, Lung, and Blood Institute. (2014). *Evidence-based management of sickle cell disease: Expert panel report 2014.* (Washington, DC: Department of Health and Human Services), 1–181.

17

Immune System/ Infectious Disease

Donna Martin, DNP, RN, CMSRN, CDE, CNE

OVERVIEW

▶ The immune system helps protect the body against foreign organisms, removes damaged cells, and destroys foreign bodies and mutated cells to help maintain homeostasis.

▶ Infections develop when the immune system is unable to provide adequate defense against microorganisms. Maintaining a healthy immune system is key to decreasing the risk of infection.

ANATOMY AND PHYSIOLOGY

▶ The immune system is composed of the:
  - Lymphatic system
  - Mononuclear phagocyte system
  - Polymorphonuclear leukocytes
  - White cells
  - Body defenses:
    - First line of defense:
      - Physical barriers—intact skin and mucous membranes
      - Chemical barriers—such as pH
      - Normal flora—indigenous/beneficial
      - Cough reflex
      - Peristalsis
      - Oils and perspiration on skin
      - Respiratory passages—cilia
    - Second line of defense:
      - Inflammatory response:
        - Response to injury
        - Local effects
        - Systemic effects
    - Third line of defense:
      - Immune responses

▶ Gerontologic considerations:
- Age-related changes:
  - Impaired immune function/decreased protective mechanisms:
    - Decreased cilia function
    - Decreased ability to forcefully cough, causing retained mucus
    - Chest-wall stiffening
    - Cartilage calcification
    - Decreased elastic recoil
    - Decreased chest-wall compliance
  - Chronic illnesses, long-term–care facilities, and hospitalizations increase risk of exposure to illness.
  - Atypical presentation of infection:
    - Afebrile
    - Cognitive changes

IMMUNE RESPONSES

▶ Antigens:
- A foreign substance that elicits an immune response in the body

▶ Antibodies:
- A protein that is produced in response to the antigen to fight off the foreign substance

▶ Natural immunity:
- Immunity that is present at birth
- Immediate response to microorganisms

▶ Acquired immunity:
- Active acquired:
  - Occurs when there is an exposure to an organism that causes antibodies to develop in response. When a future exposure to that organism occurs, the body is able to fight it off.
  - Typically results in long-term immunity
  - Results from:
    - Natural exposure to the organism
    - Immunization
- Passive acquired:
  - Receives antibodies from an external source rather than developing them on their own
  - Immunity is short term
  - Results from:
    - Mother-to-fetus through the placenta and/or colostrum
    - Injection of gamma globulin

▶ Hypersensitivity:
- Occurs when the immune system overreacts against foreign antigens or the body's own tissue, which ultimately results in tissue damage.
- Autoimmune diseases are a result of a hypersensitivity reaction that causes a reaction to the body's natural proteins and antigens.

▶ Allergies:
- Sensitivity response to foreign antigens, increased immune response
- Causes:
  - Pollen

- Dust, mold
- Food
- Insect stings, cockroaches
- Animal dander
- Medications
- Latex
- Clinical manifestations:
  - Eye redness, drainage
  - Rhinitis
  - Sinusitis
  - Skin rash
- Diagnostic studies:
  - White-cell count with differential
  - Serum IgE
  - Allergy testing:
    - Scratch test, intradermal injection, patch test
    - Blood test
- Treatment:
  - Antihistamines
  - Sensitization to allergen
- Anaphylaxis:
  - A severe systemic response that occurs because mediators are released in response to the allergen
  - Causes:
    - Medications (common allergies):
      - Aspirin
      - Antibiotics
    - Foods (common allergies):
      - Peanuts
      - Milk
      - Shellfish
    - Insect venoms:
      - Wasps, hornets, yellow jackets, bees
      - Ants
    - Animal antitoxins:
      - Rabies
      - Snake venom
  - Manifestations:
    - Respiratory:
      - Coughing
      - Wheezing
      - Stridor
      - Dyspnea
      - Respiratory arrest
    - Cardiovascular:
      - Hypotension
      - Tachycardia

Clinical Consideration
Be prepared for a possible allergic reaction when doing skin testing.

Clinical Consideration
Anaphylaxis is a life-threatening emergency!

Clinical Consideration
Bronchial constriction and airway obstruction can occur within minutes.

- Dysrhythmias
- Cardiac arrest
- Skin:
  - Edema
  - Itching
  - Rash
- Neurologic:
  - Headache
  - Dizziness
  - Paresthesia

INFECTION

▶ Colonization versus infection:

- Colonization is the presence and growth of an organism.
- Infection occurs when the organism has reproduced and causes an alteration to normal tissue.

▶ The presence of a pathogen does not indicate that there will be an infection. There are several elements involved in the process of an infection. An infection can occur if the chain of infection is not altered and the host is susceptible to the organism (Figure 17.1).

- Infectious agent:
  - Microorganisms (Table 17.1):
    - Bacteria
    - Viruses
    - Fungi
    - Protozoa
  - Virulence:
    - Number of organisms
    - Potential for spread
    - Ability to produce disease

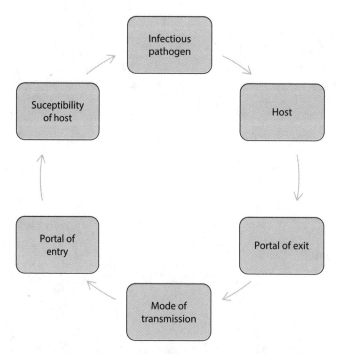

Figure 17.1 Chain of infection

TABLE 17.1	DISEASE-CAUSING ORGANISMS	
Organism Type	Description	Examples
Virus	Infectious particles with a small amount of genetic material, no cellular structure	Hepatitis A Hepatitis B Hepatitis C Ebola (hemorrhagic fever) H1N1 (swine flu) Human immunodeficiency virus (HIV) West Nile virus (West Nile fever)
Bacteria	One-celled organisms, some are normal body flora	*Staphylococcus aureus* *Escherichia coli* *Streptococcus* A and B Mycobacterium tuberculosis *Neisseria gonorrhoeae*
Fungi	Organisms similar to plants but lack chlorophyll	*Aspergillus fumigatus* (aspergillosis) *Candida albicans* (candidiasis, vaginitis, thrush) *Pneumocystis jiroveci* (Pneumocystis pneumonia) *Tinea pedis* (athlete's foot) *Tinea corpus* (ringworm)
Protozoa	Single-celled, animal-like organisms	*Plasmodium malariae* (Malaria) Amoebic dysentery
Emerging infections	International travel, population density, misuse of antibiotics, and expansion into previously uninhabited environments contribute to new and emerging infections.	Chikungunya virus (fever, muscle aches, and rash) Middle East respiratory syndrome coronavirus (MERS-CoV) Systemic inflammatory response syndrome (SIRS) Zika virus New Delhi metallo-beta-lactamase (NDM)
Reemerging infections	Infections once thought to be eradicated are now reemerging. International travel and decrease in immunization practices is thought to be the cause.	Measles Pertussis Diphtheria Tuberculosis Dengue fever
Resistant infections	Organisms that have developed a resistance to "usual" treatment. May be resistant to multiple drug therapies.	MDR-TB (multidrug-resistant tuberculosis) XDR-TB (extensively drug-resistant tuberculosis) Methicillin-resistant *Staphylococcus aureus* (MRSA) Vancomycin-resistant enterococci (VRE) *Klebsiella pneumoniae* carbapenem (KPC) Extended-spectrum beta (ß) lactamase (ESBL) Multidrug-resistant organisms (MDROs) *Pseudomonas aeruginosa*

(Lewis et al., 2017)

- Reservoir:
  - Humans
  - Animals
  - Insects
  - Food
  - Water
  - Fomites on inanimate surfaces
- Portal of exit:
  - Skin
  - Mucous membranes
  - Respiratory tract
  - Urinary tract

- Gastrointestinal tract
- Reproductive tract
- Blood
- Mode of transmission:
  - Direct contact:
    - Person to person
    - Ineffective/lack of handwashing
  - Indirect contact:
    - Sharps
    - Inanimate objects
  - Droplet:
    - Large particles
    - Can be expelled up to 3 feet
    - Example—influenza
  - Airborne:
    - Microscopic nuclei
    - Suspended in the air
    - Examples—tuberculosis, varicella
  - Vehicles:
    - Water
    - Food
    - Health care equipment/contaminated items
  - Vectors:
    - Mosquito
    - Tick
    - Flea
- Portal of entry:
  - Skin
  - Mucous membranes
  - Respiratory tract
  - Urinary tract
  - Gastrointestinal tract
  - Reproductive tract
  - Blood
- Host:
  - Age
  - Nutritional status
  - Chronic diseases
  - Susceptibility:
    - First-line-of-defense alterations
    - Second-line-of-defense alterations
    - Third-line-of-defense alterations
- Progression of infection—stages:
  - Incubation stage:
    - Time between the pathogen first entering the body and appearance of the first symptoms
  - Prodromal stage:
    - Time between nonspecific symptoms and more specific symptoms

- Illness stage:
  - Appearance of signs and symptoms related to the specific infection
- Convalescence stage:
  - Time between disappearance of acute symptoms and recovery from infection

Question	Rationale
A patient's surgical wound has become red, swollen, tender, and has a small amount of serous drainage at the distal end of the incision. When evaluating the patient's lab results you note the white-cell count has increased and the patient has a low-grade fever. Based on these findings, you suspect that a surgical site infection (SSI) is developing and is in the _____. A. illness stage B. convalescence stage C. prodromal stage D. incubation stage	Answer: A An elevated temperature and white-cell count would be indicative of nonspecific symptoms, while the change in the surgical wound is demonstrating more specific symptoms related to the specific infection (SSI).

HEALTH-CARE–ASSOCIATED INFECTIONS (HAIs)

▶ A health-care–associated infection (HAI) develops because of a visit to a health care setting or during a hospitalization. These infections were previously known as "health-care–acquired infections" or "nosocomial infections."

▶ HAIs are expensive to both the health care system and the provider. These types of infections have been identified as "never events" and health care providers are no longer able to receive reimbursement for the care and treatment of these infections.

▶ Types of HAIs:
- Iatrogenic—develops from a diagnostic or therapeutic procedure that was performed
- Exogenous—caused by a microorganism that is not native to the person
- Endogenous—caused by the patient's normal flora

▶ Risk factors:
- Age
- Nutritional status
- Chronic illness
- Acute illness
- Stress/immune response

▶ Sites of HAIs:
- Urinary tract—catheter-associated urinary-tract infection (CAUTI)
- Surgical sites—surgical-site infection (SSI)
- Gastrointestinal tract—*Clostridium difficile* (c-diff)
- Wounds
- Respiratory tract—ventilator-associated pneumonia (VAP)
- Bloodstream—central line-bloodstream associated infection (CLABSI)

▶ Common HAI organisms:
- *Escherichia coli (E. coli)*
- *Staphylococcus aureus (S. aureus)*
- *Enterobacter aerogenes*

INFECTION PREVENTION

▶ Medical asepsis—clean technique to reduce the number or minimize the spread of pathogens:
- Hand hygiene is key and should be performed:
  - Immediately before and after patient contact/care
  - Immediately after any exposure to body fluids
  - Immediately after the removal of gloves
  - When hands are visibly soiled
  - Vigorous 15-second scrub with soap or antimicrobial agent
  - Alcohol-based hand solution must come in contact with all hand surfaces
  - Nails should be short and polish-free
  - Artificial nails or extensions should not be worn by direct care providers.
- Disinfection:
  - Eliminates most microorganisms, except spores:
    - Alcohol wipes
    - Chlorhexidine solution/wipes
- Standard precautions—precautions followed whenever there is potential for contact with blood, body fluids, or skin/mucous membranes that are not intact:
  - Personal protective equipment (PPE):
    - Used based on the potential for exposure:
      - Gloves
      - Gowns
      - Mask
      - Eye protection
- Transmission-based precautions—used in addition to standard precautions for known or suspected infection or colonization:
  - Contact precautions:
    - Used for direct and indirect contact with organisms
    - Typically consists of gown and gloves
    - Example—MRSA
  - Droplet precautions:
    - Used for diseases that contain large droplets
    - Mask when within 3 feet of patient
    - May require gloves, gown, face shield
    - Example—influenza
  - Airborne precautions:
    - Minute particles suspended in the air
    - Negative-pressure room, filtered and vented to outside
    - N95 respirator mask when entering room
    - Example—tuberculosis
  - Protective environment:
    - For immunocompromised patients
    - Wear all PPE and perform excellent handwashing to protect the patient.
    - Example—neutropenia

Clinical Consideration

Hand hygiene must be performed with soap and water when caring for a patient with c-diff.

▶ Surgical asepsis:
- Requires the highest level of asepsis
- Prevents contamination of equipment or objects because of the use of sterile technique
- Used for procedures to prevent introduction of microorganisms:
  - Intentional perforation of the skin (intravenous [IV] catheter insertion)
  - Insertion of catheters into a sterile body cavity (urinary catheter)
  - When the integrity of the skin is disrupted
- Preparation:
  - Ensure sterile technique to maintain integrity of:
    - Field
    - Equipment
    - Solutions
    - Gloves
- Contamination occurs when:
  - Sterile packaging is torn or wet
  - Sterile items come in contact with nonsterile items
  - Sterile field or object is out of sight or below the waist
  - Prolonged exposure to the air

Question	Rationale
A patient with a chronic venous right leg ulcer was admitted to the acute care unit. While completing the admission history and assessment, the patient states that he has a history of methicillin-resistant *Staphylococcus aureus* (MRSA) in his leg wound. What intervention would you expect to be implemented for this patient? A. Medical asepsis will be used for dressing changes B. No special interventions, since it is only a history of MRSA C. Only use soap and water to clean hands D. The patient will be put on contact precautions	Answer: D Since the patient has a history of MRSA and is admitted with a leg wound that has been the source of the MRSA infection, it would be best to put that patient on contact precautions until a current MRSA infection is ruled out. When doing a dressing change for this leg wound, use surgical asepsis (sterile technique) to prevent introduction of microbes. Alcohol-based antiseptic hand gel is appropriate to use to clean hands when caring for patients with MRSA.

Diagnostic tests:
▶ Imaging:
- Chest x-ray:
  - Screening and evaluation of changes
- Computed tomography (CT) scan
  - Identify abscesses
▶ Laboratory:
- White-cell count (Table 17.2)
  - Total white-cell count
  - Differential
  - "Shift to the left"—significant increase in immature white cells (neutrophils)

TABLE 17. 2	WHITE-CELL COUNT REFERENCE RANGES		
	Normal Range		Elevation typically indicates
White cells—adult	4000–11,000	4.0–11.0/mm³	Inflammatory and infectious processes, leukemia
White-cell differential			
Segmented neutrophils	55–70%	2500–8000/mm³	Bacterial infection
Banded neutrophils	0–8%		Acute bacterial infection
Lymphocytes	20–40%	1000–4000/mm³	Chronic bacterial infection or acute viral infection
Monocytes	2–8%	100–700/mm³	Chronic inflammatory disorders
Eosinophils	1–4%	50–500/mm³	Allergic reaction, parasitic infection
Basophils	0.5–1.0%	25–100/mm³	Allergic reaction
(Lewis et al., 2017)			

- Cultures:
  - Blood
  - Urine
  - Wounds
- Sputum specimens:
  - Culture and sensitivity—for diagnosis and treatment of infection
  - Gram stain—classify bacteria as gram-positive or gram-negative
  - Acid-fast bacteria (AFB) culture—used to diagnose tuberculosis (TB)
  - Cytology—to determine presence of abnormal cells and malignancy
- Testing for antibodies and/or antigens
▶ Nursing diagnosis:

  Various nursing diagnoses are appropriate for patients experiencing infections and immune disorders:
- Ineffective protection related to inadequate nutrition, medications, treatments, abnormal blood profiles
- Impaired social interaction related to isolation
- Risk for infection related to immune response
- Deficient knowledge related to disease process and treatment

Question	Rationale
The provider's patient progress note related to a patient's complete blood count (CBC) shows a "shift to the left." Which assessment finding will the nurse expect? A. Elevated temperature B. Low O₂ saturation C. Cool extremities D. Pallor and weakness	Answer: A When a patient is experiencing a significant infection there is an increased demand for white cells. To meet this demand many immature cells are released; therefore, there would be a shift to more immature cells. Decreased O₂ saturation, cool extremities, pallor, and weakness are findings often associated with anemia.

AUTOIMMUNE DISORDERS

According to the American Autoimmune Related Diseases Association (AARDA) (n.d.), there are more than 100 autoimmune diseases. The immune system responds to invading microorganisms by producing antibodies for protection. Typically, the immune system does not mount an attack against the normal body cells. In autoimmune disorders, the immune response triggers the immune system to attack the person's own tissue. Some of the more common immune disorders will be discussed.

▌ Rheumatoid arthritis (see Chapter 15)

▌ Scleroderma (see Chapter 18)

▌ Systemic lupus erythematosus (SLE):

- Chronic inflammatory immune disease due to an abnormal immune response, more likely to occur in females; antigen–antibody complexes deposited in blood vessels cause destruction.

- Can affect any body system or organ; varies by individual

- *Assessment/Intervention/Education*

  - Manifestations:

    - Integumentary—alopecia (hair loss), butterfly rash over cheeks and bridge of nose, photosensitivity

    - Cardiopulmonary—dysrhythmias, endocarditis, pleural effusion, pericarditis, hypertension

    - Neurologic—seizures, peripheral neuropathy, cognitive dysfunction, headaches, stroke

    - Hematologic—anemia, leukopenia, thrombocytopenia, coagulation disorders, fatigue

    - Renal—mild proteinuria, glomerulonephritis, end-stage renal disease

    - Musculoskeletal—arthritis, increased bone loss, fractures

  - Nursing Diagnosis:

    - Fatigue related to chronic inflammation

    - Impaired skin integrity related to immune response; photosensitivity, skin rash

  - Diagnosis:

    - There is no specific diagnostic test for SLE; diagnosis is based on having four or more of the following criteria:

      - Malar rash—"butterfly-shaped" rash

      - Discoid rash—red rash with raised round or oval patches

      - Photosensitivity rash

      - Mouth sores

      - Arthritis—discomfort and swelling in two or more joints

      - Inflammation of lung tissue (pleuritis) or heart (pericarditis)

      - Renal dysfunction—proteinuria

      - Seizures, strokes, or psychosis (a mental health problem)

      - Abnormal blood tests; anemia, leukopenia, thrombocytopenia

      - Positive antinuclear antibodies (ANAs)

      - Positive anti–double-stranded DNA (anti-dsDNA), anti-Smith (anti-Sm), or antiphospholipid antibodies

  - Treatment:

    - Early monitoring and prevention of organ involvement critical to quality of life

    - Treatment may vary based on organ involvement, exacerbations, and periods of remission

- Pain management
- Medications:
  - Nonsteroidal antiinflammatory drugs (NSAIDs)
  - Methotrexate
  - Corticosteroids for exacerbations
  - Antimalarial drugs—hydroxychloroquine (Plaquenil)
  - Immunosuppressive drugs—azathioprine, cyclophosphamide
  - Topical immunomodulators
- Patient teaching:
  - Take active role in treatment and plan of care
  - Stay active to maintain mobility of joints
  - Be aware of the action, side effects, and administration of SLE medications
  - Pregnancy counseling prior to conception
  - Avoid triggers for exacerbations: stress, sun, illness

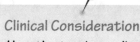

Clinical Consideration

Abruptly stopping medications may exacerbate disease.

INFECTIOUS DISEASES

▶ Human immunodeficiency virus (HIV)/acquired immunodeficiency syndrome (AIDS)
- Progressive compromise of the immune system. According to the CDC (2017) there are three stages of the disease:
  - Stage 1: Acute HIV infection—2 to 4 weeks after initially infected with HIV, flu-like symptoms develop and the patient has a large amount of the virus in the blood; very contagious.
  - Stage 2: Clinical latency (asymptomatic HIV or chronic HIV infection)—HIV still reproduces but at a slow rate, may last up to a decade or more if receiving treatment; at the end of this stage, the CD4 T-cell count declines significantly and HIV viral load increases (sometimes HIV never converts to AIDS, especially if the patient is taking medications).
  - Stage 3: AIDS—diagnosed when an HIV infected person's immune system becomes severely compromised, CD4 T-cell count drops below 200 cells/mm³ or if certain opportunistic infections develop. During this time the person has a very high viral load and is very infectious.
- Transmission of the virus:
  - Exposure to infected body fluids:
    - Sexual transmission:
      - Unprotected sex
    - Exposure to infected blood and blood products:
      - Sharing of needles/syringes
      - Transfusions (rare in countries that test donated blood)
      - Puncture wounds with infected blood exposure (rare)
      - Splash exposure of infected blood/body fluids (rare)
  - Perinatal:
    - Women can transmit the virus to their infant during pregnancy, at delivery, and during breast-feeding
    - Mothers who receive antiretroviral therapy (ART) are much less likely to transmit the virus to their infant.
    - One in four infants of infected mothers who did not receive any treatment are likely to have HIV.
  - HIV is **not** spread casually
- Pathophysiology:
  - Retrovirus (replicates in a backward manner), RNA to DNA
  - Targets the lymphocyte—fuses to the CD4 T cell

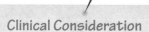

Clinical Consideration

Semen, vaginal secretions, and blood may contain HIV.

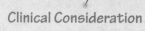

Clinical Consideration

HIV is not transmitted by casual contact, such as hugging, handholding, dry kissing, and sharing utensils.

- Destroys the CD4 T cell as it replicates
- As number of CD4 T cells decrease, immune responses decrease
- Susceptible to opportunistic diseases (Table 17.3)
- ***Assessment/Intervention/Education***
- Detailed medical history
- Clinical manifestations:
  - Stage 1—typically 2 to 4 weeks after exposure, often mistaken for a cold, flu, or infectious mononucleosis:
    - Fever
    - Enlarged lymph nodes
    - Sore throat
    - Headache
    - Muscle pain
    - Malaise
    - Joint/muscle pain
    - Rash

TABLE 17. 3	COMMON OPPORTUNISTIC INFECTIONS ASSOCIATED WITH HIV	
Organism	Type of infection	Manifestations
Candida albicans	Fungal	GI—esophagus (affects swallowing) Respiratory—trachea, bronchi, and/or lungs
Coccidioides immitis	Fungal	Respiratory—pneumonia (also called valley fever, desert fever, San Joaquin Valley fever)
Cryptococcus neoformans	Fungal	Neurologic—meningitis, cerebral edema Respiratory—pneumonia
Cryptosporidium muris	Protozoan parasite	Gastrointestinal (GI)—gastroenteritis, chronic diarrhea, intestinal cramping, weight loss
Cytomegalovirus (CMV)	Viral	Eye—retinitis, may result in blindness GI—esophagitis, gastroenteritis Neurologic—encephalitis Respiratory—pneumonitis
Herpes simplex virus (HSV)	Viral	Mucous membranes—chronic cold sores, ulcerations Respiratory—bronchitis, pneumonia GI—esophagitis
Histoplasma capsulatum	Fungal	Respiratory—pneumonia Neurologic—meningitis, central nervous system (CNS) manifestations
Human herpesvirus 8 (HHV-8) Kaposi sarcoma (KS)	Viral	Cancer that causes the capillaries to grow abnormally, causing vascular lesions on the skin
Mycobacterium avium complex (MAC)	Bacterial	GI—gastroenteritis, diarrhea, weight loss
Mycobacterium tuberculosis (TB)	Bacterial	Respiratory—causes cough, tiredness, weight loss, fever, and night sweats May also affect larynx, lymph nodes, brain, and kidney.
Pneumoncystis jiroveci	Fungal	Respiratory—pneumonia, difficulty breathing, high fever, dry cough
Toxoplasma gondii	Parasite	Neurologic—encephalitis, cognitive dysfunction, motor impairment, headache, seizures

- Diarrhea
- Neuropathy
- Meningitis
- Stage 2:
  - Typically has no symptoms
  - May not appear sick during this stage
- Stage 3:
  - Increasing number of illnesses/opportunistic infections
- Diagnosis—no one test is definitive, recommendations are for a combination of tests (WHO, 2017)
  - Antigen–antibody tests:
    - Look for both HIV antibodies and antigens
    - Antibodies may be detected as early as 28 days after exposure
  - Antibody tests:
    - Rapid antibody screening test
      - Can use blood or oral fluids
      - Results available in 30 minutes
    - Oral fluid antibody self-test
      - Oral swab
      - Results available in 20 minutes
    - Home collection kit:
      - Finger-stick blood collection
      - Results available in 24 hours
      - Any positive test has to have a repeat or follow-up test to confirm the positive result; antibody-only and the oral tests have to have a follow-up blood test to confirm
  - Nucleic acid test (NAT):
    - Looks for the actual virus in the blood
    - Not typically the test of choice:
      - Expensive
      - Preexposure prophylaxis (PrEP) and postexposure prophylaxis (PEP) may decrease accuracy of results.
- Nursing diagnosis:
  - Hopelessness related to physical condition
  - Situational low self-esteem related to chronic cobtagious illness
- Treatment:
  - No cure for HIV infection
  - Immediate ART is recommended for all individuals with HIV to reduce the morbidity and mortality associated with HIV infection (U.S. Department of Health and Human Services [USDHHS], 2017).
  - A medication regimen generally consists of two nucleoside reverse transcriptase inhibitors (NRTIs) in combination with a third from another drug class (USDHHS, 2017). (Table 17.4.)
  - PrEP:
    - Tenofovir and emtricitabine (Truvada)
    - Given to those at high risk for contracting HIV (CDC, 2017):
      - Sexual-contact risk decreased by 90%
      - IV-drug-abuse risk decreased by 70%
  - PEP
    - Used in emergency situations
    - Start within 72 hours of exposure to HIV

TABLE 17.4   HIV DRUG THERAPY

Class	Action	Medications	Side effects
Nucleoside/ nucleotide reverse transcriptase inhibitors (NRTIs)	Blocks reverse transcriptase, an enzyme HIV needs to make copies of itself	Abacavir (Ziagen) Didanosine (Videx, Videx EC) Emtricitabine (Emtriva) Lamivudine (Epivir) Stavudine (Zerit) Tenofovir disproxil fumarate (Viread) Zidovudine/azidothymidine/AZT (Retrovir)	Decrease in bone density, increased risk of MI, dyslipidemia, nausea and vomiting, hepatic effects, peripheral neuropathy, neuromuscular weakness, hyperpigmentation, Stevens–Johnson syndrome-toxic epidermal necrolysis, bone marrow suppression (with azathioprine)
Non-nucleoside reverse transcriptase inhibitors (NNRTIs)	Binds to and alters reverse transcriptase, an enzyme HIV needs to make copies of itself.	Efavirenz (Sustiva) Etravirine (Intelence) Nevirapine (Viramune, Viramune XR) Rilpivirine (Edurant)	Decrease in bone density, cardiac conduction defects, dyslipidemia, hepatic effects, insomnia, suicidal tendencies, depression, rash, Stevens–Johnson syndrome (toxic epidermal necrolysis)
Protease inhibitors (PIs)	Blocks protease, an enzyme HIV needs to duplicate	Atazanavir (Reyataz) Darunavir (Prezista) Fosamprenavir (Lexiva) Indinavir (Crixivan) Nelfinavir (Viracept) Saquinavir (Invirase) Tipranavir (Aptivus)	Bleeding, decrease in bone density, cardiac conduction defects, dyslipidemia, nausea and vomiting, hepatic effects, rash, Stevens–Johnson syndrome (toxic epidermal necrolysis), increase in body fat, hyperglycemia
Chemokine receptor 5 (CCR5) antagonist	Blocks CCR5 receptors on the surface of certain immune cells that HIV needs to enter the cells	Maraviroc (Selzentry)	Hepatotoxicity, constipation, diarrhea, flatulence, infection, nausea, vomiting, headache, fatigue, cough, rash
Fusion inhibitors	Blocks HIV from entering the CD4 T cells	Enfuvirtide (Fuzeon)	Injection site reaction, diarrhea, nausea, fatigue, weight loss, infection
Integrase inhibitors	Blocks HIV integrase, an enzyme HIV needs to duplicate	Dolutedravir (Tivicay) Raltegravir (Isentress)	Decrease in bone density, dyslipidemia, nausea and vomiting, rash, decreased renal function, Stevens–Johnson syndrome (toxic epidermal necrolysis)
Pharmacokinetic enhancer (booster) (PK)	Increases the effectiveness of an HIV medicine included in an HIV regimen	Ritonavir (Norvir) Cobicistat (COBI or c) (Tybost)	Diarrhea, parasthesia, hypercholesterolemia, nausea, vomiting, fatigue, rash
Combination medications	Two or more drugs combined into a single tablet	Efavirenz, emtricitabine, and tenofovir disoproxil fumarate (Atripla) Emtricitabine and tenofovir disoproxil fumarate (Truvada)	See above, based on medications in combination

Adapted from https://aidsinfo.nih.gov/understanding-hiv-aids/fact-sheets/

- • Medications taken daily or twice daily for 28 days
  - Lifelong ART can control the virus and slow progression of the disease process
- • Patient teaching:
  - Adherence—taking medications as prescribed
  - Avoid exposure to other infections (sexually transmitted infections [STIs], opportunistic infections)
  - Adequate nutritional intake
  - Prevent contracting/spread of HIV:
    - • Abstinence
    - • Limit sexual partners.
    - • Use condoms for protection.
    - • **Never** share needles.
    - • Avoid alcohol, smoking, and illicit drugs.

- Long-term effects of HIV/AIDS: AIDS-related dementia, AIDS wasting syndrome, peripheral neuropathy, chronic pain, lipodystrophy, and development of metabolic syndrome/coronary artery disease (CAD)

▶ Sepsis:

- Sepsis consists of a multitude of symptoms in response to an infection that leads to new organ dysfunction and has a high mortality rate (Rhodes et al., 2017). Sepsis should be treated as an emergency; early identification and initial treatment are keys to improved patient outcomes. Sepsis is often described by severity:
  - *Sepsis:* "Life-threatening organ dysfunction caused by dysregulated host response to infection." (Rhodes et al., 2017)
  - *Septic shock:* "Subset of sepsis with circulatory and cellular/metabolic dysfunction associated with higher risk of mortality." (Rhodes et al., 2017)
- *Assessment/Intervention/Education*
  - Recent illness
  - Symptoms may be vague
  - Clinical manifestations (early):
    - Fever
    - Tachycardia
    - Tachypnea
    - Mental-status changes
  - Diagnosis:
    - Identification of change in status, based on sepsis screening
    - Sepsis-related organ failure assessment (SOFA)/quick SOFA (qSOFA) screening, predictor of mortality—<u>not</u> diagnostic for sepsis; used with confirmed or suspected infection
      - Criteria:
        - Respiratory rate ≥22 breaths/min
        - Change in mental status
        - Systolic blood pressure ≤100 mg Hg
    - Organ dysfunction, new onset
    - Laboratory results:
      - Lactate level:
        - ≥2 mmol/L, repeat within 6 hours
        - ≥4 mmol/L indicates severe sepsis/septic shock
      - White cells
        - Total white-cell count >10,000 usually indicates infection, inflammation, or tissue necrosis
      - Plasma procalcitonin (elevates in 2 to 4 hours, peaks 24 to 48 hours after sepsis onset)
    - Culture results (culture suspected sources of infection)
  - Treatment:
    - Rapid response or "code sepsis" may be called on the basis of patient assessment.
    - Immediately upon presentation:
      - Broad-spectrum antimicrobials should be started within 1 hour of identification of sepsis or septic shock.
      - Appropriate antibiotics are chosen for identified/suspected source; more than one antimicrobial may be started.
      - Blood cultures should be drawn prior to initiation of antibiotics.
      - Fluid bolus of 30 mL/kg for sepsis-induced hypotension should be administered within the first 3 hours.
      - Vasopressors should be used with hypotension that is unresponsive to fluid bolus, to achieve a mean arterial pressure of 65 mm Hg.

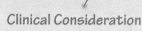

Clinical Consideration
Rapid identification and treatment is directly related to patient outcomes and recovery!

- Treat the source of infection:
  - Change antibiotics once source and sensitivity are known (if not already taking appropriate antibiotic)
  - De-escalate antibiotics as infection resolves
- Depending on severity of sepsis, intensive care unit (ICU) level of care may be appropriate:
  - May need intubation/mechanical ventilation
- Blood glucose levels maintained at <180 mg/dL
- Prophylaxis
  - Venous thromboembolism (VTE)—heparin or low-molecular-weight heparin recommended
  - Stress ulcer prevention—recommended for patients with risk factors for GI bleeding
- Remove invasive lines/tubes as soon as possible:
  - Central lines
  - IVs
  - Foley catheters
- Psychological support; counseling, cognitive therapy
- Physical support; rehabilitation necessary because of deconditioning
- Referral to hospice/palliative care if condition warrants
  - Patient teaching:
    - Sepsis prevention and awareness—will be more susceptible to sepsis in the future
    - Postsepsis syndrome (PSS) may occur in half of sepsis survivors:
      - Sleep disturbances; insomnia, nightmares
      - Extreme fatigue
      - Changes in cognitive functions
      - Posttraumatic stress disorder (PTSD) may develop.
    - Recovery may be very slow, and the person may not return to baseline—differs for each individual.

▌ Antibiotic resistance:

- Antibiotics are one of the most commonly prescribed medications; 50% of them are used inappropriately (CDC, 2017).
- Resistance occurs when bacteria are able to fight the effects of antibiotics that typically would have killed or stopped the growth of the organism. (Figure 17.2)

▌ Methicillin-resistant *Staphylococcus aureus* (MRSA)

- *Staphylococcus aureus* (staph) is a common pathogen that many people have on their skin and in their nares. Typically, this pathogen does not cause a problem when it is on/in the expected body location, which is referred to as "colonization."
- When staph migrates to other areas of the body, it usually results in an infection, requiring antibiotics.
- MRSA is a type of staph infection that is resistant to the antibiotics that are often used to treat this type of infection. (e.g., nafcillin [Nallpen], oxacillin [Bactocill], dicloxacillin, amoxicillin)
- *Assessment/Intervention/Education*
  - Risk factors for the development of MRSA:
    - Admittance to hospitals and long-term–care facilities
    - Chronic comorbidities
    - Previously treated with antibiotics
    - Acute or chronic wounds
    - Invasive medical devices, such as catheters

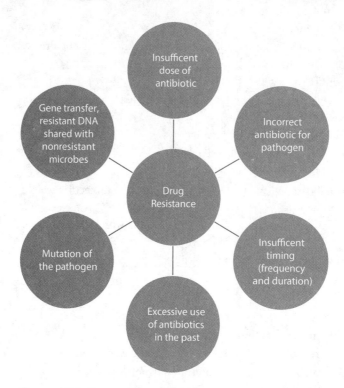

Figure 17.2 Factors That Contribute to Antibiotic Resistance

- Clinical manifestations:
  - Surgical-site infections
  - Skin and soft-tissue infections
- Diagnosis:
  - Screening is done on high-risk patients admitted to acute care settings:
    - Nasal swab
  - Culture results of suspected MRSA site
- Treatment:
  - MRSA-positive nasal swab:
    - Topical mupirocin ointment to anterior nares for 5 days
  - Culture-positive for MRSA:
    - Contact precautions/isolation
    - Determine sensitivity of the organism so correct antibiotic can be selected
    - Vancomycin, trimethoprim–sulfamethoxazole (Bactrim); possibly clindamycin (Cleocin)
- Patient teaching:
  - Complete course of antibiotics, when prescribed
  - Visitors and staff must follow contact precautions
- Vancomycin-resistant enterococci (VRE):
  - Enterococci bacteria are normally found on the skin and in the gastrointestinal tract, where they do not cause an infection.
  - When enterococci migrate to other parts of the body, an infection can develop.
  - VRE results from enterococci that fight the effects of vancomycin.
  - ***Assessment/Intervention/Education***

- Risk factors:
  - Admitted to hospitals and long-term–care facilities
  - Chronic comorbidities
  - Previously treated with antibiotics, specifically vancomycin
  - Acute or chronic wounds
  - Invasive medical devices, such as catheters
- Clinical manifestations:
  - Urinary tract infection common
  - Bloodstream infection
  - Wound or surgical-site infection
- Prevention:
  - Handwashing after using the bathroom and before preparing/eating food
  - A patient who screens positive for VRE should always be placed on VRE precautions/isolation.
  - Environmental cleanliness
- Diagnosis:
  - Culture and sensitivity
- Treatment:
  - Antibiotic based on culture and sensitivity results
- Patient teaching:
  - Handwashing
  - Complete course of antibiotics, when prescribed
  - Visitors and staff must follow contact precautions

▶ *Clostridium difficile* (*C. difficile* or c-diff):

- A spore-forming bacterium that overtakes the gastrointestinal tract when the normal flora are destroyed by antibiotics used to treat another infection
- ***Assessment/Intervention/Education***
  - Clinical manifestations:
    - Watery diarrhea (several stools per day)
    - Fever
    - Loss of appetite
    - Abdominal pain
    - Nausea
  - Diagnosis:
    - Stool culture
  - Treatment:
    - Handwashing with soap and water
    - Stop current antibiotics (if possible)
    - Medications:
      - Metronidazole (Flagyl)
      - Vancomycin (oral)
      - Fidaxomicin (Dificid)
    - Fecal transplantation may be an option to treat repeated *C. difficile* infections.
  - Patient teaching:
    - *C. difficile* can survive on inanimate surfaces for extended periods of time.
    - Excellent handwashing with soap and water
    - Complete course of antibiotics as ordered
    - Current recommendation—take probiotics or eat yogurt when on antibiotics

> **Clinical Consideration**
> Alcohol-based, waterless hand gel is not effective against *C. difficile*.

CASE STUDY

A 28-year-old African American male works as a salesman. He is married to a woman and has three children. He presents for an HIV test because several of his friends have recently tested positive. He has never had an HIV test. He is seen at the clinic today. The nurse is gathering information from him related to his history and performing his admission physical assessment.

1. **What type of test(s) will he have performed to diagnose HIV? What teaching and counseling goes with the tests? How does the provider describe these tests?**

    ▶ *HIV is the virus that causes AIDS. Being HIV-positive does not mean that the patient has AIDS, but it can progress to AIDS. ART has been proven to prevent the progression of HIV to AIDS.*

    ▶ *Antibody tests, combination tests (antibody–antigen tests), and nucleic acid tests (NATs) are the three main types of HIV tests that can be used. Each of these tests has a different window period in which they can detect the HIV infection. (The "window period" is the time between when a person contracts HIV and when the test can detect the HIV infection.)*

    - *__Antibody tests__ check for HIV antibodies in blood or fluids from the mouth. HIV antibodies are disease-fighting proteins that the body produces in response to HIV infection. It takes the body time to make antibodies in response to the HIV infection, and there may not be enough antibodies to be detected for 3 to 12 weeks. (The window period for antibody tests in most people is somewhere between 3 and 12 weeks from the time of possible exposure/infection.)*

    - *__Combination tests (antibody/antigen tests)__ can detect both HIV antibodies and HIV antigens (a part of the virus) in blood. Since it takes longer for the body to develop antibodies, the combination test can detect HIV infection before the antibody test alone. It can take 2 to 6 weeks for a person's body to make enough antigens and antibodies for a combination test to detect HIV infection. Combination tests are now recommended for HIV testing performed in labs.*

    - *__Nucleic acid tests (NATs)__ detect HIV in the blood. Although not used for routine testing, HIV infection can be detected with these tests about 7 to 28 days after a person has been infected with HIV. These tests are expensive and may be used if there was a high-risk exposure and/or if the patient is exhibiting early symptoms of HIV infection.*

    ▶ *An antibody test (oral swab or blood) or combination test will be performed first for most people. If it is positive, then a confirming testing will be done to make sure the diagnosis is correct. If the initial test is negative and it was performed during the window period, it is recommended that the individual be retested 3 months after the initial exposure to HIV. The individual must be taught to continue to use condoms and other HIV-prevention measures. If the antibody or combination test is negative, the provider should discuss whether preexposure prophylaxis (PrEP), the strategy that those at high risk of acquiring HIV may use to reduce their risk, is right for them. This includes using tenofovir/emtricitabine (Truvada) in combination with condom use, regular HIV testing, and other proven prevention strategies. With the health care provider (HCP), the patient should determine when to retest (AIDSinfo, 2018).*

2. **What else will the nurse ask this patient during the health assessment?**

    ▶ *Sexual history; number of partners; was protection used?*

    ▶ *Have you had sexual contact with a person who is HIV-positive?*

    ▶ *Have you had sexual contact with someone who has HBV or HCV?*

    ▶ *History of drug use—shared needles? Still using?*

- *Do you drink alcohol? If so, how much per day?*
- *Have you received a blood transfusion or clotting factors before 1985?*
- *Have you received a tattoo?*
- *Do you have a history of STIs, TB, hepatitis?*
- *Have you experienced any of the following symptoms?*
    - *Night sweats, insomnia, frequent illness, frequent infections, pain, and malaise?*
    - *Fatigue, memory issues, confusion, "brain fog"; attention deficit?*
    - *Blurred vision, loss of vision? Change in hearing?*
    - *Weight loss, anorexia, nausea/vomiting, lesions on lips, in mouth, in throat; difficulty swallowing, diarrhea, change in color of stool?*
    - *Change in color of skin, rashes, lesions?*
    - *Shortness of breath, cough?*
    - *Chest pain, palpitations?*
    - *Weakness in the legs? Neuropathy? Paresthesia? Gait disturbance? Falls?*
    - *Genital or anal lesions, sores, drainage? Pain with urination? Pain in rectal/anal area? Enlarged lymph nodes in groin, underarms, or neck?*
    - *Anxiety, fear, feeling out of control?*

3. **In a patient with possible HIV infection, what would be evaluated in the physical assessment?**

   The nurse would be looking for any of the following:

   - *Fatigue, lymphadenopathy, deposits of fat in trunk or abdomen; pale, dry skin; lesions, rashes, nonhealing wounds*
   - *Confusion, slurred speech, memory loss, agitation, depression, withdrawn, demeanor, apathy, inappropriate behavior, sensory loss, seizures, coma*
   - *Dry eyes, lesions, redness*
   - *Sores/lesions on lips, mucous membranes, throat; white patches on tongue or in mouth; gingivitis; tooth decay*
   - *Tachypnea, dyspnea, abnormal breath sounds, cough*
   - *Bradycardia/tachycardia, abnormal heart sounds*
   - *Diarrhea—foul-smelling, hematochezia, melena; hepatosplenomegaly; abdominal masses; abdominal pain with palpation*
   - *Muscle wasting; tremors, ataxia, foot drop, neuropathy, loss of coordination, paralysis, abnormal gait*
   - *Genital swelling, lesions, rashes, drainage, excoriation*

The provider examines the patient and does not note any worrisome physical assessment findings. His physical exam is essentially normal. His CBC, complete metabolic panel (CMP), and thyroid-stimulating hormone (TSH) are within normal limits.

He tests positive for HIV antibodies. The provider meets with him to decide on the course of treatment. The viral load comes back around 12,000 copies/mL. His CD4 count is 500. He agrees to start the ART treatment plan.

4. **What type of testing is completed prior to starting treatment for HIV/AIDS?**

   The patient will be tested for hepatitis and STIs. Baseline CMP, complete blood count (CBC), CD4 count, and viral load testing will be completed. Genotype and phenotype assays are completed to help the HCP determine which specific type of HIV the patient has and which medications to administer. The provider will use these tests to determine which medications are least likely to have resistance develop against them.

5. What must the nurse teach the patient about adherence and compliance?

▶ *If the patient is taking the medications as prescribed, this can lower the viral load by 90 to 99%.*

▶ *If the patient does not take the ART medications as prescribed, the virus can mutate and the medications may no longer be useful. Then, the viral load can increase and the CD4 count will go down.*

▶ *If he thinks he has side effects from the medications, he must notify the provider immediately. He should not stop the medication, decrease the dosage, or change the dosing interval unless told to do so. Patients should not start taking other medications, herbals supplements, or over-the-counter products without checking with the HCP. These may also influence the way the ART medications work.*

▶ *The patient will be on at least three medications (may be 2 from the same classification and 1 other drug) that may be combined in 1 pill to reduce pill burden.*

▶ *Follow-up testing also must be completed as ordered to ensure the medications are working to decrease the viral load and increase the CD4 counts.*

6. What needs to be taught to the patient about disease transmission?

▶ *He can pass HIV on to anyone who has contact with his semen, preseminal fluids, rectal fluids, or blood.*

▶ *He is unable to donate blood or organs.*

▶ *He must use a condom each time he has any type of sexual activity—anal, oral, vaginal. Oral dams and female condoms are available for use also.*

▶ *Limit the number of sexual partners.*

▶ *Get tested for STIs—these increase the risk of disease transmission.*

▶ *Insist that partner(s) gets tested for STIs and HIV.*

▶ *This patient does not have a history of IV drug use, but this would be another risk of transmission.*

▶ *HIV is mainly spread by having anal or vaginal sex without a condom and/or also by not taking medicines to prevent or treat HIV.*

▶ *It is important for the patient to know that even if his viral load test results are "nondetectable," he still may be able to pass the disease on to others with exposure of mucous membranes or blood to his blood, semen, seminal fluid, or anal fluids.*

7. What will the nurse discuss with the patient related to prevention of opportunistic infections (OIs)?

▶ *The patient must take his ART medications to keep his CD4 counts high and the viral loads low. This is the best way to prevent OIs.*

▶ *When the CD4 counts drop, the patient is susceptible to opportunistic infections.*

▶ *Maintaining adequate nutrition and getting enough sleep and exercise also help boost and maintain immune function.*

▶ *Cutting back on or eliminating alcohol, tobacco, and recreational drug use contributes to immunocompetency. In addition, patients can participate in unsafe sexual practices while under the influence of drugs.*

▶ *Avoiding exposure to new infections by using condoms, decreasing the number of sexual partners, and using less risky sexual behaviors is critical. Maintaining regular appointments and contact with the HCP and keeping the HCP informed of any new signs/symptoms, or changes in health is critical.*

▶ *The patient must get hepatitis B, influenza, tetanus–diphtheria–acellular pertussis (Tdap), and pneumococcal vaccines. (Depending on the patient's age/*

specific situation, HPV and menningococcal vaccines may be recommended.) The patient should not receive a live attenuated vaccine if the CD4 count is less than 200 cells/μl.

▶ *The HCP may also place the patient on prophylactic medications to prevent the development of opportunistic infections.*

▶ *The patient should be taught to avoid contact with animal feces and if they have touched human feces, they need to wash their hands thoroughly.*

▶ *He must not ingest raw or undercooked eggs; undercooked poultry, meat, or seafood; unpasteurized milk, cheeses, or fruit juices; raw seed sprouts such as alfalfa or mung bean sprouts.*

▶ *Water should be from the tap, filtered, or bottled.*

▶ *If the patient is traveling, he should be taught to be very careful to avoid food and water that could make him sick.*

Bibliography

American Autoimmune Related Diseases Association. (n.d.). Autoimmune diseases. Accessed March 12, 2018, from https://www.aarda.org

Aschenbrenner, D.S., and Venable, S.J. (2012). *Drug Therapy in Nursing*, 4th ed. (Philadelphia: Wolters Kluwer).

Centers for Disease Control and Prevention. (2017). HIV/AIDS basics. Accessed October 6, 2017, from https://www.cdc.gov/hiv/

Centers for Disease Control and Prevention. (2017). Infection control. Accessed October 11, 2017, from https://www.cdc.gov/infectioncontrol/index.html

Centers for Disease Control and Prevention. (2017). Zika virus. Accessed October 6, 2017, from https: https://www.cdc.gov/zika/index.html

Centers for Disease Control and Prevention. (2018). CDC health information for international travel: Advising travelers with specific needs: Immunocompromised travelers. Accessed March 17, 2018, from https://wwwnc.cdc.gov/travel/yellowbook/2018/advising-travelers-with-specific-needs/immunocompromised-travelers

Centers for Disease Control and Prevention, the National Institutes of Health, and the HIV Medicine Association of the Infectious Diseases Society of America. (n.d.). Guidelines for the prevention and treatment of opportunistic infections in HIV-infected adults and adolescents: Recommended immunization schedule for adults and adolescents with HIV infection. Accessed March 18, 2018, from https://aidsinfo.nih.gov/guidelines/html/4/adult-and-adolescent-opportunistic-infection/365/figure--immunization

Dellinger, R.P., Schorr, C.A., and Levy, M.M. (2017). A users' guide to the 2016 surviving sepsis guidelines. *Critical Care Medicine* 45, 381–385.

Lewis, S.L., Bucher, L., Heitkemper, M., and Harding, M.M. (2017). *Medical-Surgical Nursing: Assessment and Management of Clinical Problems*, 10th ed. (St. Louis: Elsevier).

Potter, P.A., Perry, A.G., Stockert, P.A., and Hall, A.M. (2016). *Fundamentals of Nursing*, 9th ed. (St. Louis: Elsevier).

Rhodes, A., Evan, L.E., Alhazzani, W., Levy, M.M., Antonelli, M., Ferrer, R., ... Dellinger, R.P. (2017). Surviving sepsis campaign: International guidelines for management of sepsis and septic shock: 2016. *Intensive Care Medicine* 43, 304–377.

Singer, M., Deutschman, C.S., Seymour, C.W., Shankar-Hari, M., Annane, D., Bauer, M., ... Angus, D.C. (2016). The third international consensus definitions for sepsis and septic shock (Sepsis-3). *JAMA* 315, 801–810.

U.S. Department of Health and Human Services. (2017). Guidelines for the use of antiretroviral agents in adults and adolescents living with HIV. Accessed March 4, 2018, from https://aidsinfo.nih.gov/guidelines/html/1/adult-and-adolescent-arv/10/initiation-of-antiretroviral-therapy

World Health Organization (WHO). (2017). HIV/AIDS. Accessed June 24, 2018, from http://www.who.int/mediacentre/factsheets/fs360/en/

18

Integumentary System

Nancy Paez, BSN, RN, CWCN, CHRN, LNC, CWS, DAPWCA
Amy Hagen, BSN, RN, CWS
Meritta Harris, BSN, RN, CWS, CHRN

OVERVIEW

▌ Covering the body's entire surface, the skin is the largest organ; it represents approximately 10% of our total body weight and receives one-third of the body's circulating blood volume.

▌ The skin is the only organ constantly exposed to a changing environment.

▌ Over the lifespan from birth to maturity, the skin undergoes a sevenfold expansion.

▌ Skin is capable of self-regeneration.

▌ Skin thickness varies from 0.5 mm in the tympanic membrane to 6 mm on the soles of the feet and palms of the hands.

ANATOMY

▌ The skin is made up of two layers (Figure 18.1):
- Epidermis (outermost layer):
  - Avascular and thin
  - Regenerates every 4 to 6 weeks
  - Functions:
    - Maintains skin integrity
    - Provides physical barrier against assault by microorganisms and the environment
    - Maintains hydration by holding moisture in
  - Made up of 5 layers:
    - Stratum corneum (horny layer):
      - Top layer
      - Made up of dead keratinized cells
      - Water barrier—regulates passage of water in and out
      - Protects against infectious microorganisms, chemicals, dirt, and the environment
    - Stratum lucidum:
      - Translucent line of cells
      - Found only on soles and palms

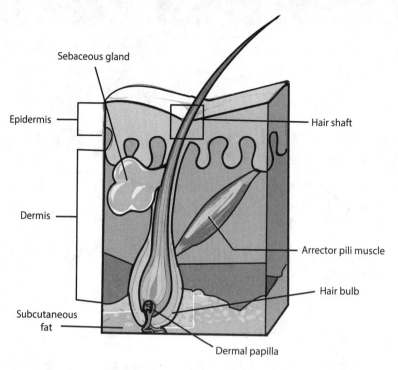

Figure 18.1 Layers of the Skin

- Stratum granulosum:
  - 2 to 3 cells thick
  - Contains keratinocytes
- Stratum spinosum:
  - Comprised of keratinocytes, which are becoming larger and flatter and contain less water as they travel to the surface of the skin
- Stratum germinativum, or stratum basale (basal):
  - Innermost layer
  - Single layer of cells
  - Basal keratinocytes that grow, divide, and differentiate to other layers of epidermis
  - Anchored to the basement membrane, which is anchored to the dermis
- Also contains melanocytes, which produce pigment; Langerhans cells, which assist in responding to and processing reactions to antigens
- Basement membrane (dermal–epidermal junction):
  - Separates epidermis and dermis
  - Layer affected in blister formation with dermatologic diseases, second-degree burns, and full-thickness wounds
- Dermis:
  - Blood vessels, hair follicles, lymphatic vessels, and sebaceous, sweat, and scent glands
  - Composed of fibroblasts, which form collagen, elastin, and other extracellular matrix proteins
  - Thickest layer of skin

FUNCTIONS OF THE SKIN

▶ Protection:
  - Physical barrier to microorganisms and other foreign matter
  - Protects against infection and excessive fluid loss

- Immune processing via Langerhans cells
▶ Sensation:
  - Nerve endings in skin enable us to feel pain, temperature, pressure
▶ Thermoregulation:
  - Regulates body temperature by vasoconstriction, vasodilation, sweating, excretion of waste products (electrolytes and water)
▶ Metabolism:
  - Synthesis of vitamin D
▶ Communication/body image:
  - Frowning, smiling, facial gestures
  - Scarring
  - Identification

Question	Rationale
As we age, our skin becomes less able to function as it did in our youth. Is this important to know? A. Yes, because it increases the risk for developing pressure ulcers and skin tears. B. Yes, because it becomes more rigid. C. Yes, because it becomes thicker and less responsive to topical moisturizers. D. No, it isn't important.	Answer: A Over time the skin undergoes many changes. As part of the aging process, the skin becomes thinner and more fragile, increasing the risk of pressure ulcers and skin changes.

SKIN LESIONS

Overview
▶ Primary lesions:
  - Physical changes in the skin caused directly by disease process
▶ Secondary lesions:
  - May evolve from primary lesions
  - May be caused by external influences—i.e., scratching, trauma
▶ Distinction between primary and secondary lesions is not always clear

Types of Skin Lesions, Primary
▶ Macule:
  - A change in color
  - <1 cm
  - Flat
  - Freckles, tattoo, erythema
▶ Patch:
  - Large macule
  - >1 cm
▶ Papule:
  - Solid
  - Raised
  - Distinct borders
  - <1 cm
  - Wart, mole

- ▶ Nodule:
  - Solid
  - Palpable
  - Raised
  - ≥ 1 cm
  - Lipoma, tumor
- ▶ Vesicle:
  - Raised
  - <1 cm
  - Filled with clear fluid
  - Herpes simplex, chickenpox
- ▶ Bullae:
  - Raised
  - >1 cm
  - Fluid-filled
  - Herpes zoster, insect-bite reaction
- ▶ Pustule:
  - Circumscribed
  - Raised
  - Filled with pus
  - Can be sterile or infected
  - Acne, folliculitis
- ▶ Plaque:
  - Solid
  - Raised
  - Flat-topped
  - >1 cm
  - Psoriasis, chronic eczematous dermatitis
- ▶ Wheal:
  - Raised
  - Flesh-colored or erythematous papule or plaque
  - Transient, generally last <24 hours
  - Hives
- ▶ Cyst:
  - Walled-off lesion
  - Filled with fluid or semisolid material
  - Pilar or epidermoid
- ▶ Eczema:
  - Most common inflammatory skin condition
  - Itchy, erythematous patches, plaques or papules that may become "juicy"
  - May dry into scabs or crusts or develop into scales
  - Treatment—topical steroid therapy

Types of Skin Lesions, Secondary

- ▶ Scales:
  - Flakes or plates
  - Desquamated layers of stratum corneum
  - Dandruff, psoriasis

▶ Crusts:
  - Formed from blood, serum, or other dried exudate
  - Honey-colored crusts indicate superficial infection
  - Infected insect bites, resolving impetigo

▶ Erosions:
  - Shallow loss of tissue, involving only the epidermis
  - Nonscarring
  - Often evolve from blisters and pustules
  - Canker sore

▶ Ulcer:
  - Deeper defect than erosion
  - Usually involves dermis or deeper layers
  - Heals with scarring

▶ Fissure:
  - Linear ulcers or cracks in the skin
  - Often painful

▶ Excoriation:
  - Traumatized or abraded skin
  - Caused by scratching

▶ Nursing Diagnosis:

Various nursing diagnoses are appropriate for patients experiencing skin and tissue disorders:

  - Impaired skin integrity related to altered epidermis and/or dermis
  - Impaired tissue integrity related to wound, debridement, presence of infection
  - Disturbed body image related to open wound, wound appearance

ULCERS AND PRESSURE INJURY

Overview

▶ In 2018, the National Pressure Ulcer Advisory Panel (NPUAP) changed the label from pressure ulcer to pressure injury, in an attempt to be more inclusive of all stages.

▶ A pressure injury is localized damage to the skin and underlying soft tissue, usually over a bony prominence, related to a medical procedure or from a medical device. The injury can be intact skin or an open ulcer and occurs as the result of intense and/or prolonged pressure or pressure in combination with shearing forces. The tolerance for pressure and shear may also be affected by the microclimate, nutrition, perfusion, comorbidities, and condition of the soft tissue. Shearing occurs from friction against the skin, resembling an abrasion (National Pressure Ulcer Advisory Panel [NPUAP]).

▶ Annual cost to treat is $9.1 billion to $11.6 billion

At-Risk Patients Have One or More of the Following Conditions

▶ Any condition requiring the patient to be in bed or a chair without the ability to shift weight (immobility, fractures, etc.) (Figure 18.2) (Figure 18.3)

▶ Dehydration

▶ Diabetes mellitus

▶ Decreased sensation

▶ Incontinence

▶ Malnutrition (obesity or underweight)

▶ Altered mental health status (coma, confusion)

▶ Multisystem trauma

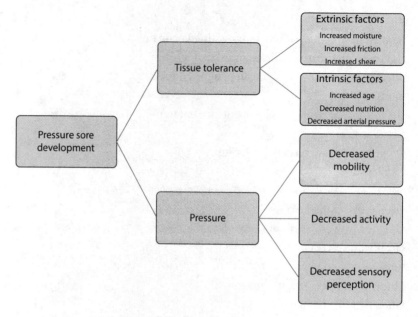

Figure 18.2 Pressure Injury Risk Factors

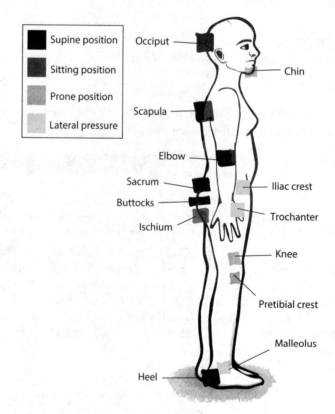

Figure 18.3 Impact of Positioning on Pressure Injury

▶ Poor circulation

▶ Previous pressure injury

Pathogenesis

▶ Soft tissue compressed between a bony prominence and an external surface

▶ Result of intensity, duration, and tissue tolerance

▶ Pressure interrupts blood flow to the capillaries and surrounding tissues, depriving them of oxygen and nutrients. This leads to local ischemia, hypoxia, edema, inflammation and cell death, which ultimately results in a pressure injury (Figure 18.4).

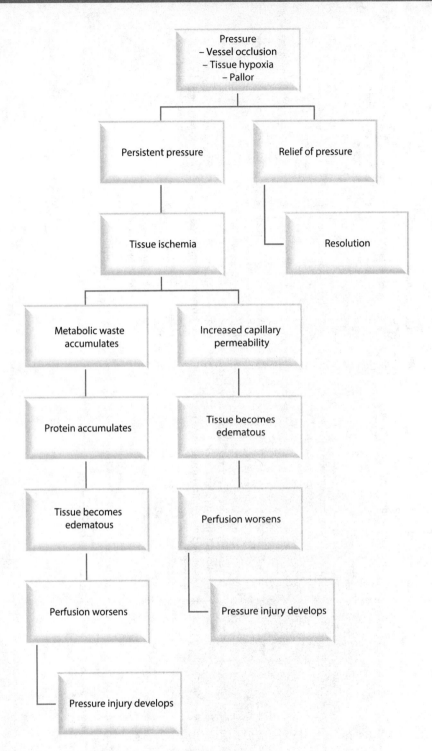

Figure 18.4 Pathogenesis of Pressure Wounds

Assessment

▶ Assess pressure injury risk using tools such as the Braden Scale (Table 18.1)

▶ Stage 1 pressure injury (Figure 18.5):

- Nonblanchable erythema of intact skin, which may appear differently in darkly pigmented skin.
- Presence of blanchable erythema or changes in sensation, temperature, or firmness may precede visual changes.
- Color changes do not include purple or maroon discoloration; these may indicate deep-tissue pressure injury.

TABLE 18.1   BRADEN SCALE FOR PREDICTING PRESSURE ULCER RISK

	1	2	3	4
Sensory Perception Ability to respond meaningfully to pressure-related discomfort	**1. Completely Limited:** Unresponsive (does not moan, flinch, or grasp) to painful stimuli, due to diminished level of consciousness or sedation, OR Limited ability to feel pain over most of body surface.	**2. Very Limited:** Responds only to painful stimuli. Cannot communicate discomfort Except by moaning or restlessness, OR Has a sensory impairment, which limits the ability to feel pain or discomfort over 1/2 of body.	**3. Slightly Limited:** Responds to verbal commands but cannot always communicate discomfort or need to be turned, OR Has some sensory impairment, which limits ability to feel pain or discomfort in 1 or 2 extremities.	**4. No Impairment:** Responds to verbal command. Has no sensory deficit which would limit ability to feel or voice pain or discomfort.
Moisture Degree to which skin is exposed to moisture	**1. Constantly Moist:** Perspiration, urine, etc. keep skin moist almost constantly. Dampness is detected every time patient is moved or turned.	**2. Moist:** Skin is often but not always moist. Linen must be changed at least once a shift.	**3. Occasionally Moist:** Skin is occasionally moist, requiring an extra linen change approximately once a day.	**4. Rarely Moist:** Skin is usually dry: linen requires changing only at routine intervals.
Activity Degree of physical activity	**1. Bedfast:** Confined to bed.	**2. Chairfast:** Ability to walk severely limited or nonexistent. Cannot bear own weight and/or must be assisted into chair or wheel chair.	**3. Walks Occasionally:** Walks occasionally during day but for very short distances, with or without assistance. Spends majority or each shift in bed or chair.	**4. Walks Frequently:** Walks outside the room at least twice a day and inside room at least once every 2 hours during waking hours.
Mobility Ability to change and control body position	**1. Completely Immobile:** Does not make even slight changes in body or extremity position without assistance.	**2. Very Limited:** Makes occasional slight changes in body or extremity position, but unable to make frequent or significant changes independently.	**3. Slightly Limited:** Makes frequent though slight changes in body or extremity position independently.	**4. No Limitations:** Makes major and frequent changes in position without assistance.
Nutrition Usual food intake pattern	**1. Very Poor:** Never eats complete meal. Rarely eats more than 1/3 of any food offered. Eats 2 servings or less of protein (meat or dairy products) per day. Takes fluids poorly. Does not take a liquid dietary supplement. OR Is NPO and/or maintained on clear liquids or IV for more than 5 days.	**2. Probably Inadequate:** Rarely eats a complete meal and generally eats only about 1/2 of any food offered. Protein intake includes only 3 servings of meat or dairy products per day. Occasionally will take a dietary supplement. OR Receives less than optimum amount of liquid diet or tube feeding.	**3. Adequate:** Eats over half of most meals. Eats a total of 4 servings of protein (meat, dairy products) each day. Occasionally will refuse a meal, but will usually take a supplement if offered, OR is on a tube feeding or TPN regimen, which probably meets most of nutritional needs.	**4. Excellent:** Eats most of every meal. Never refuses a meal. Usually eats a total of 4 or more servings of meat and dairy products. Occasionally eats between meals. Does not require supplementation.
Friction and Shear	**1. Problem:** Requires moderate to maximum assistance in moving. Complete lifting without sliding against sheets is impossible. Frequently slides down in bed or chair, requiring frequent repositioning with maximum assistance. Spasticity, contractures, or agitation leads to almost constant friction.	**2. Potential Problem:** Moves feebly or requires minimum assistance. During a move skin probably slides to some extent against sheets, chair, restraints, or other devices. Maintains relatively good position in chair or bed most of the time but occasionally slides down.	**3. No Apparent Problem:** Moves in bed and in chair independently and has sufficient muscle strength to lift up completely during move. Maintains good position in bed or chair at all times	
				TOTAL SCORE

Bergstom 1987

Stages of pressure injury

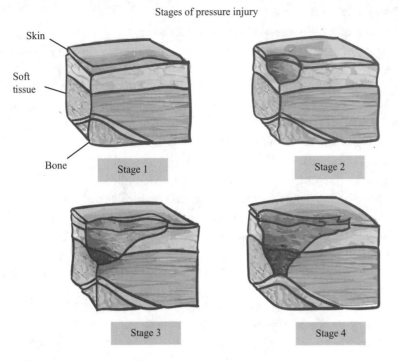

Figure 18.5 Staging of Wounds

▶ Stage 2 pressure injury (Figure 18.5):
- Partial thickness skin loss with exposed dermis.
- Wound bed is viable, pink or red, and moist.
- May present as an intact or ruptured serum-filled blister.
- Adipose tissue is not visible.
- Granulation tissue, slough, and eschar are not present.
- Most commonly the result of adverse microclimate and shear in the skin over the pelvis and shear in the heel.
- Should not be used to describe moisture-associated skin damage (MASD), including incontinence-associated dermatitis (IAD), intertriginous dermatitis (ITD), medical-adhesive–related skin injury (MARSI), or traumatic wounds (skin tears, burns, abrasions).

▶ Stage 3 pressure injury (Figure 18.5):
- Full-thickness loss of skin, in which adipose tissue is visible in the ulcer.
- Granulation tissue and epibole often present.
- Slough and/or eschar may be visible.
- Depth of tissue damage varies by anatomic location.
- Undermining and tunneling may occur.
- Fascia, muscle, tendon, ligament, cartilage, and bone are not present.
- If slough or eschar obscures the extent of tissue loss, this is an unstageable injury.

▶ Stage 4 pressure injury (Figure 18.5):
- Full-thickness skin and tissue loss.
- Fascia, muscle, tendon, ligament, cartilage, or bone exposed or directly palpable.
- Slough and/or eschar may be visible.
- Epibole may be present.
- Undermining and/or tunneling may occur.
- If slough and/or eschar obscure the extent of tissue loss, this is an unstageable pressure injury.

Clinical Consideration
Epibole is a clinical condition in which the wound edges are rolled or curled under.

▶ Unstageable pressure injury:
  - Obscured full-thickness skin and tissue loss.
  - Extent of damage is not confirmed because slough and/or eschar obscures wound bed.
  - If slough and/or eschar is removed, a stage 3 or 4 pressure injury will be revealed.
  - Stable, dry eschar on heels or ischemic limbs should not be removed or softened.
▶ Deep-tissue pressure injury:
  - Persistent nonblanchable deep red, maroon, or purple discoloration
  - Intact or nonintact skin
  - Epidermal separation—dark wound bed or blood-filled blister
  - Pain and temperature changes often precede skin-color changes.
  - Discoloration may appear differently in darkly pigmented skin.
  - Result of intense and/or prolonged pressure and shear forces at the bone–muscle interface.
  - Wound may evolve rapidly to reveal extent of tissue damage or may resolve without tissue loss.
▶ Additional pressure-injury definitions:
  - Medical-device–related pressure injury:
    - Describes an etiology
    - Results from use of devices designed and applied for diagnostic or therapeutic purposes
    - Pressure injury usually conforms to the shape and size of the device
    - Should be staged using the staging system
  - Mucosal membrane pressure injury:
    - Found on mucous membranes with a history of a medical device in use at the location of the injury.
    - Because of the anatomy of the tissue, these injuries cannot be staged.

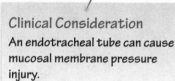

Clinical Consideration
An endotracheal tube can cause mucosal membrane pressure injury.

Intervention/Education

▶ All stages require topical care and some may need surgical intervention.
▶ First, reduce interface pressure:
  - You can put anything on a pressure injury but the patient.
  - Frequently reposition and turn.
  - Support surfaces.
  - Do not elevate the head of the bed >30 degrees.
  - Do not use donut cushions.
  - Use lifting devices when possible.
▶ Maintain and improve tissue tolerance to pressure to prevent injury:
  - Daily inspection
  - Skin care protocols
  - Reduce environmental factors
  - Minimize exposure to incontinence, wound exudate, perspiration
  - Minimize friction and shear
  - Optimize nutritional support
  - Provide activities as appropriate
  - Document all interventions
▶ Apply dressings as appropriate
▶ Teach patient and family about risk factors
▶ Teach patient and family about tensile strength

Question	Rationale
The best initial treatment for a pressure injury is: A. Antimicrobials to prevent infection B. Occlusive dressing to keep foreign bodies out of wound C. Position patient off the area D. Elevate the head of the bed	Answer: C Relieve the pressure. Remember you can put anything on a pressure injury but the patient!

VENOUS ULCERS

Overview

▶ Ulcers are caused by peripheral venous disease and are commonly located proximal to the medial or lateral malleolus, above the inner or outer ankle, or on the lower calf area of the leg. In the past, these were called "stasis ulcers."

▶ Account for 70 to 90% of all leg ulcers (Sen et al., 2009)

▶ Total cost of care for venous leg disease per patient can exceed $40,000.

▶ The United States spends an estimated $2.5 billion to $3.5 billion per year treating venous ulcers.

▶ Estimated recurrence rate is 57 to 97%.

Pathogenesis

▶ Ulcerations are a direct result of ambulatory venous hypertension from chronic venous insufficiency

▶ Contraction of the calf muscle pump and competent valves are essential to normal venous function

▶ Venous system fails to push venous blood toward the heart

▶ Valve failure changes the unidirectional blood flow into bidirectional blood flow.

▶ Blood pools in the lower extremities, increasing pressure in the legs.

▶ The end result of prolonged venous hypertension is damage to the skin and soft tissues, which makes them more susceptible to ulceration.

Assessment/Wound Characteristics

▶ Patients can experience:

- Pain, itching, tingling (stasis dermatitis)
- Leg(s) may feel heavy, cramped, or tired.
- Leg(s) may be edematous from the knee down.
- Tissue may feel hard.
- Skin may be dark purple, brown, or red:
  - Because of pooled blood
  - Brown is consistent with hemosiderin staining.
- Shallow open area on lower legs in ankle area:
  - Can be painful
  - Irregular edges
  - Surrounding skin shiny or tight from edema

▶ Drainage/exudate:

- Foul odor can be consistent with infection

Risk Factors

▶ History of deep-vein thrombosis
▶ Varicosities
▶ Age
▶ Prolonged standing
▶ Pregnancy
▶ Trauma to lower extremities
▶ Incompetent perforators
▶ Obesity
▶ Family history of venous disease
▶ Heart failure with edema

Interventions

▶ Compression therapy
▶ Limb elevation
▶ Surgical procedures:
  • Vein stripping
  • Vein ligation
  • Sclerotherapy
▶ Optimize nutrition
▶ Physical therapy
▶ Exercise
▶ Weight control
▶ Pharmacologics:
  • Pentoxifylline (Trental, Pentoxil)
  • Sulodexide (oral combination of heparin and dermatan sulfate)
  • Horse chestnut
▶ Laser treatment
▶ Elastic (Ace) bandages, thromboembolic deterrent (TED) hose, and medical compression stockings (Tubigrip) are not designed for therapeutic compression

Patient Education

▶ Maintain appropriate weight.
▶ Perform daily exercise.
▶ Wear prescribed compression for life.
▶ Elevate legs whenever possible.
▶ Seek treatment quickly when ulcers develop.
▶ Maintain blood pressure.

ARTERIAL ULCERS

Overview

▶ Occur as the result of severe tissue ischemia
▶ Extremely painful
▶ Lack of blood flow leads to cell death, tissue damage
▶ Body is slow to heal without correction

Characteristics

◗ Patient:
- Pain in legs or affected area when blockage may be present
- Cramping in legs when walking; relief with rest (claudication)
- Pain at rest during the night
- Leg(s) may be discolored.
- Leg(s) may be cool to touch.
- Leg(s) typically hairless
- Shiny skin

◗ Wound:
- Punched out
- Raised edges
- Pale wound bed
- Lack of bleeding
- Ulcer may or may not be painful
- Area may be gangrenous
- Dry wound bed

Risk Factors

◗ High blood pressure
◗ High cholesterol
◗ Smoking
◗ Diabetes mellitus
◗ Chronic kidney disease
◗ History of myocardial infarction, angina, or stroke

Interventions

◗ Bypass surgery
◗ Stent placement
◗ Angioplasty
◗ Amputation:
- Last resort
◗ Pharmacologics:
- Antiplatelets
- Vasodilators
- Antilipemics
- Analgesics
- Anticoagulants
◗ Recommend/encourage lifestyle changes

Patient Education

◗ Smoking cessation
◗ Regular exercise
◗ Optimized nutrition:
- Low fat
- Low cholesterol
◗ Maintain blood glucose levels

▶ Proper footwear:
  • Always wear shoes to protect feet.
  • Shoes must be properly fitted to prevent injury.

DIABETIC ULCERS

Overview

▶ According to recent statistics from the American Diabetes Association (2017), 9.4% of the population in the United States has diabetes. Diabetes is a major contributing factor to hardening and narrowing of large and small blood vessels, leading to poor blood flow (microvascular disease). This physiologic effect on the blood vessels also damages the nerves, causing neuropathy in many patients. Loss of sensation leaves the patient with diabetes at significant risk for ulcers, especially of the feet.

▶ Wagner grading: Evaluation and classification of diabetic foot ulcers is essential for development of an effective treatment plan. The Wagner grading scale is the most commonly used scale to consistently identify depth and infection in a diabetic foot ulcer and is essential in the development of a treatment plan to avoid amputation (Table 18.2).

Assessment

▶ Deformities causing areas of pressure:
  • Hallux valgus—bunions
  • Hammer toes—toes bent into claw-like position
  • Ankle-joint equinus—ankle-joint dorsiflexion <10 degrees
  • Charcot foot—destruction of the bones of the foot, causing deformity
▶ Callous formation—sustained areas of pressure
▶ Loss of protective sensation:
  • Semmes–Weinstein monofilament examination (SWME) (Figure 18.6)
▶ Duration of diabetes
▶ Glycemic control
▶ Previous history of ulceration
▶ Smoking history
▶ Functional abilities
▶ Peripheral vascular disease:
  • Color—rubor; cyanosis

TABLE 18.2	WAGNER DIABETIC FOOT ULCER GRADING
Grade	Description
0	Skin intact; old healed ulcer or deformity may be present
I	Superficial ulcer without penetration into the epidermis and dermis
II	Deeper ulcer that reaches the tendon, bone, or joint capsule
III	Grade II ulcer with abscess, osteitis, osteomyelitis, or tendinitis
IV	Gangrene of some portion of the toe, toes, and/or forefoot; tissue may be wet or dry, infected or not infected
V	Gangrene involves the entire foot, no local procedures are possible, minimum treatment is a below-the-knee amputation
(Wagner, 1981)	

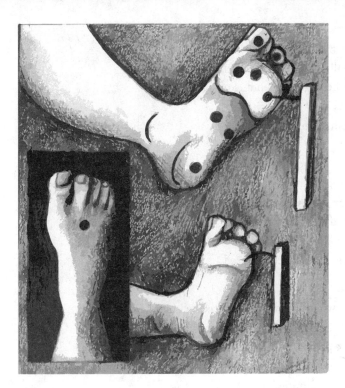

Figure 18.6 Semmes-Weinstein monofilament Examination (SWME)

- Assess arterial flow:
  - Pulse evaluation, bedside Doppler
  - Capillary refill <3 seconds
  - Arterial Doppler/duplex scans, assess arterial–brachial index (ABI)
- Radiography/x-ray of bilateral feet
- Nutritional assessment:
  - Patient history
  - Labs: Thromboplastin (TP); albumin; prealbumin; transferrin
- Lab work:
  - Ulcer/wound culture with Gram stain—assess infection
  - Cardiovascular risk panel; total cholesterol, low-density lipoproteins (LDLs), high-density lipoproteins (HDLs), triglycerides
  - Blood glucose level; hemoglobin (Hgb) A_{1c}
  - Erythrocyte sedimentation rate (ESR); C-reactive protein
  - Complete blood count (CBC) with differential
  - Blood urea nitrogen (BUN), creatinine, electrolytes

Wound Characteristics

- Formation/area of wound—sites of repetitive pressure or friction:
  - Plantar aspect of foot
  - Lateral aspect of foot
  - Metatarsal head
- Color:
  - Wound base is beefy red
  - Granulation tissue

▶ Size:
- Variable
- Usually small with well-defined margins
- Can be larger, depending on age of ulcer

▶ Drainage:
- Minimal unless infected

▶ Edema:
- Generally not present

▶ Skin temperature:
- Warm, unless associated peripheral vascular disease

▶ Surrounding skin/tissue:
- Often dry with fissures
- Wound area thick, callused

Risk Factors

▶ Risk for wound formation increases with loss of sensation:
- Undetected trauma or puncture

▶ Pressure points:
- Ill-fitting footwear
- Bony deformities
- Structural changes

Interventions

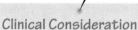

Clinical Consideration

TCC is a specially designed cast used to take weight off of the foot (off-loading).

▶ Early wound closure—primary intervention to prevent infection of tissue, bone, joint capsules

▶ Pressure relief:
- Total contact casting (TCC)—gold standard
- Removable orthotic walkers (Charcot restraint orthotic walker [CROW]) affixed to limit removal
- Consistent pressure relief through healing/wound closure process

▶ Assess/treat infection

▶ Serial/routine sharp debridement of wound bed—decrease bioburden

▶ Glycemic control

▶ Maintain moist wound bed:
- Appropriate dressing choice important

▶ Nutritional supplements:
- Enhance protein intake
- Vitamins

▶ Adjunctive hyperbaric oxygen therapy:
- Enhances healing through oxygenation
- Wagner grade 3 or higher

▶ Treatment of neuropathic pain

Patient Education

▶ Prevention is key:
- Inspection:
  - Daily foot exam for blisters, cuts, swelling, or redness
  - Use mirror if unable to see bottom of feet.
  - Keep skin moisturized after bathing.

- Bathing:
  - Wash feet daily; thoroughly dry between toes.
  - Test water with hands or elbow to prevent burns.
- Protective foot care:
  - Stockings, well-fitting with no tight elastic
  - Shoes, sufficiently wide for feet; thick flexible rubber soles
  - Never walk barefoot.
  - Use socks for warmth—never heating pad.
- Routine podiatric care, toenail care
- Smoking cessation
- Regular exercise
- Nutrition:
  - Increase protein in diet
  - Glucose control
  - Nutritional supplements
  - Dietician evaluation and treat

AUTOIMMUNE DISORDERS ASSOCIATED WITH SKIN

▶ Many chronic skin conditions can impact adults at different ages; some are less well understood and are difficult to treat.

▶ It is important to seek medical attention and obtain medical advice to avoid long-term damage and worsening of systemic symptoms.

▶ Over time, as the systemic condition or disease progresses, or goes untreated, skin damage may occur.

▶ Some of the following types of conditions cause a secondary skin condition or damage.

▶ Autoimmune disorders such as scleroderma, lupus, Sjögren syndrome, rheumatoid arthritis, and dermatomyositis can cause different skin manifestations that are very complex and not fully understood.

▶ Each disorder can become progressively more complex and develop more serious complications over time.

Scleroderma

▶ This disorder of the connective tissue causes thickened areas of skin around joints, leading to inflammation and pain.

▶ These thickened areas become tight because of the connective-tissue disorder.

▶ Affects other parts of the body:

- Blood vessels beneath the skin become hardened under the thickened patches.
- Can be diffuse to a localized area (local scleroderma) or systemic (affecting many areas)
- Scleroderma is an overproduction of collagen in the connective tissue:
  - As the main component of the connective tissue, the skin can become very rigid and restrictive to body systems depending on the severity of the disease.
- Affects women more than men.
- Skin can appear shiny and taut, and often movement is restricted.
- Systemic scleroderma can affect many body organs such as kidneys, lungs, and esophagus as the scarring creates much difficulty with movement and function.

▶ Treatment determined by presenting symptoms

Sjögren's Syndrome

▸ Evidenced by dry eyes, dry mouth

▸ Often occurs with other autoimmune conditions such as rheumatoid arthritis and lupus

▸ Can be difficult to diagnose; causes body to fight its own cells and tissues

▸ Glands seems to be targeted initially, causing the inability to secrete tears or saliva.

▸ Persistence includes vaginal dryness, yeast infections, vision problems, and dental cavities because of the lack of moisture in these areas

▸ Treatment depends on symptoms and severity

▸ Most often these patients are being treated for the symptoms they are having:

- Dry eyes, dry mouth can be treated with over-the-counter remedies
- Severe cases may require surgery of the tear ducts to seal them closed to reduce surface exposure.

Rheumatoid Arthritis

▸ An autoimmune disease that leads to raised nodules under the skin and over inflamed joints

▸ These nodules are very firm, can be painful, and are referred to as rheumatoid nodules

▸ Small purple areas, called "purpura," in the skin are also present:

- Purpura is caused by bleeding under the skin from blood vessels that have weakened from long-term steroid use.
- As with many autoimmune disorders, steroids may be included in the treatment plan, causing further risk for skin damage.

Dermatomyositis

▸ Disorder caused by inflammation of the muscles, blood vessels, and skin

▸ May present as a reddish or purple rash or even appear as a mild sunburn

▸ The areas can also be patchy and rough.

▸ The exact cause is unknown; however, there is evidence suggesting an underlying autoimmunity.

▸ Seen in women more often than in men

▸ The treatment plan is specific to the symptoms, such as itching, redness, and pain.

▸ Muscle weakness, and addition symptoms, can worsen and affect other parts of the body including:

- Esophagus
- Lungs

BURNS

Overview

▸ Another type of skin damage, more acute than chronic, are burn injuries

▸ "One civilian fire death occurs every 2 hours and 41 minutes."

▸ Burns are usually categorized into types based on the tissue damage and surface area the burn may cover on the body.

▸ Burn centers see over 200 admissions annually (American Burn Association, 2017)

Minor Burns

▸ First-degree burn anywhere on the body

▸ Second-degree burn less than 2 to 3 inches wide.

TABLE 18.3	CLASSIFICATIONS OF BURNS
Degree of Burn	Definition
Superficial (formally, first-degree burns)	Damage to the outermost layer of the skin—the epidermis; usually with signs of redness and pain.
Superficial partial-thickness (formally, second-degree burn)	Damage to both the epidermis and the dermal layer of the skin; can form blisters. These types of burns can cause pain, swelling and redness.
Deep partial-thickness (formally, third-degree burn)	Damage to the dermis, epidermis, and deeper skin tissues. A patient may experience numbness with this tissue damage.
Full-thickness (formally, fourth-degree burn)	Damage to all the layers of the skin, completely destroying tissues; will require specialty care, including skin grafts to improve healing and decrease hypertrophic scarring.

(American Burn Association, 2017)

Major Burns

▶ Third-degree burn
▶ Second-degree burn larger than 2 to 3 inches wide
▶ Second-degree burn on hands, face, feet, groin, buttocks, or over a major joint (U.S. National Library of Medicine, 2018)

Burns have traditionally been categorized as first,- second-, third-, and fourth-degree (Table 18.3).

Thermal Burns

▶ Damage to the skin by exposure to a hot or cold source that destroys cells or tissue
▶ Scalding injuries are reported as 34% of the burn injuries (American Burn Association, 2017)
▶ Can happen during everyday activities such as bathing or cooking.
▶ Treatment will vary depending on severity:
  • Topical management and small bandage
  • Complex dressing change occurring frequently, requiring medical assistance and pain management until skin begins to heal

Chemical Burns

▶ Caused when the skin comes in contact with a caustic irritant
▶ Can be acidic or alkaline, causing a reaction from the skin
▶ Should be assessed quickly and causative agent flushed away with water for at least 20 minutes
▶ Take care with flushing the area, so skin does not come into further contact with chemical and cause further harm before seeking medical attention
▶ Identification of chemical agent is important to the plan of care

Electrical Burns

▶ A burn caused by electrical current passing through the body
▶ Approximately 1000 deaths are caused annually due to electrical injuries
▶ Mortality rate of 3 to 5%.
▶ It is important for these injuries to be assessed by medical personnel and treated in the acute phase to be sure they do not get worse or go untreated.

Burn Shock Response

▶ A very complex metabolic reaction that occurs as a disruption of normal cellular process due to a major burn injury.

▶ Immediate release of cytokines and other cellular mediators at the local and systemic levels to protect the body

▶ The complex response includes an increased cellular permeability as well as a vaso-constriction to support the body system.

▶ This type of shock should be supported with fluids and intense medical management until the patient stabilizes.

▶ Most literature recommends that any burn over 20% of the total body-surface area (TBSA), all burns on face, hands and feet, groin and all children with burns should be treated in a burn center because of the complex nature, extreme pain, as well as the additional risks of infection.

SPECIAL/UNCOMMON WOUND POPULATIONS

Overview

▶ Often, uncommon wounds are intrinsic to another disease. It may be that the clinical manifestations are not consistent with the patient's history or that a wound is not responding to treatment as expected. Some of the wounds discussed are rare, but because they are associated with a higher than usual rate of morbidity and mortality, it is important to be familiar with them.

Staphylococcal Scalded Skin Syndrome (SSSS)

▶ Presents with a widespread formation of fluid-filled, thin-walled blisters that rupture easily and look much like a burn.

▶ Caused by the release of two exotoxins from toxigenic strains of *Staphylococcus aureus*.

▶ Although it is most common in children under 6 years, it can also occur in adults who are immunocompromised or have renal failure.

▶ Unlike toxic epidermal necrolysis, the mucous membranes are not involved.

Treatment

- Elimination of the primary infection
- Rehydration
- Antipyretics
- Topical treatment of the desquamated skin to include:
  - Exudate control
  - Pain management
  - Maintaining a moist environment
  - If tissue loss is massive, treat using burn therapy principles

Toxic Epidermal Necrolysis (TEN)

▶ A potentially life-threatening disorder

▶ Initially presents with a fever and flu-like symptoms

▶ A few days later the skin begins to blister and peel:
  - Painful, raw areas form
  - Mucous membranes are affected
  - Widespread erythema
  - Necrosis
  - Bullous detachment of the epidermis and mucous membranes

Complications

- Dehydration
- Sepsis
- Pneumonia
- Multiple organ failure
- Most commonly caused by certain medications
- Also caused by infections

Risk Factors

- Human immunodeficiency virus/acquired immunodeficiency syndrome (HIV/AIDS)
- Systemic lupus erythematosus

Treatment

- Eradicate/eliminate the cause
- Manage pain
- Antihistamines
- Antibiotics
- Corticosteroids
- Prevent hypothermia

Necrotizing Fasciitis

- Also known as "flesh-eating disease"
- Rare and serious bacterial infection affecting the tissue beneath the skin
- Spreads rapidly along the fascial plane
- Symptoms appear and progress rapidly.
- Frequently, the pain associated with the wound is more severe than what would be expected based on the size.
- Skin becomes red, edematous, and hot to the touch.
- Fever and chills with nausea, vomiting, and diarrhea also possible.
- More advanced symptoms can include:
  - A reddish-purple appearance of the skin
  - Large bullae form as the skin becomes necrotic and sloughs off.
  - Sometimes progresses to cutaneous gangrene
  - Can cause death in 25 to 50% of patients
- Group A streptococcus bacteria are the most common cause.
- Several other bacteria have been associated with the disease.

Risk Factors

- Predisposition to infection:
  - Immunocompromise
  - Advanced age
  - Peripheral vascular disease
  - Obesity
  - Diabetes
  - IV drug use

Treatment

- Aggressive surgical debridement of all nonviable and any suspect viable tissue
- Intravenous antibiotics
- Dressings should meet the requirements of the wound:

- Fill the dead space
- Deliver topical treatment
- Allow monitoring of the wound bed
- Absorb exudate

Pyoderma Gangrenosum (PG)

▶ Autoinflammatory skin disorder

▶ Associated with multiple autoimmune diseases such as:

- Rheumatoid arthritis
- Chronic active hepatitis
- Ulcerative colitis
- Crohn's disease

Characteristics

- Insect bites or small papules
- Progress to large, deep ulcers with necrotic tissue
- A hallmark sign of pyoderma gangrenosum is pathergy (a skin condition in which minor trauma leads to ulcers that are resistant to healing).
- Wounds are irregularly shaped, with violaceous edges.
- Exquisitely painful
- Erythematous
- Exudative
- Often filled with slough

Diagnosis

- PG is a condition that is diagnosed by exclusion; it is often misdiagnosed as vasculitis or malignancy.
- Skin biopsy shows neutrophilic inflammatory infiltrate.

Risk Factors

- Autoimmune disorders

Treatment

- Combination of systemic therapy with corticosteroids and topical wound care:
  - Protection from trauma
  - Management of exudate
  - Pain control
  - Sharp debridement is contraindicated.

Calciphylaxis

▶ Typically seen in patients with end-stage renal disease.

▶ Syndrome of calcification of the blood vessels

▶ Initial presentation is purplish mottling that progresses to bleeding tissues that become necrotic.

▶ The lesions are very painful.

Treatment

- Options are not standardized or particularly effective.
- Mortality is related to the underlying renal disease process.
- Wound care is related to the needs of the wounds:
  - Debridement as indicated
  - Dressings to manage exudate
  - Protect the wound
  - Fill any dead space

- Prevent infection
- Address pain

Sickle Cell Disease

▶ A group of inherited red blood cell disorders
▶ One symptom is leg ulcers:
  - Can be very painful
  - Ulcers possibly the result of multiple factors:
    - Trauma
    - Infections
    - Inflammation in combination with the microcirculatory environment
    - Although they present in the same area as venous ulcers and may resemble them in appearance, they are not the result of venous insufficiency.

Treatment

- Protection from insult
- Debridement
- Compression
- Pain management
- Local care
- Despite best efforts, these ulcers are likely to recur.

ADDRESSING BIOBURDEN

Overview

▶ The body's greatest defense against infection is intact skin.
▶ When skin integrity is breached, the open area hosts normal skin flora as well as contaminated body fluid.
▶ This bacterial burden, otherwise known as "bioburden," has a complex effect on wounds.
▶ Bacteria compete for limited nutrients and oxygen available, while producing endotoxins that destroy and/or alter normal cellular activity.
▶ Treating bioburden is complex, addressing the quantity of microorganisms in the wound as well as their virulence and diversity of interactions with the body.

Chronic Wounds

▶ All chronic wounds have some degree of bacterial bioburden.
▶ They have consistent elevated proinflammatory cytokines, matrix metalloproteinases (MMP's) and neutrophils.
▶ Neutrophils continue to arrive at the wound because of the elevation of cytokines, MMP's and keep the wound in the inflammatory phase of wound healing.
▶ Most common effect of this persistent chronic inflammatory phase is delayed healing.

Continuum of Bacterial Bioburden

▶ Contamination:
  - Nonreplicating microorganisms on the wound surface without a host reaction
  - Typical of all wounds to be inhabited by normal flora
  - Antimicrobials not indicated
  - Replicating microorganisms adhere to the wound surface without a host reaction.
▶ Colonization:
  - Replicating microorganisms adhere to the wound surface without a host reaction.
  - Antimicrobials not indicated

▶ Critical colonization:
- Replicating microorganisms present on the wound
- Attached to the cells and structures in the wound
- Host does not exhibit classic signs of infection.
- Level of bacteria inhibits wound healing.

Biofilm

▶ Complex community of aggregated bacteria embedded in a self-secreted extracellular polysaccharide matrix
▶ Bacteria within the biofilm respond to signals from other bacteria in the community
▶ Highly resistant to and poorly penetrated by antimicrobials
▶ Debridement indicated in conjunction with antimicrobials

Infection (Local)

▶ Invasion of tissue by microorganisms that yield a local or systemic host response
▶ Treatment with antimicrobials indicated after cultures obtained to direct therapy
- Assessment/clinical indications for wound infections:
  - Lack of healing after 2 weeks of topical therapy
  - Local signs of infection:
    - Increased erythema
    - Increased amount or changed character of exudate
    - Odor
    - Increased warmth of tissue
    - Edema or induration
    - Pain or tenderness
  - Systemic signs of infection:
    - Fever
    - Chills
    - Leukocytosis
    - Pain in neuropathic extremity
    - Elevated glucose for diabetic patients
- Lab test/cultures
  - CBC
    - Elevation of white cells with infection
  - ESR:
    - Marker of inflammation
  - C-reactive protein levels:
    - Elevate with inflammation
  - Stain cultures
  - Tissue biopsy:
    - Removal of a piece of the tissue with sharp instrument
    - Gold standard
    - Needle aspiration
      - Aspiration of fluid from tissue adjacent to the wound
    - Swab technique:
      - Most commonly performed
      - Levine technique:
        - Proven to have more specificity and sensitivity than the Z technique

- Rotate and press down on the swab when obtaining the culture to express wound fluid from 1 cm^2 area of the wound, rolling the tip of the swab on its side in one full rotation.
- Treatment:
  - Reduce bioburden without causing additional tissue injury
  - Treat infection without causing the development of drug resistance
- Local treatment:
  - Good wound cleansing techniques with appropriate cleansing solution
  - Topical/wound dressings:
    - Bactericidal:
      - Acetic acid
    - Broad spectrum:
      - Cadexomer iodine:
        - Absorb fluids to remove exudate, pus, and debris.
        - Slow release of iodine kills organisms in wound.
      - Chlorhexidine 0.02%
      - Silver dressings
  - Methylene blue and gentian violet:
    - Effective against methicillin-resistant *Staphylococcus aureus* (MRSA)
  - Chlorine—Dakin solution
- Debridement:
  - Autolytic
    - Lysis of necrotic tissue by the body's own white cells and natural enzymes
  - Chemical/enzymatic
    - Addition of exogenous enzymes to remove necrotic tissue
    - Collagenase; Dakin solution; silver nitrate
  - Biosurgical
    - Maggot therapy
    - Mechanical:
      - Wet to dry gauze
      - Hydrotherapy
      - Ultrasonic mist therapy
    - Sharp:
      - Removal of tissue with sharp sterile instrument
      - May require surgical removal

Infection (Systemic)

- Primary treatment of wound infection
- Important to obtain culture and gram stain results to determine appropriate treatment for organism.

Patient Education

- Ensure patient has clear understanding of wound cleansing technique.
- Encourage compliance with recommended appointments for serial debridement.
- Complete antibiotic therapy even if no symptoms are seen.
- Enhanced education on each specific dressing choice and what is the expectation of exudate
- Discuss patient's ability to apply dressing and adapt choice to meet patient's needs.
- Protect perineal area wounds from body fluids.

CASE STUDY

A 55-year-old male with a 20-year history of diabetes presents to the hospital with a wound on the plantar surface of his right foot and a second wound on that heel. He reports that his "sugars" are well controlled; and his blood glucose this morning was 145 mg/dL. He has a 40-year history of smoking. He lives alone and periodically skips meals but "makes up for it" at his next meal. His current weight is 325 lb. He is unkempt. He was working until 2 months ago but had to stop as he was having difficulty ambulating. Now he rarely leaves home. He is wearing soiled shorts, a tee shirt, and open-toed sandals with holes on the bottom. His legs are edematous, with significant hemosiderin staining. Although there is no wound at present, his skin is tight and oozing. He uses towels to prevent the drainage from getting on the furniture.

His vital signs are stable, lungs are clear. Blood glucose is 120 mg/dL fasting. Other physical findings are unremarkable. On assessment, the wounds have threads and pieces of fabric in them, and they are dirty. The plantar surface wound is surrounded by callus; the heel wound is black and dry. The ABI is 0.7, and pulses are diminished.

1. **What would be important information for the nurse to note?**
   - *Blood sugars may not be as consistently well controlled as he believes.*
   - *He has two significant diabetic ulcers.*
   - *He has peripheral arterial disease (PAD), as evidenced by the pale, shiny, hairless lower extremities and a 0.7 ABI.*

2. **What should be included in the initial plan of care?**
   - *Wound care consult*
   - *Daily diary to monitor food intake, both quantity and quality for 4 days*
   - *Refer for vascular workup*
     - *Need to evaluate blood flow in and out of legs*
     - *In order for wounds to heal, there must be adequate flow.*
   - *Encourage leg elevation, above heart whenever possible.*
   - *Encourage off-loading of foot.*
   - *Debride callus.*
   - *Debride necrotic tissue from wounds.*
   - *Assess for infection.*
   - *Evaluate sensation.*
   - *Measure and photograph wounds.*
   - *Apply dressing to maintain moisture balance and protection from environment.*

3. **What education would be important to provide prior to the patient's discharge home?**
   - *Keep follow-up appointments as scheduled.*
   - *Keep dressings dry; change/reinforce dressings as needed.*
   - *Ensure that the wounds stay covered with sterile dressings to prevent infection.*
   - *Elevate extremities and off-load as prescribed.*
   - *Teach signs and symptoms of infection, local and systemic.*
   - *Encourage patient to keep a log of blood glucose testing and bring to provider visits.*
   - *Topical antimicrobials to reduce bioburden while awaiting results of culture and sensitivity testing.*

Bibliography

American Burn Association. (2017). Burn incidence and treatment in the United States: 2017. Accessed March 2, 2018, from http://ameriburn.org/who-we-are/media/burn-incidence-fact-sheet/

American Diabetes Association. (2017). Accessed March 2, 2018, from http://www.diabetes.org/diabetes-basics/statistics

Ayello, E.A., et al. (2018). Survey results from the Philippines: NPUAP changes in pressure injury terminology and definitions. *Advances in Skin and Wound Care* 31, 601–606.

Bergstrom, N. (1987). The Braden Scale for predicting pressure sore risk. *Nurses* 36, 205–210.

Bryant, R.A. (2000). *Acute and Chronic Wounds: Nursing Management.* (St. Louis: Elsevier).

Hess, C. T. (2013). *Clinical Guide to Skin and Wound Care*, 7th ed. (Ambler, PA: Lippincott Williams & Wilkins).

Kumar, S., Fernando, D.J., Veves, A., Knowles, E.A., Young, M.J., and Boulton, A.J.M. (1991). Semmes-Weinstein monofilaments: a simple, effective and inexpensive screening device for identifying diabetic patients at risk of foot ulceration. *Diabetes Research and Clinical Practice* 13, 63–67.

Sen, C.K., Gordillo, G.M., Roy, S., Kirsner, R., Lambert, L., Hunt, T.K., … Longaker, M.T. (2009). Human skin wounds: a major and snowballing threat to public health and the economy. *Wound Repair and Regeneration* 17, 763–771.

Wagner, F.W. (1981). The dysvascular foot: a system for diagnosis and treatment. *Foot & Ankle* 2(2), 64–122.

U.S. National Library of Medicine. (2018). Burns. Accessed June 25, 2018, from https://medlineplus.gov/ency/article/000030.htm

19

Cancer

Donna Martin, DNP, RN, CMSRN, CDE, CNE

OVERVIEW

▶ *Cancer* is a generic term used to describe more than 200 diseases characterized by uncontrolled and unregulated growth of cells. Cancer cells can spread from their original site to other parts of the body. Cancer is the second leading cause of death worldwide (WHO, 2017) (Table 19.1).

ANATOMY AND PHYSIOLOGY

▶ Cancer development is noted by a defect in cell proliferation (growth) and cell differentiation:

- Cell growth and division is an uncoordinated, unregulated process.
- New cells are different in structure and function from tissue of origin.

▶ There are several genetic changes that contribute to cancer. These genetic changes affect three types of genes:

- Proto-oncogenes
  - Involved in cell growth and division
  - When altered they can become tumor-inducing genes (oncogenes)
  - This alteration may occur with exposure to carcinogens.
  - Oncogenes have the ability to change a normal cell to a malignant cell.

TABLE 19.1	2016 ESTIMATED CANCER DEATHS	
Cancer	Male—no. (%)	Female—no. (%)
Lung	85,920 (27%)	72,160 (26%)
Prostate	26,120 (8%)	40,450 (14%)
Colon	26,020 (8%)	23,170 (8%)
Pancreas	21,120 (7%)	20,330 (7%)
Liver	18,280 (6%)	10,270 (4%)
Leukemia	14,130 (4%)	10,270 (4%)
Esophagus	12,720 (4%)	8,890 (3%)

American Cancer Society (2016). Leading sites of new cancer cases and deaths, 2016 estimates. Retrieved from http://www.cancer.org

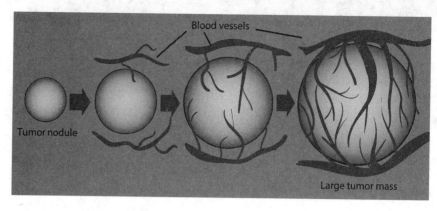

Figure 19.1 Process of Angiogenesis

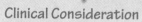

Clinical Consideration

For example, alterations in BRCA1 and BRCA2 tumor suppressor genes play a role in breast and ovarian cancers.

- Tumor-suppressor genes:
  - Involved in cell growth and division
  - Alterations can cause uncontrolled division and development of tumors
- DNA-repair genes:
  - Fix damaged DNA
  - May cause mutations that become cancerous
▶ Metastasis:
- Cancer cells from the original (primary) site travel to distant parts of the body.
- Angiogenesis (Figure 19.1):
  - The tumor has access to a blood supply
  - Speeds up cancer cell replications
  - Avenue for cancer cells to spread to distant parts of the body
- Tumor-associated antigens present because of malignant transformation of cells
▶ Carcinogens:
- Chemical:
  - Examples include:
    - Hydrocarbons:
      - Chimney soot, tars
      - Cigarette smoke
    - Industrial agents:
      - Asbestos
      - Formaldehyde
      - Benzene
      - Arsenic
      - Insecticides
- Radiation:
  - Cellular exposure to radiation causes damage to the DNA and malignancies.
  - Examples include:
    - Ultraviolet (UV) radiation—melanoma and basal-cell carcinoma (skin cancer)
    - Radiation exposures from atomic exposure—leukemia and thyroid cancers
- Viral
  - Some viruses change the DNA and RNA in the cells that have been infected, causing the cells to transform into malignant cells.
  - Examples include:
    - Human papillomavirus (HPV)—cervical squamous cell carcinoma
    - Human immunodeficiency virus (HIV)—Kaposi sarcoma

TABLE 19.2   BENIGN VERSUS MALIGNANT CHARACTERISTICS

Benign	Malignant
Expansive growth	Infiltrating growth
Generally slow growth	Generally rapid growth
Usually encapsulated	Rarely encapsulated
Well differentiated	Poorly differentiated
Fairly normal, similar to parent cell	Abnormal, very different from parent cell
Demonstrates contact inhibition	Does not demonstrate contact inhibition
Stays within their cell type	Does not stay within their cell type
Local spread	Local and distant spread
Recurrence rare	Recurrence common

- Hepatitis B virus—hepatocellular carcinoma
- Epstein–Barr virus (EBV)—Burkitt lymphoma

▶ Classifications (Table 19.2):
- Benign:
  - Well differentiated—easy to identify parent cells
  - Usually encapsulated
  - Limited vascular access
  - Recurrence rare
- Malignant:
  - Poorly differentiated—can be hard to determine parent cell
  - Rarely encapsulated
  - Seeks out vascular access, speeds up growth
  - Recurrence possible
- Anatomic classification:
  - Carcinomas—epithelial tissue
  - Sarcomas—connective tissue
  - Lymphoma—lymph tissue
  - Myeloma—plasma cells
  - Leukemia—bone marrow
- Grading—appearance of cells and differentiation from tissue or origin:
  - Grade I:
    - Mild dysplasia—slightly different from normal cell
    - Well differentiated from tissue of origin
  - Grade II:
    - Moderate dysplasia—more abnormal
    - Moderately differentiated from tissue of origin
  - Grade III:
    - Severe dysplasia—very abnormal
    - Poorly differentiated from tissue of origin
  - Grade IV:
    - Anaplasia—cells appear immature, loss of cell characteristics
    - Cell of origin difficult to determine

- Grade X:
  - Unable to grade
- Staging—extent and spread of the disease:
  - Stage 0—cancer in situ
  - Stage I—limited to tissue of origin
  - Stage II—local spread
  - Stage III—extensive local and regional spread
  - Stage IV—distant spread, metastasis:
    - Main sites of metastasis—brain, lung, liver, adrenal, bone
- Tumor–node–metastasis (TNM) system—extent of disease:
  - T—invasiveness
  - N—involvement of lymph nodes
  - M—distant metastasis
- Gerontologic considerations:
  - Age-related changes:
    - Longer exposure to carcinogens
    - Decline in physiologic functioning:
      - Multiple comorbidities
      - Decreased immune response
    - Manifestations may be mistaken as age-related changes
  - Other factors:
    - Projected life expectancy
    - Patient wishes; durable power of attorney (POA) for heath care, living will
    - Presence or absence of a support system

PREVENTION AND EARLY DIAGNOSIS

- Cancer prevention:
  - Avoid exposure to carcinogens:
    - Smoking
    - Reduction in radiation exposure: UV radiation, ionizing radiation:
      - Tanning beds
      - Sun exposure
      - Medical radiation
      - Radon gas
    - Immunosuppression
  - Lifestyle changes:
    - Regular exercise
    - Balanced diet
  - Risk-reducing procedures
  - Early detection through screening
- Early diagnosis:
  - Early identification, diagnosis, and staging:
    - Improved survival rate
    - More treatment options may be available
  - Teach patients to notify provider of early warning signs of cancer—CAUTION (American Cancer Society [ACS], 2018b)
    - Change in bladder or bowel habits
    - A sore throat that does not heal

- **U**nusual bleeding or discharge
- **T**hickening or lump in the breast or elsewhere
- **I**ndigestion, or difficulty with swallowing
- **O**bvious change in mole or wart
- **N**agging cough or hoarseness
- Screening:
  - Practice self-examination:
    - Breast
    - Testicular
  - Follow cancer screening guidelines:
    - Breast:
      - Mammogram
        - Every 12 to 24 months for average-risk women 40 years or older (ACOG, 2017a; AHRQ, 2014) and continue until age 75 (ACOG, 2017a)
    - Colon:
      - Beginning at age 50 for men and women; recommendations should be individualized based on medical history and family history (ACS, 2018c).
      - Noninvasive (any positive results should be followed up with a colonoscopy):
        - Fecal immunochemical test (FIT) every year
        - Guaiac-based fecal occult blood test (gFOBT) every year
        - Stool DNA test every 3 years
      - Invasive:
        - Colonoscopy every 10 years
        - Alternative testing options—any abnormalities must be followed up with a colonoscopy:
          - CT colonography (virtual colonoscopy) every 5 years
          - Flexible sigmoidoscopy every 5 years
          - Double-contrast barium enema every 5 years
    - Cervical:
      - Pap smear (ACOG, 2017b ; AHRQ, 2014)
        - Women 21 to 29 years of age—every 3 years
        - Women 30 to 65 years of age—every 3 to 5 years
      - HPV screening (ACOG, 2017b; AHRQ, 2014)
        - Women 21 to 29 years of age—screening not recommended
        - Women 30—65 years of age—every 5 years
    - Prostate:
      - Serum prostate-specific antigen (PSA):
        - Men 55-69 years of age—consider screening (USPSTF, 2017)
        - PSA <2.5 ng/mL—retest every 2 years.
        - PSA result >2.5 ng/mL—retest yearly

> **Clinical Consideration**
> A FIT or gFOBT done during a digital rectal exam can miss 90% of colon cancer.

> **Clinical Consideration**
> A take-home FIT or gFOBT test that uses a multiple-samples method is recommended for a more accurate screening.

DIAGNOSTIC TESTS

Definitive diagnosis is made by cell biopsy and brushings. Other diagnostic tests can be used to determine location and associated problems.

- Biopsy:
  - Fine-needle aspiration
  - Large-core needle biopsy
  - Excisional/incisional biopsy

- Cytologic studies
- Sentinel lymph node biopsy—evaluation of the first lymph node near the tumor to evaluate spread
  ▶ Imaging—depending on site or type of cancer suspected:
  - X-rays
  - Computed tomography (CT) scan
  - Magnetic resonance imaging (MRI)
  - Positron-emission tomography (PET) scan
  - Endoscopic tests
  ▶ Laboratory:
  - Complete blood count (CBC)
    - Red cells—assess for anemia
    - White cells—assess for neutropenia or infection
    - Platelets—assess for thrombocytopenia
  - Tumor markers:
    - Carcinoembryonic antigen (CEA)—increased levels are a marker of cancer, most sensitive to colon cancer
    - α-Fetoprotein (AFP)—used to screen for liver, testicular, and ovarian cancer
    - PSA—increased in cancerous and noncancerous prostate disorders
  - Genetic markers
    - BRCA1 and BRCA2—identifiy mutations in breast cancer genes
    - Adenomatous polyposis coli (APC)—tumor-suppressor gene, abnormalities often indicate colon cancer
  - Molecular receptors:
    - Estrogen receptors
    - Progesterone receptors
  - Bone marrow analysis:
    - Bone marrow aspiration:
      - Liquid portion of the bone marrow is aspirated
    - Bone marrow biopsy:
      - Large needle used to obtain a core of solid bone marrow

TREATMENT

Treatment of cancer is based on several factors; tumor type, site, extent of disease, and goal of treatment. Goals of treatment for cancer are cure, control, and palliation. Early detection usually has the best outcomes, as more treatment options may be available. Treatment is usually multimodal utilizing surgery, radiation, and/or chemotherapy.

  ▶ Definitions of treatment goals:
  - Cure—to eradicate all abnormal cancer cells
  - Control—to control the growth and spread of cancer cells
  - Palliation—to provide relief of symptoms caused by cancer, such as pain or pressure

Surgery

Indications include:

- Diagnosis:
  - Biopsy—obtain a sample of the abnormal cells
- Determine diagnostic and treatment plan:
  - Staging must be done to determine the degree of differentiation of the abnormal cells.

- Cure and/or control:
  - Removal of localized cancer tissue:
    - Primary site—site of origin of the abnormal cells
    - Metastatic site—cancer cells that have traveled through the lymph and hematologic systems to a site different from the primary site
- Palliation of symptoms:
  - Relieve pain
  - Relieve obstruction
  - Stop hemorrhage/bleeding
- Supportive care:
  - Insertion of therapeutic devices:
    - Feeding tubes
    - Suprapubic catheter
- Rehabilitation:
  - Reconstructive surgery:
    - Colostomy reversal
    - Breast reconstruction
- Prevention:
  - Removal of organs to prevent cancer development
    - Prophylactic mastectomy; women with a mutation of the *BRCA1* or *BRAC2* gene, strong family history of breast cancer, history of lobular carcinoma in situ, or who have had cancer in one breast.
    - Prophylactic oophorectomy; women with a mutation of the *BRCA1* or *BRAC2* gene are at high risk for ovarian cancer; this surgery can reduce the risk of ovarian and breast cancer in at-risk women.

Radiation

Involves the delivery of high-energy beams to interfere with cellular function, causing cell death. The goal is to target the radiation to the exact site of cancer cells to prevent excessive damage to healthy cells.

- Cure:
  - To destroy abnormal cells
- Control:
  - Shrink tumor size preoperatively
- Palliation:
  - Relieve pain
  - Relieve obstruction
  - Improve sense of well-being
- Route:
  - External beam
    - Low-energy beams (particulate radiation using electrons, neutrons, and protons)—penetrate only short distances; best used for superficial cancers.
    - High-energy beams (photons)—penetrate deeper tissues; spare surrounding tissue; full intensity of beam does not occur until the set depth is achieved.
    - Site for radiation therapy is marked on the patient's skin to ensure that the exact same spot is irradiated each time.
  - Internal:
    - Sealed:
      - Radioactive seeds, rods, or ribbons placed close to tumor or body cavity

- Can be temporary or permanent
  - The radiation in seeds gradually decays.
  - Body fluids are **not** contaminated
- Unsealed:
  - Administered orally or instilled in body cavity:
    - Private room with signage "Radioactive Material"
    - All body fluids contaminated
    - Double-flush body fluids
- Nursing care:
  - Limit exposure; follow time, distance, and shielding guidelines
- Side effects/complications—depends on location of radiation treatment (Table 19.3):
  - Fatigue
  - Skin changes:
    - Wet desquamation
    - Dry desquamation
  - Pneumonitis
  - Cardiovascular
  - Gastrointestinal
- Patient teaching:
  - Caring for radiation treatment area:
    - Do not wash off treatment markings.
    - Assess skin for changes/side effects.
    - Apply only the lotions or creams as instructed by radiation staff.
  - Monitor for adverse effects of radiation and notify provider.

TABLE 19.3	SIDE EFFECTS OF CHEMOTHERAPY AND RADIATION	
System	Problem	Nursing Interventions
Psychosocial *Experienced by most cancer patients*	Fatigue Persistent tiredness Interferes with daily activities Often persists long after treatments have ceased	Encourage periods of rest but to maintain as many of normal activities as possible Encourage exercise as tolerated

Integumentary
 	
Alterations in skin and hair cells
	Radiation
	Wet desquamation
	  Sloughing of skin cells faster than new skin cells
	Dry desquamation
	  Erythema of skin in irradiated areas
	Chemotherapy
	Hyperpigmentation
	  Patches of dark skin
	Photosensitivity
	  Itching, burning, and skin changes
	Erythrodysesthesia (hand–foot syndrome)
	  Affects hands and soles of feet; from redness and tingling to ulcerations, blistering, and severe pain
	Alopecia
	  Hair loss, usually reversible, 3–4 weeks after therapy is discontinued
		Skin alterations
		  Teach patient to clean site gently with mild soap.
		  Do not wash away radiation markings.
		  Protect skin from temperature extremes; do **not** use ice or heating pads.
		  Avoid creams and constrictive clothing.
		  Avoid direct exposure to the sun.
		  Avoid skin irritants.
		Alopecia
		  Provide resources for wigs, head scarves, and head coverings
		  Avoid excessive shampooing and brushing of hair.
		  Consider trimming hair prior to the start of treatment.
		  Use ice cap to decrease hair loss.

(continued)

TABLE 19.3   *(Continued)*

System	Problem	Nursing Interventions

Gastrointestinal
 	
Chemotherapy medications, cellular destruction
 	
Damage to the mucosal lining of the gastrointestinal (GI) tract
	Nausea/vomiting
	  Onset within hours of treatment
	  Anticipatory nausea and vomiting
	  Onset between 24 hours and weeks after treatment
	Diarrhea
	  Triggered by chemotherapy or pelvic radiation
	Dysphagia
	  Present challenge to swallowing because of irritation of mouth, throat, and esophagus
	Stomatitis, mucositis, esophagitis
	  Inflammation and irritation of the lining of the GI tract mucosa
	Anorexia
	  Poor appetite due to above GI side effects
	  Typically peaks about 4 weeks after treatment begins
		Nausea/vomiting
		  Administer antiemetics prophylactically and as needed.
		  Avoid foods with strong odors.
		  Provide diversional activities.
		Diarrhea
		  Low-residue, low-fiber diet
		  Avoid foods that aggravate diarrhea.
		  Administer antidiarrheals, antimotility medications, antispasmodics
		Stomatitis, mucositis, esophagitis
		  Provide meticulous oral care
		    Avoid commercial mouthwashes.
		    Encourage soft, nonirritating foods
		    Avoid spicy foods
		    Topical anesthetics (viscous lidocaine)
		Anorexia
		  Offer supplements to provide additional calories.
		  Increase protein, as tolerated.
		  Monitor weight.

Hematologic
 	
Bone marrow depression impacting production of red and white cells and platelets
	Anemia
	  Decreased red-cell production
	Leukopenia
	  Reduction in white blood cells, increasing risk for infection
	Thrombocytopenia
	  Risk for bleeding due to platelet count ≤20,000/µL
		Monitor hemoglobin, hematocrit, white cells, and platelet counts.
		Epogen for anemia
		Monitor for bleeding and infection (especially during the nadir).
		Teach patient about neutropenic and thrombocytopenic precautions.
		Pegfilgrastim (Neulasta Onpro) for leukocytosis

Cardiovascular
 	
Inflammation from radiation, damage to ventricles from chemotherapy
	Pericardial effusion/pericarditis
	  Thoracic radiation damage
	Heart failure
	  Use of cardiotoxic chemotherapy drugs
	    Doxorubicin (Adriamycin)
	    Daunorubicin
		Baseline electrocardiography (ECG) and echocardiography for patients with CAD
		Periodic ECG and echocardiography to assess for cardiac changes, specifically left ventricular function

Neurologic
 	
Most often occurs with chemotherapy
	"Chemo brain"
	  Decreased cognitive clarity
	  States "foggy" feeling
	  May experience poor memory
	Peripheral neuropathy
	  Paresthesias from some chemotherapy drugs
	    Plant alkaloids
	    Taxanes
	    Cisplatin
	Increased intracranial pressure
	  Due to edema from radiation
		"Chemo brain"
		  Get adequate rest/sleep.
		  Keep a detailed planner.
		  Engage in cognitive activities; puzzles, word games.
		Peripheral neuropathy
		  Monitor for paresthesias, muscle weakness
		  Administer medications to decrease neuropathic pain
		    Gabapentin (Neurontin)
		Increased intracranial pressure (ICP)
		    Closely monitor for any changes in neurologic status.
		    Corticosteroids may be ordered.

Pulmonary
 	
Lung tissue damage from radiation and some chemotherapy
	Pneumonitis
	  Inflammatory reaction associated with thoracic radiation
	Pulmonary edema
	  Inflammatory reaction that contributes to alveolar capillary destruction
		Assess and monitor for cough and shortness of breath

Reproductive
 	
Damage to reproductive organs from chemotherapy or local radiation
	Infertility
	  May be temporary or permanent
	  Impact to testes and ovaries are based on therapy type, duration, and age of person
		For patients of childbearing age, offer sperm/ova banking prior to the initiation of chemotherapy or radiation treatment.

Genitourinary
 	
Damage to lining of bladder and kidney from chemotherapy or local radiation
	Hemorrhagic cystitis
	  Side effect of radiation
	Nephrotoxicity
	  Damage to renal cells from byproduct of tumor lysis syndrome (TLS) and chemotherapy drugs
	    Cisplatin
	    Methotrexate
		Monitor for signs of urinary frequency, dysuria, hematuria.
		Encourage increased fluid intake.
		Patient may be prescribed allopurinol (Zyloprim) to prevent TLS.

Chemotherapy

The goals of chemotherapy, often called "antineoplastic therapy," are consistent with the overall treatment goals of cure, control, and palliation. The drugs used are cytotoxic; they inhibit growth and spread of malignant cells. These drugs have a systemic effect on the body, which contributes to multiple side effects.

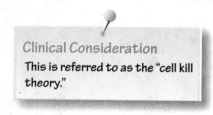

Clinical Consideration

This is referred to as the "cell kill theory."

- Chemotherapy drug types:
  - Cell-cycle-phase–specific drugs are those that work during specific phases of cell division. These drugs are typically given by infusion over a period of time.
  - Cell-cycle-phase–nonspecific drugs are not dependent on any particular phase of cell division; these antineoplastic agents work during all phases of the cell cycle. They are typically given in bolus doses.
- Cellular kinetics of chemotherapy drugs:
  - Chemotherapy is administered in courses. This is done as only a percentage of cancer cells are destroyed with each chemotherapy treatment. It is believed that the proportion of cancer cells that are destroyed with each course is dependent on the medication and dose (Figure 19.2).
- Access:
  - Chemotherapy drugs are irritants or vesicants and can cause severe tissue breakdown and necrosis if they infiltrate into the surrounding tissue.
    - Avoid using peripheral intravenous lines to avoid extravasation risk
    - Use a central venous access device, port, or peripherally inserted central catheter (PICC)

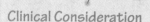

Clinical Consideration

A peripheral IV should not be used for chemotherapy because of the potential for severe tissue damage.

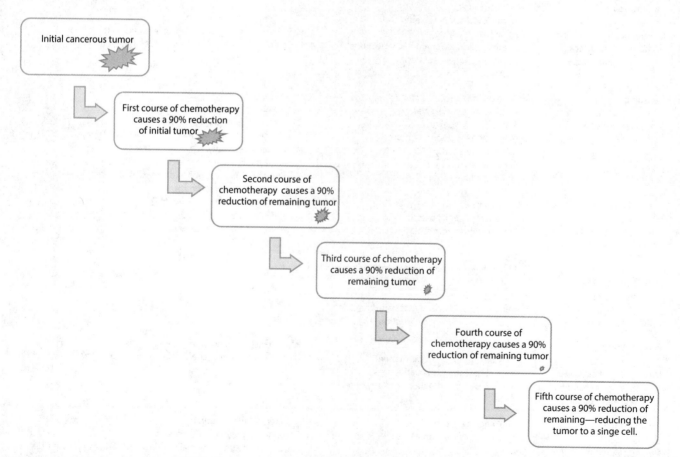

Figure 19.2 Example of the Cell Kill Theory

- Other chemotherapy administration routes:
  - Intraarterial—infusion of chemotherapy into the artery that directly supplies blood to the tumor
  - Intraperitoneal—instillation of chemotherapy into the peritoneum for 1 to 4 hours
  - Intrathecal—instillation of chemotherapy directly into the subarachnoid space
  - Intravesical—instillation of chemotherapy into the bladder for 1 to 3 hours
- Complications (Table 19.3):
  - Myelosuppression:
    - Nadir:
      - 7 to 14 days after receiving chemotherapy
      - Greatest risk for infection and bleeding
    - Neutropenia:
      - Absolute neutrophil count <1000/mm^3
    - Thrombocytopenia:
      - Platelets <20,000/mm^3
  - Anemia:
    - Suppression of red bone marrow
  - Gastrointestinal effects:
    - Nausea and vomiting (Table 19.4)
    - Anorexia
    - Mucositis
  - Integumentary effects:
    - Alopecia:
      - Begins 2 to 3 weeks after first dose
      - May lose eyebrows, lashes, and other body hair
      - New hair growth begins 4 to 6 weeks after last dose.
      - Hair may grow back a different color and texture.
    - Skin reactions:
      - Erythema
      - Hyperpigmentation
      - Photosensitivity
  - Fatigue—overwhelming, persistent feeling of being tired
  - Neurologic—peripheral neuropathy
  - Reproductive changes—sterility

> **Clinical Consideration**
>
> It is critical to vigilantly monitor for complications during the nadir.

TABLE 19.4	ANTIEMETIC MEDICATIONS
Decrease nausea and vomiting	
Metoclopramide (Reglan)	
Ondansetron (Zofran)	
Granisetron (Kytril)	
Dolasetron (Anzemet)	
Palonosetron (Aloxi)	
Dexamethasone (Decadron)	
Lorazepam (Ativan)	
Preventing nausea and vomiting	
Aprepitant (Emend)	
Rolapitant (Varubi)	
Netupitant–palonosetron (Akynzeo)	

- Chemotherapy drugs (Table 19.5)
- Nursing considerations when working with chemotherapy
  - Safe handling:
    - Should be administered only by staff who have received chemotherapy administration education.
    - Wash hands before and after handling chemotherapeutic agents.
    - Wearing chemotherapy personal protective equipment (PPE) for drug administration and handling the patient's bodily fluids for 48 hours after administration of chemotherapy.
    - Double-flush all body fluids with the bowl covered for the first 48 hours after receiving chemotherapy.
    - Spill kits need to be readily available and staff trained in proper use.
  - Proper disposal:
    - Dispose of all equipment that comes in contact with the chemotherapeutic agents in a hazardous waste container.
- Patient teaching:
  - How to store and dispose of chemotherapeutic agents if administered at home as well as how to dispose of bodily fluids for 48 hours after treatment
  - Neutropenia precautions:
    - Avoid crowds.
    - Stay away from sick people.
    - Stay away from people who have recently had immunizations for smallpox/chickenpox.
    - Protect skin against breakdown.
    - Check rectal, oral, eyes, nose, genital, and rectal areas and PICC line for redness.
    - Notify provider about chills, sweating, loose stools, fever (low grade), mouth breakdown, abdominal pain, vaginal itching, discharge.

TABLE 19.5	COMMON DRUGS USED FOR THE TREATMENT AND PREVENTION OF CANCER

Breast Cancer

Tamoxifen citrate (Nolvadex)
Raloxifene hydrochloride (Evista)
Trastuzumab (Herceptin)
Doxorubicin (Adriamycin)
Epirubicin (Ellence)
Paclitaxel (Taxol, Abraxane)
Docetaxel (Taxotere)
5-fluorouracil (5-FU)
Cyclophosphamide (Cytoxan)
Carboplatin (Paraplatin)
Cisplatin

Cervical Cancer

Prevention
  Recombinant human papillomavirus (HPV) bivalent vaccine (Cervarix)
  Recombinant HPV nonavalent vaccine (Gardasil)
  Recombinant HPV quadrivalent vaccine (Gardasil 9)

Treatment
  Cispatin
  Fluorouracil (5-FU)
  Carboplatin (Paraplatin)
  Paclitaxel (Taxol)
  Gemcitabine (Gemzar)

(continued)

TABLE 19.5 (Continued)

Colon Cancer

Bevacizumab (Avastin)
Fluorouracil (5-FU)

Hodgkin's Lymphoma

ABVD regimen is the standard chemotherapy treatment
    Doxorubicin (Adriamycin)
    Bleomycin
    Vinblastine (Velban, Velsar)
    Dacarbazine chlorambucil
BEACOPP
    Bleomycin
    Etoposide (VP-16)
    Doxorubicin (Adriamycin)
    Cyclophosphamide (Cytoxan)
    Vincristine (Oncovin)
    Procarbazine
    Prednisone
Stanford V
    Doxorubicin (Adriamycin)
    Nitrogen mustard (Mechlorethamine)
    Vincristine (Oncovin)
    Vinblastine (Velban, Velsar)
    Bleomycin
    Etoposide (VP-16)
    Prednisone

Non-Hodgkin's Lymphoma

A common combination is R-CHOP
    Rituximab (Rituxan)
    Cyclophosphamide (Cytoxan)
    Doxorubicin (also known as hydroxydaunorubicin)
    Vincristine (Oncovin)
    Prednisone.
Another common combination, CVP, leaves out doxorubicin and rituximab

Lung Cancer

Bevacizumab (Avastin)
Carboplatin (Paraplat, Paraplatin)
Cisplatin (Platinol)
Docetaxel (Taxotere)
Gemcitabine (Gemzar)
Methotrexate (Abitrexate, Folex, Mexate)
Paclitaxel (Abraxane, Taxol)
Pemetrexed (Alimta)
Vinorelbine (Navelbine)

Prostate Cancer

Docetaxel (Taxotere)
Cabazitaxel (Jevtana)
Mitoxantrone (Novantrone)
Estramustine (Emcyt)

Thyroid Cancer

Cabozantinib-s-malate (Cometriq)
Doxorubicin hydrochloride
Lenvatinib mesylate (Lenvima)
Sorafenib tosylate (Nexavar)
Vandetanib (Caprelsa)

- Thrombocytopenia precautions:
  - Floss with care.
  - Blow nose gently.
  - Avoid contact sports.
  - Increased fluid intake.
  - Avoid household injuries.
  - Use electric razor.
  - Check joints for bleeding.
  - Report dizziness.
  - Use soft toothbrush.
  - Check for bleeding gums, bruising, hemagglutination, black stools, petechiae.

Immunotherapy

- Uses the immune system to fight cancer:
  - Helps to boost the immune system to prevent infections
  - Helps to destroy cancer cells
- Medications:
  - Cytokines
    - α-Interferon (Intron A)
    - Interleukin-2 (Proleukin)
  - Vaccines:
    - Bacille Calmette–Guérin (BCG) vaccine; used for bladder cancer
  - Monoclonal antibodies:
    - Trastuzumab (Herceptin); IV route—for breast cancer
    - Lapatinib (Tykerb); oral route—for breast cancer
    - Bevacizumb (Avastin)—prevents vascularization of tumors
    - Bortezomib (Velcade)—causes cell death from protein accumulation

Hematopoietic stem-cell transplantation (HSCT)

- Indications:
  - Leukemia
  - Hodgkin and non-Hodgkin lymphoma
  - Multiple myeloma
  - Aplastic anemia
  - Thalassemia
  - Severe sickle cell disease
- Types:
  - Allogeneic:
    - Donor stem cells that are considered a human leukocyte (HLA) tissue match; many times it is a family member, but matched unrelated donors can be found through a bone marrow registry.
  - Syngeneic:
    - Donor stem cells from an identical twin
  - Autologous:
    - Patients' own stem cells are harvested prior to chemotherapy; they subsequently receive their own stem cells after treatment is completed. This option is used when there is no allogeneic match.
- Harvesting:
  - Directly from the bone marrow
  - Peripheral-blood stem cells
  - Umbilical cord blood

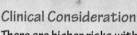

Clinical Consideration
There are higher risks with using stem cells from unrelated donors.

- Complications:
  - Infection is a significant cause of morbidity and mortality after HSCT.
  - Early noninfectious complications (within 3 months after HSCT); bacterial infections such as *Staphylococcus, Enterococcus, Pseudomonas,* and *Clostridium difficile.*
  - Late noninfectious complications (3 months after HSCT); cytomegalovirus (CMV) and reactivation of latent infections
  - Graft-verse-host disease (GvHD) is a condition that occurs after an allogeneic bone marrow transplantation when the immune cells from the donor attack the recipient's tissues.

Complementary and Alternative Therapies

- Complementary—treatments that are used along with conventional treatments to relieve symptoms experienced by patients with cancer because of the disease process or the treatment (also called "integrative therapy").
  - Examples include meditation, ginger tea, guided imagery, massage therapy
- Alternative—alternative therapies are either untested or have shown to not be an effective treatment option for cancer.

Question	Rationale
The nurse is caring for a patient who has received unsealed radiation through an oral drink. The nurse should incorporate the use of which strategy for the reduction of self-exposure? A. Limit the time with the patient and ensure a safe distance from the patient. B. Dispense the drugs that are part of the treatment regimen for the client. C. Be certified from an approved chemotherapy administration program. D. Wear a radiation meter or film badge to measure exposure.	Answer: A Caring for the patient who has received unsealed radiation requires that the nurse take special precautions. These precautions include limiting the time of exposure, maintaining an appropriate distance from the patient, and using shielding whenever possible. Each staff member must wear a dedicated radiation meter to monitor their exposure to the radiation.

ONCOLOGIC EMERGENCIES

▶ Infection:
- Cause—significant neutropenia
- Manifestations:
  - Fever >100.4° (38°C)
  - Can quickly progress to sepsis
  - May be fatal
- Treatment:
  - Aggressive treatment of infection

▶ Hypercalcemia:
  - Cause—bone destruction from tumor or secretion of parathyroid substances from tumor
  - Manifestations:
    - Serum calcium >12 mg/dL
    - Muscle weakness, fatigue
    - Seizures, coma
  - Treatment:
    - Fluids
    - Bisphosphonates:
      - Pamidronic acid
      - Zoledronic acid

▶ Superior vena cava syndrome (SVCS):
  - Cause—obstruction of the superior vena cava by tumor
  - Manifestations:
    - Facial and periorbital edema
    - Distention of neck and head veins
    - Headaches, seizures
  - Treatment:
    - Needs prompt treatment
    - Radiation to obstruction

▶ Syndrome of inappropriate antidiuretic hormone (SIADH):
  - Cause—abnormal production of antidiuretic hormone (ADH)
  - Manifestations:
    - Hypotonic hyponatremia
    - Weight gain without edema
    - Mental status changes
    - Seizures
    - Coma
  - Treatment:
    - Correct sodium–water balance
    - Fluid restriction

▶ Spinal cord compression:
  - Cause—cancer in epidural space
    - Lymphomas invade epidural space
  - Manifestations:
    - Severe and persistent back pain
    - Motor and sensory changes
    - Change in bowel and bladder function
  - Treatment:
    - Laminectomy for surgical decompression
    - Radiation therapy
    - Corticosteroids
    - Pain management

▶ Tumor lysis syndrome (TLS):
  - Cause—cell destruction causing significant release of potassium, phosphate, DNA, and RNA

- Manifestations:
  - Hyperuricemia
  - Hyperphosphatemia
  - Hyperkalemia
  - Hypocalcemia
- Treatment:
  - Hydration
  - Allopurinol
  - Sodium bicarbonate

▶ Cardiac tamponade:
- Cause—constriction of pericardium by tumor or fluid or pericarditis from radiation to chest
- Manifestations:
  - Shortness of breath
  - Chest heaviness
  - Nausea and vomiting
- Treatment:
  - Pericardial window
  - Indwelling pericardial catheter

Question	Rationale
The nurse is caring for a 65-year-old man undergoing chemotherapy treatment for lung cancer. He is neutropenic. When assessing his vital signs the nurse notes an oral temperature of 100.4° F. The most appropriate interpretation of this finding is that: A. The patient is experiencing the expected increase in metabolism that often accompanies malignancy. B. He may have a urinary-tract infection causing a low-grade fever. C. A systemic chemotherapeutic effect is probably occurring. D. He may have a serious infection, and prompt further medical attention may be needed.	Answer: D An oral temperature of 100.4°F is considered an oncologic emergency in patients who are receiving chemotherapy. Because of a decrease in white cells, these patients are very susceptible to infection. With the patient's inability to adequately fight off an infection, sepsis, a life-threatening emergency, may develop.

Nursing diagnosis:

▶ Ineffective coping related to cancer diagnosis and treatment
▶ Activity intolerance related to weakness from cancer, treatment effects
▶ Imbalanced nutrition: less than body requirements related to loss of appetite from side effects of treatment, disease process, depression
▶ Disturbed body image related to weight loss, hair loss
▶ Fatigue related to disease process treatment effects, anemia
▶ Risk for infection related to neutropenia
▶ Risk for bleeding related to thrombocytopenia

Question	Rationale
The nurse is caring for a 47 y/o with a pulmonary malignancy. She started chemotherapy yesterday and is experiencing severe nausea. The nurse makes the diagnosis of altered nutrition, less than body requirements related to chemotherapy-induced nausea. Which is the most appropriate nursing intervention related to this diagnosis? A. Encourage a high-fat snack prior to chemotherapy. B. Advise the patient to never to omit a meal. C. Administer prescribed antiemetic medication before chemotherapy and for as long as needed afterward. D. Ensure that the patient is taking a daily multivitamin.	Answer: C Administering the prescribed antiemetic medication before, during, and after treatments helps to decrease the nausea and vomiting associated with chemotherapy. A high-fat meal may contribute to nausea and vomiting.

LUNG CANCER

Lung cancer is the leading cause of cancer deaths and accounts for more cancer deaths than breast, prostate, and colon cancer combined. Many patients with lung cancer are asymptomatic and may not be diagnosed until the cancer is in an advanced stage.

- Types (ACS, 2017):
  - Non–small-cell; most common type of lung cancer (85%)—includes squamous-cell carcinoma, adenocarcinoma, and large-cell carcinoma
  - Small-cell (oat-cell) cancer—accounts for approximately 10 to 15% of lung cancers; tends to spread quickly
  - Lung carcinoid tumor (lung neuroendocrine tumors); less than 5% of lung cancers, grows slowly and typically does not spread
- Risk factors:
  - Smoking and second-hand smoke are responsible for the majority (>80%) of all lung cancers; this includes cigar and pipe smoking (ACS, 2017).
  - Exposure to high levels of radon, pollution, industrial agents, and asbestos.
- The ACS estimates for lung cancer in the United States for 2017 were:
  - About 222,500 new cases of lung cancer (116,990 in men and 105,510 in women)
  - About 155,870 deaths from lung cancer (84,590 in men and 71,280 in women)
- Manifestations:
  - Early:
    - May have no symptoms
    - Vague and nonspecific symptoms
    - Persistent cough
    - Blood-tinged sputum
    - Dyspnea or wheezing
    - Site in the lung determines how soon symptoms appear

- Late:
  - Hoarseness
  - Anorexia
  - Fatigue
  - Weight loss
  - Superior vena cava obstruction
- Diagnosis:
  - Chest x-ray may indicate an abnormality.
  - CT scan may indicate extent of abnormality.
  - Biopsy of lung tissue is necessary for definitive diagnosis:
    - Sample may be obtained with a bronchoscopy, CT-guided needle aspiration, or thoracentesis.
- Nursing diagnosis:
  - Ineffective airway clearance related to tumor
  - Ineffective breathing pattern related to presence of a lung lesion
- Treatment (Table 19.5):
  - Depends on goals of treatment; cure, control, palliation
  - May include surgery, radiation, chemotherapy, targeted therapy, and immunotherapy
- Patient teaching:
  - Education about diagnostic tests, diagnosis, treatment options, and prognosis
  - Smoking cessation
  - Provide information on community resources available to patient

BREAST CANCER

Breast cancer occurs when breast-tissue cells begin to differentiate from their typical appearance and grow out of control. Most often, breast cancer begins in the ductal tissue, and because of the close proximity of the breast to the lymph nodes, cancer cells are able to spread easily. Breast cancer can develop in both women and men, although 99% of breast cancers occur in women (ACS, 2018a).

- Risk factors:
  - The incidence of breast cancer increases with age, as hormonal regulation is associated with the development of breast cancer.
  - Hormone-replacement therapy—estrogen and progesterone
  - A personal or family history of breast cancer
  - Presence of the *BRCA1* and *BRCA2* gene mutations
  - Atypical benign breast disease
  - Early menarche, late menopause
  - Nulliparity or first pregnancy after age 30
- Manifestations:
  - A lump or thickening of the breast tissue detected by breast self-exam by patient or breast exam by provider
  - Abnormality detected on mammography
- Diagnosis:
  - Mammogram may indicate an abnormality:
    - Compare to previous mammograms.
    - Digital or three-dimensional mammography provides more details than previous technology.

- Biopsy of the abnormal breast tissue is necessary for definitive diagnosis:
  - Sample may be obtained by fine-needle aspiration, core needle biopsy, or excisional biopsy.
- Nursing diagnosis:
  - Disturbed body image related to loss of sexually significant body part
- Treatment:
  - Depends on goals of treatment; cure, control, palliation
  - Surgery:
    - Lumpectomy—removal of tumor and some tissue surrounding the tumor
    - Total mastectomy—removal of the entire breast
    - Modified radical mastectomy—removal of the breast and affected lymph nodes, as determined by a sentinel node biopsy; leaves muscle
    - Breast reconstruction may be done at time of mastectomy or at a later date.
    - Complications:
      - Delayed wound healing
      - Impaired arm mobility
      - Lymphedema due to lymph node dissection; lymph fluid unable to return to central circulation
      - Altered body image
  - Radiation—to irradiate residual cancer cells after surgery
    - External-beam radiation
      - Typically 5 days a week, for several weeks
    - Brachytherapy—internal radiation
      - Radioactive seeds are placed in the location where the tumor was removed:
        - May remain in place for several days
        - May be placed for a set time and removed between treatments
    - Complications:
      - Breast edema
      - Skin changes, including wet desquamation, redness, and darkening of the skin
  - Chemotherapy (Table 19.5):
    - May be used before surgery to shrink the tumor
    - May be used after surgery for any cells that may have been missed during surgery of for spread outside the breast tissue
    - Complications/side effects are similar to those for any patient receiving chemotherapy
  - Hormone therapy:
    - Used to block estrogen in tumors that grow in response to estrogen, with the intent of causing tumor regression
  - Immunotherapy:
    - These drugs are targeted at specific genes (such as *BRCA1* and *BRCA2*)—for example, Herceptin
- Patient teaching:
  - Provide education and support to the patient and family members or support system as desired by patient.
  - Teach about diagnosis, treatment, and prognosis. This may include long-term oral chemotherapy.
  - Importance of restoring arm function and prevention of lymphedema.

Question	Rationale
Six months ago, a patient was treated for stage II cancer of the right breast and underwent a lumpectomy and axillary lymph node dissection with radiation to the chest wall postoperatively. Today, she presents with pain, tingling, and swelling of the right hand and arm. The patient's symptoms are suggestive of: A. Peripheral neuropathy secondary to nerve damage during surgery B. Postradiation inflammation C. Lymphedema D. Posttraumatic stress syndrome	Answer: C Lymphedema can occur when axillary nodes have been removed during the treatment of breast cancer because of problems with drainage within the lymph system. Care must be taken to avoid any injury or to exacerbate this drainage problem. Precautions should be taken on the side of the mastectomy/lymph node removal—for example, no blood draws, no blood pressures, and no peripheral IV sites.

COLORECTAL CANCER

Colorectal cancer is the second leading cause of cancer deaths and affects both men and women, although rates are higher in men.

- Risk factors:
  - No single identifiable risk factor associated with colorectal cancer
  - Personal or family history of colorectal cancer
  - History of irritable bowel syndrome (IBS)
  - Presence of the *KRAS* gene
- Manifestations:
  - Early:
    - May have no symptoms
    - Fatigue
    - Weight loss
  - Late:
    - Palpable abdominal mass
    - Hepatomegaly
    - Ascites
    - Presence of blood in stool
- Diagnosis:
  - Colonoscopy is the recommended screening, with biopsy of any abnormalities and polyps
  - Biopsy of colon tissue is necessary for definitive diagnosis
  - Determination of extent of disease can be done with CT scan or MRI
- Nursing diagnosis:
  - Constipation or diarrhea related to altered bowel elimination patterns from tumor or treatment
- Treatment:
  - Depends on goals of treatment; cure, control, or palliation
  - Surgery:
    - Polypectomy or local excision of cancer

- Hemicolectomy—part of the colon, the cancer, and a small segment on either side are removed and the ends are anastomosed
- Total colectomy—removal of the entire colon
- Colostomy reversal, if indicated
- Complications:
  - Delayed wound healing
  - Temporary or permanent colostomy may be necessary.
- Radiation—to irradiate residual cancer cells after surgery:
  - Used as an adjuvant to surgery and chemotherapy
- Chemotherapy:
  - May be used before surgery to shrink the tumor
  - May be used after surgery for any cells that may have been missed
  - May be used for palliative therapy for nonsurgical tumors
  - Complications/side effects are similar to those for any patient receiving chemotherapy
- Patient teaching:
  - Provide education and support to the patient and family members or support system as desired by patient.
  - Teach about diagnosis, treatment, and prognosis; may include colostomy care.

PROSTATE CANCER

According to the American Cancer Society (2018d), prostate cancer is diagnosed in 1 of every 10 men. Prostate cancer is slow-growing and is the second leading cause of cancer deaths for men, accounting for approximately 29,400 deaths a year.

- Risk factors:
  - Age—incidence significantly increases with age
  - Ethnicity—African Americans have highest incidence
  - Family history
- Manifestations:
  - Early:
    - Typically no symptoms
  - Late:
    - Pain in lumbosacral region
    - Spontaneous pelvis, femur fracture
    - Symptoms may be similar to those of benign prostatic hyperplasia (BPH) (see Chapter 12)
- Diagnosis:
  - PSA—if elevated, further testing needed
  - Digital rectal exam (DRE)—if nodules found, further testing needed
  - Transrectal ultrasound (TRUS)—can visualize abnormalities of the prostate and a biopsy can be completed
  - Biopsy of prostate tissue is necessary for definitive diagnosis.
- Nursing diagnosis:
  - Decisional conflict related to numerous treatment choices
  - Sexual dysfunction related to treatment effects
- Treatment:
  - Depends on goals of treatment; cure, control, or palliation
  - Watchful waiting—as prostate cancer is typically slow-growing, a conservative approach may be used, monitoring the progress of the disease.

- Surgery:
  - Radical prostatectomy:
    - Removal of all prostate tissue including part of the bladder and the seminal vesicles
  - Nerve-sparing prostatectomy—robot-assisted surgery:
    - Removal of the prostate while sparing the nerves reduces the risk of erectile dysfunction
  - Cryotherapy:
    - Freezing the cancer cells with nitrogen, destroying the tissue
  - Complications:
    - Erectile dysfunction, loss of sexual function
    - Urinary incontinence
    - Damage to the urethra
- Radiation:
  - External-beam radiation
    - Typically 5 days a week for several weeks
  - Brachytherapy:
    - Permanently placing radioactive seeds into the prostate gland; effects of radiation decline over a few weeks to months.
    - Up to 100 seeds may be placed.
  - Complications:
    - Skin changes to irradiated area
    - Gastrointestinal and urinary-tract changes
    - Erectile dysfunction
- Chemotherapy (Table 19.5):
  - Typically used for palliative therapy in prostate cancer
  - Complications/side effects are similar to those for any patient receiving chemotherapy
- Hormone therapy:
  - Used to block androgen receptors in tumors that grow in response to androgen
  - Tumors tend to become resistant to hormone therapy over time.
  - A bilateral orchiectomy will eliminate androgen production.
- Patient teaching:
  - Provide education and support to the patient and family members or support system as desired by patient
  - Teach about diagnosis, treatment, and prognosis
  - Teach Kegel exercises if experiencing problems with urinary incontinence
  - Indwelling urinary catheter care, if appropriate
  - Avoid close physical contact for the first few weeks if radioactive seeds were implanted; avoid pregnant women and children.

THYROID CANCER

Most growths in the thyroid gland are benign fluid-filled nodules. Papillary cancer is the most prevalent type of thyroid cancer. These tumors are slow-growing, but tend to spread to the lymph nodes in the neck.

- Risk factors:
  - Exposure to head or neck radiation earlier in life
  - Exposure to radioactive fallout
  - Personal or family history of goiter

- Manifestations:
  - Palpable nodules on thyroid gland
  - Enlarged thyroid gland
  - May experience difficulty breathing or swallowing as the tumor grows
  - Elevated serum calcitonin level
- Diagnosis:
  - Nodular palpation on thyroid gland requires further follow-up
  - Ultrasound, CT scan, MRI may be done although not diagnostic
  - Thyroid scan may indicate whether nodule is benign or malignant by the uptake/or lack of uptake of radioactive iodine, but not diagnostic
  - Biopsy of thyroid tissue is necessary for definitive diagnosis; typically obtained by ultrasound-guided fine-needle aspiration.
- Nursing diagnosis:
  - Risk for ineffective airway clearance related to thyroid enlargement, postthyroidectomy
- Treatment:
  - Depends on goals of treatment; cure, control, palliation
  - May include surgery, radiation, chemotherapy, targeted therapy, and immunotherapy
  - Surgery:
    - Affected lobes of the thyroid gland are removed—partial or total thyroid lobectomy.
    - Neck lymph nodes may be removed.
    - Complications:
      - Hypocalcemia
      - Airway obstruction
      - Tetany due to manipulation or removal of the parathyroid gland
      - Thyroid storm if patient does not get adequate radioactive iodine to shrink size and vascularity of thyroid preoperatively
      - (See Chapters 6 and 11)
  - Radiation:
    - Radioactive iodine (radioiodine) is taken in a liquid or capsule form. The thyroid gland will take up the radioactive iodine, allowing for targeted radiation. There must be a high level of thyroid-stimulating hormone (TSH) in order for the thyroid gland to take up the iodine.
      - Special precautions will need be to be followed by the patient as this is typically done as an outpatient procedure.
    - External-beam radiation to eradicate any remaining cancer cells after surgery or that may extend beyond the thyroid gland
    - Complications:
      - Skin changes to irradiated area
      - Men may have low sperm counts; women may have an irregular menstrual cycle for up to a year.
      - There is a slight risk that leukemia may develop after treatment with radioactive iodine.
  - Chemotherapy (Table 19.5):
    - Typically used for advanced thyroid cancer
    - Complications/side effects are similar to those for any patient receiving chemotherapy.
  - Thyroid hormone therapy:
    - Higher than normal doses may stop remaining cancer cells from growing if tumor is dependent on the TSH.

- Patient teaching:
  - Provide education and support to the patient and family members or support system as desired by patient.
  - Teach about diagnosis, treatment, and prognosis.
  - Importance of taking thyroid hormone therapy as prescribed.
  - Follow-up with endocrinologist, oncologist, and lab levels—TSH, serum calcitonin, thyroglobulin
  - Voice rest, humidity, neck support with cervical (C) collar after surgery; prolonged hoarseness may indicate laryngeal-nerve damage; tracheostomy tray/suture removal tray/suction at bedside or nearby.

LEUKEMIA

Leukemia is a malignancy of the blood and bone marrow and is fatal if left untreated. Most often it is associated with cancer of the white cells but can also be found in other types of blood cells. Acute types of leukemia are fast-growing and chronic types are slow-growing. The type of leukemia plays a role in determining treatment options and prognosis.

- Types (ACS, 2018e):
  - Acute lymphocytic leukemia (ALL)
  - Acute myeloid leukemia (AML)
  - Chronic lymphocytic leukemia (CLL)
  - Chronic myeloid leukemia (CML)
  - Chronic myelomonocytic leukemia (CMML)
- Risk factors:
  - Chemical agents
  - Chemotherapy agents
  - Viruses; human T-cell leukemia virus type 1 (HTLV-1)
  - Radiation:
    - Occupational exposure
    - Environmental; nuclear bomb sites, radiation leaks
- Manifestations:
  - Increased abnormal white-cell count
  - Chronic medical problems—splenomegaly, hepatomegaly, bone pain
  - Chloromas—solid mass of white cells
  - White-cell count >100,000 cells/μL
  - Leukostasis—thickening of the blood due to excessive white cells
- Diagnosis:
  - Peripheral-blood testing
  - Bone marrow biopsy
- Nursing diagnosis:
  - Ineffective protection related to abnormal white cells
  - Fatigue related to abnormal labs, side effect of chemotherapy
- Treatment:
  - Depends on goals of treatment; cure, control, palliation
  - Watchful waiting with supportive care with asymptomatic chronic leukemia
  - Chemotherapy—typically done in three stages:
    - Induction stage:
      - Aggressive treatment, with the goal of remission
      - Bone marrow severely depressed; monitor for and treat thrombocytopenia, neutropenia, and anemia

> **Clinical Consideration**
> Leukostasis can be life-threatening.

- Postinduction/postremission stage:
  - Other high-dose chemotherapy agents may be given.
  - Continue high-dose therapy once remission has been achieved to ensure eradication of cancer cells.
- Maintenance stage:
  - Lower dose of chemotherapy drugs every 3 to 4 weeks for an extended duration to prevent leukemia cells from relapsing
- HSCT (discussed earlier in this chapter)
- Patient teaching:
  - Provide education and support to the patient and family members or support system as desired by patient.
  - Teach about diagnosis, treatment, and prognosis.
  - Teach patient how to manage chemotherapy side effects.
  - Provide patient with community resources.
  - Stress the importance of ongoing follow-up care.

Question	Rationale
In caring for a patient receiving chemotherapy in whom mucositis has developed, the nurse should: A. Assist the patient in cleansing the mouth before and after meals with a commercial mouthwash, because of its antibacterial qualities. B. Teach the patient to brush teeth and tongue with a toothbrush to remove plaques caused by candidiasis. C. Monitor for redness, white lesions, difficulty swallowing and low-grade fever. D. Provide lemon glycerin swabs for mouth care.	Answer: C Mucositis is an inflammation and irritation of the lining of the oral mucous membranes, usually accompanied by open sores. It is important to avoid commercial mouthwashes and lemon glycerin swabs, as they may be irritating to the open areas. It would be important for the nurse to monitor the oral mucous membranes for redness, white lesions, difficulty swallowing, and a low-grade fever, as these may indicate an infection.

LYMPHOMA

Lymphoma is characterized by malignant tumors that originate in the bone marrow and in the lymphatic system. There are two types of lymphoma;

- Types (ACS, 2018f):
  - Hodgkin's lymphoma:
    - Originates in the B lymphocytes
    - Typically is localized or regional
    - Patient experiences fever, night sweats, weight loss
    - Other manifestations:
      - Small amount of alcohol can cause pain at tumor site
  - Non-Hodgkin's lymphoma (NHL):
    - Originates in the B and T lymphocytes
    - Disease is disseminated
    - Uncommon to experience fever, night sweats, weight loss
    - Symptoms are based on where the disease has spread.

Clinical Consideration

A fever >100.4°F, drenching night sweats, and weight loss of greater than 10% from baseline are associated with a poor prognosis.

- Risk factors:
  - Hodgkin's lymphoma:
    - Previous infection of the Epstein–Barr virus, often referred to as "infectious mononucleosis"
    - Family history of Hodgkin's lymphoma
    - HIV infection
  - Non-Hodgkin's lymphoma:
    - Exposure to certain chemicals and drugs
    - Radiation exposure
    - Transplant recipients
    - HIV
    - Autoimmune diseases
- Diagnosis:
  - Peripheral-blood analysis
  - Lymph node biopsy
  - Bone marrow biopsy
  - PET and CT scans are used to determine the extent of the disease.
- Nursing diagnosis:
  - Powerlessness related to treatment, progression of disease
  - Ineffective protection related to cancer suppressing immune system
- Treatment:
  - Hodgkin's lymphoma:
    - Chemotherapy—aggressive therapy is key (Table 19.5)
    - Radiation—typically done after chemotherapy treatments
    - HSCT—may be indicated once disease is in remission
  - Non-Hodgkin's lymphoma:
    - Chemotherapy (Table 19.5)
    - Radiation—may be used sometimes, but not the standard
- Patient teaching:
  - Provide education and support to the patient and family members or support system as desired by patient.
  - Teach about diagnosis, treatment, and prognosis.
  - Teach patient how to manage chemotherapy side effects.
  - Provide patient with community resources.
  - Stress the importance of ongoing follow-up care.

CASE STUDY

A 60–year-old female presents to her provider with a worsening persistent cough. She has a 40-year history of smoking a pack of cigarettes each day, has been feeling pressure in her chest when she breathes deeply, and becomes short of breath if she speaks more than a sentence or two. Her medical history includes osteoarthritis and chronic obstructive pulmonary disease (COPD). Her primary care provider orders a chest x-ray, which shows a large pleural effusion. She then undergoes thoracentesis.

1. Why would the provider order a thoracentesis?

▷ *A thoracentesis is done to remove excess fluid from the pleural space. This is done by inserting a needle into the pleural space. The fluid removed is typically sent for pathology testing to determine its cause.*

2. What teaching would be provided to the patient?

▶ *The patient will need to sit on the edge of the bed with their arms resting on a table.*

▶ *A local anesthetic will be used to numb the area.*

▶ *She may feel pressure or discomfort during the insertion of the needle and while the fluid is being removed.*

▶ *Potential risks include pneumothorax, bleeding, and infection.*

Pathology studies on the thoracentesis fluid indicate small-cell carcinoma. A CT scan is ordered; it identifies several lesions in the right lung, and a CT-guided biopsy of one of the lung lesions reveals poorly differentiated small cell carcinoma, consistent with a primary lung tumor. No sites of metastasis are found. She is diagnosed with stage III small-cell carcinoma. It is decided that this patient is not a candidate for surgery because the malignant cells in her thoracentesis fluid indicate spread to the pleural cavity.

3. What are some risk factors for lung cancer?

▶ *Smoking, tuberculosis, environmental carcinogens*

4. What manifestations might a patient with lung cancer exhibit?

▶ *There may be no early symptoms*

▶ *Later symptoms may include cough; blood or rust-colored sputum; chest, shoulder, back or arm pain; pleural effusion; wheezing; stridor; pericardial effusion; weight loss; and shortness of breath.*

It was decided that the patient would be treated with combination chemotherapy of paclitaxel (Taxol) and cyclophosphamide (Cytoxan).

5. For which side effects will she need to be monitored?

▶ *Taxol is a cell-cycle–specific chemotherapy medication; adverse effects include nausea, vomiting, alopecia, and myelosuppression.*

▶ *Cytoxan is cell-cycle–nonspecific chemotherapy medication; adverse effects include more severe myelosuppression, hemorrhagic cystitis, SIADH, cardiomyopathy, alopecia, nausea and vomiting*

Discussion:

When a patient has a pleural effusion, a thoracentesis is performed to drain excess fluid from the pleural cavity. Pleural fluid is routinely sent to the lab for pathologic testing, which would determine whether there are abnormal cells. Chemotherapy is a common choice of treatment for patients with lung cancer.

Bibliography

Agency for Healthcare Research and Quality. (June 2014). *2014 guide to clinical preventative services.* Retrieved February 13, 2018 from https://www.ahrq.gov/sites/default/files/publications/files/cpsguide.pdf

Aschenbrenner, D.S., and Venable, S.J. (2012). *Drug Therapy in Nursing*, 4th ed. (Philadelphia: Wolters Kluwer).

American Cancer Society. (2017). Key statistics for lung cancer. Accessed September 27, 2017, from https://www.cancer.org/cancer/non-small-cell-lung-cancer/about/key-statistics.html

American Cancer Society. (2018a). Breast cancer. Accessed April 8, 2018, from https://www.cancer.org/cancer/breast-cancer/about.html

American Cancer Society. (2018b). Cancer. Retrieved July 26, 2018 from https://www.cancer.org/cancer/cancer-basics/signs-and-symptoms-of-cancer.html

American Cancer Society. (2018c). Colorectal cancer. Retrieved July 26, 2018 from https://www.cancer.org/latest-news/american-cancer-society-updates-colorectal-cancer-screening-guideline.html

American Cancer Society. (2018d). Key statistics for prostate cancer. Accessed April 8, 2018, from https://www.cancer.org/cancer/prostate-cancer/about/key-statistics.html

American Cancer Society. (2018e). Leukemia. Accessed April 8, 2018, from https://www.cancer.org/cancer/leukemia.html

American Cancer Society. (2018f). Lymphoma. Accessed April 8, 2018, from https://www.cancer.org/cancer/lymphoma.html

American College of Obstetricians and Gynecologists. (July 2017a). *ACOG practice bulletin: Breast cancer risk assessment and screening in average-risk women.* Retrieved February 13, 2018 from https://www.acog.org/-/media/Practice-Bulletins/Committee-on-Practice-Bulletins----Gynecology/Public/pb179.pdf?dmc=1&ts=20180218T2153314300

American College of Obstetricians and Gynecologists. (September 2017b). *ACOG FAQ085: Cervical cancer screening.* Retrieved February 13, 2018 from https://www.acog.org/-/media/For-Patients/faq085.pdf?dmc=1&ts=20180218T2253239218

Grossman, S., and Porth, C.M. (2013). *Pathophysiology: Concepts of Altered Health States*, 9th ed. (Philadelphia: Lippincott Williams & Wilkins).

Hatzimichael, E., and Tuthill, M. (2010). Hematopoietic stem cell transplantation. *Stem Cells and Cloning: Advances and Applications* 3, 105–117.

Lewis, S.L., Bucher, L., Heitkemper, M., and Harding, M.M. (2017). *Medical-Surgical Nursing: Assessment and Management of Clinical Problems*, 10th ed. (St. Louis: Elsevier).

National Comprehensive Cancer Network. (2017). Clinical practice guidelines. Accessed November 16, 2017, from https://www.nccn.org/professionals/physician_gls/default.aspx

U.S. Preventive Services. (2017). Prostate cancer screening. Retrieved February 13, 2018 from https://www.uspreventiveservicestaskforce.org/Page/Document/draft-recommendation-statement/prostate-cancer-screening1

World Health Organization. (2018). Cancer. Retrieved July 27, 2018 from http://www.who.int/cancer/en/

20

End-of-Life Care

Stacie J. Elder, PhD, RN, CNE

OVERVIEW

Whatever the specialty, most nurses will likely care for a patient who dies. Yet nurses are often ill-prepared to manage end-of-life issues (Herbert, Moore, and Rooney, 2011). The American Nurses Association (ANA) (2016) recognizes this and has revised a position statement that reflects their belief that "the US health system is ill-designed to meet the needs of patients near the end-of-life and their families." In recognition of this stance, the ANA mandates that "Nurses are obliged to provide comprehensive and compassionate end-of-life care." This end-of-life care includes interdisciplinary collaboration in communicating with patients and families, clinical treatment of symptoms, decision making, respect for patient autonomy, and treatment of physical problems as well as emotional and spiritual needs of both patients at the end-of-life and their families.

Similar statements and suggestions are made by other organizations, such as the American Society for Pain Management (Reynolds, Drew, and Dunwoody, 2013), End-of-Life Nursing Education Consortium (ELNEC, 2009), World Health Organization (WHO, 2004), and the Institute of Medicine (IOM, 2016). Shared aims include, but are not limited to, patient autonomy, standards of care, symptom management, education of health care workers, holistic treatment of patients, retention of dignity, ethical principles, coping with dissent, and withdrawal of life-prolonging therapies (when this is the patient's desire).

DEFINITIONS

- *End-of-life care:* Support and health care given during the time surrounding death, whether sudden, gradual, in a chronic or acute disease and whether the death be sudden, gradual, or with extensive suffering (Reynolds, Drew, and Dunwoody, 2013).

- *Palliative care:* Model of care for the ill, especially focusing on relief of symptoms and the stress of serious illness while supporting the best possible quality of life for patients and their families or significant others. The goal is to increase the comfort level but not to treat the underlying illness(es) (Reynolds et al., 2013; Carr, 2006).

- *Hospice care:* A team-oriented approach to expert medical care, pain management, and emotional and spiritual support expressly tailored to the patient's needs and wishes. Support is provided to the patient's loved ones as well. At the center of hospice and palliative care is the belief that each of us has the right to die pain-free and with dignity, and that our families will receive the necessary support to allow us to do so (https://www.nhpco.org/about/hospice-care).

Question	Rationale
Palliative care includes all but which one of the following? A. Providing psychosocial support B. Increasing comfort level of the patient while not continuing regular treatment for the disease process C. Developing goals for the patient D. Supporting the patient's wishes through partnership with the physician and the family.	Answer: C The patient develops their own goals. The nurse advocates for those goals.

COMMUNICATION

In order to ascertain the needs of end-of-life patients and their families, taking into account their beliefs and perceptions of end-of-life care and decision making, and employing the appropriate communication techniques are essential for the nurse. Therapeutic communication is of the utmost importance. One of the first steps is to understand that there are stages of grief that guide communication with those involved in end-of-life situations. There are many models, but the one used most is that of Elisabeth Kubler-Ross (2014). It is a five-stage linear process, as outlined below.

▶ Stage I: Denial:
- Patients and family do not accept the diagnosis/prognosis.
- A belief is that there is a mistake and the patient will get better and live longer
- Those affected will choose to not talk about it and do not want to hear any details or make any decisions:
  - Nurses must be good listeners.
  - Open-ended questions must be asked to help the patient/families.
  - What issues can I clarify for you? How can I help you?

▶ Stage II: Anger:
- Blame is placed on a situation, person, or self.
- Why me? What did I do to deserve this? I cannot die now!
  - Help the patient to identify fears/hurt and start to heal.
  - Encourage openness and forgiveness.

▶ Stage III: Bargaining:
- Patient or family member barters for favors from God.
- Demonstrates a belief in God or spirituality.
  - Open the conversation about spirituality and what it means to the patient.

▶ Stage IV: Depression:
- Most common step; indicates recognition of mortality
- Involves emotional responses such as crying, withdrawing, refusing visitors
- Asks, "Why bother with anything now?"
  - Pastoral request
  - Counseling
  - Antidepressants
  - Allow and encourage patient to verbalize
  - Be a good listener; sometimes just sit quietly with patient.

- Stage V: Acceptance:
  - Accepts the fact of mortality
  - Ready to die but does not indicate a suicide wish
  - Makes end-of-life final plans willingly
  - Tries to comfort family:
    - Allow patient to verbalize feelings
    - Assist with end-of-life wishes of patient
    - Educate patient and family on possible signs/symptoms that patient may experience during the final days
- Nursing communication tips regarding patients/families at end of life
  - The steps of grief do not always happen in order. It is different for every situation. Assess the characteristics, and do not assume which stage the patient is experiencing.
  - The steps of grief do not apply to everyone.
  - Be an active listener.
  - Never ask "yes" or "no" questions.
  - Use phrases such as, "Tell me about…", "What makes you say that?", "What is bothering you at this time?", "Is there anything that I can do for you?"
  - NEVER say that you understand or know what or how the patient is feeling.
  - Do not give your personal opinions or impose your beliefs on someone else.
  - Keep patient autonomy your first priority.
  - Sit at eye level with the patient.
  - Speak slowly and deliberately, not in a hurried manner.
  - Never tell anyone that they are wrong.

Question	Rationale
Mr. and Mrs. S. have just been told that Mr. S.'s left ventricular ejection fraction is only 25%. He is now experiencing multisystem organ failure as a result of his cardiomyopathy. Mr. S. remains stoic but Mrs. S. screams at her husband and asks, "How can you do this to me? I can't take it! I can't take it! I can't take it!" and runs from the room. Mr. S. turns to his side with tears in his eyes. The best thing for you to do is: A. Stay by Mr. S. and tell him it is not his fault and everything will be okay. B. Go after Mrs. S. and sit with her, telling her that you understand how she feels but it is time to concentrate on her husband and his condition. C. Leave the room and wait to see what happens next, checking for his advance directive information. D. Sit with Mr. S. quietly, hold his hand and if he responds in any way to you, ask him how he is feeling right now.	Answer: D In "A," you are not telling him the truth—everything will not be okay. You cannot tell him it is not his fault as it is not for you to judge. In "B," you cannot tell Mrs. S. you understand; it is inappropriate to ever say that as you do not know how another person feels and what they have personally have experienced. In "C," you are avoiding the issue and not helping anyone.

EARLY AND MIDDLE END-OF-LIFE SIGNS AND SYMPTOMS

When assessing a dying patient, always assess using airway, breathing, and circulation (the ABCs) as you would for any other patient. It is important to prioritize the care of the patient using those criteria. Care never ends. End-of-life care does not mean end of all care. This is one of the most important times to make certain that the patient is as comfortable as possible and that all possible comfort measures are taken. Families state that one of the things that they recall the most is how comfortable the nurse made the patient and their families at such a stressful time.

Many times, the patients' significant others notice obvious and sometimes subtle changes in the patient's condition. The following signs and symptoms are common and are part of the dying process. The nurse should begin to discuss this with the family so that they do not become alarmed when changes such as these occur. The teaching should include the palliative treatments and interventions that can lessen the discomfort of the patient. The next section will detail the final symptoms preceding imminent death of which the family and friends should be taught are signaling the end of life.

- Breathing:
  - Congestion
  - Secretions
  - Change in breathing pattern
  - Atelectasis
- Neurologic:
  - Confusion
  - Insomnia
  - Restlessness
  - Change in vital signs: decrease in blood pressure, change in pulse rate/pattern, hyperthermia
- Urologic:
  - Decrease in urine output
  - Incontinence
- Cardiac:
  - Arrhythmias
  - Bradycardia
  - Peripheral edema
  - Cool and mottled extremities
- Gastrointestinal (related to treatment of symptoms):
  - Constipation
  - Diarrhea
  - Nausea and vomiting
- Lack of thirst and appetite are common, yet can be upsetting and worrisome for the family. It should be taught that lack of food and water has been found to not be uncomfortable for the patient and many times results in a feeling of euphoria.

Question	Rationale
Mr. L. is an 80-year-old gentleman with a history of prostate cancer that was treated with radiation and chemotherapy several years ago. He has recently been reporting severe leg pain and a cough. A CT scan reveals a recurrence of his cancer in his left pleural cavity and left femur. He was admitted to the telemetry unit after being found at home, lethargic. Now he is reporting severe pain in his leg, has a very wet, productive cough, and is dyspneic. His vital signs are: blood pressure 150/96 mm Hg, heart rate 116 beats/min, respiratory rate 36 breaths/min, oxygen saturation (SaO2) 86%, and temperature 99.9°F. Your first action should be to: A. Finish your complete history and physical prior to doing anything else. B. Have him rate his pain on the pain scale. C. Call the provider for orders, stat. D. Administer oxygen per nasal cannula and attach an SaO$_2$ monitor.	Answer: D The best answer is D. You must address his breathing status immediately. Regardless of his prognosis, Mr. L. should be not in psychologic or physical distress, if possible. Breathlessness produces increased anxiety and affects vital signs and oxygenation. Oxygenation takes precedence over all other issues. A complete history and physical can be done at any time and should not take priority over his breathing. The patient will not be able to respond appropriately if he is in pain, is coughing, and cannot breathe. He may be able to rate pain once he is not gasping for breath and anxious. The nurse must address the dyspnea immediately. Breathing takes precedence over everything else. Then the nurse can call the provider for further orders.

FINAL SYMPTOMS PRECEDING IMMINENT DEATH

▶ Hypotension
▶ Glassy eyes, half-open eyes
▶ Weak pulse
▶ Increase in internal body temperature
▶ Gasping for breath
▶ Irregular heart beats
▶ Increase in restlessness
▶ Skin mottling and decrease in temperature of skin
▶ Anuria
▶ Unable to awaken
▶ Increased sleeping

▶ Hallucinations such as visions of angels, what the patient perceives as heaven, or visions of family members/friends who have preceded them in death. They are generally comforting, realistic, meaningful, and reassuring in nature.

Soon before these symptoms start to manifest, the patient, if awake, will most likely begin to withdraw from everyone. He/she may wish to say goodbye to loved ones. It is acceptable to let family members know that they can give their loved one "permission" to let go and that they will be all right. There is never a timetable that indicates when the patient will die. It may be seconds, minutes, hours, or days. It is impossible to predict. As the above signs and symptoms start manifesting, the family can expect that the end of life is imminent. It should be communicated to the family that they can continue to give comfort measures such as hand-holding, continuously speaking to the patient, applying moist swabs to the mouth, keeping the patient warm/cool as needed, etc. The nurse may offer to give a small amount of an opioid to decrease gasping for breath.

TREATMENT OF RESPIRATORY SYMPTOMS

There are a variety of reasons for respiratory decline at the end of life. Anxiety is one of the main reasons for respiratory changes. It can be a secondary effect of depression, which is caused by lack of motivation, anger, denial, guilt, isolation, and self-blame. Other causes include pneumonia, chronic obstructive pulmonary disease (COPD), heart failure (HF), or a cold, among other reasons (Table 20.1).

TABLE 20.1	RESPIRATORY SYMPTOM TREATMENT/INTERVENTION	
Cause	Pharmacologic	Nonpharmacologic
Anxiety	Oxygen per nasal cannula, mask Anxiolytic medication—buspirone (Buspar) preferred over lorazepam (Ativan) Antidepressants—selective serotonin-reuptake inhibitors (SSRIs), tricyclic antidepressants with caution related to contraindicated drugs	Fan Calm, quiet environment Music, distraction Hand-holding Quiet atmosphere
Pneumonia	Antibiotics per sensitivity Antipyretic (acetylsalicylic acid [aspirin, ASA]; acetaminophen [Tylenol]) Oxygen	Head of bed elevated Fluids Incentive spirometer
Bronchospasm	Bronchodilators (albuterol) Oral steroids (prednisone) Oxygen	
Rales	Oxygen Decrease intravenous (IV) fluids Diuretic furosemide (Lasix)	Elevate head of bed (HOB)
Effusions	Opioids (morphine)	
Airway obstruction		Swallow test Pureed or thickened foods
Thick Secretions	Anticholinergic (scopolamine, subcutaneously or transdermally) Antitussive (guaifenesin) Opioids (morphine) Bronchodilators (terbutaline)	Incentive spirometer Nebulized saline or humidifier Cool air HOB up and turn patient on side
Decreased hemoglobin	Opioids if not transfusing	

WHO, 2004; Kochar, 2015; AACN, 2007.

TREATMENT OF PAIN

At least half of patients experience significant pain at the end of life. It can be a variety of types of pain. Regardless of whether it is neuropathic (neuropathies) or nociceptive (somatic or visceral), it affects the quality of life and causes anxiety and distress. The nurse must take several steps prior to treating the pain:

▶ Consider the cause.

▶ Assess whether it is acute or chronic.

▶ Take a thorough medication history.

▶ Assess whether the patient is able to verbalize pain or has a fear of the medication causing death or addiction.

▶ Consider cultural practices with pain identification, tolerance, and control.

The WHO (2004) developed a pain ladder that rates pain in three categories using a standard pain scale of 1 to 10:

- Mild pain: rating of 1 to 3
- Moderate pain: rating of 4 to 6
- Severe pain: rating of 7 and above

There are a number of generally agreed-upon guidelines regarding the use of pain medication at the end of life:

▶ There is a preference for oral, intravenous, transdermal, and rectal medications.

▶ Subcutaneous injections and sublingual delivery are not preferred but can be done.

▶ Intramuscular injections are highly discouraged.

▶ Pain medications should be administered at fixed intervals, every 2 hours, 4 hours, etc., around the clock in order to keep the medication at the desired level in the blood.

▶ If the pain medication effects wear off, there should be a breakthrough dosage ordered that is approximately 10 to 20% of the original oral dose and 50 to 75% of the intravenous dose, or a nonopioid or adjuvant analgesic may be administered.

▶ Opioids are ordered in conjunction with nonopioids and adjuvant drugs.

▶ Be very cautious about interactions between antidepressants and other medications as well as delayed metabolism of the drugs related to age and cause of pain.

▶ Opioids do not cause death at recommended dosages. They relax the muscles and enable the patient to breathe more easily while decreasing the pain.

▶ Types of pain medication used at the end of life include:
  - Nonopioids
    - Acetaminophen (Tylenol)—antipyretic and analgesic:
      - Assess for liver damage.
    - Nonsteroidal antiinflammatory drugs (NSAIDs) for bone pain, inflammation; analgesics:
      - Assess for bleeding and renal dysfunction.
  - Opioids:
    - Morphine (MS Contin, Roxanol):
      - Constipation develops in almost 100% of opioid users.
      - Respiratory depression is not frequent with appropriate dosage, but it is possible.
      - Beware of overmedicating with opioids, as elderly and compromised patients have a slower metabolism that could result in a delayed bolus effect of the drug.
      - Naloxone (Narcan) reverses confirmed respiratory distress that may occur after an initial dose of a narcotic being used for pain. It can also be used if there is a drop in the oxygenation level during sleep resulting in unconsciousness that is related to use of a narcotic.

- Hydromorphone (Dilaudid)
- Codeine
- Fentanyl
- Oxycodone (Oxycontin)
- Meperidine (Demerol), highly discouraged by ELNEC:
  - Renal dysfunction
- Opioid agonists— propoxyphene (Darvon/Darvocet), highly discouraged by ELNEC:
  - Renal dysfunction
  - Tremors and seizures
- Mixed agonist–antagonist—buprenorphine (Buprenex), moderately discouraged by ELNEC:
  - Psychomimetic effects
- Adjuvant analgesics:
  - Antidepressants—used for neuropathic pain
    - Tricyclic antidepressants have many side effects and contraindications.
    - SSRIs reduce anxiety and pain but are not a first-line drug.
  - Anticonvulsants—used for neuropathic pain
  - Local anesthetics—local pain and pruritus
  - Corticosteroids—used for bone and visceral pain:
    - Increase appetite and energy
    - Psychosis with some dosages

Nonpharmacologic treatment of pain includes options such as:

- Relaxation techniques:
  - Meditation
  - Breathing exercises
  - Heat/cold massage
- Guided imagery
- Distraction
- Music therapy
- Support groups
- Pastoral care and consultation
- Acupuncture

Question	Rationale
When the provider orders pain medication within wide parameters, such as morphine 2 to 10 mg IV, every 4 hours, the least important assessment prior to determining the initial dose you will give is: A. Asking the patient to rate the pain on a pain scale B. Looking at recent pain medication records for time and strength of previous doses C. Asking the patient how much pain medication he/she needs right now D. Finding the patient's allergies and looking for any contraindications with other medications that are ordered	Answer: C The patient may or may not know how much was last given or may wish to determine the strength himself/herself, which is inappropriate. Always: - Ask the patient to rate the pain on a pain scale. - Note the dose, time, and strength of the last dose to avoid overdosing. - Keep in mind that elderly patients metabolize drugs at a slower rate. - Know that the patient is not the best judge of how much pain medication should be given.

SIDE EFFECTS OF THE PHARMACOLOGIC PAIN TREATMENTS

There are many side effects of drugs given for pain. Some can be long-standing and others are preventable. All side effects should be considered prior to administering medications, with the intent of maintaining the best quality of life possible.

▶ Constipation occurs with almost 100% of patients taking opioids as well as for those who have limited activity and decreased fluid intake.
  • Senna (Senokot)—stimulates bowel activity:
    • Watch for liver damage
  • Dioctyl sulfosuccinate (Docusate)—stool softener, sometimes used in conjunction with Senna
  • Milk of Magnesia—osmotic shift of fluid into intestines:
    • Overdose or prolonged use may cause electrolyte imbalances.
  • Sorbitol or lactulose—osmotic frequently used for opioid-induced constipation
    • May be given in enema form if other routes unavailable
  • Metoclopramide (Reglan)—prokinetic drug:
    • Observe for extrapyramidal symptoms
  • Encourage fruits and high-fiber foods
  • Dried paw paw seeds can be mixed in water to drink.
  • Encourage fluids, if not contraindicated
  • Physical activity:
    • Not always possible with end-of-life patients
▶ Diarrhea:
  • Atropine
  • Diphenoxylate/atropine (Lomotil)
  • Psyllium (Metamucil):
    • Must be able to drink at least 6 glasses of water
  • Metronidazole (Flagyl) if caused by infection
▶ Fatigue:
  • Corticosteroids
  • Antidepressants
    • SSRIs are first–line treatment—paroxetine (Paxil).
    • Tricyclics are discouraged in elderly.
▶ Delirium:
  • Low-dose diazepam (Valium)
  • Haloperidol (Haldol):
    • Watch for disorientation
  • Lorazepam (Ativan) or midazolam (Versed):
    • Highly discouraged
  • Listen to patient carefully.
  • Provide emotional support.
  • Decrease noise.
  • No caffeine
  • Keep environment static and familiar.
  • Keep similar time patterns.
  • Use simple sentences and talk slowly.
▶ Nausea and vomiting:
  • Haloperidol (Haldol) if anxiety is adding to the nausea and vomiting:
    • Dystonia, dyskinesia

- Cannabinoids are second-line antiemetics:
  - Domperidone
- Phenothiazines may cause excessive drowsiness; use with caution:
  - Metoclopramide (Reglan)
- Antihistamines:
  - Diphenhydramine (Benadryl)
- Anticholinergics:
  - Scopolamine (Transderm Scop):
    - Dry mouth
    - Urinary retention
    - Possible agitation
    - Also effective for treating "death rattle"
- Benzodiazepines:
  - Watch for sedation, amnesia
- Serotonin-blocking agent
  - Ondansetron (Zofran):
    - Headache
    - Dry mouth
- Relaxation
- Imagery
- Distraction
- Music therapy

▶ Pruritus:

- Corticosteroid creams
- Chlorhexidine:
  - Diluted in bath and put on after bath (0.05%)
- Moisturize skin frequently:
  - Aqueous cream

▶ Decubitus ulcer:

- Turn patient frequently or reposition in chair/bed.
- Assess for reddened areas at pressure points.

Examples of End-of-Life Care for Specific Patient Conditions

▶ Initial steps:

- Assess patient status and prognosis.
- Communicate with the patient regarding his/her expected or preferred outcomes, goals, feelings, and treatment options:
  - Research reveals that patients want timely and clear communication with their goals considered and treatment delivered maintaining dignity and comfort (ELNEC, 2007; Holmes, 2011; Kastenbaum, 2001; Kochhar, 2015; Kuebler et. al, 2002; WHO, 2004; Wingate and Wiegand, 2008).
  - Understanding the patient's wishes, or the surrogate's in some cases, is paramount.
  - The surrogate is a decision maker only when the patient is unable to make decisions alone.
  - Remember, you are a patient advocate; the care planning is based wholly on the patient's wishes.

▶ If receiving palliative care, all treatments to alleviate or cure the cancer are terminated:

- Medications:
  - Opioids:
    - Assess latest pain medication administration and dose status.

- Anxiolytics
- Antidepressants
- Antiemetics
- Medications for whatever other complications occur
- Discuss end-of-life directives.

Heart Failure

▶ Initial steps:
- Assess for respiratory status.
- Assess for cardiac status.
- Assess for pain:
  - 78% of heart failure patients state they have inadequate pain control
▶ Symptoms would most likely include dyspnea, pain, confusion, weakness, edema, fatigue, anxiety, productive cough, and cachexia.
▶ Medications/treatments:
- Diuretics
- Oxygen to keep SaO2 >92%.
- Scopolamine
- Digoxin (Lanoxin)
- Opioids:
  - Morphine
  - Codeine
- Tricyclics
- Anxiolytics
- Buspirone (Buspar)
- Fans
- Head of bed (HOB) elevated
- Spiritual needs
▶ Discuss advance directives

Chronic Obstructive Pulmonary Disease

▶ Assess for symptoms such as air hunger, pursed-lip breathing
▶ Other likely symptoms:
- Hypoxia
- Fatigue
- Insomnia
- Cough: productive, mucous production
- Anxiety
- Depression
- Fear
- Pain
- Cachexia
▶ Medications/treatments:
- Bronchodilators
- Oxygen
- Mucolytic
- Opioids
- Anxiolytics
- Antidepressants
- HOB elevated

- Fans
- Cool temperature in room
- Physiotherapy
▷ Discuss advance directives

FINAL HOURS

Sometimes, the final hours are the most difficult for both the patient's family and the nurse. The ability to help the patient or make them better is not a possibility. It can be very stressful to wait for the death and be totally helpless. The patient may exhibit:

▷ A brief initial surge in energy

▷ A consistent drop in blood pressure

▷ Heart rate that is irregular, appearing to stop and then suddenly reappearing:

- Sometimes it is best to turn off the monitor because it becomes something that everyone stares at, watching the rhythm and rate change. It can be deceiving, confusing, and distracting at times.

▷ Inability to communicate

▷ Allow the family to be present if they wish to be.

▷ Do not force your beliefs and wishes on the family.

▷ Maintain privacy for the patient and the family.

▷ Dim the lights.

▷ Be present only if the patient and family wish you to be; there is nothing more you can do.

▷ *If the family is not present in the room at this time,* remove all of the equipment, lines, and any attachments the patient might have. Note that if this is a coroner's case or the death was unusual, the equipment, lines, and tubes cannot be touched or removed. Make certain to determine this first before doing any postmortem care or preparation. Clean the patient, change the gown, and make sure the eyes are closed. Invite the family in to see the patient after making the patient look as normal as possible by reinserting dentures, combing hair, having the sheet over the lower extremities, and having the side rails down. Provide tissue for the family and friends.

CASE STUDY

Mr. M. is a 78-year-old male with a 10-year history of prostate cancer that has metastasized to his liver, bones, and lungs. He has undergone countless chemotherapy regimens and has decided that he wants no more treatment. Gradually, he has lost his appetite, appears gaunt and pale, experiences frequent drowsiness, and is isolating himself from family and friends. Because of his new onset of dizziness, he is brought to the hospital for evaluation. Current medications include a 25 mcg/hr fentanyl transdermal (Duragesic) patch, change every 3 days; docusate sodium (Colace) 50 mg at bedtime; and naproxen (Naprosyn) 500 mg twice daily for bone pain.

Physical examination reveals the following: blood pressure BP 86/48 mm Hg, heart rate 120 beats/min, respiratory rate 30 breaths/min, sodium 160 mEq/L; potassium 5.4 mEq/L; hemoglobin 13.5 g/dL; white-cell count 11.0 mm^3, blood urea nitrogen (BUN) 30 mg/dL, creatinine 1.5 mg/dL; SaO$_2$ 86%, and urine output 40 mL/6 hours. The patient is lethargic, drowsy, and noncommunicative. He appears disoriented to time and reports generalized, acute pain that he rates at an 8 when he is awake. Has had no bowel movement for 3 days and urination is infrequent.

1. **What does the assessment of Mr. M. most probably indicate?**

   a. *His electrolytes are abnormal: hypernatremia and hyperkalemia are present. His BUN and creatinine are elevated, indicating dehydration and impaired kidney function.*

   b. *His vital signs are indicative of hypovolemia with hypotension, tachypnea, and tachycardia.*

   c. *Disorientation might be a result of the hypernatremia or be symptomatic of a steady decline in his health.*

   d. *He is most probably dehydrated.*

   e. *SAO2 is low, signifying hypoxia and possibly fluid in the lungs or heart failure.*

   f. *Increased white-cell counts are indicative of a possible evolving infectious process as well.*

Mr. M. is given 2 L of lactated Ringers and is showing improvement in his cognition and responsiveness. He still reports sharp, aching bone pain and abdominal discomfort. He is admitted for 24 hour observation. A geriatric specialist, oncologist, and hospice representative are consulted. CT scanning shows that his metastatic prostate cancer is spreading and there is no change in his renal function. Mr. M. reports that he is just tired, in pain, and "wants to be left alone so he can go home." His family is close and they support him in his decision but are very concerned that he will suffer even more after declining further treatment.

2. **How can the nurse advocate for Mr. M?**

   a. *The nurse should speak with Mr. M. and ask him how he feels and what his wishes are at this point. Sit quietly and allow him to talk. Ask for clarification but do not lead the conversation. The nurse may state the following: "Tell me how you are feeling." "Explain what you mean about being left alone to go home." "What kind of treatment do you want?"*

   b. *Encourage him to tell his family how he is feeling and what he wants. Let him know that he is able to decide his own plan of care. This is patient autonomy.*

   c. *Explain hospice to Mr. M., and ask if he is interested in hearing more about it.*

3. **How does the nurse explore the family's concerns about his suffering?**

   a. *Ask them what they know about palliative care/hospice care.*

   b. *Explain that it does not mean no treatment at all, but is meant to keep the patient comfortable while providing no curative measures.*

   c. *Have the family discuss this with the patient and the hospice nurse.*

4. **What changes in treatment might be made to treat his symptoms?**

   a. *Adding Senna to the docusate to help treat the constipation.*

   b. *Changing the pain medication to an opioid that can be given around the clock but adjusted as needed—for example, morphine sulfate—to avoid overdosing.*

   c. *Starting an adjuvant medication for anxiety or depression.*

Mr. M. is receiving hospice care at his daughter's house and his condition begins to decline. She has questions about how she will know when the end is near for him. Her brother is very concerned about his father's shortness of breath and refusal to eat or drink anything and wonders if he needs to be there when his father passes away.

5. **How does the nurse address these concerns and questions?**

   a. *It is not possible to determine when a person will die. It can be very sudden or take hours to days. Certain signs signal the final hours:*

      i. *A consistent drop in blood pressure*

      ii. *Slow, irregular breathing with periods of apnea*

      iii. Audible chest sounds—"death rattle"

      iv. Irregular heart rate or heart rate that seems to stop and start

      v. Inability to communicate

      vi. Bluish tint to the upper and lower extremities

      vii. Cool body temperature

  b. The family should try to be present if the patient has expressed that he does not want to die alone or if the family member wishes to be there. There is no right or wrong answer.

  c. Dim the lights and make the patient as comfortable as possible.

  d. Lack of food and water is not painful for the patient.

  e. A low concentration of oxygen via nasal cannula and a low dose of morphine can ease breathing.

Discussion

While a person retains his/her cognitive capabilities and mental capacity, the decision regarding treatment and direction of end-of-life care is their own. It is a nurse's job to ensure that every person with these characteristics understands that they have the right of autonomy—the right to determine end-of-life wishes. The nurse, however, must avoid the pitfall of trying to impose his/her own beliefs on the patient. Objectivity must be maintained as well as the duty to safeguard the ethical patient right of autonomy. Communication with the patient and the family is an essential component of end-of-life care.

While patient wishes and treatments vary, the goals of end-of-life care are to provide comfort, both physical and spiritual, as well as end-of-life dignity and privacy for the patient. Of course, that should involve consulting with interdisciplinary colleagues such as pastors, spiritual leaders, hospice specialists, geriatric physicians, etc. Understanding the expectations of end-of-life signs and symptoms assists health care professionals to anticipate and help the family to accept the final steps in each patient's life. There are palliative treatments for every symptom that a nurse can anticipate at the end-of-life, from nausea and depression to pain and dyspnea and many more. The utilization of these treatments can help ensure that no one spends the "final hours" in discomfort and misery.

Families have been found to remember the nurse as the most important person during the end-of-life experience. The nurse's job is to treat the families as well as the patient and keep them informed about the status of the dying patient and the comfort measures taken to ease the process. This is what they will remember when recalling their loved one's final hours.

Bibliography

American Association of Colleges of Nursing, City of Hope End-of-Life Nursing Education Consortium. (2007). End-of-life core curriculum. Accessed June 29, 2018, from www.aacn.nche.edu/ELNEC

ANA Center for Ethics and Human Rights. (2016). ANA position statement: Nurses' roles and responsibilities in providing care and support at the end of life. Accessed June 29, 2018, https://www.nursingworld.org/~4af078/globalassets/docs/ana/ethics/endoflife-positionstatement.pdf.

Carr, T.K. (2006). *Introducing Death and Dying.* (Upper Saddle River, NJ: Pearson Prentice Hall).

Cross Roads Hospice. (2018). *A guide to understanding end-of-life signs and symptoms.* Accessed June 29, 2018, https://www.crossroadshospice.com/caregiver-guidance/physical-emotional-changes/

Herbert, K., Moore, H., and Rooney, J. (2011). The nurse advocate in end-of-life care. *The Ochsner Journal* 11, 325.329. Accessed June 29, 2018, https://www.ncbi.nlm.nih.gov/pmc/articles/PMC3241064/

Holms, J., Milligan, S., and Kydd, A. (2011). A study of lived experiences of registered nurses who have provided end-of-life care within an intensive care unit. *International Journal of Palliative Nursing, 20*(11), 549–556. doi:10.12968/ijpn.2014.20.11.549

Institute of Medicine (IOM). (2014). *Dying in America: IOM committee's proposed core components of quality end-of-life care*. Accessed June 29, 2018, http://nationalacademies.org/hmd/~/media/Files/Report%20Files/2014/EOL/Table%20-%20Core%20Components%20of%20Quality%20Care.pdf

Jansen, K., Schaufel, M.A., and Ruths, S. (2014). Drug treatment at end of life: an epidemiological study in nursing homes. *Scandinavian Journal of Primary Health Care* 32, 187–192.

Kastenbaum., R.J. (2001). *Death, Society, and Human Experiences*, 7th ed. (Needham Heights, MA.: Pearson Education).

Kochhar, S. (2015, February). Discussing end-of-life care with COPD patients. *Independent Nurse*. Accessed June 29, 2018, www.independentnurse.co.uk

Kubler-Ross, E. (2014). *On death and dying: What the dying have to teach doctors, nurses, clergy and their own families*. (New York, NY: Simon & Schuster, Inc.)

Kuebler, K.K., Berry, P.H., and Heidrich, D.E. (2002). *End-of-Life Care: Clinical Practice Guidelines*. (Philadelphia: Saunders).

Registered Nurses' Association of Ontario. (2001). *End-of-Life Care during the Last Days and Hours*. Toronto: Registered Nurses' Association of Ontario.

Reynolds, J., Drew, D., and Dunwoody, C. (2013). American Society for Pain Management nursing position statement: pain management at the end of life. *Pain Management Nursing* 14(3), 172–175.

Roijmakers, J.J.H., vanZuylen, L., Furst, C.J., Becarro, M., Marorana, L., Pilastri, C., …Costantini, M. (2013). Variation in medication use in cancer patients at end of life: a cross-sectional analysis. *Support Care Cancer* 21, 1003–1011.

Wingate, S., and Wiegand, L.-M. (2008). End-of-life care in the critical care unit for patients with heart failure. *Critical Care Nurse* 28(2), 84–94. Accessed June 29, 2018, http://ccn.aacnjournals.org

World Health Organization (WHO). (2004). Palliative care: symptom management and end-of-life care. Accessed June 29, 2018, http://www.who.int/hiv/pub/imai/primary_palliative/en/

Behavioral Health and the Medical-Surgical Patient

Aliesha Emerson, MSN, RN-C

OVERVIEW

Many hospitalized patients are in crisis regardless of what type of nursing unit they are admitted to. An individual does not always need to be admitted to a behavioral health unit to treat their behavioral health issues. It is important to understand that this patient population is getting older and is increasingly complex to manage because they usually have multiple comorbidities. Any patient, regardless of diagnosis, can exhibit or experience behavioral symptoms. With various demands on nurses, caring for these patients can prove difficult, and may result in burnout and feelings of being overwhelmed and of helplessness. Understanding behavioral health disorders and signs of escalation is important in order to recognize how to better treat the medical and psychiatric needs of patients. This will help keep patients and caregivers mentally and physically safe.

ANXIETY

Anatomy

▶ The brain's amygdala controls fear and anxiety
▶ Patients with anxiety disorders often show intensified amygdala responses to anxiety cues.

Etiology

▶ Anxiety is manifested from a source of:
- Significant stress:
  - Hospitalization
  - Illness
  - Fear of death
  - Unfamiliar environment
- Loss of control
- Separation from family, friends, or support system
- Overwhelming questions from hospital staff

Escalation Assessment

▶ Pacing:

- Continuously coming out to the nurse's station
- Repetitive questioning
- For the nonverbal or elderly patient may consist of grimacing or rocking back and forth in chair or bed

▶ Yelling, or increasing tone of voice

▶ Crying

▶ Verbalizing that they are anxious

▶ Hypertension

▶ Cardiac arrhythmias

▶ Hyperventilation

▶ Increase in pain

▶ Diaphoresis

Nursing Diagnosis

▶ Anxiety related to unfamiliar environment, understanding of diagnosis, diagnostic tests, and treatments

▶ Ineffective breathing pattern related to panic and worrisome or irrational thoughts

▶ Powerlessness related to unfamiliar environment and loss of control of one's own body

Interventions

▶ Communicate using a calm tone:

- Do **not** match your voice pitch with that of the patient.

▶ Keep your patient informed:

- Use understandable terms.
- Give information in short sessions in order to avoid the patient becoming psychologically crowded or overwhelmed.
- If available, use communication boards and keep up to date with plan of care or activities.
- An informed patient is a less anxious patient.

▶ Try your best to have all providers involved in the care *physically* see the patient:

- During interdisciplinary rounds, or treatment team meeting, inform providers that the patient is increasingly anxious.
- Patients get more anxious the less they see, get to talk to, or ask questions of a provider, especially when it involves tests, labs, results, or discharge.

▶ Allow patient to verbalize fear or anger :

- Take a time-out from the computer or other documentation responsibilities, if possible, to allow the patient to verbalize anxiety.
- Ensure privacy and remove "audience" (e.g., other patients, providers, staff).

▶ Do **not** confront or argue with the patient.

▶ Use distraction:

- If possible, let the patient have his or her own music, movies, laptop, etc.
- Journaling
- Drawing or adult coloring

Plan of Care

▶ Maintain a safe environment for patient and staff:

- Begin to remove dangerous objects from room if escalation increases.
- Know your exit and stay close to it at all times.

Question	Rationale
Which intervention will best help reduce anxiety in a 36-year-old patient who has been hospitalized for ectopic pregnancy? A. Ask all members of the health care team to assess the quality of care the patient is receiving frequently. B. Assign the patient to a talkative, optimistic roommate similar in age. C. Explain to the patient what will happen during the hospitalization. D. Check on the patient frequently and encourage talk about future plans.	Answer: C Educating and explaining clearly what will happen during this traumatic time for the patient will help to clarify any questions the patient may be too scared or distracted to ask. This will ease any fears or additional anxiety. Asking health care members to constantly assess the quality of care has the potential to exacerbate anxiety—seeing more health care providers in and out of the room may lead the patient to think that something else is wrong. Having a talkative roommate will not allow the patient to fully rest or have the private time needed with the family or support system. Finally, encouraging the patient to talk about the future at this time is premature because the event is relatively new and the patient hasn't had the time to fully heal mentally or physically. Avoid "psychologically crowding" the patient.

> Keep environment as quiet as possible.
> Assess for depression at the beginning of admission.
> Communicate with the care team that the patient is anxious.
> Do not make demands.
> Medicate as needed.

Medication/Treatment (Table 21.1)

> **Clinical Consideration**
>
> Geriatric medication considerations:
> - Give smaller doses.
> - These medications can cause greater sedation at times.
> - Effects of antianxiety medications can also mimic symptoms of dementia.
> - Place patient on fall precautions.

TABLE 21.1	ANTIANXIETY DRUGS AND THEIR ACTIONS
Medication	**Action**

Selective serotonin-reuptake inhibitors (SSRIs)
    Citalopram (Celexa)
    Escitalopram (Lexapro)
    Fluoxetine (Prozac)
    Paroxetine (Paxil)
    Sertraline (Zoloft)
	Relieve symptoms by blocking the reabsorption, or reuptake, of serotonin by certain nerve cells in the brain.

Serotonin–norepinephrine-reuptake inhibitors (SNRIs)
    Venlafaxine (Effexor)
    Duloxetine (Cymbalta)
	Increase the levels of the neurotransmitters serotonin and norepinephrine by inhibiting their reabsorption into cells in the brain.

Benzodiazepines
    Alprazolam (Xanax)
    Clonazepam (Klonopin)
    Diazepam (Valium)
    Lorazepam (Ativan)
	Frequently used for short-term management of anxiety; highly effective in promoting relaxation and reducing muscular tension and other physical symptoms of anxiety. Long-term use may require increased doses to achieve the same effect, which may lead to problems related to tolerance and dependence.

Tricyclic antidepressants
    Amitriptyline (Elavil)
    Imipramine (Tofranil)
    Nortriptyline (Pamelor)
	With Concerns about long-term use of benzodiazepines, tricyclic antidepressants may be utilized; can cause significant side effects, including orthostatic hypotension, constipation, urinary retention, dry mouth, blurry vision.

Patient Education

▶ Encourage patient to talk to someone:
  - Someone whom the patient trusts who is already nearby, or call someone
  - The sooner the better
▶ Encourage the patient to take slow, deep breaths:
  - Hyperventilation leads to arrhythmia; it also causes other symptoms, such as chest pain and light-headedness.
▶ Understand that anxiety is a normal human response
▶ Regular exercise can counteract physical symptoms of anxiety
▶ Avoid caffeine and alcohol
▶ Lack of sleep can aggravate anxiety; promote proper sleep hygiene.

BIPOLAR DISORDER

Anatomy

▶ Biologic differences:
  - Some people with this disorder have physical changes in their brains.
  - The significance of these changes is still uncertain.
▶ Neurotransmitters:
  - An imbalance in naturally occurring brain chemicals (neurotransmitters) plays a significant role in bipolar disorder.:
▶ Inherited traits:
  - Common in people who have a first-degree relative, such as a sibling or parent, with the condition.
  - Research continues to try to isolate the gene that causes this disorder.

Escalation Assessment

▶ Is the patient feeling grandiose?
  - No fear. No consequences.
▶ Is the patient talking fast? Are the eyes darting? Is he or she questioning everything and unable to listen? Is there no rational thought?
▶ Is the patient beginning to have auditory or visual hallucinations?
▶ Observe your patient silently:
  - Listen to phone conversations if you are in the room or in the hallway.
    - What is the content of the conversation?
    - Is there:
      - Escalating volume?
      - Yelling?
      - Slamming of phone?
▶ How is the patient sleeping?
  - Lack of sleep, or no sleep at all?
  - Constantly moving
▶ Is there a history of substance abuse?
  - Substance abuse can exacerbate manic symptoms and violent outbursts
▶ Has there been recent or past trauma or a stressful situation?
  - Being hospitalized
  - Receiving a poor diagnosis or prognosis
  - Change in environment

Nursing Diagnosis

▶ Risk for injury related to:
  • Extreme hyperactivity
  • Irrational thoughts and decision making
▶ Risk for self-directed violence related to:
  • Impulsivity
  • Manic excitement
  • Rage reaction
  • Restlessness
▶ Ineffective individual coping related to:
  • Inadequate level of perception of control
  • Ineffective problem-solving strategies or skills

Interventions

▶ Encourage expression of feelings:
  • Venting can avoid an explosion.
  • Relieves anxiety, tension, and often fear
▶ Maintain personal space
▶ KNOW YOUR EXIT:
  • Assess area for possible items that may present a hazard.
▶ Keep tone of voice low and calm:
  • Use simple terms.
  • Avoid matching tone or volume.
▶ Distract patient, if possible.
▶ Keep patient in a quiet environment with little stimulation:
  • The patient is already overstimulated.
▶ Do not take the patient's words personally.
▶ Maintain the patient's dignity:
  • Avoid confrontational situations.
▶ Do not reinforce attention-seeking or "entertaining" behaviors.
▶ If possible, offer medications.
▶ Offer choices when possible—the patient needs some kind of control:
  • For example, before medicating the patient: "Mr. S. would you like some medication to take the edge off? Do you want it in your arm or buttock?"
▶ Communicate with your team constantly:
  • Once you leave the room, be sure you inform someone else of the escalating behaviors while you get medication ready.

Plan of Care

▶ Set limits and boundaries from the beginning of admission:
  • Must stay consistent
▶ Keep a uniform and structured day if possible:
  • If there are tests and lab work that must be done, give patient a general idea of when and where particular activities will occur.
▶ Communicate the plan with health care team.
▶ Guide the patient as much as possible:
  • The patient is unable to control internally, so assistance and redirection from the nurse is necessary.
▶ Maintain a safe environment and decrease stimulation.

Medication/Treatment (Table 21.2)

TABLE 21.2	DRUGS USED FOR BIPOLAR DISORDER
Medication	Action

Mood stabilizers
  Lithium (Lithobid)
  Valproic acid (Depakene)
  Divalproex sodium (Depakote)
  Carbamazepine (Tegretol)
  Lamotrigine (Lamictal)
	Balance certain brain chemicals (neurotransmitters) that control emotional states and behavior

Antipsychotics
  Olanzapine (Zyprexa)
  Risperidone (Risperdal)
  Quetiapine (Seroquel)
  Aripiprazole (Abilify)
  Ziprasidone (Geodon)
	Thought to block certain chemical receptors in the brain, which results in relieving symptoms of psychotic disorders

Selective Serotonin Reuptake Inhibitors (SSRIs)
  Citalopram (Celexa)
  Escitalopram (Lexapro)
  Fluoxetine (Prozac)
  Paroxetine (Paxil)
  Sertraline (Zoloft)
	Relieve symptoms by blocking the reabsorption, or reuptake, of serotonin by certain nerve cells in the brain.

Benzodiazepines
  Alprazolam (Xanax)
  Clonazepam (Klonopin)
  Diazepam (Valium)
  Lorazepam (Ativan)
	Enhance the action of the neurotransmitter, GABA (gamma aminobutyric acid); the function of GABA is to slow or calm things down.

Clinical Consideration

Be aware of lithium toxicity—nystagmus, hypotension, ataxia, seizures, cardiovascular collapse
Depakote: Monitor liver function and complete blood count:
Obesity can be a common side effect of these drugs:
- Sedation causes patients to exercise less frequently.
- Dry mouth causes patients to take in more sweet drinks.

Patient Education
- Emphasize the need for medication adherence:
  - Both patient and patient's support system should be educated.
- Effective coping mechanisms:
  - Keep a regular schedule.
  - Practice healthy sleep habits.
  - Encourage the patient to keep a journal to note stresses, triggers, or thoughts.
- Lifestyle changes:
  - Regular exercise
  - Avoid caffeine, alcohol, and drugs.

BORDERLINE PERSONALITY DISORDER

Anatomy
- No conclusive labs or imaging
- Often have issues with psychological testing such as the Rorschach test

Etiology
- Borderline personality disorder:
  - Has no single cause or risk factor
  - Has a genetic predisposition:
    - No single, specific gene for borderline disorder
  - Can be due to poor parenting as a result of not having guidance or a positive role model on which to base parenting skills:
    - Early separation from one or both parents

Question	Rationale
An extremely agitated patient is pacing in front of the nurse's station and states, "I'm more than capable of purchasing all of the property of this company." His mood varies from outbursts of laughter to punching the walls in his room angrily. Which is the most accurate documentation of this client's behavior? A. Patient disoriented and euphoric; will continue to monitor. B. Exhibiting fairytale thinking in relation to hallucinations; restless. C. Mood inappropriate; exhibiting manic symptoms. D. Agitated and pacing; demonstrating ideas of grandeur; mood labile.	Answer: D This answer clearly states physically what the patient is exhibiting as well as the current state of thinking. While the patient perhaps is euphoric as well as manic, he is still aware of where he is so he is not disoriented, nor does he show any evidence of visual or auditory hallucinations.

- Can result from repeated emotional, physical, or sexual abuse by someone within or outside of the family itself
- Can result from inconsistent, unsupportive care

Escalation Assessment

▶ Triggers:
  - Ask patient about triggers.
  - Invasive procedures may be a trigger:
    • Keep patient informed about plan of care.
    • Has there been a change in testing times, or disagreement ?
    • Is there disagreement, conflict or uncertainty related to a procedure or intervention?
▶ Does the patient feel rejected?
  - Abnormal lab or test result
  - Moving rooms
  - Isolation precautions
▶ Patient may be sarcastic or threatening.
▶ Evidence of self-mutilation

Nursing Diagnosis

▶ Risk for self-mutilation related to:
  - Need for attention
  - Feelings of depression, rejection, self-hatred, separation anxiety, and guilt
  - Impulsive behavior
  - Inability to verbally express feelings
▶ Impaired social interaction related to:
  - Unstable or abusive family background
  - Unacceptable social interaction, behaviors, or values
▶ Ineffective coping related to:
  - Extreme emotional state
  - Lack of motivation
  - Trauma—history of physical, emotional, or sexual abuse

Interventions

▶ Be mindful of your body language, attitude, and tone of voice.

▶ Listen actively and be sympathetic:
- Do not get distracted by electronics (cell phones, computers, etc.).
- Avoid interrupting the patient.
- Make the patient feel heard.

▶ Focus on the emotions the patient is displaying, not the words:
- How is the patient conveying the message?
- Is he or she getting angrier or louder?
- Do not argue.

▶ History of substance abuse:
- Medicate when possible

▶ Distract:
- Music, movies, journaling

▶ Set boundaries from the beginning of admission, and communicate with health care team:
- Make it clear that there is structure; however, circumstances can change.
- Boundaries must be clear, firm, and to a degree, flexible.
- Be consistent

▶ Give patient alternatives or choices when available.

▶ Avoid threats and ultimatums.

▶ If the patient threatens, give him or her time and space.

Plan of Care

▶ Establish therapeutic trusting, open, and honest relationship from the beginning of admission.

▶ Identify triggers that may set off the patient:
- Report triggers thoroughly to care team.

▶ Keep a safe environment for patient:
- Determine suicidal gestures, attempts, or current thoughts
- If necessary, place patient in the room closest to nurses' station.

▶ Set boundaries and communicate these boundaries to the team.

▶ Administer medication as indicated.

Medication/Treatment (Table 21.3)

> **Clinical Consideration**
>
> Because of the side effects of prescribed drugs, including weight gain, increased appetite, and lethargy, these patients are prone to cardiovascular issues. Smoking and alcohol use, which are prevalent among this population, also can affect the patient's cardiovascular health.

TABLE 21.3	BORDERLINE PERSONALITY DISORDER DRUGS AND THEIR ACTIONS
Medication	**Action**
Mood Stabilizers 　Lithium (Lithobid) 　Valproic acid (Depakene) 　Divalproex sodium (Depakote) 　Carbamazepine (Tegretol) 　Lamotrigine (Lamictal)	Balances certain brain chemicals (neurotransmitters) that control emotional states and behavior
Antipsychotics 　Olanzapine (Zyprexa) 　Risperidone (Risperdal) 　Quetiapine (Seroquel) 　Aripiprazole (Abilify) 　Ziprasidone (Geodon)	Thought to block certain chemical receptors in the brain which results in the relief of symptoms of psychotic disorders

Patient Education

◗ Encourage counseling and therapy:
- It is important for patients to find a provider that they can trust.
◗ Medication compliance
◗ Healthy habits:
- Sleep hygiene
- Eating healthy foods
- Regular exercise
◗ Avoid drugs and alcohol

Question	Rationale
A patient is admitted with heart failure and also is diagnosed with borderline personality disorder. He is constantly ordering pizza to be delivered directly to his room for himself and his girlfriend. His last nurse allowed him to do so. This is detrimental to the patient's health. Having delivery service come directly into the room where there is a roommate is a privacy issue. This behavior should be addressed to: A. Reduce complaints made to patient relations by the roommate B. Set realistic boundaries C. Guide the patient to make better dietary choices D. Reduce angry outbursts	Answer: B Realistic boundaries must be set at the beginning of the admission with patients who have this disorder. Communicating clearly to the patient why pizza delivery is inappropriate is paramount. Additionally, these communication points must be made to all health care team members in order to maintain consistency and decrease the patient's chances of reverting to the same behavior.

SCHIZOPHRENIA

Anatomy
◗ Family history
◗ Computed tomography (CT) scans do show atrophy of cortex
◗ Positron-emission tomography (PET) scans have determined diminished glucose and oxygen metabolism in the frontal lobe.
◗ Imbalance of dopamine and serotonin

Escalation Assessment
◗ Body movements getting tighter—clenching fists and jaw
◗ Pacing
◗ Talking faster
◗ Talking to themselves
◗ Staring off and not making eye contact

Nursing Diagnosis
◗ Altered thought process related to:
- Delusional thinking
- Inability to stay on topic

Clinical Consideration
These patients can be poor historians: Ask family, or friends about baseline behavior. If you have access to belongings, ask if they can show you their medications.

Clinical Consideration
Neurologic disorders such as, epilepsy, brain tumors, and encephalitis can often mimic schizophrenia.

- Unable to focus
- Escalating behaviors in reaction to normal stimuli
- Hallucinations
- Difficulty problem solving

▶ Social isolation related to:

- Depression
- Limited interaction with others
- Dependence on nonverbal communication
- Avoidance of social situations

▶ Ineffective coping related to:

- Feelings of loneliness or rejection
- Inability to perform daily self-care tasks
- Physical and emotional withdrawal

Interventions

▶ Obtain patient's permission to touch:

- May strike out to protect themselves

▶ Approach them in a calm, unhurried manner

▶ Avoid crowding the patient physically and psychologically

▶ Respond neutrally to condescending remarks

▶ If the patient wants to be left alone, give them space, but make sure you return soon.

▶ Consider postponing procedures that require physical contact with hospital personnel if patient becomes suspicious or agitated.

▶ Explore the content of hallucinations:

- Validate that you know that what they are hearing is real to them.

Plan of Care

▶ Set limits firmly but without anger:

- Avoid punitive attitude

▶ Be flexible:

- Give the patient as much control as possible

▶ Maintain safe environment:

- Always assess room for possible dangerous objects.
- Know your exit.

▶ Communicate plan of care to other members of health care team.

▶ Encourage autonomy.

▶ Establishing trust from beginning of admission:

- Show patient medications and read labels out loud; this encourages medication compliance.

Medication/Treatment (Table 21.4)

Clinical Consideration

Noncompliance is prevalent, as is toxicity from mediations. Patients may experience exacerbation of symptoms.

TABLE 21.4	SCHIZOPHRENIA DRUGS AND THEIR ACTIONS
Medication	Action

Antipsychotics
    Olanzapine (Zyprexa)
    Risperidone (Risperdal)
    Quetiapine (Seroquel)
    Aripiprazole (Abilify)
    Ziprasidone (Geodon)
	Thought to block certain chemical receptors in the brain, which results in the relief of symptoms of psychotic disorders.

Antimanic Lithium (Lithobid, Lithate)	Alters sodium transport in nerve and muscle cells. Inhibits the activity of hyperactive neurologic circuits involved in producing mania

Patient Education

▶ Medication education

▶ Thought-stopping and focus techniques

▶ Alternative ways to express feelings in nonthreatening ways

▶ Teach distraction techniques and involve patient in current activities:

- Watching a movie on TV

- Journaling in the moment

▶ Encourage verbalization of feelings and let patient know that it is acceptable to talk about the hallucinations.

▶ Encourage patient to make note of personal triggers to avoid escalation.

> **Clinical Consideration**
>
> These medications can affect weight, blood sugar, triglycerides, and cardiac rhythm.

Question	Rationale
A patient with schizophrenia has been admitted to the acute care unit with an infected decubitus ulcer. The patient verbalizes that he's hearing voices telling him to leave the hospital immediately. He then begins to stare off, avoiding eye contact. Which response to this patient is the best? A. "I don't hear anything—I may have to check your temperature to make sure you're not septic." B. "You know those voices aren't real, right?" C. "I know what you're hearing is real to you but I don't know what it's saying—can you tell me more about what you're hearing?" D. "Let's check your blood sugar to make sure you're not hypoglycemic."	Answer: C When a known schizophrenic patient has hallucinations, the nurse should not play into the situation (e.g., nodding, and agreeing), but should also not deny that it is happening to the patient. The nurse must instead provide support and help the patient if he is having other feelings of anxiety or fear by exploring the contents of the hallucinations. Before checking temperature or blood sugar, assess for additional symptoms that would be associated with those two interventions before performing them. By putting off assessment of the current hallucinations, exacerbation of agitation may occur.

ALCOHOL WITHDRAWAL

Anatomy

▶ Alcohol decreases overall brain excitability.

▶ Stopping consumption suddenly causes hyperexcitability or delirium tremens (DTs).

▶ Patients can be completely unaware of behaviors during withdrawal.

▶ Hallucinations, both auditory and visual, can occur.

▶ Alcohol withdrawal can result in death.

Escalation Assessment

▶ When was the patient's last drink, and are they able to tell you?

▶ Use the Clinical Institute Withdrawal Assessment of Alcohol Scale (CIWA-Ar) (Table 21.5)

- This scale is meant to warn about increasing symptoms of withdrawal and of escalating behaviors.

- Focus on the "Anxiety" and "Agitation" portions.

TABLE 21.5	CLINICAL INSTITUTE WITHDRAWAL ASSESSMENT OF ALCOHOL SCALE (CIWA-AR)

Mild risk, CIWA-Ar <8; moderate risk, 9–15; severe risk, >15

Nausea/vomiting	0 No nausea/vomiting 1 Mild nausea with no vomiting 2 3 4 Intermittent nausea with dry heaves 5 6 7 Constant nausea, frequent dry heaves and vomiting
Tremors	0 No tremor 1 Tremor not visible but can be felt fingertip to fingertip 2 3 4 Moderate tremor with arms extended 5 6 7 Severe tremor even with arms extended
Diaphoresis	0 No sweat visible 1 Rarely perceptible sweating-palms moist 2 3 4 Beads of sweat obvious on forehead 5 6 7 Drenching sweats
Anxiety	0 Normal activity 1 Mildly anxious 2 3 4 Moderately anxious or guarded 5 6 7 Acute panic states—i.e., severe delirium/schizophrenic reactions
Agitation	0 Normal activity 1 2 3 4 Moderately fidgety and restless 5 6 7 Paces back/forth during interview or constantly thrashes about
Tactile disturbances	0 None 1 Very mild itching, pins/needles sensation/burning/numbness 2 Mild itching, pins, needles, burning, numbness 3 Moderate itching/pins/needles/burning/numbness 4 Moderately severe hallucinations 5 Severe hallucinations 6 Extremely severe hallucinations 7 Continuous hallucinations
Auditory disturbances	0 Not present 1 Very mild harshness or ability to frighten 2 Mild harshness or ability to frighten 3 Moderate harshness or ability to frighten 4 Moderate severe hallucinations 5 Severe hallucinations 6 Extremely severe hallucination 7 Continuous hallucinations

(continued)

TABLE 21.5	(Continued)
Visual disturbances	0 Not present 1 Very mild sensitivity 2 Mild 3 Moderate 4 Moderately severe 5 Severe 6 Very severe 7 Extremely severe
Headache, fullness in head	0 Not present 1 Very mild 2 Mild 3 Moderate 4 Moderately severe 5 Severe 6 Very Severe 7 Extremely severe
Orientation and clouding of sensorium	0 Oriented and can do serial additions 1 Cannot do serial additions or is uncertain about date 2 Disoriented about date by no more than two calendar days 3 Disoriented about date by more than two calendar days 4 Disoriented about place and/or person

(Naranjo et al., 1989)

- Elevated vital signs
- Auditory and visual hallucinations:
  - Grabbing at invisible objects
  - Increasing restlessness

Nursing Diagnosis

- Risk for injury related to:
  - Environmental conditions interacting with the individual's adaptive and protective means
- Risk for decreased cardiac output related to:
  - Inadequate blood pumped by heart to meet metabolic demands of the body
  - Direct effect of alcohol on heart muscle
  - Altered systemic vascular resistance
  - Electrical alterations in rate, rhythm, conduction
- Risk for ineffective breathing pattern related to:
  - Direct effect of alcohol withdrawal on respiratory center or sedatives given to reduce withdrawal symptoms
  - Tracheobronchial obstruction
  - Chronic respiratory problems and inflammatory process
  - Decreased energy or fatigue

Interventions

- Maintain calm environment, minimize noise, if possible.
- Establish nonjudgmental relationship.
- Reorient and obtain CIWA-Ar score immediately:
  - Treat as needed
- Determine anxiety needs.
- Assess even at night in order to medicate patient appropriately.
- Patient safety and careful assessment of patient's respiratory status, level of consciousness, and ability to swallow must be monitored. These patients may aspirate and often have to go to the intensive care unit.

Plan of Care

▶ Diligent assessment of the patient:
  - Determine stage or phase of withdrawal
▶ Communicate with all staff regarding patient's withdrawal symptoms
▶ Medicate throughout all shifts:
  - Consistent medication will help to prevent the occurrence of violent situations.
▶ Keep patient close to the nurse's station; equip with bed alarm.

Medication/Treatment (Table 21.6)

TABLE 21.6	ALCOHOL WITHDRAWAL DRUGS AND THEIR ACTIONS
Medication	Action

Benzodiazepines
  Alprazolam (Xanax)
  Clonazepam (Klonopin)
  Diazepam (Valium)
  Lorazepam (Ativan)
	Frequently used for short-term management of anxiety. Benzodiazepines are highly effective in promoting relaxation and reducing muscular tension and other physical symptoms of anxiety. Long-term use may require increased doses to achieve the same effect, which may lead to problems related to tolerance and dependence.

Vitamins
  Thiamine (vitamin B$_1$)
  Multivitamin/multimineral
	Replete nutritional deficiencies related to alcohol withdrawal to restore healthy body chemistry.

Patient Education

▶ Medication compliance:
  - Keep a list of medication and include amounts:
    - Bring that list to follow-up visits
▶ Activity and rest:
  - Plenty of sleep
  - Quiet environment
▶ Avoid alcohol:
  - Set goals for self
  - Healthy diet and noncaffeinated, nonalcoholic beverages
▶ Avoid caffeine
▶ Avoid stress:
  - Explore calming therapies such as journaling, music therapy, and talk therapy.

Question	Rationale
The patient is experiencing alcohol withdrawal and starts to exhibit diaphoresis, tremors, as well as "picking" at the air. The blood pressure is 187/90 mm Hg and the pulse 102 beats/min. Which medication would the nurse expect to administer in order to control these withdrawal symptoms? A. Benztropine (Cogentin) B. Lorazepam (Ativan) C. Haloperidol (Haldol) D. Ziprasidone (Geodon)	Answer: B The medication most likely to be administered to the patient who is experiencing these symptoms is a benzodiazepine, such as lorazepam (Ativan). These symptoms of hyperactivity are rebound effects when the sedation from alcohol begins to decrease.

OPIOID WITHDRAWAL

Anatomy

▶ Opioids affect multiple systems of the body, as they bind with all opioid receptor sites.

▶ Withdrawal occurs in all of these systems in various ways:

- Pain, stress, gastrointestinal system, temperature regulation, respiratory system, endocrine system, and mood

Escalation Assessment

▶ Violence is a possibility just before the patient begins withdrawal:

- Patient aware of what is coming within the first few hours of withdrawal; wants to prevent it
- May threaten staff
- Threaten to leave against medical advice (AMA) in order to obtain opioids to halt withdrawal symptoms

▶ Determine when patient last used opioids

▶ Use Clinical Opioid Withdrawal Scale (COWS) Assessment (Table 21.7)

- Assess level of withdrawal and need for medication.

TABLE 21.7	CLINICAL OPIATE WITHDRAWAL SCALE (COWS)	
Assessment	Scoring criteria	
Mild, 5–12; moderate, 13–24; moderately severe, 25–36; severe, >36		
Resting pulse rate: record beats per minute *Measured after patient is sitting or lying for one minute.*	Pulse rate, ≤80	0
	Pulse rate, 81–100	1
	Pulse rate, 101–120	2
	Pulse rate >120	4
Sweating: over past half hour not accounted for by room temperature or patient activity	No report of chills or flushing	0
	Subjective report of chills or flushing	1
	Flushed or observable moistness on face	2
	Beads of sweat on brow or face	3
	Sweat streaming off face	4
Restlessness observed during assessment	Able to sit still	0
	Reports difficulty sitting still, but is able to do so	1
	Frequent shifting or extraneous movements of legs/arms	3
	Unable to sit still for more than a few seconds	5
Pupil size	Pupils pinpoint or normal size for room light	0
	Pupils possibly larger than normal for room light	1
	Pupils moderately dilated	2
	Pupils so dilated that only the rim of the iris is visible	5
Bone or joint aches; if patient was having pain previously, only the additional component attributed to opiate withdrawal is scored	Not present	0
	Mild diffuse discomfort	1
	Patient reports severe diffuse aching of joints/muscles	2
	Patient is rubbing joints or muscles and is unable to sit still because of discomfort	4

(continued)

TABLE 21.7 (*Continued*)

Assessment	Scoring criteria	
Runny nose or tearing not accounted for by cold symptoms or allergies	Not present	0
	Nasal stuffiness or unusually moist eyes	1
	Nose running or tearing	2
	Nose constantly running or tears streaming down cheeks	4
Gastrointestinal upset: over past 1/2 hour	No symptoms	0
	Stomach cramps	1
	Nausea or loose stool	2
	Vomiting or diarrhea	3
	Multiple episodes of diarrhea or vomiting	5
Tremor observation of outstretched hands	No tremor	0
	Tremor can be felt, but not observed	1
	Slight tremor observable	2
	Gross tremor or muscle twitching	4
Yawning observation during assessment	No yawning	0
	Yawning once or twice during assessment	1
	Yawning three or more times during assessment	2
	Yawning several times per minute	4
Anxiety or irritability	None	0
	Patient reports increasing irritability or anxiousness	1
	Patient obviously irritable/anxious	2
	Gross tremor or muscle twitching	4
Gooseflesh skin	Skin is smooth	0
	Piloerection of skin can be felt or hairs standing up on arms	3
	Prominent piloerection	5

(*Wesson & Ling, 2003*)

Nursing Diagnosis

▶ Anxiety related to:
  - Cessation of opioid use and physiologic withdrawal
  - Situational crisis or being hospitalized
  - Threat of intense pain or discomfort
▶ Denial related to:
  - Situational crisis
  - Ineffective coping with substitution of opioid use
  - Cultural factors or personal value systems
▶ Ineffective individual coping related to:
  - Personal vulnerability

- Inadequate support systems
- Previous use of opioids in order to cope

Interventions

▶ Continuously evaluate the level of withdrawal.

▶ Establish a nonjudgmental relationship and ask about opioid abuse:
  - Once treated, the medical diagnoses can then be treated as well
  - Ask what works for them when they are going into withdrawal

▶ If they are trying to leave or becoming agitated, offer or obtain medications to help calm them

Plan of Care

▶ Begin assessment of phase of withdrawal at admission.

▶ Inform all staff; continue to assess as well as medicate throughout shifts

▶ Around-the-clock medication will help to prevent situations from escalating.

▶ Keep close to nurse's station, if possible; use bed alarm.

▶ Be aware of visitors:
  - Using in the hospital
  - Oversedation

Medication/Treatment (Table 21.8)

TABLE 21.8	OPIOID WITHDRAWAL DRUGS AND THEIR ACTIONS
Medication	**Action**
Methadone	Relieves withdrawal symptoms Assists with detox and reduces intensity of symptoms Can be used long term Can be titrated slowly over a long period of time
Buprenorphine (Subutex, Suboxone)	Shortens length of detox Can be used long term Prevents dependence and misuse
Clonidine	Reduces anxiety, agitation, muscle aches, sweating, runny nose, and cramping
Naltrexone (Vivitrol)	Helps prevent relapse Used with long-term treatment after detox

Patient Education

▶ Medication compliance:
  - Keep a list of medication and include amounts:
    - Detox medication education
▶ Activity and rest:
  - Get plenty of sleep
  - Maintain quiet environment
▶ Avoid opioids:
  - Set goals for self.
  - Avoid unhealthy relationships.
  - Notify care provider of opioid detox or current use.
▶ Avoid stress:
  - Explore calming therapies like journaling, music therapy, and talk therapy.

Clinical Consideration

Do not be fooled by "intractable vomiting"; often CT scans of the abdomen yield negative results. Subsequently, diarrhea may develop; collect stool to rule out *Clostridium difficile* (C-diff) infection—may be negative. These may be symptoms of opioid withdrawal.

Question	Rationale
A patient with a history of heroin abuse is admitted with intractable abdominal pain. Which of the following symptoms would the nurse assess if the patient is exhibiting late signs of opioid withdrawal? A. Yawning and irritability B. Diaphoresis and restlessness C. Gooseflesh skin and increasing temperature D. Severe vomiting and diarrhea	Answer: D Vomiting and diarrhea are usually late symptoms of opioid withdrawal, as are intense muscle/joint pain, nausea, and continuous abdominal cramps. Yawning, irritability, gooseflesh skin, diaphoresis and restlessness are present during almost all phases of opioid withdrawal and get more intense over time.

CASE STUDY

A 21-year-old woman is admitted to the acute care unit with intractable vomiting. After performing a skin assessment you notice self-inflicted, superficial cuts on both arms as well as both thighs. She confides to the nurse that her mother and father sexually abused her for years until she ran away at 15 years of age. Recently, her mother passed away and she was contacted by her father, and she saw him at the funeral. Thereafter, she has begun to cut herself in order to cope with the emotions from seeing her father as well as the recent death of mother. When exploring further about the cutting, she admits that she does this often despite the events that have occurred. She says that when she's depressed or angry, she self-mutilates, especially after ruminating over the abuse in her past. After speaking with her about this, she then tells you that you are the kindest nurse ever and that the other nurse, who was caring for her earlier, was "lazy and obviously not as smart as you." She then states that the only medications that work for her vomiting are Phenergan and Xanax, requesting that you obtain an order for these within the next hour before lunch.

1. **Based on the assessment findings what personality disorder diagnosis does the nurse expect?**

   ▶ This patient is demonstrating the traits of borderline personality disorder, which is characterized by poor interpersonal relationships, abusive past, poor self-image, and impulsive behavior. She copes with any severe conflicts (such as the death of her mother and seeing her father again) with self-mutilation or self-inflicted wounds. These patients can sometimes idealize one caregiver, verbalizing that to them, over the other in order to obtain desired outcomes, such as receiving the Phenergan or Xanax in this case.

2. **What other information would be important to know?**

   ▶ Current medications for her borderline personality disorder as well as compliance.

   ▶ Does the patient have a current support system?

   ▶ What are the patient's triggers that would lead to self-mutilation?

   ▶ Are there other episodes of agitated behavior while hospitalized?

3. **What education would you want to provide this patient?**

   ▶ Encourage counseling and therapy if not already in such care

   ▶ Medication compliance

   ▶ Healthy habits:

   · Sleep hygiene

   · Eating healthy foods

- Regular exercise
- Avoid drugs and alcohol
- Alternative coping skills:
  - Adult coloring books
  - Music therapy
  - Watching a movie

Discussion:

Patients with borderline personality disorder can be a challenge to care for, especially with medical comorbidities that must be addressed while hospitalized in order to prevent exacerbation and rehospitalization. It is important to establish trust and the willingness to communicate to fully address the patient's triggers. This will avoid agitating events from occurring and facilitate successful treatment of the other medical diagnoses.

Bibliography

Bhatt, N.V. (2017). Anxiety disorder. Accessed November 17, 2017, from https://emedicine.medscape.com/article/286227-overview#a3.

Davis-Evans, C. (2013). Special needs populations: alleviating anxiety and preventing panic attacks in the surgical patient. *AORN Journal* 97, 354–364. doi: 10.1016/j.aorn.2012.12.012

Fishkind, A. (2002). Calming agitation with words, not drugs: 10 commandments for safety. Accessed July 30, 2018 from https://www.mdedge.com/sites/default/files/Document/September-2017/0104_Fishkind.pdf

Friedel, R.O. (2012). Borderline personality disorder demystified. Accessed July 3, 2018, from http://www.bpddemystified.com/what-is-bpd/causes/.

Lee, A.M., Galynker, I.I., Kopeykina, I., Kim, H., and Khatun, T. (2014). Violence in bipolar disorder. Accessed July 3, 2018, from http://www.psychiatrictimes.com/bipolar-disorder/violence-bipolar-disorder/page/0/1.

Marsh, A.A., Adams, B.R., Jr., and Kleck, R.E. (2005). Why do fear and anger look the way they do? Form and social function of facial expressions. *Personality and Social Psychology Bulletin* 31, 73–86.

McLaren, K.D., and Marangell, L.B. (2004). Special considerations in the treatment of patients with bipolar disorder and medical co-morbidities. *Annals of General Psychiatry* 3, 7.

Nadler-Moodie, Marlene. (2010). Psychiatric emergencies in med-surg patients: are you prepared? Accessed July 1, 2016, from https://americannursetoday.com/psychiatric-emergencies-in-med-surg-patients-are-you-prepared/

Naranjo, C.A., Sellers, E.M., Schneiderman, J., Sullivan, J.T., Sykora, K. (1989). Assessment of alcohol withdrawal: the revised clinical institute withdrawal assessment for alcohol scale (CIWA-Ar). *British Journal of Addiction* 84, 1353–1357. Accessed July 30, 2018 from https://s3.amazonaws.com/academia.edu.documents/41350134/Assessment_of_alcohol_withdrawal_The_rev20160120-32134-6118vt.pdf?AWSAccessKeyId=AKIAIWOWYYGZ2Y53UL3A&Expires=1532956046&Signature=NxeB1hSVD%2FU%2BKu5TRbnX1Kmyn1k%3D&response-content-disposition=inline%3B%20filename%3DAssessment_of_Alcohol_Withdrawal_the_rev.pdf

Roy-Byrne, P., Veitengruber, J.P., Bystritsky, A., et. al. (2009). Brief intervention for anxiety in primary care patients. *Journal of the American Board of Family Medicine* 22, 175–186.

The Mayo Clinic Staff. (2017). Bipolar disorder. Accessed November 17, 2017, from https://www.mayoclinic.org/diseases-conditions/bipolar-disorder/diagnosis-treatment/drc-20355961.

The Mayo Clinic Staff. (2017). Borderline personality disorder. Accessed July 30, 2018 from https://www.mayoclinic.org/diseases-conditions/borderline-personality-disorder/diagnosis-treatment/drc-20370242

Wesson, D.R., and Ling, W. (2003). The Clinical Opiate Withdrawal Scale (COWS). *Journal of Psychoactive Drugs* 35, 253–259.

22

Practice Exam

Jane Trainor, MS, RN
Laura Brennan, MS, RN
Barbara Bostelmann, MS, RN

QUESTIONS

1. The nurse is reviewing the electrocardiogram (ECG) rhythm strip, from 2 years ago, of a patient with a history of a myocardial infarction. The nurse notes that the PR interval is 0.16 second. The nurse should:
   A. Contact the health care provider (HCP) immediately
   B. Administer the as-needed (PRN) antiarrhythmic medication
   C. Document the finding
   D. Prepare the patient for a temporary pacemaker

2. A patient has been brought to the emergency room and diagnosed with hyperosmolar hyperglycemic nonketotic syndrome (HHNS) coma. Which one of the following assessment findings would the nurse expect the patient to exhibit?
   A. Rapid and deep respirations
   B. A fruity, sweet breath odor
   C. Dry mucous membranes
   D. Bradycardia

3. To assess a patient's swallowing ability following a stroke diagnosis, the nurse should **first** ask the patient to do which of the following?
   A. Swallow some water.
   B. Produce an audible cough.
   C. Suck on a piece of hard candy.
   D. Swallow a teaspoon of applesauce.

4. A patient with tuberculosis is to begin Rifater (combination of isoniazid [INH], rifampin [RIF], and pyrazinamide [PZA]), and streptomycin therapy). The patient says, "I've never had to take so many different medications for an infection before." The nurse should explain:
   A. "This type of organism is difficult to destroy."
   B. "Streptomycin prevents side effects of Rifater."
   C. "You will need multiple medications for a couple of weeks."
   D. "Aggressive therapy is needed when the infection is well advanced."

5. The nurse caring for a patient following a bowel resection notes that the patient is restless. Further assessment reveals a significant decrease in blood pressure and an increase in the pulse since the last vital sign assessment. Which action should the nurse take **next**?
   A. Recheck the vital signs in an hour.
   B. Place the patient in a reverse Trendelenburg position.

C. Slow the rate of the intravenous (IV) fluid infusing.

D. Check the patient's oxygen saturation level.

6. A patient has undergone a transsphenoidal hypophysectomy for removal of a pituitary gland tumor. Which one of the following is an appropriate postoperative nursing intervention?

A. Keeping the head of bed (HOB) elevated to 30 degrees at all times.

B. Encouraging vigorous coughing and deep breathing.

C. Instructing the patient to brush teeth every 4 to 6 hours.

D. Avoiding checking pupillary response.

7. A 76-year-old patient with chronic obstructive pulmonary disease (COPD) asks the nurse about the benefit of palliative care. The nurse tells the patient that the goal of palliative care is to:

A. Assess coping with the disease.

B. Provide all needed care.

C. Improve quality of life.

D. Treat the underlying disease.

8. When mentoring a new nurse, which of the following would be a responsibility of the mentor:

A. Monitoring attendance

B. Offering constructive feedback

C. Disciplining for frequent tardiness

D. Determining the new nurse's pay scale

9. An older adult recently diagnosed with an infection displays a **sudden onset** of confusion. The patient most likely is experiencing:

A. Dementia

B. Social isolation

C. Delirium

D. Functional decline

10. During a mass disaster drill simulating a terrorist attack, the nurse must triage many severely ill individuals. The patient who should receive care **first** is:

A. Cyanotic and not breathing

B. Gasping for breath and semiconscious

C. Apneic and has an apical rate of 50

D. Having a seizure and is incontinent of urine and stool

11. When a patient who had an above-the-knee amputation (AKA) has symptoms of phantom limb sensations, the nursing staff should:

A. Medicate the patient.

B. Explain that the pain will diminish over time.

C. Remind the patient that the limb is no longer there.

D. Offer diversional activities.

12. The nurse is providing care to a Latino patient who is hospitalized with an exacerbation of COPD. Numerous family members are present most of the time, and many of the family members are very emotional. What is the most appropriate nursing action for this patient?

A. Restricting the number of family members visiting at one time

B. Informing the family that emotional outbursts are to be avoided

C. Making the necessary arrangements so family members can visit

D. Moving the patient to a room at the end of the hallway

13. The nurse is caring for a patient in whom diabetes insipidus (DI) may be developing. The nurse would assess for which one of the following?
    A. Decreased thirst
    B. Decreased insulin levels
    C. Increased blood glucose
    D. Increased urinary output

14. All of the following should be included in the discharge teaching for a patient with urinary calculi (kidney stones) in whom a temporary stent was placed **except**:
    A. Importance of increasing fluid intake
    B. Avoidance of foods that may cause stone formation
    C. Symptoms of a urinary tract infection (UTI)
    D. Urinary catheter care until the stent is removed

15. Which one of the following instructions should be included in the teaching plan for a patient with viral hepatitis?
    A. Consume three large meals daily.
    B. The diet should be low in protein.
    C. Activity should be limited to prevent fatigue.
    D. Alcohol intake should be limited to 2 oz (60 ml) per day.

16. A patient has recently had a decrease in fluid intake and the eGFR has fallen below 60 mL/min. The nurse should perform situation, background, assessment, and recommendation (SBAR) and request that the HCP change which of the following medications?
    A. Glimepiride (Amaryl)
    B. Acarbose (Precose)
    C. Metformin (Glucophage)
    D. Stagliptin (Januvia)

17. Postoperative care for the patient who has undergone an abdominal hysterectomy includes:
    A. Ambulating the day of surgery
    B. Maintaining nothing-by-mouth (NPO) status for 24 hours
    C. Assessing the nasogastric (NG) tube output
    D. Changing the perineal pad every shift due to expected heavy bleeding

18. A patient diagnosed with Addison's disease has presented to the emergency department in Addisonian crisis. Which one of the following medications should be administered **immediately** for this life-threatening situation?
    A. Regular insulin (Humulin R)
    B. Ketoconazole (Nizoral)
    C. Hydrocortisone (Solu Cortef)
    D. Metoprolol (Lopressor)

19. The nurse is assessing an African American patient who was diagnosed with sickle cell crisis. Which assessment finding is **most** pertinent when assessing for cyanosis in patients with dark skin?
    A. Metatarsals
    B. Sclera
    C. Capillary refill time
    D. Oral mucosa

20. A patient who has undergone a colonoscopy is recovering in the postprocedure area. Which one of the following signs would be considered an emergency and require an immediate response?
    A. Blood pressure 90/40 mm Hg, heart rate 130 beats/min
    B. Hyperactive bowel sounds
    C. Watery rectal discharge
    D. Occasional abdominal cramping

21. On admitting a patient, the nurse asks about advance directives. The patient requests the advance directives form and after filling it out, requests the nurse to serve as a witness on the form. The appropriate action by the nurse would be:
    A. Signing the form
    B. Asking the unlicensed assistive personnel (UAP) to sign the form
    C. Requesting the hospital chaplain to sign the form
    D. Explaining that no hospital employee can sign the form

22. A 50-year-old patient with type II diabetes mellitus is now on both an oral diabetes medication and insulin. The patient is having difficulty with the subcutaneous injections. Which one of the following is an appropriate patient advocacy intervention?
    A. Telling the patient, "With practice, it will work out fine."
    B. Notifying the health department about the patient's situation.
    C. Asking the HCP to increase the oral diabetic medication rather than start insulin.
    D. Determining whether the patient would be willing to have a family member help.

23. The nurse is supervising an UAP who is performing mouth care on an unconscious patient. The nurse should **intervene** if the nurse noted the UAP performing which of the following actions?
    A. Turning the head to one side
    B. Placing the bed in a flat position
    C. Using an oral suction catheter
    D. Placing an emesis basin under the patient's mouth

24. The charge nurse is supervising a new graduate nurse who is performing discharge teaching on iron deficiency anemia for a female Amish patient. The charge nurse determines that the new nurse is displaying culturally sensitive behaviors in her approach to the family when she observes which of the following behaviors?
    A. The nurse is speaking only to the husband.
    B. The nurse is using complex medical terminology.
    C. The nurse is avoiding using scientific or medical jargon.
    D. The nurse is standing close to the patient and speaking loudly.

25. A patient on long-term corticosteroids is receiving medication education from the nurse. In order to minimize the occurrence of one of the adverse effects of this medication, the nurse teaches the patient to:
    A. Know the signs of a decreased blood sugar
    B. Maintain calcium intake of at least 1500 mg/day
    C. If nausea occurs stop the medication for a few days
    D. Take the medication on an empty stomach

26. The nurse is caring for a patient who had a tracheostomy tube inserted 24 hours ago. The tube becomes dislodged. What is the **initial** nursing action?
    A. Calling the HCP to reinsert the tube
    B. Ventilating the patient using a manual resuscitation bag and face mask
    C. Covering the tracheostomy site with a sterile dressing to prevent infection
    D. Calling the respiratory therapy department to reinsert the tracheostomy tube

27. Which is the priority assessment for a patient with a cervical spinal cord injury?
    A. Respiratory status
    B. Skin breakdown
    C. Emotional status
    D. Bowel sounds

28. One of the greatest challenges for the nurse caring for older adults is ensuring safe medication use. One way to reduce the risks associated with medication usage is to:
    A. Periodically review the patient's list of medications.
    B. Inform the patient that polypharmacy is to be avoided at all costs.
    C. Be aware that medication is absorbed the same way regardless of patient age.
    D. Focus only on prescribed medications.

29. Which of the following patients should the nurse assess **first**? A patient with:
    A. Multiple sclerosis (MS) who is due for a dose of prednisone
    B. Amyotrophic lateral sclerosis (ALS) who needs help with eating
    C. Descending Guillain–Barré syndrome (GBS) who was just admitted
    D. Huntington disease (HD) who is being discharged to a long-term facility

30. A patient being treated for hypertension reports having a persistent hacking cough. What class of antihypertensive should the nurse identify as a possible cause of this response when reviewing a list of this patient's medications?
    A. Angiotensin-converting enzyme (ACE) inhibitors
    B. Thiazide diuretics
    C. Calcium-channel blockers
    D. Angiotensin-receptor blockers

31. A patient has been started on a thyroid medication, and the nurse is educating the patient to note the following adverse effects: a fast heart beat or heart palpitations, difficulty sleeping, tremors, and weight loss. The nurse is teaching the patient about which of the following medications?
    A. Propylthiouracil (PTU)
    B. Levothyroxine (Synthroid)
    C. Methimazole (Tapazole)
    D. Propranolol (Inderal)

32. All of the following are appropriate nursing assessments or interventions when caring for a patient in alcohol withdrawal **except:**
    A. Monitoring vital signs
    B. Maintaining a safe environment
    C. Providing stimulation
    D. Addressing hallucinations

33. A patient has presented to the emergency department. The HCP orders 5 units of regular insulin IV and 50% dextrose IV. The patient is not diabetic. The nurse is aware that this intervention is to treat a
    A. Glucose that is 350 mg/dL
    B. Potassium of 7.8 mEq/L
    C. Respiratory acidosis
    D. DKA

34. Pertinent background information to be included when using SBAR to communicate patient information would include:
    A. Family history
    B. Insurance information

    C. Allergies

    D. Vaccinations received

35. After educating a patient who has undergone pacemaker insertion, which statement indicates further teaching is necessary?

    A. "I should place my cell phone on the side opposite to the generator."

    B. "I need to wear a medical alert device at all times indicating that I have a pacemaker."

    C. "I need to wear loose clothing over the area of my pacemaker."

    D. "When I am in the airport it is okay for me to walk through the scanner."

36. What is the **most** important action for the nurse to implement when irrigating the bladder of a patient with an indwelling urinary catheter?

    A. Using sterile equipment

    B. Instilling antibiotic solution

    C. Warming the solution to body temperature

    D. Aspirating immediately after instillation

37. A patient has taken an overdose of acetaminophen. Which of the following lab results may occur from this overdose?

    A. Increased hemoglobin

    B. Increased potassium

    C. Elevated creatinine

    D. Elevated bilirubin

38. A nurse is caring for a patient who has undergone the removal of a parathyroid tumor. The nurse suspects that the patient is experiencing postsurgical hypocalcemia if which of the following occurs:?

    A. Facial muscle contraction when the facial nerve is tapped

    B. Heart rate greater than 100 beats/min

    C. Bounding peripheral pulses

    D. Shallow, slow breathing

39. A patient who is scheduled to undergo a modified radical mastectomy decides to have family members donate blood in the event it is needed. The patient has type A-negative blood. Blood can be used from relatives whose blood is:

    A. O-positive

    B. AB-positive

    C. A- or O-negative

    D. A- or AB-negative

40. The nurse would anticipate that a temporary pacemaker would be considered for which type of dysrhythmia?

    A. Heart block

    B. Ventricular tachycardia

    C. Ventricular fibrillation

    D. Atrial fibrillation

41. Decision making in a decentralized leadership hierarchy would occur:

    A. At the senior level.

    B. At the point of care.

    C. With the board of directors.

    D. Within the nursing department only.

42. Which of the following is the **priority** nursing diagnosis for a patient with anxiety?
    A. Anxiety related to unfamiliar environment, understanding of diagnosis, diagnostic tests, and treatments
    B. Powerlessness related to unfamiliar environment and loss of control of one's own body
    C. Defensive coping related to overwhelming feelings of dread
    D. Ineffective breathing pattern related to panic and worrisome or irrational thoughts

43. A nurse is caring for a postsurgical patient. The nurse is aware that which of the following procedures leads to the highest risk of dehydration?
    A. Ileostomy
    B. Colostomy
    C. Nephrostomy
    D. Cholecystectomy

44. The nurse determines a patient is in a coma when the Glasgow Coma Scale score is:
    A. 6
    B. 9
    C. 12
    D. 15

45. The nurse has assessed an enlarged thyroid and exophthalmos on a 30 year-old woman. Laboratory testing indicates Graves' disease. Which one of the following would be an important nursing intervention?
    A. Teaching the patient to restrict calories
    B. Encouraging the patient not to nap during the day
    C. Minimizing the use of pain medications
    D. Providing artificial tears to prevent corneal ulceration

46. The nurse assesses a 73-year-old patient with peripheral vascular disease characterized by arterial insufficiency. The nurse will expect to find:
    A. Normal pedal and tibial pulses.
    B. Brownish discoloration around the ankles.
    C. Deep circular necrotic ulcers on the toes.
    D. Moderate to severe edema of the lower extremities.

47. A patient who underwent transurethral resection of the prostate (TURP) returns from the postanesthesia care unit (PACU) and accidentally pulls out the urethral catheter. What should the nurse do **first**?
    A. Reinsert a new catheter.
    B. Notify the HCP.
    C. Assess the patient's ability to void.
    D. Apply pressure to the penis.

48. After 2 weeks of IV antibiotic therapy, a patient with acute osteomyelitis of the tibia is prepared for discharge from the hospital. The nurse determines that additional instruction is needed when the patient makes which statement?
    A. "I will need to continue antibiotic therapy for 4 to 6 weeks."
    B. "I shouldn't bear weight on my affected leg until healing is complete."
    C. "I can use a heating pad on my lower leg for comfort and to promote healing."
    D. "I should notify the HCP if the pain in my leg becomes worse."

49. The nurse is reviewing discharge teaching with an African American patient who is starting lisinopril (Prinivil) therapy. The nurse should instruct the patient to notify the HCP if which of the following occurs?
    A. Dizziness when first standing up
    B. Trouble sleeping
    C. Constipation
    D. Swelling of lips

50. A patient with kidney failure states "I feel tingling around my lips." The nurse should assess for which complication?
    A. Metabolic alkalosis
    B. Hypocalcemia
    C. Hypernatremia
    D. Hypokalemia

51. An 82-year-old patient is diagnosed with pneumonia. Which white-cell (leukocyte) count level is indicative of a viral infection?
    A. 25,000 per microliter
    B. 4000 per microliter
    C. 8200 per microliter
    D. 40,000 per microliter

52. A patient is being prepared for removal of a pheochromocytoma from one of the adrenal glands. The nurse anticipates that the patient will be treated preoperatively for 7 to 10 days with which of the following medications?
    A. Broad-spectrum antibiotics
    B. Angiotensin-receptor blockers
    C. Alpha-adrenergic receptor blockers
    D. Beta-adrenergic receptor agonists

53. A patient has undergone pericardiocentesis to treat cardiac tamponade. Which sign/symptom would indicate a possible recurrence of the tamponade?
    A. Facial flushing
    B. Decreasing pulse
    C. Paradoxical pulse
    D. Rising blood pressure

54. The nurse should teach the patient with a *Chlamydia* infection to abstain from sexual activity for:
    A. 24 hours after starting antibiotics
    B. 7 days after antibiotics have been completed
    C. Until the symptoms have cleared
    D. At least 6 months after diagnosis

55. Risk factors for developing type 2 diabetes include all of the following **except:**
    A. Obesity
    B. Smoking
    C. Family history
    D. Race

56. Which instruction should the nurse include in the teaching plan for a patient taking iron supplements to correct iron deficiency anemia?
    A. Eat a low-fiber diet.
    B. Limit the intake of fluids.

    C. Limit the intake of meat, fish, and poultry.

    D. Avoid taking the iron supplements with milk or antacids.

57. An elderly patient who was admitted to the acute care unit with pneumonia has the following arterial blood gas (ABG) values: pH 7.32, PCO_2 53 mm Hg, and HCO_3 25 mEq. Which action should be taken by the nurse?

    A. Obtain an order and administer a diuretic

    B. Have the patient breathe into a rebreather bag at a slow rate

    C. Ask the patient to cough productively and take deep breaths

    D. Obtain an order for the administration of sodium bicarbonate

58. The nurse is preparing written discharge materials for a COPD patient. What readability level would be most appropriate in order to ensure that the patient understands the instructions?

    A. 12th-grade

    B. 9th-grade

    C. 6th-grade

    D. 3rd-grade

59. It is suspected that a patient is having problems with the pituitary gland. Which one of the following tests would be ordered for this patient?

    A. Ionized calcium

    B. Growth hormone

    C. Aldosterone

    D. Glycosylated hemoglobin

60. Quinapril hydrochloride (Accupril) is prescribed as an adjunctive therapy in the treatment of heart failure. After administering the first dose, the nurse should specifically monitor which parameter as the priority?

    A. Respirations

    B. Urine output

    C. Lung sounds

    D. Blood pressure

61. The nurse is assessing a patient with a closed head injury. Which of the following is an **early sign** of increased intracranial pressure (ICP)?

    A. Confusion

    B. Change in pupil reaction

    C. Seizures

    D. Coma

62. After being admitted with a diagnosis of acute diverticulitis, a patient is reporting symptoms of severe abdominal pain. The nurse assesses the abdomen and finds it to be rigid. The patient's temperature is 103°F. Which one of the following interventions should the nurse implement?

    A. Administer the antipyretic that was ordered on admission

    B. Notify the HCP

    C. Reassess vital signs in 1 hour

    D. Assess the cardiac system

63. What is the **priority** nursing intervention during a tonic–clonic seizure?

    A. Establishing a patent airway

    B. Protecting the patient from injury

    C. Restraining the patient

    D. Gaining IV access

64. When talking with a patient who is in crisis, the crisis intervention nurse should **first:**
    A. Assist the patient in deciding what will be done and how it will be done.
    B. Identify problems for the patient, putting them in the proper perspective.
    C. Explain that your institution has helped many patients with the same problem.
    D. Explore religious and cultural beliefs so the interventions support the patient's values.

65. The nurse suspects that acute respiratory distress syndrome (ARDS) is developing in a patient admitted after a near-drowning. Which information supports the nurse's suspicion?
    A. The patient has intercostal retractions and is using accessory muscles.
    B. The patient's ABGs are within normal limits.
    C. The patient's lung sounds have crackles and rhonchi.
    D. The patient appears anxious, has dyspnea, and is tachypneic.

66. The nurse is assessing the thyroid gland. Part of the appropriate technique is to:
    A. Percuss the thyroid to define the size of the gland.
    B. Darken the room to avoid glare on the neck.
    C. Have the patient turn the head to the left.
    D. Have the patient swallow during inspection and palpation.

67. The nurse is reviewing the preprocedure care for a patient scheduled to undergo echocardiography after a myocardial infarction. The nurse determines that the student nurse understands the preprocedure instructions if the student nurse makes which statement?
    A. "The patient needs to sign an informed consent form."
    B. "The procedure is painless and takes 30 to 60 minutes to complete."
    C. "The patient cannot eat or drink anything for 4 hours before the procedure."
    D. "An allergy to iodine or shellfish is a contraindication to having the procedure."

68. The nurse is caring for a patient with a diagnosis of heart failure and a secondary diagnosis of depression. When the nurse walks into the patient's room, the nurse finds the patient crying. What is the nurse's most therapeutic response?
    A. "Does crying help?"
    B. "I know you are upset."
    C. "Tell me what you are feeling now."
    D. "Do you want to tell me why you are crying?"

69. A nurse includes which of the following statements when counseling a patient who has gonorrhea?
    A. It is easily cured.
    B. It occurs very rarely.
    C. It can produce sterility.
    D. It is a viral infection.

70. The primary purpose of hospice care is:
    A. Allowing a patient to die at home
    B. Providing all care for the dying patient
    C. Coordinating care for the dying patient and family
    D. Providing comfort and support for the dying patient and family

71. The nurse is preparing to discharge an 81-year-old patient from the hospital. The nurse recognizes that the **majority** of older adults:
    A. Require institutional care.
    B. Are unable to afford any medical treatment.

C. Are capable of taking charge of their own lives.

D. Have no social or family support.

72. A nurse is mentoring a new graduate nurse who is to administer phenytoin (Dilantin) suspension to a patient receiving a continuous enteral feeding. The mentoring nurse should intervene if the new graduate nurse:

A. Flushes the tube with water before and after the phenytoin (Dilantin) administration.

B. Assesses for gastric residual before administering the phenytoin (Dilantin).

C. Raises the head of the bed to 45 degrees before administering the phenytoin (Dilantin).

D. Restarts the enteral feeding right after administering the phenytoin (Dilantin).

73. The nurse finds a patient with a spinal cord injury at T3 to be diaphoretic and flushed and with a blood pressure of 210/100 mm Hg. What should the nurse do **first**?

A. Assess for a full bladder.

B. Administer a beta-blocker.

C. Place the patient in a supine position.

D. Monitor vital signs.

74. The nurse is caring for a patient who underwent a laparoscopic cholecystectomy yesterday. Which one of the following tasks can the nurse delegate to the UAP?

A. Checking the surgical site

B. Taking the patient's vital signs

C. Auscultating the patient's abdomen for bowel sounds

D. Increasing oxygen if oxygen saturation is below 92%.

75. The patient has reported an increase in blood glucose in the morning for the past week, waking up with night sweats, and morning headaches. The nurse teaches the patient to:

A. Assess blood glucose between 2 and 4 a.m.

B. Increase the evening insulin.

C. Increase the evening snack.

D. For a week, check for ketones in the urine daily.

76. A patient in renal failure has an arteriovenous fistula (AV) and has started hemodialysis three times a week. The nurse is doing discharge teaching. Which statement indicates that **further teaching** is necessary?

A. "I will feel the AV fistula each day for a vibration."

B. "It is important that I attend my dialysis treatments as prescribed."

C. "I will check the pulse at my wrist in both arms every day."

D. "I will take my blood pressure on the arm with the fistula daily."

77. The nurse administers a fatal dose of morphine sulfate to a patient. During the subsequent investigation of the error, it is determined that the nurse did not check the patient's respiratory rate before administering the medication. Failure to adequately assess the patient is addressed under which function of the nurse practice act?

A. Defining the specific educational requirements for licensure in the state.

B. Describing the scope of practice of licensed and unlicensed care providers.

C. Identifying the process for disciplinary action if standards of care are not met.

D. Recommending specific terms of incarceration for nurses who violate the law.

78. A patient with moderate Alzheimer's disease (AD) has a nursing diagnosis of impaired memory related to the effects of dementia. What is an appropriate nursing intervention for this patient?

A. Putting a clock in the room

B. Consistently following a daily schedule

C. Engaging the patient in stimulating conversations

D. Monitoring the patient's activities

79. A patient who speaks only Mandarin is admitted with a fractured hip. Which pain rating scale would be best for the nurse to use to assess this patient's pain?

A. Verbal rating scale (VRS)

B. Visual analog scale (VAS)

C. Wong–Baker faces scale

D. 1 to10 rating scale

80. A patient with rheumatoid arthritis tells the nurse that although the physician has prescribed enteric-coated aspirin (Ecotrin), the patient has changed to acetaminophen (Tylenol). The nurse includes which of the following to educate the patient on the intended action of the Ecotrin for a patient with rheumatoid arthritis. The aspirin is given:

A. For its antiinflammatory action.

B. To decrease platelet aggregation.

C. For antipyretic action.

D. To assist with vitamin K deficiency.

81. Which finding should the nurse **most likely** expect to note for a patient with **new-onset** glomerulonephritis?

A. Hypotension

B. Smoky urine

C. Low serum potassium

D. Decreased protein in the urine

82. A patient with cancer no longer wants to continue with chemotherapy. The nurse should **first:**

A. Explain what may happen if chemotherapy is stopped.

B. Have the patient's family convince the patient to continue chemotherapy.

C. Have a person from a cancer support group come to speak with the patient.

D. Document the patient's wishes.

83. Which of the following is the **priority** assessment for a patient in alcohol withdrawal?

A. Fall risk

B. Nutrition

C. Weight

D. Aspiration risk

84. A patient is newly admitted to the medical-surgical unit. Appropriate delegation to the UAP would be:

A. Taking the initial vital signs

B. Assessing skin for breakdown

C. Obtaining a blood glucose

D. Evaluating the effectiveness of pain medication

85. A patient had a total knee replacement several days ago and has been receiving warfarin sodium (Coumadin) therapy. The nurse assesses the patient's international normalized ratio (INR) prior to administering the daily dose and notes that the INR is 2.7. The nurse will:

    A. Administer the prescribed dose of warfarin sodium (Coumadin).

    B. Assess the partial thromboplastin time (PTT) prior to administering the dose.

    C. Communicate with the provider utilizing the SBAR format and request vitamin K.

    D. Maintain the patient on bed rest until the INR value decreases.

86. The nurse should suspect the onset of peritonitis in a patient with peritoneal dialysis if which of the following is observed?

    A. Cloudy dialysate output

    B. Mild abdominal discomfort

    C. Oral temperature of 99.0°F

    D. Hematuria

87. Which of the following lab values should the nurse teach a patient with cancer of the prostate to monitor to evaluate the treatment for the disease?

    A. Blood urea nitrogen (BUN)

    B. Serum creatinine

    C. B-type natriuretic peptide (BNP)

    D. Prostate-specific antigen (PSA)

88. PICO is used to:

    A. Develop a plan of care for a patient

    B. Benchmark best practice

    C. Identify standards of care

    D. Formulate a clinical question

89. All of the following immunizations are recommended for the elderly population **except:**

    A. Meningitis

    B. Influenza

    C. Shingles

    D. Pneumococcal

90. Important teaching for the patient scheduled to undergo a radiofrequency catheter ablation procedure should include:

    A. The procedure will destroy areas of the conduction system that are causing rapid heart rhythms.

    B. The procedure has a very high complication rate.

    C. The patient will be able to go home within 3 hours after the procedure.

    D. A catheter will be placed in both femoral arteries.

91. The nurse is providing education for a group of nurses about hepatitis. Which one of the following statements will the nurse correctly include in the presentation?

    A. Hepatitis B virus (HBV) carriers continue to be infectious for life.

    B. Detection of HBV occurs 4 to 6 months after exposure.

    C. Patients should restrict protein and carbohydrates in the diet.

    D. Patients should restrict donating blood to once a year.

92. A nurse administers albuterol to a patient with asthma. For which common side effect should the nurse monitor?
    A. Flushing
    B. Dyspnea
    C. Tachycardia
    D. Hypotension

93. The nurse is monitoring a patient who is receiving a blood transfusion when the patient reports diaphoresis, warmth, and a backache. Which action should the nurse take **first**?
    A. Removing the IV catheter
    B. Documenting the occurrence
    C. Stopping the blood transfusion
    D. Hanging 0.9% sodium chloride solution

94. A patient has been diagnosed with peptic ulcer disease. The nurse will teach the patient to avoid which one of the following over-the-counter medications?
    A. Acetaminophen (Tylenol)
    B. Ibuprofen (Advil)
    C. Famotidine (Pepcid)
    D. Magnesium hydroxide/aluminum hydroxide (Maalox)

95. A patient has been admitted for a possible bowel obstruction. The patient reports pain, nausea, and feeling "bloated." The HCP orders hydrocodone/acetaminophen (Norco) 2.5mg/325mg by mouth for pain every 4 hours. Which one of the following actions should the nurse take?
    A. Asking the HCP to change the route to rectal.
    B. Giving the medication with sips of water or orange juice.
    C. Calling the HCP to suggest that the medication be changed to a different drug class.
    D. Withholding the medication until the patient no longer has nausea.

96. An 80-year-old patient, who is in frail health, is being treated for numerous health conditions, including type 1 diabetes. The HCP notes that the A1c is 7.8%. The nurse would:
    A. Remind the HCP that the insulin dose needs to be increased since the A1c is >7%.
    B. Inform the patient that the A1c is in the recommend range.
    C. Change the patient's diet to help lower the A1c.
    D. Start the patient on an oral diabetes medication.

97. A patient with inflammatory bowel disease has been started on sulfasalazine (Azulfidine). The nurse will instruct the patient regarding which of the following related to an **adverse reaction** of this medication?
    A. Use precautions when exposed to sunlight.
    B. Take medication in the evening on an empty stomach.
    C. If the urine turns blue, this is a normal reaction to the drug.
    D. If the patient is having difficulty swallowing tablets, crush and put in applesauce.

98. A patient with esophageal varices has undergone an esophagogastroduodenoscopy (EGD) and is found to have some bleeding of the varices. The nurse expects an order for which one of the following medications that will help control the bleeding?
    A. Captopril (Capoten)
    B. Vasopressin (Pitressin)

C. Interferon (Pegintron)

D. Methylprednisolone (Solu-Medrol)

99. A nurse is educating a woman who has recurrent urinary-tract infections (UTIs). Which information should be included to explain why women are more susceptible to UTIs than men?

A. Inadequate fluid intake

B. Higher body-fat content

C. Monthly menses

D. Length of the urethra

100. A 52-year-old male who is 6 hours postoperative is exhibiting signs of a pulmonary embolism. Which test/procedure provides the best diagnostic information?

A. Arterial blood gases

B. Spiral computed tomography (CT)

C. Chest x-ray

D. Angiography

101. A patient diagnosed with gastroesophageal reflux disease (GERD) is being prepared for discharge after undergoing EGD. Which one of the following statements indicates to the nurse that the patient **understands** the discharge instructions?

A. "I feel good enough to drive myself to the store after I leave here."

B. "Now I don't have to wait to lie down after I eat like I used to."

C. "I should avoid coffee and orange juice until I heal."

D. "I should expect to have a fever today and tomorrow."

102. A 24-year-old African American patient who has been living with sickle cell disease (SCD) since birth is admitted with pulmonary hypertension. The patient states, "I am so tired of being different than my friends." The best response that the nurse can give the patient is:

A. "Tell me what concerns you have."

B. "Let me turn on the TV so that you have something else to focus on."

C. "Would you like something for pain?"

D. "You are still very young, you will think differently when you get older."

103. A patient has received 10 units of regular insulin at 0630. At 1000, the UAP tells the RN that the patient is reporting feeling dizzy and has a headache. Which one of the following interventions should the nurse do **first**?

A. Instruct the UAP to obtain a blood glucose level

B. Ask the UAP to give the patient 8 ounces of orange juice

C. Assess the patient for hypoglycemia

D. Prepare to give 50% dextrose intravenously

104. When caring for a patient with a new diagnosis of syphilis, the nurse implements all of the following **except:**

A. Reporting the disease to the health department

B. Assuring the patient that confidentiality will be maintained

C. Placing the patient on contact precautions

D. Insisting that the patient report all sexual contacts

105. A patient with an acute exacerbation of systemic lupus erythematosus (SLE) has been prescribed prednisone (Deltasone). The nurse should **question** which order?

A. Assessing blood glucose daily

B. Discontinuing prednisone at discharge

C. Administering ibuprofen (Advil) 800 mg by mouth daily

D. Checking electrolyte panel daily

106. Which values should the nurse assess to evaluate the effectiveness of dialysis treatment?
    A. Blood pressure and weight
    B. Weight and blood urea nitrogen
    C. Potassium level and creatinine levels
    D. Blood urea nitrogen and creatinine levels

107. When auscultating the chest of a patient with pneumonia, the nurse should expect to hear which type of sounds over areas of consolidation?
    A. Bronchial
    B. Bronchovesicular
    C. Vesicular
    D. Bronchophony

108. Which assessment finding would help differentiate a hemorrhagic stroke from a thrombotic stroke?
    A. Sensory disturbance
    B. History of hypertension
    C. Sudden onset of a headache
    D. Motor weakness

109. A male patient with a history of chronic kidney disease is hospitalized. The nurse assesses him for signs of chronic kidney disease which include:
    A. Facial flushing
    B. Pruritus
    C. Diminished urinary stream
    D. Dribbling after voiding

110. A new graduate nurse is administering packed red cells to a patient with a hemoglobin of 6.4. The mentoring nurse should **intervene immediately** if the new graduate does which of the following?
    A. Primes the tubing with normal saline
    B. Identifies the blood band with a second nurse
    C. Takes the blood pressure, pulse, and respiratory rate 15 minutes after the blood has started
    D. Tells the patient that a transfusion reaction could occur

111. A patient with a new colostomy has arrived on the postsurgical unit. The nurse would call the HCP if which one of the following was noted when assessing the surgical site?
    A. Mild discomfort at the surgical site
    B. Stoma color dark red/purple
    C. Small amount of bleeding from stoma
    D. Mild edema of stoma

112. A patient has been diagnosed with DKA, with a blood sugar of 850 mg/dL. Which one of the following orders would be **most important to administer first** for this patient?
    A. Regular insulin IV push
    B. Regular insulin subcutaneously
    C. 50% dextrose
    D. 0.9% sodium chloride

113. When locating the Erb's point to hear aortic and pulmonic sounds, the nurse should place the stethoscope at the:
    A. Fifth intercostal space near the midclavicular line.
    B. Second intercostal space at the left sternal border.
    C. Fifth intercostal space at the left sternal border.
    D. Third intercostal space at the left sternal border.

114. Despite the nurse's best efforts at therapeutic communication, a patient refuses hemodialysis and threatens to leave the hospital. What should the nurse do **first**?
    A. Explain the "against medical advice" (AMA) form.
    B. Have a family member persuade the patient to continue dialysis.
    C. Notify the HCP
    D. Document the patient's wishes.

115. What surgical treatment will the nurse prepare the patient for in the presence of compartment syndrome?
    A. Fasciotomy
    B. Amputation
    C. Internal fixation
    D. Release of tendons

116. A patient newly diagnosed with cirrhosis has been started on propranolol (Inderal) to reduce portal venous pressure. Which one of the following should be a nursing consideration related to propranolol?
    A. The drug can mask signs of shock and hypoglycemia.
    B. Instruct patient to immediately discontinue the drug if having side effects.
    C. Patients with asthma need an increased dose.
    D. For an overdose, of propranolol (Inderal) give a cardioselective beta-blocker.

117. A nurse is instructing a patient regarding the administration of glargine (Lantus) insulin. Which one of the following strategies for subcutaneous administration should be included in the plan of care?
    A. Rotate sites by using the arm one day, abdomen next day, and the thigh the day after.
    B. Select one injection site for insulin injections and use it exclusively.
    C. Administer this medication 30 to 60 minutes after a meal.
    D. Select an appropriate area on the body and rotate injection sites within that area.

118. Which instructions should the nurse include in the teaching plan for a patient who will be taking simvastatin (Zocor) when discharged?
    A. Increase the dietary intake of potassium.
    B. Take the medication in the morning with breakfast.
    C. Notify the prescriber if unexplained muscle tenderness or pain occurs.
    D. Take the medication at least a half hour after meals.

119. A nurse is caring for a patient with glomerulonephritis. What should the nurse instruct the patient to do to prevent recurrent attacks?
    A. Avoid swimming in lakes.
    B. Take showers instead of baths.
    C. Seek early treatment for possible throat infections.
    D. Restrict fluid intake.

120. The nurse is reviewing discharge teaching with a 75-year-old woman with osteoporosis. The patient refuses to eat or drink dairy items. Which food, high in calcium, can the nurse suggest?

A. Eggs

B. Potatoes

C. Apples

D. Salmon

121. A 34-year-old patient has been newly diagnosed with Crohn's disease. The patient states to the nurse, "I'm just miserable. How long will it be until this goes away?" The **best** response by the nurse would be:

A. "I think I know how you feel."

B. "Just keep positive thoughts in your mind."

C. "Are you thinking about harming yourself?

D. "You sound very frustrated. Can you tell me your concerns?"

122. A patient has been diagnosed with end-stage liver disease. Which one of the following assessments would be **most important** to observe for?

A. Visual changes

B. Blood in stool

C. Hair loss

D. Increased albumin

123. A 32-year-old patient with the diagnosis of pernicious anemia and GERD (gastroesophageal reflux disease) is getting ready to be discharged. The patient is distraught and concerned over what will happen after discharge. Which statement below is **inaccurate** to tell the patient?

A. "Your hemoglobin and hematocrit values are low."

B. "Your reticulocyte count may run low."

C. "At this point in time, there is not a cure for this condition."

D. "It is appropriate to take omeprazole for your GERD."

124. The nurse is providing dietary instructions for an Asian patient with chronic kidney disease. As the nurse explains the instructions, the patient continuously turns away. Which nursing action is **most appropriate**?

A. Continue the instructions, verifying patient understanding.

B. Stop the verbal instructions and give the patient written instructions.

C. Stress the importance of the instructions with the patient.

D. Ask the patient why he turns away when being instructed.

125. The nurse explains to the family of a patient who has had a stroke that the purpose of a cerebral angiography is to:

A. Differentiate between a hemorrhagic stroke and a thrombotic stroke.

B. Assess patency of cerebral blood vessels.

C. Measure the amount of increased intracranial pressure (ICP).

D. Determine the amount of brain activity.

126. A patient has been admitted for acute pancreatitis. Which one of the following assessments is **most important** related to one of the **main systemic complications** of acute pancreatitis?

A. Palpating the lower abdomen

B. Checking for the Trousseau sign

C. Assessing pedal pulses

D. Auscultating bowel sounds

127. A nurse is caring for a patient with a diagnosis of right ventricular failure. Which condition **unrelated** to cardiac disease is the major cause of right ventricular failure?

   A. Renal disease

   B. Hypovolemic shock

   C. Severe systemic infection

   D. Chronic obstructive pulmonary disease (COPD)

128. Which data are significant when assessing a patient diagnosed with rule-out Legionnaires' disease?

   A. Decreased bilateral lung sounds in the upper lobes

   B. Symptoms of aching muscles, high fever, malaise, and coughing

   C. Exposure to a saprophytic water bacterium transmitted into the air

   D. The amount of cigarettes smoked per day and the age when smoking started

129. A patient has undergone open reduction and internal fixation (ORIF) of a fractured hip. The nurse monitors this patient for which **initial** sign of a fat embolism?

   A. Confusion

   B. Decreased pedal pulse on the affected side

   C. Petechiae over the chest

   D. Fever

130. The nurse is preparing to administer trimethoprim–sulfamethoxazole (Bactrim) to a patient with a urinary-tract infection (UTI) and notes that the dose prescribed is higher than that recommended. The nurse calls the HCP to clarify the prescription, and the HCP instructs the nurse to administer the dose as prescribed. Which action should the nurse take **next**?

   A. Call the pharmacy

   B. Contact the nursing supervisor

   C. Call the medical director on call

   D. Administer the dose as prescribed

131. Anasarca develops in a patient as a result of nephrotic syndrome. Which of the following would be an appropriate nursing diagnosis, related to the anasarca, for this patient?

   A. Risk for fluid volume deficit

   B. Acute pain

   C. Disturbed body image

   D. Urinary retention

132. A patient has had surgery for diverticulitis and now has a loop stoma to allow the bowel to rest. The nurse correctly instructs the patient that:

   A. the loop stoma has one opening.

   B. the loop stoma is going to be temporary.

   C. the rectum will not have any stool or discharge.

   D. a clear liquid diet is to be followed until the next surgery.

133. A patient admitted to the hospital for severe gastritis states that she has not been able to eat or drink for 3 days. After an assessment, the nurse identifies the problem of fluid volume deficit. Which one of the following interventions **is most appropriate** to include in the plan of care?

   A. Having the patient on a low-residue diet

   B. Obtaining an order for total parental nutrition (TPN)

   C. Monitoring lung sounds every 4 to 6 hours

   D. Assessing and maintaining the current IV site

134. Which of the following is the antihypertensive agent of choice for patients with diabetes and no other contraindications?
    A. Calcium-channel blocker
    B. A potassium sparing diuretic
    C. Angiotensin-converting enzyme (ACE) inhibitor
    D. A loop diuretic

135. Which clinical manifestation would the nurse expect for a patient diagnosed with Parkinson's disease?
    A. 4 + deep tendon reflexes
    B. Muscle flaccidity
    C. Tremors when sleeping
    D. Bradykinesia

136. When caring for a patient with acute kidney injury, which of the following clinical manifestation would cause the **greatest** concern?
    A. Decreased urine output
    B. Increased white-cell count
    C. Increased serum potassium
    D. Increased blood urea nitrogen (BUN)

137. The recommended treatment for an initial VTE (venous thromboembolism) in an otherwise healthy patient with no significant comorbidities would include:
    A. Subcutaneous unfractionated heparin as an outpatient.
    B. Subcutaneous low-molecular-weight heparin (LMWH) as an outpatient.
    C. IV Argatroban as an inpatient.
    D. IV unfractionated heparin as an inpatient.

138. An elderly patient is being discharged to home following a myocardial infarction. His elderly spouse will be his primary caregiver. The couple have no children but have a nephew who checks in on them occasionally. The nurse, collaborating with the social worker, should suggest which of the following for discharge planning?
    A. Arranging for placement in an extended care facility for the patient
    B. Suggesting that both the patient and the spouse be placed in an extended care facility
    C. Insisting that the nephew take a more active role in the care of the patient and spouse
    D. Arranging for a referral for home care

139. The patient has a nursing diagnosis of activity intolerance related to anemia. The nurse can help the patient with which of the following outcomes related to this diagnosis?
    A. Sleeping 14 hours per day
    B. Balancing activity with rest throughout the day
    C. Increasing hemoglobin within 1 month
    D. Increasing intake of iron-rich foods

140. During a physical assessment of a patient with anemia, which finding most concerns the nurse?
    A. Dyspnea at rest
    B. Pallor
    C. Poor appetite
    D. Bone pain

141. A patient hospitalized with thrombocytopenia strikes his knee on the bed frame when returning to bed. The nurse should:
    A. Assess for blood in the urine
    B. Apply ice to the knee
    C. Request a stat platelet count
    D. Splint the knee

142. The nurse is providing discharge teaching for a patient with heart failure who is receiving spironolactone (Aldactone). What dietary teaching should be included for this patient?
    A. Increase consumption of sodium-rich foods.
    B. Use salt substitute instead of regular table salt.
    C. Increase calcium intake.
    D. Adhere to moderate to low intake of potassium-rich foods.

143. The nurse is teaching a patient about modifiable risk factors for hypertension. Which of the following is a modifiable risk factor?
    A. Age
    B. Ethnicity
    C. Obesity
    D. Genetics

144. The family of a patient dying from cancer refuses to consider hospice care. What is the nurse's priority?
    A. Assessing the family's understanding of hospice care
    B. Accepting their decision
    C. Asking someone who has used hospice care to speak with the family
    D. Seeking assistance from the hospital chaplain

145. A patient with a venous thromboembolism (VTE) is receiving heparin intravenously and warfarin (Coumadin) orally. The morning lab results are as follows: activated partial thromboplastin time (aPTT) 43 seconds; internationalized normalized ratio (INR) 1.8. The nurse should collaborate with the HCP to:
    A. Discontinue the heparin and increase the warfarin dose.
    B. Increase the heparin and keep the warfarin dose the same.
    C. Discontinue both the heparin and warfarin.
    D. Discontinue the warfarin and keep the heparin dose the same.

146. A patient with a spontaneous pneumothorax asks, "Why did they put this tube into my chest?" The nurse explains that the purpose of the chest tube is to:
    A. Check for bleeding in the lung.
    B. Monitor the function of the lung.
    C. Drain fluid from the pleural space.
    D. Remove air from the pleural space.

147. A nurse is assigned to care for a patient who has just returned from Beijing with pneumonia and a cough. The nurse observes the UAP putting on the protective clothing before entering the patient's room. Which option indicates that the UAP understands what protective clothing must be worn to reduce the risk of acquiring an infection?
    A. Gown and gloves
    B. Gown, mask, cap, and gloves
    C. Gloves, barrier mask, and gown
    D. Gloves, gown, N-95 mask, and eye shield

148. A patient has just been diagnosed with obstructive sleep apnea (OSA) following a sleep study. Which statement is most accurate when providing patient teaching?

   A. "You will need to wear an oral appliance (mouth guard) at night to keep your airway open."

   B. "You will need to come back in a month and schedule the bariatric surgery."

   C. "It is acceptable for you to sleep on your back or stomach."

   D. "It is acceptable to take a sedative prior to going to sleep."

149. A 25-year-old patient with a history of asthma is brought to the emergency department because of respiratory distress. The nurse immediately places the patient in a bed with the head of the bed elevated and administers oxygen via a facemask. The HCP performs a physical assessment, writes orders, and admits the patient. Which order should the nurse carry out **first**?

   A. Administer the nebulizer treatment to facilitate breathing.

   B. Obtain a blood specimen to send to the laboratory for tests.

   C. Notify the respiratory therapist to perform chest physiotherapy.

   D. Obtain an incentive spirometer and review proper technique with the patient.

150. Which patient should the nurse see **first**? A patient:

   A. Admitted with pneumonia with a pulse oximetry reading of 92%.

   B. Being discharged to an extended care facility.

   C. Who has undergone abdominal surgery and is reporting jaw pain radiating to the ear.

   D. Who had a stroke 3 days ago and needs assistance with feeding.

ANSWERS

1. Answer: C

   Rationale: The PR interval range is 0.12 to 0.2 second; therefore, the finding is normal.

2. Answer: C

   Rationale: Dry mucous membranes are assessed in both HHNS and diabetic keto-acidosis (DKA) due to hyperglycemia. Rapid and deep breathing (Kussmaul respirations) occurs with DKA. A sweet breath occurs with DKA because of the breakdown of fat, producing ketones.

3. Answer: B

   Rationale: If the patient can produce an audible cough, no harm is done. Once an audible cough is established, the nurse should then have the patient attempt to swallow water. If water, hard candy, and/or applesauce are given to a patient with dysphagia, they may be aspirated.

4. Answer: A

   Rationale: Multiple drugs are administered because of the concern regarding drug resistance. Streptomycin is an antibiotic; it does not prevent the side effects of Rifater therapy. Multiple antituberculosis drugs are necessary for an extended period, approximately 6 to 8 months depending on the individual. The infection may not be advanced and this statement and may increase the patient's anxiety.

5. Answer: D

   Rationale: The patient may be going into shock. Gather further assessment data and notify the HCP. Rechecking vital signs in an hour is a do-nothing response—shock will worsen. Raise the legs higher than the heart; do not put in reverse Trendelenburg. Increase the rate of the IV fluids to replace fluids; do not decrease the fluids.

6. Answer: A

Rationale: HOB elevation prevents pressure on the incision and prevents postoperative headaches. The patient should avoid vigorous coughing, sneezing, or straining to have a bowel movement to prevent cerebral spinal fluid leakage at the surgical site. Brushing the teeth should be avoided for 10 days after surgery to preserve the suture site. Neurologic assessments, including pupillary response, should be done to detect complications.

7. Answer: C

Rationale: The goal of palliative care is to improve the quality of life for the patient; it focuses on the relief of symptoms. The goal is to increase comfort but not to treat the underlying disease.

8. Answer: B

Rationale: The nurse manager will monitor attendance and tardiness. The human resources department determines pay. The mentor will help with skills, give constructive feedback, and perform the peer evaluation.

9. Answer: C

Rationale: Most older adults do not manifest the typical signs/symptoms of infection such as fever and high white-cell counts. Delirium or acute confusion is often the first sign of an infection.

10. Answer: B

Rationale: Disaster triage is based on the principle of the greatest good for the greatest number; those who have a likelihood of survival are treated first. People who are gasping for breath and are conscious have priority over those who are cyanotic and not breathing. Patients who are not breathing and cyanotic have low priority because survival requires multiple time-consuming interventions that detract from the care needed by others. Patients having a seizure have low priority because a seizure is not life-threatening.

11. Answer: A

Rationale: Phantom pain is real and the patient should be medicated after the nurse uses a pain rating scale. Phantom pain may or may not diminish over time, but the patient should be treated immediately. The patient knows the limb is gone. Diversional activities may help but the patient needs to be medicated also.

12. Answer: C

Rationale: In the Latino/Hispanic culture, loud crying and other physical manifestations of grief are socially acceptable. Making the necessary arrangements provides a culturally sensitive approach to the patient's family, as long as they are not interfering with patient care. Restricting the number of visitors and warning against emotional outbursts are inappropriate interventions. Moving the patient may or may not be appropriate; it may be safer to have the patient closer to the nurses' station.

13. Answer: D

Rationale: Symptoms of DI are polyuria, decreased urine specific gravity, and excessive thirst. These can be due to the reduction of antidiuretic hormone (ADH) in patients who have had the pituitary gland removed.

14. Answer: D

Rationale: Pushing fluids will help flush any small stones and may prevent formation of certain types of stones. Once a stone is removed, the stone type will be determined and the patient will be taught to avoid foods that may precipitate stone formation. UTIs can be common with urinary calculi, and the patient should seek medical attention with signs and symptoms of UTIs. Catheters are not used for urinary calculi. Patients will be treated with pain medication and increased fluid intake to assist with passing of calculi.

15. Answer: C

Rationale: The patient with viral hepatitis needs rest to heal. The patient should have up to six small meals that are high in calories, protein, and carbohydrates. Alcohol should be eliminated.

16. Answer: C

Rationale: metformin (Glucophage) is contraindicated for patients with decreased fluid intake/dehydration and renal failure.

17. Answer: A

The patient should ambulate and do leg exercises to prevent venous thromboembolism (VTE). The patient will be allowed to eat and drink as long at he or she is not nauseated. The patient will not have a nasogastric (NG) tube and most likely will have no or minimal vaginal bleeding.

18. Answer: C

Rationale: Addisonian crisis is caused by insufficient adrenocortical hormone levels that have decreased sharply. The treatment is IV hydrocortisone. The patient can also be treated with IV infusions of 0.9% sodium chloride, glucose (patient is at risk for hypoglycemia), and electrolyte replacement. Ketoconazole (Nizoral) is used for Cushing's syndrome. Metoprolol (Lopressor) would lower the blood pressure and is contraindicated.

19. Answer: D

Rationale: The oral mucosa and the conjunctivae should be assessed in patients with dark skin because cyanosis cannot be assessed in the lips or fingertips.

20. Answer: A

Rationale: Decreased blood pressure and increased heart rate can indicate impending shock due to a perforated colon. Hyperactive bowel sounds and some abdominal cramping are to be expected because of stimulation of the bowel during the procedure. Watery discharge is also expected because of the bowel prep.

21. Answer: D

Rationale: The witness cannot be an employee or an official hospital volunteer. The patient will have to find someone who is not an employee of the hospital.

22. Answer: D

Rationale: Further assessment is needed, and the patient should be included in the choice of intervention.

23. Answer: B

Rationale: The head of the bed needs to be elevated to prevent aspiration. The UAP should turn the head to one side, use an oral suction catheter, and use an emesis basin when doing oral care.

24. Answer: C.

Rationale: When providing information to the Amish couple, avoid using scientific or medical jargon (as with any patient).When educating or counseling a female Amish patient, most couples will want to discuss health care options together. The nurse should never use complex medical terminology with any patient. Standing close and speaking loudly is inappropriate in most counseling situations.

25. Answer: B

    Rationale: Long-term corticosteroid use can cause osteoporosis; therefore, the patient needs adequate calcium in the diet. Corticosteroid use can cause elevated blood sugars. The medication should not be discontinued abruptly (adrenal crisis may occur if stopped), and should be taken with food to decrease gastrointestinal irritation.

26. Answer: B

    Rationale: If the tracheostomy tube is dislodged, the initial nursing action is to ventilate the client using a manual resuscitation bag and face mask. A fresh tracheostomy tract typically takes about a week to mature. Nobody should attempt reinsertion of a dislodged tube via the surgical stoma because this can create a false lumen, which can be very harmful to the patient. Covering the site is incorrect because this action will block the airway.

27. Answer: A

    Rationale: Cervical injuries can cause respiratory depression so it is the priority. The other assessments are also important, but they do not take priority over respiratory status.

28. Answer: A

    Rationale: Reviewing the patient's medications will ensure that there are no duplicates or interactions. While polypharmacy should be monitored, it may not be possible to eliminate it. Elderly patients absorb medication more slowly. All of the patient's medications (both prescribed and the over the counter) should be assessed, as there may be drug–drug interactions.

29. Answer: C

    Rationale: Guillain–Barré syndrome can cause paralysis and can affect the lungs, necessitating possible intubation. This patient should be seen first. The other three patients are stable. The patient with MS should be seen second to receive the medication on time. The nurse should assist with feeding the patient with ALS because of the risk of aspiration, so this should not be delegated. The nurse will have to facilitate the discharge for the patient with HD, but this can wait.

30. Answer: A

    Rationale: ACE inhibitors increase the sensitivity of the cough reflex, leading to the common adverse effect sometimes referred to as an ACE cough. A cough is not a side effect of the other categories of medication.

31. Answer: B

    Rationale: Levothyroxine (Synthroid) is given to patients with hypothyroidism. The side effects could be increased heart rate and blood pressure, insomnia, tremors, and weight loss. Propylthiouracil (PTU) and methimazole (Tapazole) are used for hyperthyroidism. Propranolol is a beta-blocker and will slow the heart rate.

32. Answer: C

    Rationale: Stimulation should be kept to a minimum while the patient is withdrawing from alcohol. Monitoring vital signs and addressing hallucinations are part of the CIWA scale, and maintaining a safe environment is important for all patients, especially those withdrawing from alcohol.

33. Answer: B

    Rationale: Insulin will attach to potassium and bring it back into the red cells. This can be done quickly if the patient needs to wait for renal dialysis to be started. IV regular insulin with 50% dextrose are not used to treat the other conditions.

34. Answer: C

Rationale: The patient's allergies may determine what the HCP may order. Family history may be important to know for a full history and physical but is not needed to give an SBAR report for a specific problem. Insurance and vaccinations would not be priority background information.

35. Answer: D

Rationale: Hand scanning should be requested at the airport as the patient should avoid all situations involving electromagnetic fields. Radiofrequency energy from cell phones can interact with some electronic devices; this type of interference is called "electromagnetic interference," and a simple precaution to avoid interference is to add distance between the cell phone and the pacemaker. A medic alert ID and/or carrying a pacemaker information card at all times is important for the patient's safety in case of an emergency. Loose clothing over the site initially is important as it is more comfortable than pressure being applied to the site.

36. Answer: A

Rationale: The bladder is sterile; therefore, care must be taken to use sterile equipment and sterile technique. Sterile saline is used to irrigate a catheter, not antibiotic solution. The solutions should be at room temperature, and the irrigation should drain by gravity.

37. Answer: D

Rationale: An overdose of acetaminophen (Tylenol) will cause liver damage; therefore, bilirubin will be increased on the liver-function test. Acetaminophen can decrease hemoglobin and potassium and has no effect on creatinine.

38. Answer: A

Rationale: Low calcium will cause irritability of nerves and muscles. Trousseau's and Chvostek's sign (tapping the facial nerve) should be monitored for 72 hours after surgery. Other signs of hypocalcemia are bradycardia, prolonged QT interval, cardiac dysrhythmias, and diminished pedal pulses.

39. Answer: C

Rationale: Both A- and O-negative blood are compatible with the client's blood. A-negative is the same as the client's blood type and is preferred; in an emergency, type O-negative blood also may be given. Although type O blood may be used, it will have to be Rh-negative; Rh-positive blood is incompatible with the client's blood and will cause hemolysis. AB-positive blood is incompatible with the client's blood and will cause hemolysis. A-negative blood is compatible with the client's blood, but AB-negative is incompatible and will cause hemolysis.

40. Answer: A

Rationale: The use of a temporary pacemaker is considered a lifesaving measure for patients who are experiencing heart block. A temporary pacemaker is used until the heart block is resolved using medical interventions or a permanent pacemaker is inserted. Ventricular tachycardia is treated with intravenous medications and possibly cardioversion or defibrillation. Ventricular fibrillation necessitates immediate cardiopulmonary resuscitation (CPR) and the use of a defibrillator. Atrial fibrillation is initially treated with medications and possibly electrical cardioversion.

41. Answer: B

Rationale: Decentralized leadership hierarchy is a flat organizational structure, meaning that authority for action is at the point of care. Self-governance is emphasized and more satisfaction is seen. The senior level and the board of directors' decision making is centralized, emphasizing top-down decision making. While the nursing department is at the point of care, the point of care involves more than just nursing.

42. Answer: D

    Rationale: While all are appropriate, the physiologic diagnosis takes precedence. The patient with anxiety can hyperventilate; therefore, breathing assessment should be the priority.

43. Answer: A

    Rationale: An ileostomy can initially have an output of up to 2000 mL/day.

44. Answer: A

    Rationale: The Glasgow Coma Scale score ranges from 3 to 15—the lower the score, the more severe the condition. A score of 9 and above indicate more meaningful responses.

45. Answer: D

    Rationale: Patients with Graves' disease can be at risk for corneal ulceration if they have exophthalmos. These patients may need 4000 to 5000 calories a day and should not be on calorie restriction. Patients should take rest periods and control pain.

46. Answer: C

    Rationale: Peripheral arterial insufficiency is characterized by deep circular necrotic ulcers on the toes and other pressure areas, cool shiny skin, decreased peripheral pulses, pain at rest, and minimal to no edema. Peripheral venous insufficiency is characterized by brownish discoloration around the ankles, presence of pulses, and moderate to severe edema.

47. Answer: B

    Rationale: The HCP must reinsert the catheter because of the trauma from surgery. The patient will need the catheter reinserted to allow for the continuous bladder irrigation. The bleeding is coming from the urethra; therefore, pressure on the penis will not stop the bleeding.

48. Answer: C

    Rationale: Activities such as exercise or heat application, which increase circulation and serve as stimuli for the spread of infection, should be avoided by patients with acute osteomyelitis. Oral or IV antibiotic therapy is continued at home for 4 to 6 weeks, weight bearing is contraindicated to prevent pathologic fractures, and it is necessary to notify the HCP if increased pain occurs.

49. Answer: D

    Rationale: African Americans are at risk for developing angioedema; therefore, the nurse should instruct the patient about early signs of angioedema. The other three choices are side effects of lisinopril, but the nurse can teach the patient how to manage these side effects.

50. Answer: B

    Rationale: Hypocalcemia can cause tingling around the lips and twitching of fingers and toes. If the calcium gets too low, the patient can experience seizure. Metabolic alkalosis, hypernatremia, and hypokalemia will not cause tingling.

51. Answer: B

    Rationale: Viral infections generally do not cause a rise in the white-cell count as found with bacterial infections. With viral infections, the white-cell count is often 4000 or lower. Anything over 10,000 is indicative of an acute bacterial infection.

52. Answer: C

    Rationale: The goal of patient preparation for this surgery is to control high blood pressure and tachycardia caused by the epinephrine and norepinephrine being secreted from the tumor. Alpha-adrenergic receptor blockers will block the release of epinephrine and norepinephrine. None of the other medications has this mechanism of action.

53. Answer: C

Rationale: Hypotension, tachycardia, jugular vein distention, cyanosis of the lips and nails, dyspnea, muffled heart sounds, diaphoresis, and paradoxical pulse (a decrease in systolic arterial pressure by more than 10 mm Hg during inspiration) are indications of this emergency situation. The other choices are not indications of cardiac tamponade.

54. Answer: B

Rationale: 24 hours is too soon. The patient will not yet be symptom-free. Patients should be taught to take the entire dose of antibiotics and to still abstain from sexual activity until 7 days after antibiotic treatment is completed and the patient is asymptomatic. The symptoms may clear prior to 7 days after the antibiotics are complete. The patient does not have to wait 6 months.

55. Answer: B

Smoking is a not a risk factor for type 2 diabetes. All of the rest are risk factors.

56. Answer: D

Rationale: The patient should avoid taking the iron supplements with milk or antacids because these decrease the absorption of iron. The patient should eat a high-fiber diet and increase fluid intake to prevent the side effect of constipation. The patient should increase the intake of natural sources of iron, such as meats, fish, and poultry.

57. Answer: C

Rationale: Normal ABG values are pH 7.35 to 7.45, PCO_2 35 to 45 mm Hg, and HCO_3 22 to 26 mEq. Because the PCO_2 is high, the nurse should instruct the patient to "blow off" the PCO_2 by coughing and deep breathing. There is no indication for a diuretic. Breathing into a bag will increase the PCO_2. HCO_3 is normal so no need to give sodium bicarbonate.

58. Answer: C

Rationale: The best readability level in the United States is 6th-grade level. The average American reads effectively at the 6th- to 8th-grade level (regardless of education achieved). Even people with much higher reading levels learn medical and health information when the material is presented at the 6th- to 8th-grade readability level.

59. Answer: B

Rationale: Growth hormone (somatotropin) is secreted by the pituitary gland. Calcium would be related to the parathyroid gland, aldosterone to the adrenal glands. Glycosylated hemoglobin is related to pancreatic studies.

60. Answer: D

Rationale: Quinapril hydrochloride (Accupril) is an ACE inhibitor. It is used in the treatment of hypertension and as adjunctive therapy in the treatment of heart failure. Excessive hypotension ("first-dose syncope") can occur in patients with heart failure or in those who are severely salt- or volume-depleted. Although respirations, urine output, and lung sounds should be monitored, the nurse should specifically monitor the client's blood pressure

61. Answer: A

Rationale: Confusion, headache, nausea and vomiting are early signs. The other three are later signs.

62. Answer: B

Rationale: Patient is exhibiting signs of peritonitis, which is an emergency.

63. Answer: B:

Rationale: Safety is the priority. Never restrain a patient who is having a seizure. The airway can be accessed after the seizure—do not put anything in the patient's mouth.

64. Answer: A

Rationale: Although problem-solving potential is increased when clients are involved in exploring alternatives that will affect the direction of their own lives, clients in crisis may be overwhelmed and initially need assistance in making decisions. The patient, not the crisis intervention practitioner, should identify the problem; the practitioner facilitates the process. The information that others have been helped is useless because the patient is unable to empathize with others at this time. Identifying the client's religious and cultural beliefs is not the priority at this time.

65. Answer: D

Rationale: Many respiratory conditions exhibit these same symptoms, not just ARDS. The ABGs would not be normal because the patient's pO_2 would be low. Breath sounds are usually clear in the early stages of ARDS.

66. Answer: D

Rationale: In order to see or palpate an enlarged thyroid, it helps to have the patient swallow during assessment in order to watch the upward movement. Cross-lighting will help visualize any shadows from the thyroid. Patients should have their neck in neutral or slightly extended position. The thyroid gland is not percussed during assessment.

67. Answer: B

Rationale: Echocardiography is a noninvasive, risk-free, pain-free test that involves no special preparation. It is commonly done at the bedside or on an outpatient basis. The client must lie quietly for 30 to 60 minutes while the procedure is being performed. The other choices are not preprocedure preparations.

68. Answer: C

Rationale: Use open-ended questions. Do not use yes/no questions. (However, if the patient is suicidal, asking if the patient is going to hurt himself or herself and if the patient has a plan are two appropriate yes/no questions.) Do not use "I"—focus on the patient.

69. Answer: C

Rationale: Patients take antibiotics for this bacterial (not viral) infection and follow-up testing is recommended 3 months after treatment completion, as it is not easily cured. It is the most common sexually transmitted disease. For females, it can cause pelvic inflammatory disorder, which can lead to sterility.

70. Answer: D

Rationale: Hospice is not a place but a concept of care that provides compassion and support for the dying patient and family. The care is provided by the family or by hospital or extended-care personnel with support from hospice personnel.

71. Answer: C

Rationale: The majority of older adults are capable of taking care of their own lives. They may live in homes/apartments either alone, with a significant other or family, can afford medical treatment, and have social or family support.

72. Answer: D

    Rationale: Enteral feeding should be withheld for 1 hour prior to and 1 hour after administration of phenytoin (Dilantin). The tube should be flushed with 20 ml of water before and after the dose is given. The gastric residual should be checked prior to administering any medication, and the nurse should follow the policy of the institution regarding when to return the residual and when to discard the residual. The head of the bed needs to be at least 30 degrees but can be higher.

73. Answer: A

    Rationale: Autonomic dysreflexia is often precipitated by a full bowel or full bladder. First, the cause of the dysreflexia needs to be addressed. Medication for the high blood pressure that accompanies autonomic dysreflexia may be given but not a beta-blocker, as the patient may also be bradycardic. The head of the bed should be raised. Vital signs should be taken but only after raising the head and taking care of the full bladder.

74. Answer: B

    Rationale: Taking vital signs is within the UAP scope of practice so long as it is not the first set of vital signs when a patient is admitted or changing level of care. The other activities are in the nursing scope of practice.

75. Answer: A

    Rationale: The Somogyi effect is manifested by hypoglycemia during sleep and hyperglycemia (due to the body's response to the hypoglycemia) when the patient wakes up. It is caused by too much insulin. The patient should check the blood glucose between 2 and 4 a.m. to assess for a drop. The nurse would need to contact the provider for a change in insulin dose; also, the patient probably needs a decrease in insulin.

76. Answer: D

    Rationale: Taking a blood pressure in the arm with the fistula could damage the fistula. The patient should assess for a thrill each day. The patient should understand the importance of not missing dialysis. Comparing bilateral pulses each day is important to ensure that the fistula is not impeding circulation.

77. Answer: C

    Rationale: Acceptable standards of care were not met (the nurse failed to adequately check the patient's respiratory rate before administering the medication). This has nothing to do with education or UAPs. The nurse will not be incarcerated.

78. Answer: B

    Rationale: Adhering to a regular, consistent daily schedule helps the patient to avoid confusion and anxiety and is important both during hospitalization and at home. Clocks may be useful in early AD, but they have little meaning to a patient as the disease progresses. The patient may not be able to engage in stimulating conversations. Monitoring the patient's activities is important but does not change the disturbed thought processes.

79. Answer: C

    Because the patient does not speak the same language as the nurse evaluating the pain, the Wong–Baker scale would be the most objective measurement. The other three scales require some explanation in order to be used properly.

80. Answer: A

    Rationale: Aspirin reduces inflammation by inhibiting prostaglandin synthesis. Aspirin does decrease platelet aggregation and has antipyretic effects, but these are not the intended actions for a patient with rheumatoid arthritis. Assisting with vitamin K deficiency is not a mechanism of action for aspirin.

81. Answer: B

Rationale: Hematuria will result in dark or smoky, tea-colored urine and is a classic sign of glomerulonephritis. Blood pressure and potassium may rise because of inadequate glomerular filtration. The patient will exhibit proteinuria.

82. Answer: A

Rationale: The patient has the right to health care decisions; however, the decision has to be an informed one. The nurse should explain to the patient what may happen if hemodialysis is discontinued, call and inform the HCP, and then document.

83. Answer: D

Rationale: Aspiration risk is related to breathing and therefore is the priority. The other parameters should also be assessed and monitored.

84. Answer: C

The initial vital signs should be obtained by an RN and if stable can then be performed by a UAP. RNs should not delegate assessment, evaluation, or teaching. Obtaining a blood glucose is within the scope of practice for the UAP.

85. Answer: A

Rationale: The INR should be between 2 and 3 for most patients after total knee replacement, so the dose is therapeutic. PTT is used to assess IV heparin. Vitamin K is an antidote for warfarin if the INR is too high. The patient should be up and about, as the INR is at a therapeutic level.

86. Answer: A

Rationale: The dialysate output should be clear—cloudy would indicate the presence of white cells. The patient may experience some mild abdominal discomfort from the peritoneal dialysis procedure. The temperature elevation is slight and may not be indicative of an infection. Hematuria is not related to peritoneal dialysis.

87. Answer: D

Rationale: Increased PSA levels can be an indication of cancer and the higher the level, the greater the tumor burden. BUN and creatinine may increase because of impaired renal function but are not specific to prostate cancer. BNP is specific for heart failure.

88. Answer: D

Rationale: PICO stands for patient population, intervention, comparison, and outcome and is a way to formulate a clinical question for evidenced-based research.

89. Answer: A

Rationale: The Centers for Disease Control and Prevention (CDC) recommends the administration of meningococcal conjugate vaccine for all preteens and teens. Influenza vaccine should be administered yearly for all ages. Shingles vaccine should be administered to adults 50 or over. Pneumococcal vaccine is recommend for all adults over the age of 65 and for those who have certain chronic health conditions.

90. Answer: A

This procedure uses electrical energy to "burn" or ablate areas of the conduction system. It has a low complication rate. Patients go to a recovery area for 4 to 6 hours after the procedure and may go home later the same day or the next day. The catheter is inserted through the femoral vein.

91. Answer: A

Rationale: Hepatitis B carriers have this for life. The virus can be present before and after symptoms occur. Patients should eat a well-balanced diet with the appropriate number of calories per day. Patients with hepatitis cannot donate blood.

92. Answer: C

Rationale: Albuterol produces sympathetic nervous system side effects such as tachycardia and hypertension. Pallor, not flushing, is a common side effect. Dyspnea is not a common side effect; this medication is given to decrease respiratory difficulty. Hypertension, not hypotension, is a common side effect.

93. Answer: C

Rationale: If a patient experiences diaphoresis, warmth, and a backache, a transfusion reaction is suspected. The nurse stops the transfusion and prevents the infusion of any additional blood; then the nurse hangs a bag of 0.9% sodium chloride solution. This maintains IV access and helps maintain the client's intravascular volume. The primary HCP is notified, as is the blood bank. The nurse also documents the occurrence, the actions taken, and the patient's response. To preserve the IV access, the nurse should not remove the catheter and discontinue the IV site.

94. Answer: B

Rationale: Nonsteroidal antiinflammatory drugs such as ibuprofen are contraindicated in patients with gastrointestinal (GI) lesions or GI bleeding. Acetaminophen is not contraindicated for patients with GI issues. Famotidine might be used as a treatment, since it decreases gastric secretions. Magnesium hydroxide/aluminum hydroxide will also decrease HCl and is used as a GI medication.

95. Answer: C

Rationale: Opioids can cause constipation and would be contraindicated with a bowel obstruction.

96. Answer: B

Rationale: The A1c recommendation for patients older than 65 years of age who have multiple comorbidities is <8%. No change in medication or diet is indicated.

97. Answer: A

Rationale: This medication can cause photosensitivity, Stevens–Johnson syndrome, and the urine can turn orange-yellow. Do not crush the medication.

98. Answer: B

Rationale: Vasopressin will cause vasoconstriction and help control bleeding.

99. Answer: D

Rationale: The length of the urethra is shorter and therefore microorganisms can reach the bladder more easily. Fluid intake does not account for the difference in infections between men and women. Menses does not put the women at risk for an UTI, nor does body fat.

100. Answer: B

Rationale: The spiral CT provides a definitive diagnosis for pulmonary embolism. Blood gases provide supporting information (hypoxemia, hypocarbia, and respiratory alkalosis). A chest x-ray can rule out other disorders. but it is not adequate for a definitive diagnosis, and it may yield a false negative result. Angiography also provides a definitive diagnosis, but it is more invasive and is associated with more complications.

101. Answer: C

Rationale: Patients should avoid acidic foods/liquids that could harm the esophagus. Patients should not drive for 24 to 48 hours after the procedure because of the sedation used. The patient should not develop a fever; this could indicate perforation. The patient still needs to sleep with the HOB elevated. An EGD does not cure GERD.

102. Answer: A

Rationale: The nurse should validate what the patient is saying and ask an open-ended question to further explore the topic with the patient. The other choices are ineffective responses, as they avoid the cue received from the patient.

103. Answer: C

Rationale: The nurse needs to assess the patient before any intervention can be performed. The other interventions might be appropriate depending on the result of the glucose test, which the UAP can obtain.

104. Answer: D

Rationale: The nurse cannot insist but can encourage the patient to report all sexual contacts. The health department will be notified of the disease, but confidentiality will be maintained. Health care staff should use contact precautions while caring for the patient.

105. Answer: B

Rationale: Prednisone is typically not stopped abruptly, as adrenal crisis could occur. Prednisone can cause hyperglycemia, so blood glucose should be checked. SLE can cause pain, so high doses of NSAIDs may be used. Prednisone can cause hypernatremia, hypokalemia, and hypocalcemia, so electrolytes should be monitored.

106. Answer: A

Rationale: Both the blood pressure and weight will decrease after dialysis. The BUN and creatinine will remain elevated in a patient with kidney disease. The potassium may decrease, but the creatinine will not. Both parts of the choice have to be correct for the answer to be correct.

107. Answer: A

Rationale: Chest auscultation reveals bronchial breath sounds over areas of consolidation. Bronchovesicular sounds are heard normally over midlobe lung regions. Vesicular breath sounds are commonly heard in the lung bases. Bronchophony is the increased transmission/change in character of the spoken voice due to atelectasis, infarction, or compression of lung tissue.

108. Answer: C

Rationale: A hemorrhagic stroke is often precipitated by a sudden, severe headache. The other three findings may be seen with either a hemorrhagic stroke or thrombotic stroke.

109. Answer: B

Rationale: The accumulation of metabolic wastes in the blood (known as "uremia") may cause pruritus. The patient typically becomes pale, not flushed, with chronic kidney disease related to anemia. Diminished urinary stream and dribbling after voiding are related to prostate issues, not chronic kidney disease.

110. Answer: C

Rationale: The new graduate also needs to take the patient temperature 15 minutes after the blood is started. Priming the tubing and verifying with another nurse are correct interventions. The nurse does need to inform the patient of the risks of blood transfusion, but this is not the best response.

111. Answer: B

Rationale: A dark red/purple stoma can indicate compromised blood supply to stoma. A pink/red stoma is normal. Mild edema and a small amount of bleeding is expected. Some discomfort near the sugical site is also an expected finding.

112. Answer: D

Rationale: Prompt replacement of fluids and electrolytes is important to prevent cerebral edema. Insulin will be needed, but this is not the first intervention.

113. Answer: D

Rationale: The Erb's point is located at the third intercostal space at the left sternal border, where aortic and pulmonic sounds can be auscultated. The fifth intercostal space near the midclavicular line is used to listen to the mitral area. The second intercostal space at the left sternal border is the pulmonic area. The fifth intercostal space at the left sternal border is the tricuspid area. Sounds from the tricuspid valve can be heard best here.

114. Answer: C

Rationale: The HCP will need to talk with the patient, explain the eventual outcome if the patient refuses dialysis, and explain the AMA form. Neither the nurse nor the HCP can force the patient to have dialysis if the patient is of sound mind. If the patient is confused, then a guardian with the power of attorney (POA) can make the decision for the patient. The patient's family may attempt to persuade the patient, but if the patient is of sound mind, the nurse's role is to give the facts but not persuade. Documentation should occur but is not the first thing the nurse does.

115. Answer: A

Rationale: Compartment syndrome is a medical emergency. The patient will need a fasciotomy—a surgical procedure in which the fascia is cut to relieve pressure; this is commonly done to treat loss of circulation to an area of tissue or muscle. Amputation may be necessary if compartment syndrome is not treated promptly.

116. Answer: A

Rationale: Beta-blockers mask the tachycardia seen with hypoglycemia and shock. The drug should not be stopped abruptly. The drug can cause bronchospasm in patients with asthma. For overdose of beta blockers, give isoproterenol or atropine.

117. Answer: D

Rationale: To promote the absorption of glargine (Lantus) insulin, one anatomic area should be selected, then serial locations within that site should be rotated. Using different anatomical sites each day can result in significant change in absorption rates of the insulin and the patient's blood glucose levels. Using one injection site regularly may lead to lipodystrophy. Regular insulin is administered before eating a meal, not after.

118. Answer: C

Rationale: Simvastatin (Zocor) does not affect levels of potassium. The patient should be monitored for unexplained muscle tenderness or pain. Mild muscle injury can occur in 5-10% of patients that take statins. This can progress to myositis (muscle inflammation), with increased CK levels. The medication is most effective when taken at bedtime because cholesterol synthesis is highest at night.

119. Answer: C

Rationale: streptococci, common in throat infections, can cause glomerulonephritis. Baths and possibly swimming in lakes can cause urethritis but not glomerulonephritis. Fluid restriction will not prevent recurrent attacks, and fluid would help prevent urinary stasis.

120. Answer: D

Rationale: Salmon is high in calcium. Other nondairy foods high in calcium are white beans, sardines, kale, bok choy, dried figs, almonds, and oranges.

121. Answer: D

Rationale: The nurse should encourage the patient to express concerns and feelings. Telling the patient to think positive thoughts or saying you know how the patient feels does not address the patient's concerns. The patient's statement does not indicate plans for self-harm.

122. Answer: B

Rationale: Coagulation factors in end-stage liver disease would be depleted; therefore, the most important assessment would be for bleeding. Hair loss may occur with liver failure although it is not the most important assessment. End-stage liver disease does not affect vision and may decrease albumin.

123. Answer: D

Rationale: This condition causes malabsorption of vitamin B_{12} because of the absence of the intrinsic factor in gastric secretions. Protein-pump inhibitors such as omeprazole may impair vitamin B_{12} absorption. Hemoglobin and hematocrit are low. Reticulocyte counts are low. There is no cure for this condition, and treatment is lifelong.

124. Answer: A

Rationale: The nurse needs to consider the characteristics of the Asian culture, so it would be appropriate for the nurse to continue the conversation. Some in the Asian culture are uncomfortable with direct eye contact. Direct eye contact is also less common in some Latin American cultures, some Middle Eastern cultures, and Native American cultures.

125. Answer: B

Rationale: Angiography can detect abnormality of vessels. CT scanning is used to differentiate between hemorrhagic stroke and thrombotic stroke. An intraventricular catheter is used to measure increased ICP. Functional magnetic resonance imaging (fMRI) can measure brain activity.

126. Answer: B

Rationale: Tetany caused by hypocalcemia is one of the main systemic complications of pancreatitis and can be assessed by checking for Trousseau's sign. This will elicit spasm of the hand and forearm when a blood pressure cuff is inflated, if hypocalcemia is present.

127. Answer: D

Rationale: COPD causes destruction of the capillary beds around the alveoli, interfering with blood flow to the lungs from the right side of the heart. As the heart continues to strain against this resistance, heart failure eventually results. Renal disease causes stress on the left side of the heart. Hypovolemic shock will not cause stress on the right side of the heart. Severe systemic infection will produce greater stress on the left side of the heart.

128. Answer: C

Rationale: Legionnaires' disease is caused by a saprophytic water bacterium that is transmitted through the air from places where the bacteria are found (e.g. rivers, lakes, water distribution centers, and respiratory apparatuses). Abnormal breath sounds can be heard in many respiratory diseases. Aching muscles, high fever, malaise, and coughing are typical of many respiratory diseases; they are not specific to Legionnaires' disease. Cigarette smoking is important to assess in any respiratory illness.

129. Answer: A

Confusion is the initial symptom of a fat embolism due to hypoxemia. Petechiae are a sign, but not the initial one, of a fat embolism. Petechiae are caused by occlusion of small vessels within the skin. The risk for a fat embolism is greatest in the first 36 hours after the fracture of a large bone, after fracture of the pelvis, or after multiple fractures. Fever occurs with a fat embolism, but not initially. A decrease in the pedal pulse is not related to a fat embolism.

130. Answer: B

Rationale: Nurses should follow the nursing chain of command. Calling the pharmacy may help verify the dosage, but the dose was already determined to be higher than recommended. The nurse should not call the medical director, as the nurse should stay within the nursing chain of command. The nurse should not administer a higher-than-recommended dose without further investigation.

131. Answer: C

Rationale: Anasarca is characterized by widespread edema (face, extremities, trunk). The patient will have fluid volume overload due to the widespread edema. The patient may or may not have pain related to the edema, and there is no urinary retention.

132. Answer: B

Rationale: The loop stoma has two openings, is used to rest the bowel, and it can be reversed a number of months later. It has an opening for stool to exit the body and an opening for the excretion of mucous. The resting bowel still secretes mucus, which can be passed through the rectum. The patient should follow a nutritious diet.

133. Answer: D

Rationale: The patient needs fluids, which is the correct treatment for dehydration. TPN could provide nutrition, but it is not first-line choice for fluid volume deficit. Lung sounds are important, but they are more so with fluid volume overload.

134. Answer: C

Rationale: An ACE inhibitor is indicated as the primary medication of hypertensive therapy in diabetes management, as these offer renal protection.

135. Answer: D

Rationale: Clinical manifestations of Parkinson's disease include bradykinesia, cogwheel rigidity, and resting tremors; however, when sleeping, the tremors are absent. The patient may also have a mask-like appearance.

136. Answer: C

Rationale: While all four options are expected, hyperkalemia can cause the most immediate, life-threatening complications.

137. Answer: B

Rationale: LMWHs have a more predictable dose response and fewer bleeding complications than other agents, and they typically do not require ongoing anticoagulant monitoring and dose adjustment. The balance of benefit versus harm must be assessed. Heparin can increase the risk of bleeding. Argatroban is used primarily in patients at risk for or with HIT (heparin-induced thrombocytopenia). LMWH is a better option, as it can provide more clinical and economic benefits versus the inpatient IV infusion.

138. Answer: D

Rationale: Nothing indicates that the patient and the spouse need 24-hour care. Home health can assess the patient's needs and help keep the patient in his own home. The nurse cannot insist on someone providing care.

139. Answer: B

    Rationale: Because the diagnosis is activity intolerance, the nurse should help the patient with a balance of rest and activity; 14 hours may be too much sleep. The other choices are appropriate outcomes for the patient, but they are not directly related to the diagnosis of activity intolerance.

140. Answer: A

    Rationale: Airway and breathing take priority. The patient may exhibit pallor, poor appetite, and bone pain, but the dyspnea at rest needs to be addressed immediately.

141. Answer: B

    Think RICE: rest, ice, compression, and elevation. While the patient is at greater risk for bleeding, the local injury will not cause systemic bleeding. The nurse should fill out an occurrence report and the HCP should be notified. Icing the location of the injury will help reduce swelling. The injury will not cause the platelets to drop further, so there is no need for a stat platelet count. The knee should not be splinted.

142. Answer: D

    Rationale: Spironolactone is a potassium-sparing diuretic; therefore, moderate to low levels of potassium intake should be maintained. Sodium should be restricted. Salt substitutes contain potassium and therefore should be avoided. Calcium intake should not be increased.

143. Answer: C

    Rationale: Obesity can be modified. Age, ethnicity, and genetics cannot be modified.

144. Answer: A

    Rationale: The family may not understand what hospice care involves. First assess before implementing. The patient and family do have the right to refuse hospice care but the decision has to be an informed one.

145. Answer: B

    Rationale: Both the aPTT (most facilities use 60 to 80 seconds as the therapeutic range for a patient taking IV heparin) and INR (usually 2 to 3 for treatment of a VTE) are below therapeutic levels. The patient will receive both heparin and warfarin until the INR is therapeutic (between 2 and 3). Although the INR is still below the therapeutic range, the dose usually remains the same, as the INR takes time to become therapeutic.

146. Answer: D

    Rationale: With a pneumothorax, a chest tube attached to a closed chest drainage system removes trapped air and helps to reestablish negative pressure within the pleural space; this results in lung reinflation. A closed chest drainage system may be inserted to remove the blood that results from a hemothorax, not to assess for bleeding. The reason for use of a closed chest drainage system is to drain fluid from the pleural space.

147. Answer: D.

    Rationale: Gloves, gown, N-95 mask, and eye shield protect the UAP from airborne transmission. The patient's recent travel and clinical diagnosis suggest that the patient may have severe acute respiratory syndrome (SARS), which is spread by airborne transmission (droplets) and has been known to infect health care workers through exposure of the eyes.

148. Answer: A

Rationale: The patient may need a mouth guard and perhaps even a continuous positive airway pressure (CPAP) mask or bilevel positive airway pressure (BiPAP) mask to prevent obstruction of the airway. Bariatric surgery is a last option, indicated only if all other treatments fail. The side-lying position is the best option for keeping the airway unobstructed. Sedatives can further depress the respiratory system.

149. Answer: A

Rationale: Albuterol (Proventil) relaxes smooth muscles in the respiratory tract, resulting in bronchodilation. The priority is to facilitate respirations. This intervention follows the ABCs of emergency care—airway, breathing, circulation. Obtaining a blood specimen is not the priority. Notifying the respiratory therapist is not the priority; chest physical therapy is performed after the respiratory airways are opened. The use of an incentive spirometer can be taught after the acute episode of respiratory distress; it should be used after the respiratory airways are opened.

150. Answer: C

Rationale: Patient C could be experiencing a myocardial infarction and should be assessed first. The patient with pneumonia has a pulse oximetry reading of 92% and should be assessed second. The other two patients are stable.

Bibliography

Ackley, B.J., Ladwig, G.B., and Makic, M.B. (2017). *Nursing Diagnosis Handbook: An Evidence-Based Guide to Planning Care,* 11th ed. (St. Louis: Mosby).

Burchum, L., and Rosenthal, L. (2016). *Lehne's Pharmacology for Nursing Care,* 9th ed. (St. Louis: Saunders Elsevier).

Centers for Disease Control and Prevention. (2018, January 25). What vaccines are recommended for you. Accessed July 4, 2018 https://www.cdc.gov/vaccines/adults/rec-vac/index.html

Center for Disease Control and Prevention. (2007). Guidelines for isolation precautions: Preventing transmission of Infectious agents in health setting. Accessed July 4, 2018, https://www.cdc.gov/infectioncontrol/guidelines/isolation/appendix/index.html

Colgrove, K. C. (2017). *Med-Surg Success: A Q & A Review Applying Critical Thinking to Test Taking,* 3rd ed. (Philadelphia: Davis).

Finkelman, A., and Kenner, C. (2016). *Professional Nursing Concepts: Competencies for Quality Leadership,* 3rd ed. (Sudbury, MA: Jones and Bartlett).

Lewis, S.L., Bucher, L., Heitkemper, M., and Harding, M.M. (2017). *Medical-Surgical Nursing: Assessment and Management of Clinical Problems,* 10th ed. (St. Louis: Elsevier).

Mayo Clinic. (2018, January 3). Cardiac ablation. Accessed July 4, 2018, https://www.mayoclinic.org/tests-procedures/cardiac-ablation/about/pac-20384993

National Heart, Lung, and Blood Institute. (n.d.). COPD. Accessed July 4, 2018, https://www.nhlbi.nih.gov/health-topics/copd

National Institutes of Health. (n.d.). Emergency preparedness. Accessed July 4, 2018, www.ors.od.nih.gov/ser/dem/emergencyPrep/Pages/emergencyPrep.aspx

Nugent, P. (2011). *Mosby's Comprehensive Review of Nursing for the NCLEX-RN Examination,* 20th ed. (St. Louis: Elsevier).

Potter, P.A., Perry, A.G., Stockert, P.A., and Hall, A.M. (2016). *Fundamentals of Nursing,* 9th ed. (St. Louis: Elsevier).

Wilson, S.F., and Giddens, J.F., eds. (2017). *Health Assessment for Nursing Practice,* 6th ed. (St. Louis: Elsevier Mosby).

Index